Hemostasis and Thrombosis

Hemostasis and Thrombosis

Editor: Nicholle Newman

AMERICAN
MEDICAL PUBLISHERS
www.americanmedicalpublishers.com

AMERICAN
MEDICAL PUBLISHERS
www.americanmedicalpublishers.com

Cataloging-in-Publication Data

Hemostasis and thrombosis / edited by Nicholle Newman.
p. cm.
Includes bibliographical references and index.
ISBN 979-8-88740-178-2
1. Hemostasis. 2. Thrombosis. 3. Blood--Coagulation. 4. Protein C deficiency.
5. Protein S deficiency. I. Newman, Nicholle.
RC647.C55 H46 2023
616.157--dc23

American Medical Publishers,
41 Flatbush Avenue,
1st Floor, New York,
NY 11217, USA

ISBN 979-8-88740-178-2 (Hardback)

Contents

Preface IX

Chapter 1 **The use of direct oral anticoagulants for thromboprophylaxis or treatment of cancer-associated venous thromboembolism** 1
Norah S. Alsubaie, Shahad M. Al Rammah, Reema A. Alshouimi, Mohammed Y. Alzahrani, Majed S. Al Yami, Abdulaali R. Almutairi, Osamah M. Alfayez, Ghazwa B. Korayem and Omar A. Almohammed

Chapter 2 **The evolution of clot strength in critically-ill COVID-19 patients: A prospective observational thromboelastography study** 11
Colette Neethling, Gregory Calligaro, Malcolm Miller and Jessica J. S. Opie

Chapter 3 **Thromboembolic and hemorrhagic risks after vaccination against SARS-CoV-2** 22
Noppacharn Uaprasert, Krissana Panrong, Ponlapat Rojnuckarin and Thita Chiasakul

Chapter 4 **Cardiovascular risk factors are associated with augmented thrombogenicity in healthy individuals: Analysis using the Total Thrombus-formation Analysis System** 32
Yuu Oda, Takashi Ito, Yoichiro Yamada, Tadashi Koga, Tomoka Nagasato, Tomoko Ohnishi-Wada, Kazuya Hosokawa, Hiroyuki Fukase, Teruto Hashiguchi and Ikuro Maruyama

Chapter 5 **Endovascular revascularization strategies using catheter-based thrombectomy versus conventional catheter-directed thrombolysis for acute limb ischemia** 39
Maofeng Gong, Xu He, Boxiang Zhao, Jie Kong, Jianping Gu and Guoping Chen

Chapter 6 **Morphologic change in deep venous thrombosis in the lower extremity after therapeutic anticoagulation** 50
Tanapong Panpikoon, Wisanu Phattharaprueksa, Tharintorn Treesit, Chinnarat Bua-ngam, Kaewpitcha Pichitpichatkul and Apichaya Sriprachyakul

Chapter 7 **D-dimer for risk stratification and antithrombotic treatment management in acute coronary syndrome patients** 57
Flavio Giuseppe Biccirè, Alessio Farcomeni, Carlo Gaudio, Pasquale Pignatelli, Gaetano Tanzilli and Daniele Pastori

Chapter 8 **Coexistence of antithrombin deficiency and suspected inferior vena cava atresia in an adolescent and his mother** 71
M. Müller-Knapp, C. F. Classen, R. Knöfler, C. Spang, C. Hauenstein, T. Heinrich, F. L. P. Gabriel, J. Däbritz, D. A. Reuter and J. Ehler

Chapter 9 **Incidence and characteristics of arterial thromboemboli in patients with COVID-19** 77
Nancy Glober, Lauren Stewart, JangDong Seo, Christopher Kabrhel, Kristen Nordenholz, Carlos Camargo and Jeffrey Kline

Chapter 10 **Replacement of traditional prothrombin time monitoring with the new Fiix prothrombin time increases the efficacy of warfarin without increasing bleeding** ... 83
Pall T. Onundarson, Ragnar Palsson, Daniel M. Witt and Brynja R. Gudmundsdottir

Chapter 11 **Changes of antithrombotic prescription in atrial fibrillation patients with acute coronary syndrome or percutaneous coronary intervention and the subsequent impact on long-term outcomes** ... 92
Chiao-Chin Lee, Chiao-Hsiang Chang, Yuan Hung, Chin-Sheng Lin, Shih-Ping Yang, Shu-Meng Cheng, Fan-Han Yu, Wei-Shiang Lin and Wen-Yu Lin

Chapter 12 **Anticoagulation may contribute to antimicrobial treatment of Lemierre syndrome** ... 102
Jie Ge, Peipei Zhou, Yifei Yang, Tianshu Xu and Xu Yang

Chapter 13 **Impact of oral anticoagulation therapy on postoperative atrial fibrillation outcomes** ... 107
Mariana Fragão-Marques, Francisco Teixeira, Jennifer Mancio, Nair Seixas, João Rocha-Neves, Inês Falcão-Pires and Adelino Leite-Moreira

Chapter 14 **Intermediate-to-therapeutic versus prophylactic anticoagulation for coagulopathy in hospitalized COVID-19 patients** ... 117
Sirui Zhang, Yupei Li, Guina Liu and Baihai Su

Chapter 15 **The impact on renal function after long-term use of anticoagulants in atrial fibrillation patients** ... 130
Wei-Chieh Lee, Pai-Wei Lee, Po-Jui Wu, Yen-Nan Fang, Huang-Chung Chen, Yu-Sheng Lin, Hsiu-Yu Fang, Shang-Hung Chang, Ping-Yen Liu and Mien-Cheng Chen

Chapter 16 **An optimal window of platelet reactivity by LTA assay for patients undergoing percutaneous coronary intervention** ... 140
Jing Wang, Jing Wang, Zhou Dong, Jiazheng Ma, Jianzhen Teng, Tong Wang, Xiaofeng Zhang, Qian Gu, Zekang Ye, Inam Ullah, Chuchu Tan, Samee Abdus, Lu Shi, Xiaoxuan Gong and Chunjian Li

Chapter 17 **Clopidogrel versus ticagrelor in the treatment of Chinese patients undergoing percutaneous coronary intervention: Effects on platelet function assessed by platelet function tests and mean platelet volume** ... 148
Yang Zhang, Rui Peng, Xiaojuan Li, Gaowa Cheng, Ximing Wang, Jinxing Yu, Muxing Hua, Xi Chen and Zhou Zhou

Chapter 18 **Fibrinolytic markers could be useful predictors of severity in patients with pulmonary arterial hypertension** ... 160
Makoto Shoji, Taiju Matsui, Hideaki Tanaka, Kosuke Nomura, Hiroaki Tsujita, Yusuke Kodama, Shinji Koba, Youichi Kobayashi and Toshiro Shinke

Chapter 19 **Monitoring coagulation-fibrinolysis activation prompted timely diagnosis of hemophagocytic lymphohistiocytosis-related disseminated intravascular coagulation** ... 166
Liqin Ling, Xunbei Huang, Chaonan Liu, Juan Liao and Jing Zhou

Chapter 20 **Association of circulating proprotein convertase subtilisin/kexin type 9 concentration, prothrombin time and cardiovascular outcomes** ... 171
Jia Peng, Ming-Ming Liu, Hui-Hui Liu, Yuan-Lin Guo, Na-Qiong Wu, Qian Dong, Jie Qian, Ke-Fei Dou, Cheng-Gang Zhu and Jian-Jun Li

Contents

Preface IX

Chapter 1 **The use of direct oral anticoagulants for thromboprophylaxis or treatment of cancer-associated venous thromboembolism** 1
Norah S. Alsubaie, Shahad M. Al Rammah, Reema A. Alshouimi, Mohammed Y. Alzahrani, Majed S. Al Yami, Abdulaali R. Almutairi, Osamah M. Alfayez, Ghazwa B. Korayem and Omar A. Almohammed

Chapter 2 **The evolution of clot strength in critically-ill COVID-19 patients: A prospective observational thromboelastography study** 11
Colette Neethling, Gregory Calligaro, Malcolm Miller and Jessica J. S. Opie

Chapter 3 **Thromboembolic and hemorrhagic risks after vaccination against SARS-CoV-2** 22
Noppacharn Uaprasert, Krissana Panrong, Ponlapat Rojnuckarin and Thita Chiasakul

Chapter 4 **Cardiovascular risk factors are associated with augmented thrombogenicity in healthy individuals: Analysis using the Total Thrombus-formation Analysis System** 32
Yuu Oda, Takashi Ito, Yoichiro Yamada, Tadashi Koga, Tomoka Nagasato, Tomoko Ohnishi-Wada, Kazuya Hosokawa, Hiroyuki Fukase, Teruto Hashiguchi and Ikuro Maruyama

Chapter 5 **Endovascular revascularization strategies using catheter-based thrombectomy versus conventional catheter-directed thrombolysis for acute limb ischemia** 39
Maofeng Gong, Xu He, Boxiang Zhao, Jie Kong, Jianping Gu and Guoping Chen

Chapter 6 **Morphologic change in deep venous thrombosis in the lower extremity after therapeutic anticoagulation** 50
Tanapong Panpikoon, Wisanu Phattharaprueksa, Tharintorn Treesit, Chinnarat Bua-ngam, Kaewpitcha Pichitpichatkul and Apichaya Sriprachyakul

Chapter 7 **D-dimer for risk stratification and antithrombotic treatment management in acute coronary syndrome patients** 57
Flavio Giuseppe Biccirè, Alessio Farcomeni, Carlo Gaudio, Pasquale Pignatelli, Gaetano Tanzilli and Daniele Pastori

Chapter 8 **Coexistence of antithrombin deficiency and suspected inferior vena cava atresia in an adolescent and his mother** 71
M. Müller-Knapp, C. F. Classen, R. Knöfler, C. Spang, C. Hauenstein, T. Heinrich, F. L. P. Gabriel, J. Däbritz, D. A. Reuter and J. Ehler

Chapter 9 **Incidence and characteristics of arterial thromboemboli in patients with COVID-19** 77
Nancy Glober, Lauren Stewart, JangDong Seo, Christopher Kabrhel, Kristen Nordenholz, Carlos Camargo and Jeffrey Kline

Chapter 10 **Replacement of traditional prothrombin time monitoring with the new Fiix prothrombin time increases the efficacy of warfarin without increasing bleeding** 83
Pall T. Onundarson, Ragnar Palsson, Daniel M. Witt and Brynja R. Gudmundsdottir

Chapter 11 **Changes of antithrombotic prescription in atrial fibrillation patients with acute coronary syndrome or percutaneous coronary intervention and the subsequent impact on long-term outcomes** 92
Chiao-Chin Lee, Chiao-Hsiang Chang, Yuan Hung, Chin-Sheng Lin, Shih-Ping Yang, Shu-Meng Cheng, Fan-Han Yu, Wei-Shiang Lin and Wen-Yu Lin

Chapter 12 **Anticoagulation may contribute to antimicrobial treatment of Lemierre syndrome** 102
Jie Ge, Peipei Zhou, Yifei Yang, Tianshu Xu and Xu Yang

Chapter 13 **Impact of oral anticoagulation therapy on postoperative atrial fibrillation outcomes** 107
Mariana Fragão-Marques, Francisco Teixeira, Jennifer Mancio, Nair Seixas, João Rocha-Neves, Inês Falcão-Pires and Adelino Leite-Moreira

Chapter 14 **Intermediate-to-therapeutic versus prophylactic anticoagulation for coagulopathy in hospitalized COVID-19 patients** 117
Sirui Zhang, Yupei Li, Guina Liu and Baihai Su

Chapter 15 **The impact on renal function after long-term use of anticoagulants in atrial fibrillation patients** 130
Wei-Chieh Lee, Pai-Wei Lee, Po-Jui Wu, Yen-Nan Fang, Huang-Chung Chen, Yu-Sheng Lin, Hsiu-Yu Fang, Shang-Hung Chang, Ping-Yen Liu and Mien-Cheng Chen

Chapter 16 **An optimal window of platelet reactivity by LTA assay for patients undergoing percutaneous coronary intervention** 140
Jing Wang, Jing Wang, Zhou Dong, Jiazheng Ma, Jianzhen Teng, Tong Wang, Xiaofeng Zhang, Qian Gu, Zekang Ye, Inam Ullah, Chuchu Tan, Samee Abdus, Lu Shi, Xiaoxuan Gong and Chunjian Li

Chapter 17 **Clopidogrel versus ticagrelor in the treatment of Chinese patients undergoing percutaneous coronary intervention: Effects on platelet function assessed by platelet function tests and mean platelet volume** 148
Yang Zhang, Rui Peng, Xiaojuan Li, Gaowa Cheng, Ximing Wang, Jinxing Yu, Muxing Hua, Xi Chen and Zhou Zhou

Chapter 18 **Fibrinolytic markers could be useful predictors of severity in patients with pulmonary arterial hypertension** 160
Makoto Shoji, Taiju Matsui, Hideaki Tanaka, Kosuke Nomura, Hiroaki Tsujita, Yusuke Kodama, Shinji Koba, Youichi Kobayashi and Toshiro Shinke

Chapter 19 **Monitoring coagulation-fibrinolysis activation prompted timely diagnosis of hemophagocytic lymphohistiocytosis-related disseminated intravascular coagulation** 166
Liqin Ling, Xunbei Huang, Chaonan Liu, Juan Liao and Jing Zhou

Chapter 20 **Association of circulating proprotein convertase subtilisin/kexin type 9 concentration, prothrombin time and cardiovascular outcomes** 171
Jia Peng, Ming-Ming Liu, Hui-Hui Liu, Yuan-Lin Guo, Na-Qiong Wu, Qian Dong, Jie Qian, Ke-Fei Dou, Cheng-Gang Zhu and Jian-Jun Li

Chapter 21 **Prognostic value of characteristics of plaque combined with residual syntax score among patients with STEMI undergoing primary PCI: An intravascular optical coherence tomography study** 183
Xiaoxiao Zhao, Ying Wang, Runzhen Chen, Jiannan Li, Jinying Zhou, Chen Liu, Peng Zhou, Zhaoxue Sheng, Yi Chen, Li Song, Hanjun Zhao and Hongbing Yan

Chapter 22 **A catastrophic seronegative anti-phospholipid syndrome** 200
Vanda Pinto, Augusto Ministro, Nuno Reis Carreira, Ana Cardoso, Catarina Sousa Gonçalves, Mickael Henriques, João Rato, Emanuel Silva and Luís Mendes Pedro

Chapter 23 **COVID19 infection in a patient undergoing treatment for Paroxysmal Nocturnal Hemoglobinuria (PNH) with Ravulizumab** 207
Sufana Shikdar, Azra Borogovac, Elabdallah Mohamad and Mohamad Khawandanah

Chapter 24 **The disulfide bond Cys2724-Cys2774 in the C-terminal cystine knot domain of von Willebrand factor is critical for its dimerization and secretion** 211
Yuxin Zhang, Fengwu Chen, Aizhen Yang, Xiaoying Wang, Yue Han, Depei Wu, Yi Wu and Jingyu Zhang

Chapter 25 **Low FXIII activity levels in intensive care unit hospitalized COVID-19 patients** 218
Yael Lichter, Tanya Badelbayov, Irina Shalev, Reut Schvartz, Yishay Szekely, Dan Benisty, Ilana Goldiner, Maxim Kagarlyk, Keren Asraf, Ram Doolman, Efrat Luttwak, Ilya Kirgner, Irit Avivi, Nimrod Adi and Ben-Zion Katz

Permissions

List of Contributors

Index

Preface

I am honored to present to you this unique book which encompasses the most up-to-date data in the field. I was extremely pleased to get this opportunity of editing the work of experts from across the globe. I have also written papers in this field and researched the various aspects revolving around the progress of the discipline. I have tried to unify my knowledge along with that of stalwarts from every corner of the world, to produce a text which not only benefits the readers but also facilitates the growth of the field.

Hemostasis refers to body's natural reaction that stops bleeding and initiates the repair of an injury. There are three principal steps involved in the mechanism of hemostasis. These include vasoconstriction, platelet plug formation and blood coagulation. Thrombosis is a condition that develops when blood clots block the blood vessels. It is of two main types, namely, venous thrombosis and arterial thrombosis. Some common causes of thrombosis are obesity, certain medicines, disease or injury to the leg veins, and autoimmune disorders. Its treatment includes medicines such as blood thinners to prevent blood clots. It also involves the placement of stents or catheters to reopen the blockage in the vessels. Losing weight and quitting smoking can help in preventing medical complications related to thrombosis. This book outlines the processes of hemostasis and thrombosis in detail. It will also provide interesting topics for research, which the interested readers can take up. The book will prove to be immensely beneficial to students and researchers in the field of hematology.

Finally, I would like to thank all the contributing authors for their valuable time and contributions. This book would not have been possible without their efforts. I would also like to thank my friends and family for their constant support.

Editor

1

The use of direct oral anticoagulants for thromboprophylaxis or treatment of cancer-associated venous thromboembolism

Norah S. Alsubaie[1], Shahad M. Al Rammah[1], Reema A. Alshouimi[1], Mohammed Y. Alzahrani[1], Majed S. Al Yami[1], Abdulaali R. Almutairi[2], Osamah M. Alfayez[3], Ghazwa B. Korayem[4] and Omar A. Almohammed[5*]

Abstract

Background: Venous thromboembolism (VTE) is a common complication among patients with cancer and is one of the most common causes of increased morbidity and mortality. The use of direct oral anticoagulants (DOACs) for thromboprophylaxis and treatment of cancer-associated venous thromboembolism (CA-VTE) has been evaluated in several randomized clinical trials (RCTs). The aim of this meta-analysis was to assess efficacy and safety of using DOACs for thromboprophylaxis and treatment of CA-VTE and provide a summary for available guidelines' recommendations.

Methods: MEDLINE was searched to identify studies evaluating the use of DOACs for thromboprophylaxis or treatment in patients with cancer. Search was limited to peer-reviewed studies published in English. Studies were excluded if they were not RCTs or subgroup analyses of data derived from RCTs, if they did not report efficacy and safety data on patients with active cancer, or if they were published as an abstract. New VTE or VTE recurrence, and major or clinically relevant non-major bleeding (CRNMB) were used to assess the efficacy and safety, respectively. The Mantel-Haenszel random-effects model risk ratios (RRs) and the corresponding 95% confidence intervals (CIs) were calculated to estimate the pooled treatment effects of DOACs.

Results: Four studies evaluating DOACs use for thromboprophylaxis and four – for treatment of CA-VTE were included. Thromboprophylaxis with DOACs was associated with a significant reduction in the risk of symptomatic VTE (RR = 0.58; 95%CI 0.37,0.91) but with an incremental risk of major bleeding or CRNMB (RR = 1.57; 95%CI 1.10,2.26). CA-VTE treatment with DOACs was linked with a significant reduction in VTE recurrence (RR = 0.62; 95%CI 0.44,0.87) but with an incremental risk of CRNMB (RR = 1.58; 95%CI 1.11,2.24).

* Correspondence: oalmohammed@ksu.edu.sa
[5]Department of Clinical Pharmacy, College of Pharmacy, King Saud University, P.O. Box 2457, Riyadh 11451, Saudi Arabia

Conclusions: The DOACs are associated with a lower risk of symptomatic VTE and VTE recurrence, but the risk of bleeding remains a considerable concern. Clinical decisions should be made by assessing individual patient's risk of VTE and bleeding.

Keywords: Direct oral anticoagulants, Venous thromboembolism, Thromboprophylaxis, Treatment, Cancer

Introduction

Venous thromboembolism (VTE), including deep vein thrombosis (DVT) and pulmonary embolism (PE), is a common complication among patients with cancer and is one of the most common causes of increased morbidity and mortality [1]. The risk factors for VTE are multifactorial and include cancer itself, chemotherapeutic agents, and patient-specific characteristics [2], such as female sex, older age, and comorbidities like diabetes and atherosclerosis [3].

The management of VTE in patients with cancer is challenging due to an increased risk of bleeding and VTE recurrence [4]. Low-molecular-weight heparin (LMWH) has been the gold standard treatment for cancer-associated VTE (CA-VTE) and is recommended over vitamin K antagonist (VKA) on the basis of evidence from several randomized controlled trials (RCTs) [5, 6]. However, considering the patient preference, availability of oral anticoagulants, cost, and the risk of thrombocytopenia, the use of this agent might not be the best option in cancer patients with VTE [7, 8].

Direct oral anticoagulants (DOACs), including apixaban, edoxaban, rivaroxaban, betrixaban, and dabigatran, have been approved for use in medical patients for VTE prophylaxis or treatment [9–11]. Since the original RCTs evaluating DOACs for VTE management included a limited number of cancer patients, separate studies were designed to investigate the use of DOACs specifically for CA-VTE. Since then, multiple RCTs have been conducted among cancer patients to evaluate the safety and efficacy of DOACs for thromboprophylaxis and treatment of CA-VTE [7, 12–17].

The PHACS trial, which assessed the use of dalteparin for the prevention of CA-VTE, provided inconclusive results because patients were noncompliant with treatment (once-daily subcutaneous injections) [18]. On the other hand, the AVERT trial concluded that apixaban significantly reduced the incidence of VTE in cancer patients, as opposed to the CASSINI trial, which showed that rivaroxaban did not lower the incidence of VTE events during the study period [12, 13]. Later on, The International Initiative on Thrombosis and Cancer (ITAC) and the American Society of Hematology (ASH) updated their guidelines to recommend the use of rivaroxaban or apixaban for thromboprophylaxis in ambulatory patients with cancer [19], and the American Society of Clinical Oncology (ASCO) guidelines stated that apixaban, rivaroxaban, or LMWH may be offered to cancer patients for thromboprophylaxis [20]. Regarding the management of CA-VTE, apixaban, edoxaban, and rivaroxaban were found to be noninferior to LMWH [15–17]. Recently, the ASCO and ITAC guidelines have added rivaroxaban and edoxaban as the first-line agents next to LMWH for the treatment of CA-VTE [20, 21]. Furthermore, the 2021 ASH guideline recommended apixaban, rivaroxaban or LMWH for initial treatment of CA-VTE [19]. The latest American College of Chest Physicians (ACCP) guidelines also recommend DOACs over LMWH for the initiation and treatment of CA-VTE [22].

The aim of this systematic review and meta-analysis was to assess the efficacy and safety of using DOACs for thromboprophylaxis and treatment of CA-VTE. We also summarized the recommendations from guidelines regarding the use of DOACs in patients with cancer for the management of CA-VTE.

Methods

Data sources and study selection

A systematic review was conducted using MEDLINE (from January 1st 2009 through July, 31st 2020) to identify studies evaluating the use of DOACs for thromboprophylaxis or treatment in patients with cancer and reporting VTE and bleeding events. The following search terms were used: cancer, venous thromboembolism, pulmonary embolism, low-molecular-weight heparin, enoxaparin, dalteparin, tinzaparin, factor Xa inhibitors, apixaban, betrixaban, dabigatran, edoxaban, and rivaroxaban. For CA-VTE treatment, RCTs were included, and for thromboprophylaxis, RCTs and studies with subgroup analyses reporting efficacy and safety data on patients with active cancer as well as post-hoc analyses of RCTs were included. The search was limited to peer-reviewed studies published in English. Studies were excluded if they were not RCTs or subgroup analyses of data derived from RCTs, if they did not report efficacy and safety data on patients with active cancer, or if they were published as an abstract. Each study was screened for eligibility independently by two authors.

Outcomes

The efficacy outcomes in the meta-analysis were VTE recurrence in treatment studies (within up to 6 months of follow-up from the start of treatment) or a new VTE event in thromboprophylaxis studies (within up to 6 months of follow-up from the start of thromboprophylaxis). The safety outcomes were the incidence of major bleeding, clinically relevant nonmajor bleeding (CRNMB), and major bleeding or CRNMB events during the follow-up. Definitions of the efficacy and safety outcomes from the original trials were included in Supplementary Table S1.

Data extraction

Data were extracted and assessed for accuracy independently by two authors (NSA and SMA) and verified by the third author (MYA). Data were extracted on a predefined data extraction form. For each study, the following data were extracted: VTE recurrence (for treatment studies) or VTE events (for thromboprophylaxis studies), symptomatic VTE, major bleeding, CRNMB, and major bleeding or CRNMB events.

Statistical analysis

The Mantel-Haenszel random-effects model risk ratios (RRs) and the corresponding 95% confidence intervals (CIs) were calculated using the metan routine in Stata software, version 14.2 (StataCorp LLC, College Station, Texas, United States) to estimate the pooled treatment effects of DOACs. Heterogeneity was assessed using the I^2 statistics, and the values of < 40, 30–60%, 50–90% and 75–100% were defined as low, moderate, substantial, and considerable heterogeneity, respectively [23]. The risk-of-bias assessment was conducted for each study using the Cochrane Collaboration's tool, and a funnel plot was used to assess publication bias.

Results

Characteristics of the included studies

The literature search yielded a total of 887 publications. All studies matching the inclusion criteria were reviewed and screened for inclusion, and any duplicates or discrepancies were resolved by consensus. A total of 879 articles were excluded based on the date of publication, the language of publication other than English, and non-RCT design. Only eight studies (four regarding thromboprophylaxis and four regarding CA-VTE treatment), including a total of 5360 cancer patients, met the inclusion criteria (Fig. 1) [7, 12, 13, 15–17, 24, 25]. Apixaban for CA-VTE treatment was evaluated in two studies and for thromboprophylaxis in one study [7, 13, 15]; rivaroxaban for CA-VTE treatment was evaluated in two studies and for thromboprophylaxis in one study [12, 16, 24]; edoxaban for CA-VTE treatment was evaluated in one study [17]; and betrixaban for thromboprophylaxis was evaluated in one study [25]. All the included studies were RCTs except for the APEX trial, which reported data on cancer patients in a post-hoc analysis [14], and the MAGELLAN trial, in which data for cancer patients were pooled from a published meta-analysis [26]. In all included studies, VTE and VTE recurrence were confirmed by using compression ultrasonography or *computerized tomography* (*CT*) venography to confirm DVT and CT pulmonary angiography or ventilation/perfusion lung scan (VQ scan) to confirm PE. The characteristics of the included studies were summarized in Table 1. The quality of the studies was presented in Supplementary Fig. S1, while the funnel plots for efficacy and safety outcomes were reported in Supplementary Figs. S2-S10.

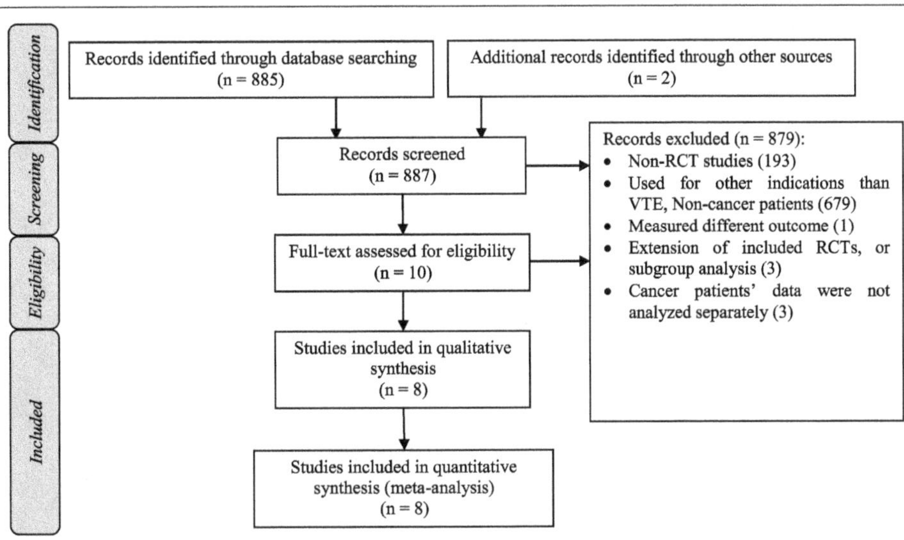

Fig. 1 PRISMA flow diagram of the included trials

Table 1 Characteristics of studies included in the meta-analysis

Study Type	Name	Year	Age (years) mean ± SD	Male sex n (%)	DOACs drug	Comparator	Follow-up (months)	Cancer patients (%)	Main efficacy outcome	Main safety outcome	Phase	Study design
Thromboprophylaxis	MAGELLAN [24]	2013	NR	NR	Rivaroxaban	Enoxaparin	3 months	7.3%	Composite of asymptomatic proximal DVT, symptomatic proximal or distal DVT, symptomatic nonfatal PE, and death from VTE	Clinically relevant bleeding	Phase 3	Subgroup analysis
	APEX [14]	2016	76.8 ± 9.3	240 (48.1)	Betrixaban	Enoxaparin	1 month	12.8%	Composite of asymptomatic proximal DVT, symptomatic proximal or distal DVT, symptomatic nonfatal PE, or fatal PE	Major bleeding	Phase 3	Subgroup analysis
	CASSINI [12]	2019	63[a]	222 (52.9)	Rivaroxaban	Placebo	6 months	100%	Composite of symptomatic or asymptomatic proximal DVT in a lower limb, symptomatic DVT in an upper limb or distal DVT in a lower limb, symptomatic or incidental PE, and death from VTE	Major bleeding	Phase 3	RCT
	AVERT [13]	2019	61.2 ± 12.4	121 (41.6)	Apixaban	Placebo	6 months	100%	VTE	Major bleeding	Phase 3	RCT
Treatment	SELECT-D [16]	2018	67[a]	116 (57)	Rivaroxaban	Dalteparin	24 months	100%	Recurrent VTE	Major bleeding	Pilot	RCT
	Hokusai VTE Cancer [17]	2018	64.3 ± 11	277 (53.1)	Edoxaban	Dalteparin	12 months	100%	Recurrent VTE	Major bleeding	Phase 3	RCT
	ADAM VTE [7]	2019	64.4 ± 11.3	72 (48)	Apixaban	Dalteparin	6 months	100%	Recurrent VTE	Major bleeding	Phase 3	RCT
	Caravaggio [15]	2020	67.2 ± 11.3	292 (50.7)	Apixaban	Dalteparin	7 months	100%	Recurrent VTE	Major bleeding	Phase 3	RCT

Abbreviations: *DOAC* direct oral anticoagulant, *DVT* deep vein thrombosis. *PE* pulmonary embolism, *VTE* venous thromboembolism, *RCT* randomized clinical trial

[a] Median age

Thromboprophylaxis results

Efficacy outcomes

VTE events There was no difference between DOACs and LMWH or placebo with regard to the occurrence of VTE events (RR = 0.69; 95%CI 0.48, 1.00) (Fig. 2).

Symptomatic VTE events The use of DOACs was associated with a 42% reduction in symptomatic VTE events when compared with LMWH or placebo (RR = 0.58; 95%CI 0.37, 0.91; number needed to treat [NNT] = 45), with no significant heterogeneity (I^2 = 0%) (Fig. 2).

Safety outcomes

Major bleeding The use of DOACs was associated with an approximately two-fold increase in the risk of major bleeding (RR = 2.13; 95%CI 1.03, 4.42; number needed to harm [NNH] = 111), with no significant heterogeneity (I^2 = 0%) (Fig. 2).

CRNMB There was no difference between DOACs and LMWH or placebo in terms of CRNMB (RR = 1.36; 95%CI 0.89, 2.08) (Fig. 2).

Major bleeding or CRNMB The use of DOACs was associated with an incremental risk of major bleeding or CRNMB when compared with LMWH or placebo (RR = 1.57; 95%CI 1.10, 2.26; NNH = 56), with no significant heterogeneity (I^2 = 0%) (Fig. 2).

Treatment results

Efficacy outcomes

VTE recurrence The use of DOACs was associated with a 38% reduction in VTE recurrence as compared with LMWH (RR = 0.62; 95%CI 0.44, 0.87; NNT = 29), with no significant heterogeneity (I^2 = 26%; p = 0.256) (Fig. 3).

Safety outcomes

Major bleeding There was no difference between the use of DOACs or LMWH with regard to major bleeding events (RR = 1.33; 95%CI 0.84, 2.11) (Fig. 3).

CRNMB The rate of CRNMB was significantly higher with the use of DOACs compared with LMWH (RR = 1.58; 95%CI 1.11, 2.24; NNH = 26), with no significant heterogeneity (I^2 = 41.8%; p = 0.161) (Fig. 3).

Major bleeding or CRNMB There was no difference between the use of DOACs or LMWH with regard to major bleeding or CRNMB (RR = 1.36; 95%CI 0.94, 1.97) (Fig. 3).

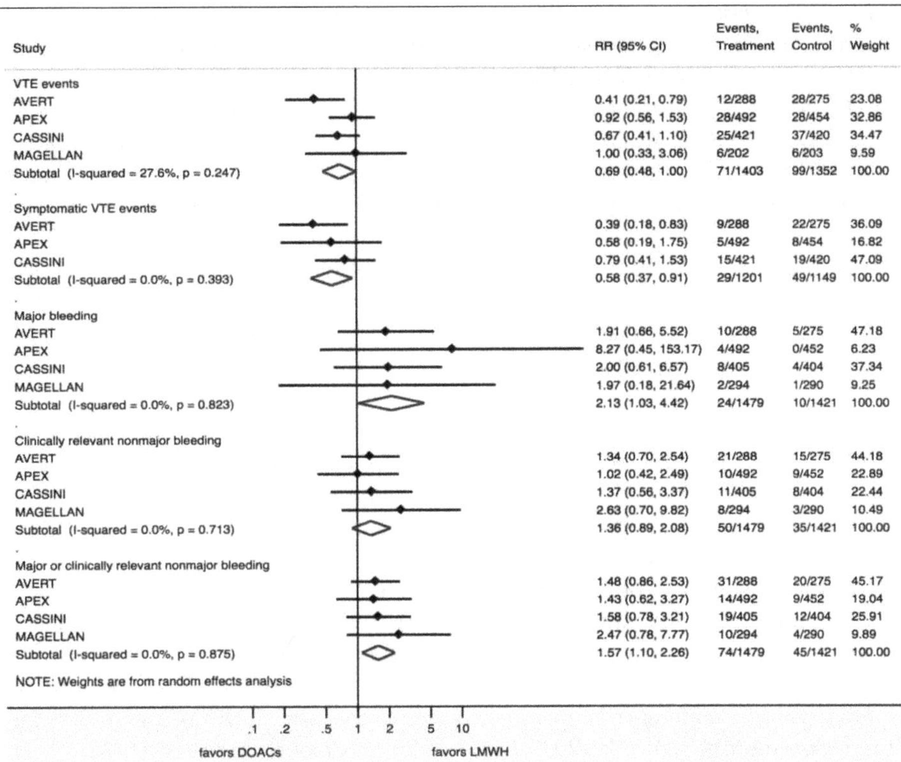

Fig. 2 Thromboprophylaxis results of the meta-analysis

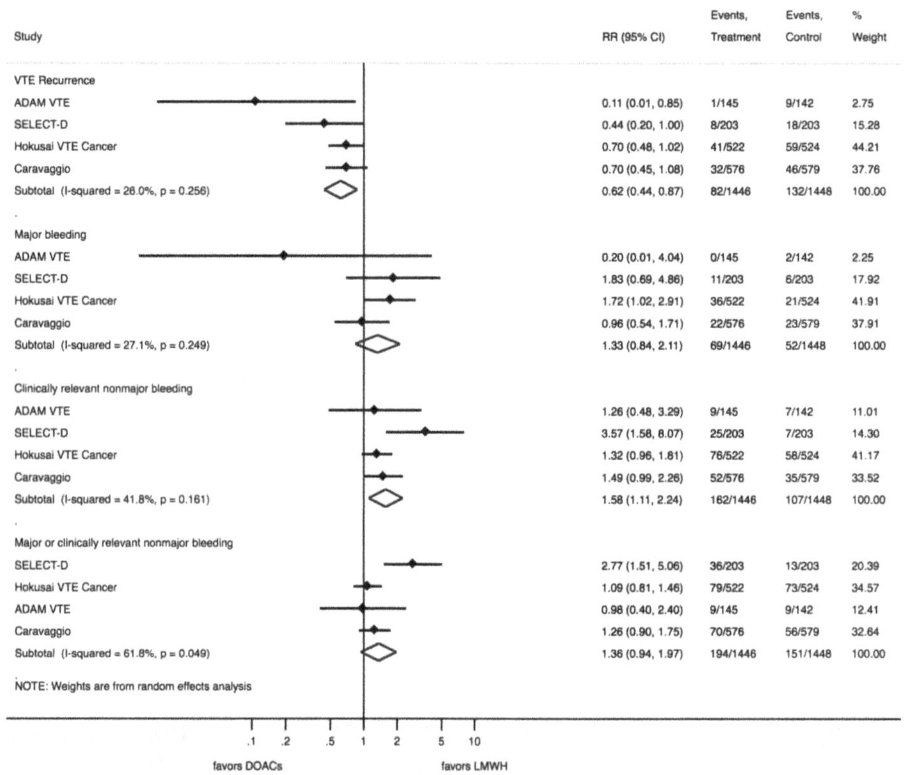

Fig. 3 Treatment results of the meta-analysis

Summary of guideline recommendations

The available guidelines provide controversial recommendations on CA-VTE treatment and prophylaxis in patients with cancer (Table 2). The 2018 guidelines of the International Society on Thrombosis and Haemostasis (ISTH) suggest DOACs for CA-VTE treatment if the bleeding risk is low and there is no risk of drug-drug interactions with anticoagulation, while LMWH is indicated as an alternative option or if there is a high-risk of bleeding or significant drug-drug interactions with anticoagulation. Rivaroxaban or edoxaban is considered as an alternative therapy to LMWH in patients with high bleeding risk with no significant drug-drug interaction [27]. The 2019 European Society of Cardiology (ESC) guidelines recommend LMWH as the first-line option for CA-VTE treatment, and edoxaban or rivaroxaban can be used as alternatives in patients without gastrointestinal (GI) cancer [10]. The 2019 ASCO guidelines recommend the use of LMWH, unfractionated heparin (UFH), fondaparinux, or rivaroxaban for initial CA-VTE treatment, while LMWH, edoxaban, or rivaroxaban is recommended over warfarin for long-term anticoagulation for up to 6 months, with no preference of one over the other beyond the first 6 months [20]. The 2020 National Comprehensive Cancer Network (NCCN) guidelines provide their recommendations on the basis of cancer site. LMWH is recommended as first-line treatment in patients with gastric or gastroesophageal lesions, while apixaban, edoxaban, or rivaroxaban are recommended for patients with other types of cancer [28]. The 2020 ITAC guidelines recommend LMWH if CrCl greater than 30 mL/min; rivaroxaban or edoxaban can be used in these patients if they do not have a high risk of GI or genitourinary bleeding. Fondaparinux is indicated as an alternative option to LMWH, rivaroxaban or edoxaban with the advantage of easier use as compared to UFH. Whereas UFH is indicated in case of contraindication to LMWH, rivaroxaban or edoxaban [21]. In the 2021 ASH guidelines, only rivaroxaban and apixaban were recommended for the initial treatment of CA-VTE, while edoxaban was added to the mentioned DOACs for the short-term treatment of CA-VTE over LMWH in patients with normal renal function. While for Long-term anticoagulation treatment of CA-VTE, the ASH recommended using DOAC, without specifying agents, or LMWH. Nonetheless, the guideline emphasized the cautious use of DOACs in patients with GI cancer [19]. Lastly, the latest ACCP guidelines (2021) now recommend the use of DOACs as a first-line option for CA-VTE treatment over LMWH [22].

For thromboprophylaxis, the ASCO, NCCN, ITAC, and ASH guidelines recommend the use of

Table 2 Summary of guideline recommendations for CA-VTE treatment and thromboprophylaxis in patients with cancer

Guideline	Year	CA-VTE Treatment		Thromboprophylaxis
		Preferred or first-line option	Alternative or second-line options	
ISTH [27]	2018	*If low risk of bleeding and no drug–drug interactions:* **DOACs**	**LMWH**	NA
ESC [10]	2019	**LMWH**	**Edoxaban or rivaroxaban**	NA
ASCO [20]	2019	*Initial treatment:* **LMWH, UFH, fondaparinux, or rivaroxaban** *Up to six months:* **LMWH, edoxaban, or rivaroxaban** *Long term anticoagulation:* **LMWH, DOAC, or VKA**	*If unable to obtain LMWH, edoxaban, or rivaroxaban:* **VKA**	*High-risk ambulatory patients (Khorana score ≥ 2):* **LMWH, apixaban, or rivaroxaban**
NCCN [28]	2020	*Patients without gastric or gastrointestinal lesions:* **Apixaban, rivaroxaban, or edoxaban** *Patients with gastric or gastrointestinal lesions:* **Dalteparin or enoxaparin**	Dabigatran (with LMWH or UFH for at least 5 days), fondaparinux, UFH, or warfarin	*High risk ambulatory patients (Khorana score ≥ 2):* **Apixaban or rivaroxaban**
ITAC [21]	2020	*Initial treatment and for up to six months:* • *if CrCl ≥ 30 mL/min:* **LMWH** • *if CrCl ≥ 30 mL/min, patient has low risk of GI or genitourinary bleeding, and no drug–drug interactions:* **Edoxaban, or rivaroxaban**	*If no contraindications:* **Fondaparinux** *If patient has contraindication for LMWH or DOACs:* **UFH**	*If hospitalized with reduced mobility and CrCl ≥ 30 mL/min:* **LMWH or fondaparinux**, or **UFH** *For patients with pancreatic cancer or Khorana score ≥ 2 while receiving systemic anticancer therapy at intermediate-to-high risk of VTE and not actively, or at a high-risk of, bleeding:* **Rivaroxaban, apixaban, or LMWH** *Immunomodulatory drugs combined with steroids or other systemic anticancer therapies:* **VKA (at low or therapeutic dose), LMWH, or low-dose aspirin**
ASH [19]	2021	*Initial treatment:* **LMWH** *Up to six months:* **DOACs** *Long term anticoagulation:* **DOACs or LMWH**	*If patient has contraindication for LMWH or DOACs:* **UFH**	*If hospitalized:* **LMWH** *High risk ambulatory patients receiving systemic therapy:* **Rivaroxaban or apixaban**
CHEST [22]	2021	**DOACs**	**LMWH**	NA

Abbreviations: *CA-VTE* cancer-associated VTE, *DOACs* direct oral anticoagulants, *LMWH* low-molecular-weight heparin, *UFH* unfractionated heparin, *VKA* Vitamin K Antagonist. *ISTH* International Society on Thrombosis and Haemostasis, *ESC* European Society of Cardiology, *ASCO* American Society of Clinical Oncology, *NCCN* National Comprehensive Cancer Network, *ITAC* International Initiative on Thrombosis and Cancer, *CHEST* American College of Chest Physicians, *NA* no specific recommendation for DOACs is available

thromboprophylaxis with apixaban or rivaroxaban (or LMWH in the ASCO) for moderate to high-risk ambulatory cancer patients with a Khorana score of two or higher [19–21, 28]; the ITAC guideline extend this recommendation to patients with intermediate-risk or pancreatic cancer, but limit it to patients with no active, or at a high risk of, bleeding [21]. Most of the guidelines' recommendations for CA-VTE treatment and thromboprophylaxis were summarized in Table 2.

Discussion

This systematic review and meta-analysis evaluated the efficacy and safety of using DOACs compared with LMWH or placebo for thromboprophylaxis and LMWH for CA-VTE treatment. By pooling the data from RCTs and post-hoc analyses of RCTs, more than 5300 patients from eight trials were analyzed. The use of DOACs was associated with about 40% lower risk of VTE recurrence and symptomatic VTE when used for CA-VTE treatment and thromboprophylaxis, respectively. However, when DOACs were used for thromboprophylaxis, the risk of major bleeding was twice higher when compared with placebo or LMWH. When thromboprophylaxis data were analyzed separately based on the comparator (i.e., placebo or LMWH), no difference was found between DOACs and LMWH in both efficacy and safety outcomes (Supplementary Fig. S11), while in studies that use placebo as a comparator, DOACs showed a significant reduction in VTE events with no difference in the other efficacy and safety outcomes (Supplementary Fig.

S12). On the other hand, when DOACs were used for CA-VTE treatment, the risk of major bleeding was not significantly higher than that for LMWH.

The use of DOACs for thromboprophylaxis in patients with cancer reduced the risk of symptomatic VTE events (RR = 0.58; 95%CI 0.37, 0.91). This result is in contrast to a previous meta-analysis, in which patients with cancer who received DOACs for thromboprophylaxis showed a nonsignificant reduction in the risk of symptomatic VTE (RR = 0.57; 95%CI 0.29, 1.12) [29]. This discrepancy is mainly due to the fact that the previous meta-analysis included only the AVERT and CASSINI trials. In the present study, the efficacy of DOACs was compared against placebo in patients who mostly had a Khorana score of two or higher [12, 13, 29]. However, the AVERT trial utilized a modified Khorana risk score, which led to the inclusion of patients with more types of cancer [13]. Even though the Khorana scores for patients included in the subgroup analysis of the MAGELLAN and APEX trials were not reported [14, 24], the addition of data from their subgroup analyses provided significant evidence supporting the use of DOACs for thromboprophylaxis to reduce the risk of VTE in patients with cancer. The majority of those trials included high-risk patients with cancer, including GI, lung, pancreatic, and metastatic cancer. In contrast, a limited number of patients with brain malignancies were included only in the AVERT trial, which may weaken the evidence supporting the use of DOACs for thromboprophylaxis in this population.

Similar to previous systematic reviews and meta-analyses that assessed the use of DOACs for CA-VTE treatment [30–32], our meta-analysis showed that DOACs were associated with a 38% risk reduction of VTE recurrence compared with LMWH. This rate was comparable to the rates reported in previous meta-analyses, which ranged from 32 to 55% [30–32]. Mulder et al. found the risk of VTE recurrence in patients using DOACs to be nonsignificantly lower than that for the LMWH group (RR = 0.68; 95%CI 0.39, 1.17) [30]. However, the most recent meta-analysis reported DOACs to be associated with a significantly lower risk of VTE recurrence compared with LMWH in patients with cancer [32], even though it did not include data from the Caravaggio trial, one of the largest trials that demonstrated the efficacy of DOACs in preventing VTE recurrence in patients with CA-VTE. The overall risk reduction of VTE recurrence observed in our meta-analysis was mainly driven by the results from the ADAM VTE trial, in which the VTE recurrence was a secondary outcome that was barely observed [7]. Moreover, the ADAM VTE was an open-label RCT that included a small sample of patients ($n = 300$) compared with the Caravaggio trial ($n = 1155$); however, the percentage of patients with upper GI cancer was similar in both trials [7, 16].

In this meta-analysis, the use of DOACs for CA-VTE treatment or thromboprophylaxis was associated with a higher risk of bleeding than LMWH or placebo. The risk of major bleeding was nonsignificantly higher with DOACs when used for CA-VTE treatment (RR = 1.33, 95%CI 0.84, 2.11), while it was twice higher when DOACs were used for thromboprophylaxis (RR = 2.13, 95%CI 1.03, 4.42). Since the definition of major bleeding was almost consistent across the studies, the differences in the risk of major bleeding can be attributed to the heterogeneity of the cancer patient population. Compared with other trials, betrixaban in the APEX trial and rivaroxaban in the CASSINI trial were associated with a higher risk of major bleeding [12, 14]. Nonetheless, the number of patients with GI and metastatic malignancies in the APEX and CASSINI trials was higher than in the AVERT trial, which might explain the increase in bleeding risk [12–14]. Here, the risk of CRNMB did not differ between the DOACs and LMWH or placebo when used for thromboprophylaxis. However, the risk of CRNMB was significantly higher among patients receiving DOACs for CA-VTE treatment. This increase was mainly driven by the SELECT-D trial, as it reported a higher risk of CRNMB in patients receiving rivaroxaban than in those on dalteparin [16]. It is also worth mentioning that the SELECT-D trial subsequently excluded patients with GI malignancies due to the increased risk of bleeding [16].

Until recently, most of the previous guidelines recommended LMWH as the first-line therapy for CA-VTE treatment over VKAs and DOACs [9, 33, 34]. This was due to insufficient evidence that supported the efficacy and safety of DOACs in patients with cancer, especially that DOAC approval trials only included a small proportion of patients with a history of active cancer [34]. However, numerous RCTs and observational studies have been published recently that used DOACs for the treatment or prevention of CA-VTE [7, 12, 13, 15–17, 25]. Also, several meta-analyses supported the lower risk of VTE recurrence and bleeding with DOACs as compared with LMWH and VKAs [30–32]. This body of evidence from RCTs and meta-analyses prompted some of the large organizations to add DOACs as a viable option for CA-VTE treatment or thromboprophylaxis in their latest guidelines [20, 21]. The ACCP, ASCO, ITAC, NCCN, and ASH have recently updated their guidelines to recommend the use of edoxaban, apixaban, or rivaroxaban as initial therapy for CA-VTE treatment in patients without gastric lesions or GI malignancies due to the increased risk of bleeding in these patients [19–22, 28]. Clinical guidelines do not recommend the routine use of pharmacological thromboprophylaxis in all patients with cancer [9, 10, 20, 21, 28]. This is mainly due to the relatively low risk of VTE in ambulatory patients with cancer and the increased risk of bleeding with the use of anticoagulants [20, 21]. The use of validated VTE risk prediction tools such as the Khorana VTE risk assessment tool can help identify patients with cancer receiving chemotherapy who are at greater risk for VTE [34]. The use of those tools prompted the development of newer guidelines supporting the use of DOACs in high-risk patients who are not at increased risk of bleeding. Thus, the current guidelines recommend the use of rivaroxaban and apixaban in patients at intermediate-to-high-risk of VTE, identified by cancer type (i.e., pancreatic) or a Khorana score of two or higher in the absence of active bleeding or not at high-risk of bleeding [20, 21]. The convenience of oral administration of DOACs provides an easier, yet effective, therapeutic alternative for subcutaneous anticoagulation, which may increase patient adherence. However, caution should be warranted with the use of DOACs in patients with high-risk of bleeding and brain malignancies due to limited safety data.

To our knowledge, this is the first systematic review and meta-analysis that assessed the efficacy and safety of DOACs for both primary and secondary prevention of CA-VTE. Nevertheless, as any other meta-analysis, it is not free of limitations. There was a variation among the included trials in terms of patient population and follow-up duration, but this does not seem to have impacted the results as no significant heterogeneity was observed in the analysis. Although we included only high-quality RCTs to assess the efficacy and safety of DOACs for CA-VTE treatment, limited RCTs were available to assess the efficacy of DOACs for thromboprophylaxis. Therefore, data from subgroup or post-hoc analyses of large RCTs were included and the heterogeneity between these studies was low. The LMWH comparator included in our analysis was limited to dalteparin, as in all previous trials starting with the CLOT trial [6]. Also, some included studies excluded patients with hematological, brain, and metastatic brain tumors, so caution is needed when generalizing our results to those populations. Finally, this analysis did not include all DOACs for both thromboprophylaxis and treatment of CA-VTE, since there were no studies that assessed the use of edoxaban for thromboprophylaxis, betrixaban for treatment, or dabigatran for both.

Conclusions

This meta-analysis highlighted the efficacy and safety of DOACs for thromboprophylaxis and treatment of CA-VTE. DOACs demonstrated a lower risk of VTE recurrence than LMWH and a lower risk of symptomatic VTE than LMWH or placebo. However, the risk of bleeding remains an important concern. Clinical decisions on the use of DOACs for CA-VTE treatment or prophylaxis should be based on individual assessment of the patient's risk for VTE and bleeding, using validated risk assessment tools. The findings can provide an additional insight into the development of future guidelines and protocols aimed to optimize anticoagulation therapy in patients with cancer.

Supplementary Information

Additional file 1 Table S1. Definitions of the outcomes for included studies. **Fig. S1.** Quality assessment of included randomized controlled trials. **Fig. S2.** Funnel plot for the VTE events outcome in the thromboprophylaxis studies. **Fig. S3.** Funnel plot for the symptomatic VTE events outcome in the thromboprophylaxis studies. **Fig. S4.** Funnel plot for the major bleeding events outcome in the thromboprophylaxis studies. **Fig. S5.** Funnel plot for the clinically relevant nonmajor bleeding events outcome in the thromboprophylaxis studies. **Fig. S6.** Funnel plot for the major or clinically relevant nonmajor bleeding events outcome in the thromboprophylaxis studies. **Fig. S7**. Funnel plot for the VTE recurrence outcome in the treatment studies. **Fig. S8.** Funnel plot for the major bleeding events outcome in the treatment studies. **Fig. S9.** Funnel plot for the clinically relevant nonmajor bleeding events outcome in the treatment studies. **Fig. S10.** Funnel plot for the major or clinically relevant nonmajor bleeding events outcome in the treatment studies. **Fig. S11**. Thromboprophylaxis results (DOACs vs. LMWH). **Fig. S12.** Thromboprophylaxis results (DOACs vs. placebo).

Acknowledgements
The authors would like to extend their appreciation to King Saud University for funding this work through the Researcher Supporting Project (RSP-2020/77), King Saud University, Riyadh, Saudi Arabia. They would also like to thank Editage® for English language editing of this manuscript.

Authors' contributions
Conceptualization, M.S.A, S.M.A., and N.S.A.; methodology, M.S.A. and A.R.A.; software, M.S.A.; validation, O.A.A. and O.M.A..; formal analysis, M.S.A.; investigation, M.Y.A.; resources, O.A.A.; data curation, N.S.A and S.M.A.; writing—original draft preparation, N.S.A., G.B.K. and R.A.A.; writing—review and editing, O.A.A., O.M.A. and M.S.A.; visualization, A.R.A. and M.Y.A.; supervision, M.S.A.; project administration, M.S.A.; funding acquisition, O.A.A. All authors have read and agreed to the published version of the manuscript. The author(s) read and approved the final manuscript.

Author details
[1]Department of Pharmacy Practice, College of Pharmacy, King Saud bin Abdulaziz University for Health Sciences, Riyadh, Saudi Arabia. [2]Saudi Food and Drug Authority, Riyadh, Saudi Arabia. [3]Department of Pharmacy Practice, College of Pharmacy, Qassim University, Qassim, Buraydah, Saudi Arabia. [4]Department of Pharmacy Practice, College of Pharmacy, Princess Nourah bint Abdulrahman University, Riyadh, Saudi Arabia. [5]Department of Clinical Pharmacy, College of Pharmacy, King Saud University, P.O. Box 2457, Riyadh 11451, Saudi Arabia.

References

1. Khorana AA, Francis CW, Culakova E, Kuderer NM, Lyman GH. Thromboembolism is a leading cause of death in cancer patients receiving outpatient chemotherapy. J Thromb Haemost. 2007;5(3). https://doi.org/10.1111/j.1538-7836.2007.02374.x.
2. Giustozzi M, Curcio A, Weijs B, Field TS, Sudikas S, Katholing A, et al. Variation in the association between antineoplastic therapies and venous thromboembolism in patients with active cancer. Thromb Haemost. 2020;120(5). https://doi.org/10.1055/s-0040-1709527.
3. Elyamany G, Alzahrani AM, Bukhary E. Cancer-associated thrombosis: an overview. Clin Med Insights Oncol. 2014;8:S18991. https://doi.org/10.4137/cmo.

4. Prandoni P, Lensing AW, Piccioli A, Bernardi E, Simioni P, Girolami B, et al. Recurrent venous thromboembolism and bleeding complications during anticoagulant treatment in patients with cancer and venous thrombosis. Blood. 2002;100(10). https://doi.org/10.1182/blood-2002-01-0108.
5. Lee AY, Kamphuisen PW, Meyer G, Bauersachs R, Janas MS, Jarner MF, et al. Tinzaparin vs warfarin for treatment of acute venous thromboembolism in patients with active cancer: a randomized clinical trial. JAMA. 2015;314(7). https://doi.org/10.1001/jama.2015.9243.
6. Lee AY, Levine MN, Baker RI, Bowden C, Kakkar AK, Prins M, et al. Low-molecular-weight heparin versus a coumarin for the prevention of recurrent venous thromboembolism in patients with cancer. N Engl J Med. 2003; 349(2). https://doi.org/10.1056/NEJMoa025313.
7. McBane RD 2nd, Wysokinski WE, Le-Rademacher JG, Zemla T, Ashrani A, Tafur A, et al. Apixaban and dalteparin in active malignancy-associated venous thromboembolism: The ADAM VTE trial. J Thromb Haemost. 2020; 18(2). https://doi.org/10.1111/jth.14662.
8. Seaman S, Nelson A, Noble S. Cancer-associated thrombosis, low-molecular-weight heparin, and the patient experience: a qualitative study. Patient Prefer Adherence. 2014;8. https://doi.org/10.2147/PPA.S58595.
9. Kearon C, Akl EA, Ornelas J, Blaivas A, Jimenez D, Bounameaux H, et al. Antithrombotic therapy for VTE disease: CHEST guideline and expert panel report. Chest. 2016;149(2). https://doi.org/10.1016/j.chest.2015.11.026.
10. Konstantinides SV, Meyer G, Becattini C, Bueno H, Geersing G-J, Harjola V-P, et al. ESC guidelines for the diagnosis and management of acute pulmonary embolism developed in collaboration with the European Respiratory Society (ERS). Eur Heart J. 2019, 2020;41(4). https://doi.org/10.1093/eurheartj/ehz405.
11. Witt DM, Nieuwlaat R, Clark NP, Ansell J, Holbrook A, Skov J, et al. American Society of Hematology 2018 guidelines for management of venous thromboembolism: optimal management of anticoagulation therapy. Blood Adv. 2018;2(22). https://doi.org/10.1182/bloodadvances.2018024893.
12. Khorana AA, Soff GA, Kakkar AK, Vadhan-Raj S, Riess H, Wun T, et al. Rivaroxaban for thromboprophylaxis in high-risk ambulatory patients with cancer. N Engl J Med. 2019;380(8). https://doi.org/10.1056/NEJMoa1814630.
13. Carrier M, Abou-Nassar K, Mallick R, Tagalakis V, Shivakumar S, Schattner A, et al. Apixaban to prevent venous thromboembolism in patients with cancer. N Engl J Med. 2019;380(8). https://doi.org/10.1056/NEJMoa1814468.
14. Ageno W, Lopes RD, Yee MK, Hernandez A, Hull R, Goldhaber SZ, et al. Extended prophylaxis of venous thromboembolism with betrixaban in acutely ill medical patients with and without cancer: insights from the APEX trial. J Thromb Thrombolysis. 2020;49(2). https://doi.org/10.1007/s11239-019-01943-5.
15. Agnelli G, Becattini C, Meyer G, Muñoz A, Huisman MV, Connors JM, et al. Apixaban for the treatment of venous thromboembolism associated with cancer. N Engl J Med. 2020;382(17). https://doi.org/10.1056/NEJMoa1915103.
16. Young AM, Marshall A, Thirlwall J, Chapman O, Lokare A, Hill C, et al. Comparison of an oral factor Xa inhibitor with low molecular weight heparin in patients with cancer with venous thromboembolism: results of a randomized trial (SELECT-D). J Clin Oncol. 2018. https://doi.org/10.1200/JCO.2018.78.8034.
17. Raskob GE, van Es N, Verhamme P, Carrier M, Di Nisio M, Garcia D, et al. Edoxaban for the treatment of cancer-associated venous thromboembolism. N Engl J Med. 2018;378(7). https://doi.org/10.1056/NEJMoa1711948.
18. Khorana AA, Francis CW, Kuderer NM, Carrier M, Ortel TL, Wun T, et al. Dalteparin thromboprophylaxis in cancer patients at high risk for venous thromboembolism: a randomized trial. Thromb Res. 2017;151. https://doi.org/10.1016/j.thromres.2017.01.009.
19. Lyman GH, Carrier M, Ay C, Di Nisio M, Hicks LK, Khorana AA, et al. American society of hematology 2021 guidelines for management of venous thromboembolism: prevention and treatment in patients with cancer. Blood Adv. 2021;5(4). https://doi.org/10.1182/bloodadvances.2020003442.
20. Key NS, Khorana AA, Kuderer NM, Bohlke K, Lee AY, Arcelus JI, et al. Venous thromboembolism prophylaxis and treatment in patients with cancer: ASCO clinical practice guideline update. J Clin Oncol. 2020;38(5). https://doi.org/10.1200/JCO.19.01461.
21. Farge D, Frere C, Connors JM, Ay C, Khorana AA, Munoz A, et al. International clinical practice guidelines for the treatment and prophylaxis of venous thromboembolism in patients with cancer. Lancet Oncol. 2019, 2019;20(10). https://doi.org/10.1016/s1470-2045(19)30336-5.
22. Stevens SM, Woller SC, Baumann Kreuziger L, Bounameaux H, Doerschug K, Geersing G-J, et al. Antithrombotic therapy for VTE disease: second update of the CHEST guideline and expert panel report - executive summary. Chest. 2021. https://doi.org/10.1016/j.chest.2021.07.056.
23. Higgins JPT, Thomas J, Chandler J, Cumpston M, Li T, Page MJ, Welch VA (editors). Cochrane Handbook for Systematic Reviews of Interventions. 2nd Edition. Chichester (UK): Wiley; 2019.
24. Cohen AT, Spiro TE, Büller HR, Haskell L, Hu D, Hull R, et al. Rivaroxaban for thromboprophylaxis in acutely ill medical patients. N Engl J Med. 2013;368. https://doi.org/10.1056/NEJMoa1111096.
25. Cohen AT, Harrington RA, Goldhaber SZ, Hull RD, Wiens BL, Gold A, et al. Extended thromboprophylaxis with betrixaban in acutely ill medical patients. N Engl J Med. 2016;375(6). https://doi.org/10.1056/NEJMoa1601747.
26. Vaidya SR, Gupta S, Devarapally SR. Treatment of cancer-associated venous thromboembolism by new oral anticoagulants: a meta-analysis. J Xiangya Med. 2017. https://doi.org/10.21037/jxym.2017.07.04.
27. Khorana AA, Noble S, Lee AYY, Soff G, Meyer G, O'Connell C, et al. Role of direct oral anticoagulants in the treatment of cancer-associated venous thromboembolism: guidance from the SSC of the ISTH. J Thromb Haemost. 2018;16(9). https://doi.org/10.1111/jth.14219.
28. Streiff MB, Holmstrom B, Angelini D, Ashrani A, Elshoury A, Fanikos J et al. Cancer-associated venous thromboembolic disease (Version 1. 2020). (2020). https://www.nccn.org/professionals/physician_gls/pdf/vte.pdf Accessed July 27, 2020.
29. Li A, Kuderer NM, Garcia DA, Khorana AA, Wells PS, Carrier M, et al. Direct oral anticoagulant for the prevention of thrombosis in ambulatory patients with cancer: a systematic review and meta-analysis. J Thromb Haemost. 2019;17(12). https://doi.org/10.1111/jth.14613.
30. Mulder FI, Bosch F, Young AM, Marshall A, McBane RD, Zemla T, et al. Direct oral anticoagulants for cancer-associated venous thromboembolism: a systematic review and meta-analysis. Blood. 2020. https://doi.org/10.1182/blood.2020005819.
31. Sabatino J, De Rosa S, Polimeni A, Sorrentino S, Indolfi C. Direct oral anticoagulants in patients with active cancer: a systematic review and meta-analysis. JACC CardioOncol. 2020. https://doi.org/10.1016/j.jaccao.2020.06.001.
32. Sidahmed S, Abdalla A, Kheiri B, Bala A, Salih M, Bachuwa G, et al. Anticoagulants for the treatment of venous thromboembolism in patients with cancer: A comprehensive systematic review, pairwise and network meta-analysis. Crit Rev Oncol Hematol. 2020;152. https://doi.org/10.1016/j.critrevonc.2020.103005.
33. Farge D, Bounameaux H, Brenner B, Cajfinger F, Debourdeau P, Khorana AA, et al. International clinical practice guidelines including guidance for direct oral anticoagulants in the treatment and prophylaxis of venous thromboembolism in patients with cancer. Lancet Oncol. 2016; 17(10). https://doi.org/10.1016/s1470-2045(16)30369-2.
34. Lyman GH, Kuderer NM. Clinical practice guidelines for the treatment and prevention of cancer-associated thrombosis. Thromb Res. 2020;191. https://doi.org/10.1016/S0049-3848(20)30402-3.

2

The evolution of clot strength in critically-ill COVID-19 patients: A prospective observational thromboelastography study

Colette Neethling[1*], Gregory Calligaro[2], Malcolm Miller[1] and Jessica J. S. Opie[3]

Abstract

Background: Few studies detail the evolution of COVID-19 associated coagulopathy. We performed serial thromboelastography (TEG) and laboratory coagulation studies in 40 critically-ill, mechanically ventilated COVID-19 patients over a 14-day period and analysed differences between 30-day survivors and non-survivors.

Methods: Single-center prospective, observational study including 40 patients with severe COVID-19 pneumonia admitted to the intensive care unit (ICU) for mechanical ventilation. TEG analysis was performed on days 1, 7 and 14 of ICU admission and laboratory coagulation studies were performed on days 1 and 14. Coagulation variables were evaluated for change over the 14-day observation period. Differences between survivors and non-survivors at 30-days were analysed and compared.

Results: On admission, TEG maximum amplitude (MA) with heparinase correction was above the upper limit of the reference range in 32 (80%) patients while 33 (82.5%) presented with absent clot lysis at 30 min. The functional fibrinogen MA was also elevated above the upper limit of the reference range in 37 (92.5%) patients. All patients had elevated D-dimer and fibrinogen levels, mildly prolonged prothrombin times (PT), normal platelet counts and normal activated partial thromboplastin times (aPTT). The heparinase MA decreased significantly with time and normalised after 14 days ($p = < 0.001$) while the increased fibrin contribution to clot strength persisted with time ($p = 0.113$). No significant differences in TEG analysis were noted between 30-day survivors and non-survivors at all time points. No patients developed disseminated intravascular coagulopathy (DIC) after 14-days, however thrombosis and bleeding were each reported in 3 (7.5%) patients.

Conclusion: Critically-ill patients with COVID-19 present in a hypercoagulable state characterised by an increased clot strength. This state normalises after 14 days despite a persistently increased fibrin contribution to clot strength. We were unable to demonstrate any significant differences in TEG parameters between 30-day survivors and non-survivors at all time points.

Keywords: Corona virus disease 2019 (COVID-19), Thromboelastography (TEG), Acute respiratory distress syndrome (ARDS), Hypercoagulability, COVID-19 coagulopathy, Critically-ill

* Correspondence: neethling.colette@gmail.com
[1]Department of Anaesthesia & Perioperative Medicine, University of Cape Town, Groote Schuur Hospital, Anzio Drive, Observatory, Cape Town 7925, South Africa

Background

In December 2019 a pneumonia-like illness emerged in Wuhan, Hubei Province in Central China. This was caused by the novel coronavirus Severe Acute Respiratory Syndrome Coronavirus 2 (SARS-CoV-2) [1]. Coronavirus disease 2019 (COVID-19) has since spread rapidly across the globe, affecting most nations worldwide. At the time of writing, global confirmed cases exceed 238 million with over 4.8million recorded deaths [2]. COVID-19 is associated with increased risk of venous thromboembolism (VTE) [3–7] and a hypercoagulable state characterised by increased clot strength and hypofibrinolysis on viscoelastic tests (VET) [8–11]. The four key mechanisms regarded to be responsible for this prothrombotic state include widespread endothelial damage, activation of coagulation and platelets, and suppression of fibrinolysis [12].

Thromboelastography (TEG) is a point of care VET which demonstrates clotting and fibrinolytic activity of whole blood in vitro. It was first used to identify bleeding abnormalities and guide blood transfusion strategies [13, 14]. More recently TEG has been validated to identify hypercoagulable states and evaluate risk for thromboembolic events [14, 15]. Most studies have evaluated VET in critically-ill COVID-19 patients at a single time point [8–11]. A minority have evaluated patients at various time points with all demonstrating a persistent hypercoagulable state [16–22], however differences between survivors and non-survivors are unclear. It is known that COVID-19 associated coagulopathy plays an integral role in morbidity and mortality with more pronounced derangements in the severely ill [23, 24]. We therefore hypothesise that hypercoagulability lessens in time, especially in those who survive. This prospective, observational study therefore aimed to describe the evolution of coagulopathy over a 14-day period and to identify any differences in coagulation parameters between 30-day survivors and non-survivors.

Methods

Study design and subjects

This was a single center, prospective, observational study which included 40 consecutive patients admitted to the intensive care unit (ICU), between July 19, and August 13, 2020 at Groote Schuur Hospital, a tertiary academic center in Cape Town, South Africa. Ethics approval was obtained from the Human Research and Ethics Committee of the Faculty of Health Sciences of the University of Cape Town (HREC 400/2020). Delayed informed consent was obtained for survivors and proxy consent for non-survivors. All patients admitted to ICU during the study period with severe COVID-19 pneumonia, as defined by the World Health Organisation, were eligible for enrolment [25]. Study patients were intubated and mechanically ventilated and had laboratory confirmed SARS-CoV-2 by reverse transcription-polymerase chain reaction. Patients were excluded if they were younger than 18 years of age, pregnant, known with active cancer or an underlying bleeding disorder.

Standard of care

As per local institutional guidelines, all patients with severe COVID-19 pneumonia with ratios of arterial oxygen partial pressure to fractional inspired oxygen ($Pa0_2/Fi0_2$) < 100 were first placed on high flow nasal oxygen (HFNO) therapy in a high care ward owing to severe constraints on ICU beds. Patients on HFNO were initiated on glucocorticoid therapy (6 mg dexamethasone) once daily for 10 days and therapeutic anticoagulation with either enoxaparin 1 mg/kg twice daily or unfractionated heparin (UFH) infusion, depending on the clinical scenario, and in the absence of contraindications [26]. Enoxaparin was monitored using anti-Factor Xa levels, targeting a therapeutic range of 0.6–1.0 IU/ml. UFH was monitored targeting an activated clotting time (ACT) of 180-220 s. If patients deteriorated clinically on HFNO therapy, they were intubated and transferred to ICU for mechanical ventilation. Glucocorticoid and anticoagulation therapy continued in the ICU. Laboratory coagulation studies included D-dimer and fibrinogen (ACL TOP 500 CTS, HemosIL reagents), platelet count (Sysmex XN-10 with Fluorocell WNR, Lysercell WNR, Cellpak DCL reagents), prothrombin time (PT) (ACL TOP 500 CTS, HemosIL RecombiPlasTin 2G reagents) and activated partial thromboplastin time (aPTT) (ACL TOP 500 CTS, HemosIL SynthASil reagents). Imaging for VTE was performed at the discretion of the treating physician when clinically indicated.

Data and sample collection

Laboratory coagulation studies were performed on day 1 and 14 of ICU admission using samples collected from an arterial line. TEG analysis was performed on day 1, 7 and 14 of ICU admission using blood from 3.2% sodium citrate Vacutainer® tubes, as per manufacturers recommendations. TEG analysis was performed within 30 min of sample collection and not specifically timed to heparin dosing. The same operator conducted the TEG analysis in all cases to prevent inter-operator variability. Patient information collected included: age, sex, body mass index (BMI),comorbidities, anticoagulation use/dosage, glucocorticoid use/dosage, date of symptom onset and ICU admission. Disease severity scores included the $Pa0_2/Fi0_2$ ratio to classify severity of acute respiratory distress syndrome (ARDS) [27], the sequential organ failure assessment (SOFA) score to quantify organ involvement [28], and the International Society on Thrombosis and Haemostasis (ISTH) disseminated intravascular coagulation (DIC) score to determine rate of DIC [29]. Outcomes measured included survival or death at 30 days and bleeding or thrombotic complications. Bleeding events were included if they met the criteria for major bleeding according to the Control of Anticoagulation Subcommittee of the ISTH [30]. Thrombotic complications included those confirmed on radiological imaging, where requested by the treating physician.

Thromboelastography

TEG analysis was performed using the TEG®6 s analyser (Haemonetics®, Braintree, MA).

Results from two TEG reagents were recorded. The first TEG was performed with citrated kaolin in heparinase to neutralise the effect of heparin. The second, TEG functional fibrinogen, contains tissue factor and a glycoprotein IIb/IIIa platelet receptor inhibitor to isolate the contribution of fibrinogen to clot strength [31]. TEG parameters recorded included the R-time, K-time, α-angle, heparinase maximum amplitude (HMA), functional fibrinogen maximum amplitude (FFMA) and clot-lysis at 30 min (LY30). Hypercoagulability was defined as an HMA above the upper limit of the reference range (> 68 mm) [32]. Patient values were compared to the reference ranges provided by the TEG 6 s operating manual.

Statistical analysis

Statistical analysis was performed using STATA/SE. Data for descriptive analysis was reported as mean (standard deviation [SD]), median (interquartile range [IQR]) or number (%) as appropriate. Differences between 30-day survivors and non-survivors at all time points were analysed using the Student t-test, Mann-Whitney U test, χ^2 test or Fisher's exact test as appropriate. Data were tested for differences at various time points using a Friedman, Wilcoxon, ANOVA and Paired t-test as appropriate. A p-value of less than 0.05 was deemed statistically significant.

Results

Forty patients were included in the study. All patients presented with severe ARDS requiring mechanical ventilation with median admission SOFA scores of 4 [4–6] and PaO_2/FiO_2 ratios of 95 (64–124). One patient developed acute kidney injury (AKI) requiring renal replacement therapy and one required extracorporeal membrane oxygenation (ECMO). The mean age was 55 years (±8) and 26 patients (65%) were male. Thirty-four patients (85%) were overweight or obese with a BMI > 25 kg/m^2 [33], 28 (70%) had hypertension and 27 (67.5%) diabetes. The median time from onset of symptoms to ICU admission was 11.5 days [8–14]. Thirty-nine patients (97.5%) received therapeutic anticoagulation; 37 (92.5%) of these received enoxaparin and 2 (5%) UFH due to acute renal failure and ECMO therapy respectively. One patient (2.5%) received prophylactic dose heparin, due to a perceived increased bleeding risk by the treating physician. Clinically significant bleeding events occurred in three patients (7.5%) whilst receiving therapeutic anticoagulation. These included pulmonary haemorrhage requiring massive blood transfusion, intracranial haemorrhage leading to brain stem death and epistaxis requiring cauterization and blood transfusion. Anticoagulation was discontinued in all these patients due to uncontrolled bleeding complications. Confirmed large vessel thrombosis occurred in 3 (7.5%) patients despite therapeutic anticoagulation. These included one case each of pulmonary embolus, cardiac thrombus and lower limb deep venous thrombosis. All patients with a bleeding or thrombotic event did not survive and no patients experienced simultaneous thrombosis and haemorrhage. Detailed TEG analysis of the bleeding and thrombotic group can be found in the supplementary figures.

At 30-day follow up, 6 patients (15%) remained in ICU, one (2.5%) patient had been discharged to the medical ward, 6 (15%) had been discharged home and 27 (67.5%) had demised with a median time from ICU admission to death of 11 days [4–19]. Figure 1 details the 14-day follow up and 30-day outcomes of study patients.

Table 1 displays baseline characteristics, laboratory coagulation and TEG values of the study patients. Admission laboratory coagulation studies demonstrated a mildly prolonged PT, elevated D-dimer and fibrinogen level, normal platelet counts and normal aPTT. The median DIC score on admission was 3 [2, 3] with only one patient meeting the ISTH criteria for DIC [29]. Admission TEG analysis confirmed a hypercoagulable state, with an HMA above the upper limit of the reference range in 32 (80%) patients and absent clot lysis at 30-min in 33 (82.5%). FFMA was also above the upper limit of reference range in 37 (92.5%) patients. The only significant differences noted between the 30-day survivor and non-survivor groups on admission were BMI (p = 0.02) and urea level (p = 0.02).

Of the 40 patients recruited, 11 died within 7 days of ICU admission and could not be followed up over the 14-day observation. Comparisons of the admission characteristics, laboratory coagulation and TEG values for the early death group (N = 11) and 30-day survivors (N = 13) are shown in Table 2.

Due to the early deaths and discharges, only 21 of the 40 patients could be evaluated for evolution of coagulopathy over the 14-day observation. Figure 2 illustrates temporal changes in disease severity scores, laboratory coagulation and TEG values over the 14-day observation for these 21 patients. Elevated D-dimer, fibrinogen levels

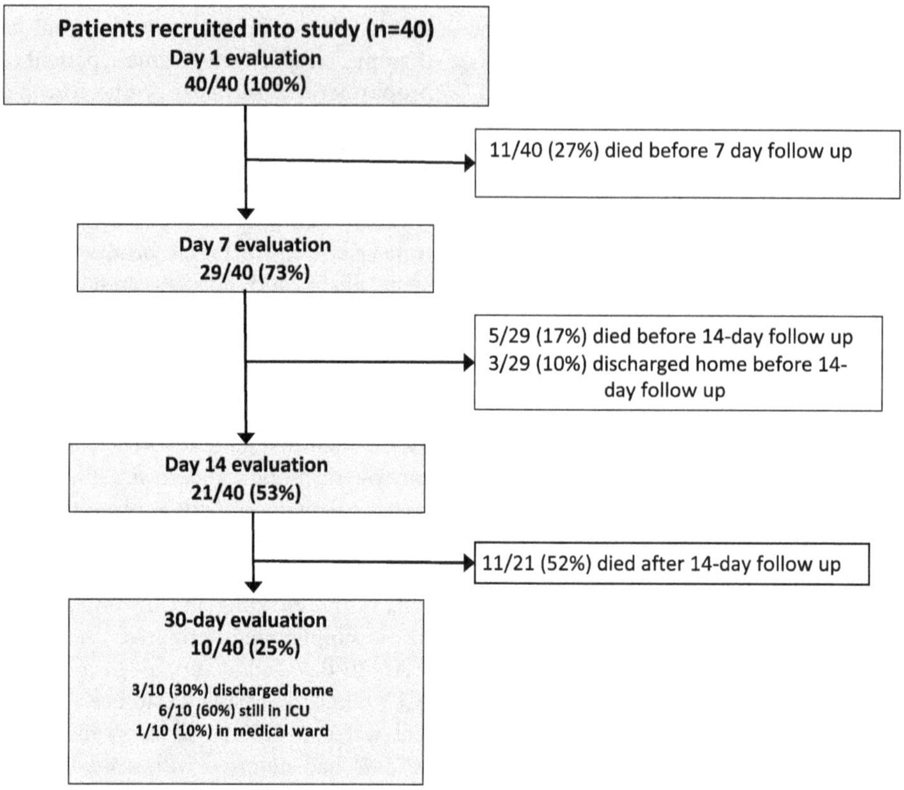

Study cohort flow diagram detailing 14-day follow up and 30-day outcomes

Fig. 1 Study cohort flow diagram

and mildly prolonged PT persisted with time. Platelet counts and aPTT remained within normal reference ranges. HMA decreased significantly over the 14-day period returning to the normal reference range ($p = < 0.001$) while the increased FFMA persisted ($p = 0.113$). The PaO_2/FiO_2 ratios improved significantly with time ($p = 0.020$). Table 3 details differences between 30-day survivors and non-survivors at all timepoints. No significant differences were noted except for aPTT and SOFA on day 14 ($p = < 0.01$, $p = 0.01$).

Discussion

Our study describing the evolution of COVID-19 associated coagulopathy in a group of critically-ill, mechanically ventilated patients using TEG demonstrates four main findings. The first is a hypercoagulable state on ICU admission, with increased fibrin contribution to clot strength. The second is impaired fibrinolysis with 82.5% showing no clot lysis at 30-min on ICU admission. The third is that the hypercoagulable state evolved in time with overall clot strength returning to normal after 14-days. Lastly, no significant differences in TEG parameters were noted at all time points between 30-day survivors and non-survivors. Standard laboratory coagulation studies demonstrated markedly elevated D-dimer and fibrinogen levels on admission which persisted over the observation period. Although the PT was marginally prolonged throughout, the platelet count and aPTT always remained within the reference range over the 14-day observation period.

COVID-19 is associated with an increased rate of VTE in critically-ill patients despite adequate dose thromboprophylaxis, in keeping with an underlying hypercoagulable state [3–7]. Standard laboratory coagulation tests are limited in their ability to reveal the complexities of this hypercoagulable state. Platelet counts are generally within the normal reference range with PT and aPTT only mildly prolonged [34]. The D-dimer, a fibrin degradation product and marker of disease severity [23, 24], is elevated in severe cases indicating increased clot formation. Postmortem findings have demonstrated platelet-fibrin microthrombi in the lungs [35] regarding it to be the source of the raised D-dimer levels [36]. The D-dimer, however, is non-specific and can be raised in various other conditions. Fibrinogen, an acute phase reactant, is also elevated in hospitalised COVID-19 patients; however, the absolute value offers little information on fibrinogen function and interaction with platelets. These limitations have sparked heightened interest in VET such as ROTEM®, TEG®, ClotPro® and

Table 1 Baseline clinical characteristics, laboratory coagulation and thromboelastography parameters on admission to the intensive care unit

Variable on admission	Reference ranges	Total ($N = 40$)	30-day Survivor ($N = 13$)	30-day Non-survivor ($N = 27$)	*P* value
Age, years (SD)		55 (±8)	52 (±9)	56 (±8)	0.09
Sex					0.08
Female n (%)		14 (35)	7 (54)	7 (26)	
Male n (%)		26 (65)	6 (46)	20 (74)	
Comorbidities					
Hypertension n (%)		28 (70)	9 (69)	19 (70)	0.94
Diabetes n (%)		27 (68)	8 (62)	19 (70)	0.58
BMI (kg/m^2)					0.02
Normal weight (18–24.9) n (%)		6 (15)	0 (0)	6 (22)	
Overweight (25–29.9) n (%)		13 (33)	2 (15)	11 (41)	
Obese (> 30) n (%)		21 (52)	11 (85)	10 (37)	
Disease Severity Scores					
SOFA score (IQR)		4 (4–6)	4 (4–4)	4 (4–6)	0.55
PaO_2/FiO_2 ratio (IQR)	200 > – ≤ 300 Mild ARDS 100 > – ≤ 200 Moderate ARDS ≤ 100 Severe ARDS	95(64–124)	95 (60–103)	96 (66–130)	0.61
DIC score (IQR)	< 5 not suggestive of DIC ≥ 5 is suggestive of DIC	3 (2–3)	3 (2–3)	3 (2–4)	0.55
Laboratory Values					
Platelet count, × 10^9/L (IQR)	171–388	354 (267–448)	352 (263–466)	356 (270–438)	0.86
Urea, mmol/L (IQR)	2.1–7.1	9.5 (7.3–11.6)	7.7 (5.8–8.5)	10.2 (9.1–13.0)	0.02
Creatinine, μmol/L (IQR)	64–104	72 (61.5–117.0)	67 (64–81)	85 (61–136)	0.32
Prothrombin time, s (IQR)[a]	11–12.5	13.7 (13.0–15.3)	13.3 (12.8–13.5)	14.2 (13.2–15.7)	1.00
Activated partial thromboplastin time, s (IQR)	25.1–36.5	30.1 (28.6–32.8)	29.9 (28.9–32.6)	30.2 (28.4–32.8)	1.00
D-Dimer, mg/L (IQR)	< 0.25	1.2 (0.6–3.1)	0.9 (0.6–2.5)	1.4 (0.6–4.0)	1.00
Fibrinogen, g/L (IQR)	2–4	5 (5–5)[b]	5 (5–5)[b]	5 (5–5)[b]	0.59
TEG Heparinase					
R-time, min (IQR)	4.3–8.3	7.7 (5.8–9.8)	7.7 (7.5–8.2)	7.8 (5.8–10.7)	0.87
K-time, min (IQR)	0.8–1.9	1.1 (0.9–1.7)	1.1 (0.9–1.4)	1.2 (0.9–1.8)	0.46
α-angle, degree (IQR)	64–77	75.4 (69.6–77.9)	75.0 (71.3–78.9)	75.9 (69.6–77.9)	0.87
Maximum amplitude, mm (IQR)	52–68	70.3 (68.5–72.1)	71.1 (69.5–72.6)	70.2 (68.5–71.7)	0.30
LY-30, % (IQR)	0–8	0 (0)	0 (0–0.1)	0 (0)	0.70
TEG Functional Fibrinogen					
Maximum amplitude, mm (IQR)	15–32	47.0 (41.2–52.6)	48.3 (41.4–50.4)	44.9 (40.2–52.6)	0.88

Table 1. Demographics, laboratory coagulation studies and thromboelastography (TEG) results for all study patients on admission to the intensive care unit (ICU). Differences between admission characteristics for overall 30-day survivors ($N = 13$) and non-survivors ($N = 27$) are shown with corresponding *p*-values. Data are reported as mean (±SD), median (IQR), n (%). Reference ranges were established by the local laboratory and TEG 6 s operating manual.

BMI Body mass index, *SOFA* Sequential organ failure assessment, *PaO_2/FiO_2* Ratio of arterial oxygen partial pressure to fractional inspired oxygen, *DIC* Disseminated intravascular coagulopathy, *PT* Prothrombin time, *aPTT* Activated partial thromboplastin time

[a]PT laboratory control for the duration of the study was 11.7 s

[b]Value is above the upper measurable limit of fibrinogen in local laboratory

Table 2 Baseline characteristics of the 30-day survivors and early death group (died before 7 days)

Variable on admission	Normal reference ranges	30-day Survivor ($N = 13$)	Died before 7 days ($N = 11$)	*P* value
Age, years (SD)		52 (±9)	57 (±9)	0.171
Female, n (%)		7 (54)	1 (9)	0.046
Comorbidities				
Hypertension, n (%)		9 (69)	7 (64)	0.556
Diabetes, n (%)		8 (62)	8 (73)	0.444
Overweight, (BMI > 25 kg/m^2) n (%)		2 (15)	6 (55)	0.055
Obese, (BMI > 30 kg/m^2) n (%)		11 (85)	2 (18)	0.002
Disease Severity Scores				
SOFA score (IQR)		4 (4–4)	5 (4–7)	0.360
PaO_2/FiO_2 ratio (IQR)		95 (60–103)	101 (81–122)	0.450
DIC score (IQR)		3 (2–3)	3 (3–4)	0.113
Laboratory Values				
Platelet count, × 10^9/L (IQR)	171–388	352 (263–466)	358 (255–438)	0.776
Urea, mmol/L (IQR)	2.1–7.1	7.7 (5.8–8.5)	9.3 (6.1–12.8)	0.296
Creatinine, μmol/L (IQR)	64–104	67 (64–81)	65 (56–136)	0.943
Prothrombin time, s (IQR)[a]	11–12.5	13.3 (12.8–13.5)	15.0 (13.6–15.8)	0.013
Activated partial thromboplastin time, s (IQR)	25.1–36.5	29.9 (28.9–32.6)	30.2 (28.7–33.3)	0.809
D-Dimer, mg/L (IQR)	< 0.25	0.9 (0.6–2.5)	3.0 (0.9–5.3)	0.096
Fibrinogen, g/L (IQR)	2–4	5 (5–5)[b]	5 (5–5)[b]	0.399
TEG Heparinase				
R time, min (IQR)	4.3–8.3	7.7 (7.5–8.2)	6.6 (5.4–9.7)	0.579
K time, min (IQR)	0.8–1.9	1.1 (0.9–1.4)	1.0 (0.8–2.0)	0.830
α-angle, degree (IQR)	64–77	75.0 (71.3–78.9)	77.3 (66.6–78.7)	0.679
Maximum amplitude, mm (IQR)	52–68	71.1 (69.5–72.6)	70.5 (69.1–71.7)	0.503
LY-30, % (IQR)	0–8	0 (0–0.1)	0 (0–0.6)	0.529
TEG functional fibrinogen				
Maximum amplitude, mm (IQR)	15–32	48.3 (41.4–50.4)	42.1 (39.4–49.1)	0.353

Table 2 Demographics, laboratory coagulation studies and thromboelastography (TEG) results for the overall 30-day survivors ($N = 13$) compared to the early death group ($N = 11$) with corresponding *p*-values provided. Data are reported as mean (±SD), median (IQR), n (%). Reference ranges were established by the local laboratory and TEG 6 s operating manual.

BMI body mass index, *SOFA* Sequential organ failure assessment, PaO_2/FiO_2 Ratio of arterial oxygen partial pressure to fractional inspired oxygen, *DIC* Disseminated intravascular coagulopathy, *PT* Prothrombin time, *aPTT* Activated partial thromboplastin time

[a]PT laboratory control for the duration of the study was 11.7 s

[b]Value is above the upper measurable limit of fibrinogen in local laboratory

Quantra® which provide a comprehensive overview of coagulation in vitro from clot initiation, formation and lysis. Many studies have evaluated VET in critically-ill COVID-19 patients at one time point and have described a profound hypercoagulable state [8–11]. However serial VET would provide deeper insight into the complex interaction between inflammation and thrombosis over time.

There is little data on the evolution of coagulopathy using VET. Hulshof et al. [16] enrolled 36 critically-ill patients and followed them up over a 6-week period using ROTEM®. They reported a persistence in hypercoagulability and hypofibrinolysis over time. Cordier et al. [20] followed up 10 patients using the TEG 5000. On admission patients with COVID-19 had increased clot strength compared to the control group. These 10 patients were followed up and TEG was repeated at ICU discharge, revealing a further increase in clot strength. They concluded that the hypercoagulable state persists, even in patients with good outcomes. Correa et al. [21] evaluated 30 patients on day 0,1,3,7 and 14 of ICU admission using ROTEM and confirmed that increased clot strength persisted over time. These previous three studies show a persistence in hypercoagulability, which is contrary to our findings. Here we report a significant trend toward normal clot strength in those that survived

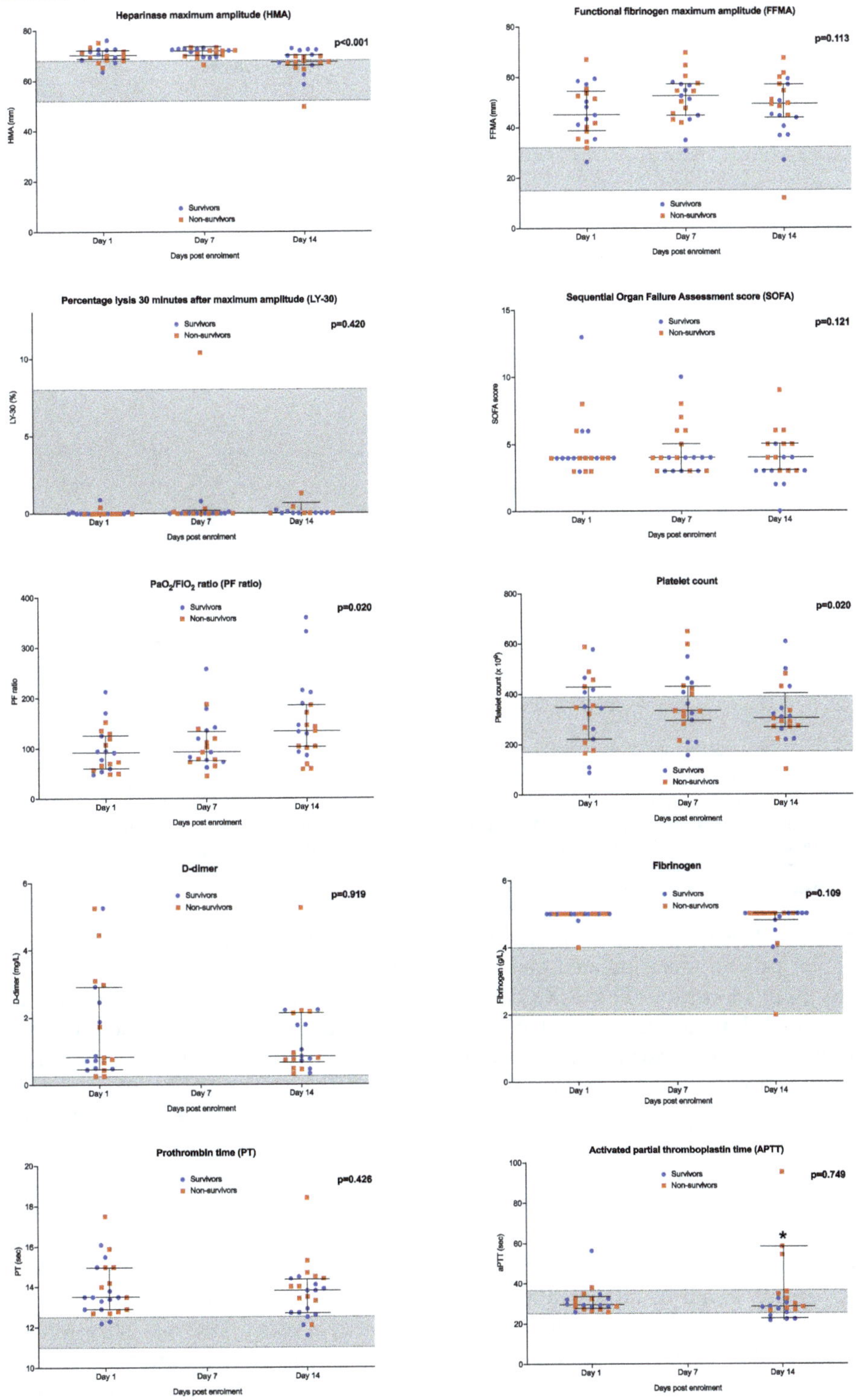

Fig. 2 Evolution in laboratory coagulation tests, thromboelastography parameters and disease severity scores over 14-day period. Figure shows temporal changes in laboratory coagulation studies, thromboelastography (TEG) parameters and disease severity scores for 21 patients that survived to 14-day evaluation. 30-day survivors and non-survivors are represented as blue and red respectively. Coloured dots represent individual measurements. Grey band represents normal reference ranges as established by the local laboratory and the TEG 6 s operating manual. Asterix (*) indicates significant differences noted between survivors and non-survivors at specific time points. Data is presented as median (IQR), *p*-values shown in graphs represent changes over 14-day observation for all patients followed up. ULN = upper limit of normal, LLN = lower limit of normal

Table 3 Differences in coagulation tests, thromboelastography parameters and disease severity scores for 30-day survivors and non-survivors

Parameter	Reference ranges	Survivors ($N = 10$)			Non-survivors ($N = 11$)			*P*-value		
		Day 1	*Day 7*	*Day 14*	*Day 1*	*Day 7*	*Day 14*	*Day 1*	*Day 7*	*Day 14*
D-dimer, mg/L (IQR)	< 0.25	0.80 (0.5–2.46)		0.93 (0.7–1.77)	0.82 (0.44–3.1)		0.79 (0.47–2.17)	0.88		0.94
Fibrinogen, g/L (IQR)	2–4	5 (5–5)[b]		4.95 (4.5–5)	5 (5–5)[b]		5 (5–5)[b]	1.00		1.00
Prothrombin time[a], s (IQR)	11–12.5	13.45 (12.9–13.8)		12.8 (12.5–13.9)	14 (12.8–15)		14 (13.4–14.7)	0.36		0.12
Activated partial thromboplastin time, s (IQR)	25.1–36.5	29.7 (28.9–32.6)		26.45 (22.4–28.6)	28.8 (27.2–32.7)		32.5 (27.8–54.4)	0.45		< 0.01
Platelet count, X10^9/L (IQR)	171–388	348.5 (223–418)	342.5 (209–444)	316 (261–429)	348 (208–458)	334 (311–432)	291 (271–334)	0.76	0.50	0.39
HMA, mm (IQR)	52–68	71.3 (68.5–72.6)	72.3 (69.5–72.8)	70.05 (66.1–72.3)	70.1 (68.2–71.8)	71.3 (69.9–72)	67.3 (65.1–69.4)	0.62	0.46	0.19
FFMA, mm (IQR)	15–32	46.65 (41.2–57.3)	51.95 (43.1–56.7)	44.15 (36.9–50.6)	41.7 (35.5–53.7)	54.4 (45.6–60.4)	51.1 (48.5–59.9)	0.70	0.40	0.07
SOFA score (IQR)		4 (4–6)	4 (3–4)	3 (2–4)	4 (3–4)	4 (3–6)	5 (3–6)	0.37	0.29	0.01
PaO_2/FiO_2 ratio (IQR)		94 (60–126)	106.5 (77–142)	168 (129–215)	73 (57–130)	93 (73–120)	104 (68–146)	0.80	0.48	0.06

Table 3: Differences in laboratory coagulation studies, thromboelastography (TEG) parameters and disease severity scores for the 30-day survivors ($N = 10$) and non-survivors ($N = 11$) over the 14-day observation. Differences at all time points between 30-day survivors and non-survivors are shown with *p*-values provided. Data presented as median (IQR). Reference ranges as established by the local laboratory and TEG 6 s operating manual.
HMA Maximum amplitude with citrated kaolin and heparinase, *FFMA* Functional fibrinogen maximum amplitude, *SOFA* Sequential organ failure assessment, *PaO_2/FiO_2* Ratio of arterial oxygen partial pressure to fractional inspired oxygen; *PT* Prothrombin time, *aPTT* Activated partial thromboplastin time
[a]PT laboratory control for the duration of the study was 11.7 s
[b]Value is above the upper measurable limit of fibrinogen in local laboratory

to the 14-day evaluation. This could be for various reasons. In our cohort, all patients were initiated on dexamethasone prior to ICU admission. The RECOVERY collaborative group revealed a decrease in 28-day mortality in mechanically ventilated patients treated with dexamethasone [37]. The routine use of dexamethasone in all our patients may have played an integral role in abating the inflammatory response and contributing to the subsequent decrease in hypercoagulability seen after 14 days. The normalisation of clot strength in our group compared to the literature could also be attributed to the timing of our patients admission to ICU. In a resource rich setting, patients would be intubated and enrolled into VET studies at an earlier stage of the disease process. In our setting, due to severe resource constraints, patients with severe ARDS were first placed on HFNO, and thus were evaluated at a more advanced stage of disease. Although we did not demonstrate any significant changes in D-dimer and fibrinogen over time, the normalisation of clot strength on TEG could correspond with clinical recovery.

The anticoagulation strategy adopted locally at our institution could also impact our findings. All patients admitted to our ICU had been fully anticoagulated with enoxaparin or UFH. Apart from its anticoagulation properties, heparin has anti-inflammatory and potentially anti-viral properties too [38]. Some VET studies support this improvement in hypercoagulability after initiation of anticoagulation. Ranucci et al. [19] recruited 10 patients into their study, performing VET with the Quantra® analyser. They initiated aggressive anticoagulation with LMWH 6000-8000 IU BD and clopidogrel and reported an improvement in hypercoagulability after 14 days of increased anticoagulation. Bocci et al. [17] embarked on a similar study to evaluate the effect of full therapeutic anticoagulation on 40 critically-ill COVID-19 patients using TEG®6 s. They found that therapeutic anticoagulation had no impact on TEG parameters over 7 days. We also did not demonstrate significant differences between admission and day 7 clot strength; however, there was a significant difference on day 14. Similar findings may have been demonstrated had Bocci et al. continued their follow up to 14 days.

Despite the overall clot strength normalising in our study patients, we did find that the increased contribution of fibrin to clot strength persisted in time, confirming many previous reports [16, 17, 19, 21]. However, our findings contradict with those of Pavoni et al. [22] who reported a decreased contribution of fibrin to clot strength over time and normalisation on day 10. The main assays used to determine fibrin contribution to clot strength are FIBTEM (which uses tissue factor and cytochalasin D) and TEG functional fibrinogen (which uses tissue factor and abiximab) [39]. The FIBTEM assay has been shown to correlate with fibrinogen levels ($r = 0.74$) [16] and relies largely on fibrinogen for clot formation [16]. Despite this, overall clot strength correlates with platelet count and not fibrinogen levels [16]. We demonstrated similar findings as our HMA correlated with platelet count ($r = 0.54$, $p < 0.001$) and fibrinogen to FFMA ($r = 0.41$, $p = 0.01$). This indicates that although fibrinogen plays an important role in increased clot strength, other factors such as platelets are also important. Studies have revealed that SARS-CoV-2 induces platelet hyperreactivity with increased activation and aggregation [40]. Platelets have also shown greater adhesion and spread on fibrinogen and collagen in those with severe COVID-19 disease [40]. The TEG functional fibrinogen however has limitations as cytochalasin D has been proven to be far superior at inhibiting platelets than abiximab [39]. Also, in the presence of thrombocytosis, which is frequently seen in COVID-19 patients, abiximab is less successful at inhibiting platelets resulting in an over-estimation of fibrin contribution to clot strength [41]. Detailed platelet function analysis would prove more instructive. We were unable to demonstrate any significant differences in TEG parameters between 30-day survivors and non-survivors at all time points. This questions the usefulness of TEG in the clinical setting to risk stratify critically-ill COVID-19 patients and improve their care.

This novel serial VET study shows improvement in hypercoagulability in critically-ill COVID-19 patients as denoted by clot strength after 14-days and compares TEG parameters in 30-day survivors and non-survivors. The main study limitation is the relatively small sample size. Only 21 patients could be evaluated for VET changes over time which limits generalisability of the results. A further limitation is that our laboratory could only measure D-dimer and fibrinogen levels up to 5.25 mg/L and 5 g/L respectively. Therefore, the true fibrinogen and D-dimer values could not be measured and are likely to be underestimated. The expensive running cost of the TEG 6 s instrument further restricted the frequency with which patients could be evaluated. Ideally, we would have performed follow up TEG testing until the outcome of death or discharge was reached. Further study would include a larger patient cohort, with more frequent and prolonged follow up of TEG to clearly illustrate the trends identified in this study. Comprehensive evaluation of platelet function would also provide better insights into the relative contributions of platelets and fibrinogen in overall clot strength.

Conclusion

Our study demonstrates that the increased clot strength seen in critically-ill COVID-19 patients normalises after 14-days, implying clinical recovery. The increased fibrin contribution to clot strength however appears to persist over time. We were unable to demonstrate any significant differences in TEG parameters between 30-day survivors and non-survivors. Further study is needed to assess the utility of TEG in identifying those at risk of poor outcomes.

Abbreviations

SARS-CoV-2: Severe acute respiratory syndrome coronavirus 2; TEG: Thromboelastography; R: Reaction; K: Kinetic; HMA: Heparinase maximum amplitude; FFMA: Functional fibrinogen maximum amplitude; MA: Maximum amplitude; α: Alpha; LY-30: Lysis of clot at 30 min; COVID-19: Coronavirus disease 2019; ICU: Intensive care unit; PT: Prothrombin time; aPTT: Activated partial thromboplastin time; IQR: Interquartile range; SD: Standard deviation; VTE: Venothromboembolism; VET: Viscoelastic test; ULN: Upper limit of normal; LLN: Lower limit of normal

Supplementary Information

Additional file 1: Figure 1. Detailed thromboelastography tracings for the pulmonary haemorrhage patient. **Figure 2.** Detailed thromboelastography tracings for the epistaxis patient. **Figure 3.** Detailed thromboelastography tracings for the intracranial haemorrhage patient. **Figure 4.** Detailed thromboelastography tracing for the patient with a deep venous thrombosis. **Figure 5.** Detailed thromboelastography tracing of the patient with a cardiac thrombus. **Figure 6.** Detailed thromboelastography tracing for the pulmonary embolus patient.

Acknowledgements

Patients and their families.
Staff of the COVID intensive care unit at Groote Schuur hospital.
Lizel Loo for her assistance in procuring equipment for the study.
Wisdom Basera for statistical support.
Haemonetics for their humanitarian donation of TEG consumables.

Authors' contributions

CN: Was responsible for conception of the research idea, study design and performed all data collection and capturing. CN was involved in the analysis and interpretation of results and the write-up of the manuscript. GC: Assisted in the statistical analysis and drafting of digital artwork for the manuscript. GC also involved in the critical review of the work. MM: Was responsible for development of research idea and study design. MM was involved in data analysis and interpretation of results. MM also responsible for the write-up and critical review of the manuscript. JO: Was responsible for development of research idea and study design. JO was involved in the data analysis and interpretation of the results. JO also responsible for the write-up and critical review of the manuscript. All authors read and approved the final manuscript.

Author details

[1]Department of Anaesthesia & Perioperative Medicine, University of Cape Town, Groote Schuur Hospital, Anzio Drive, Observatory, Cape Town 7925, South Africa. [2]Division of Pulmonology, Department of Medicine, University of Cape Town, Groote Schuur Hospital, Cape Town, South Africa. [3]Division of Haematology, Department of Pathology, University of Cape Town & National Health Laboratory Service, Groote Schuur Hospital, Cape Town, South Africa.

References

1. Li H, Liu SM, Yu XH, Tang SH, Tang CK. Coronavirus disease (COVID-19): current status and future perspectives. Int J Antimicrob Agents. 2020;55(5): 105951. https://doi.org/10.1016/j.ijantimicag.2020.105951.
2. Johns Hopkins University. Johns Hopkins University Coronavirus Resource Centre. 2021 https://coronavirus.jhu.edu/map.html. Accessed on October 12, 2021.
3. Klok FA, Kruip MJHA, van der Meer NJM, Arbous MS, Gommers DAMPJ, Kant KM, et al. Incidence of thrombotic complications in critically ill ICU patients with COVID-19. Thromb Res. 2020;191:145–7. https://doi.org/10.1016/j.thromres.2020.04.013.
4. Kruse JM, Magomedov A, Kurreck A, Munch FH, Koerner R, Kamhieh-Milz J, et al. Thromboembolic complications in critically ill COVID-19 patients are associated with impaired fibrinolysis. Crit Care. 2020;24(1):676. https://doi.org/10.1186/s13054-020-03401-8.
5. Maatman TK, Jalali F, Feizpour C, Douglas A, McGuire SP, Kinnaman G, et al. Routine venous thromboembolism prophylaxis may be inadequate in the hypercoagulable state of severe coronavirus disease 2019. Crit Care Med. 2020;48(9):783–90. https://doi.org/10.1097/CCM.0000000000004466.
6. Hippensteel JA, Burnham EL, Jolley SE. Prevalence of venous thromboembolism in critically ill patients with COVID-19. Br J Haematol. 2020;190(3):134–7. https://doi.org/10.1111/bjh.16908.
7. Trigonis RA, Holt DB, Yuan R, Siddiqui AA, Craft MK, Khan BA, et al. Incidence of venous thromboembolism in critically ill coronavirus disease 2019 patients receiving prophylactic Anticoagultion. Crit Care Med. 2020; 48(9):805–8. https://doi.org/10.1097/CCM.0000000000004472.
8. Yuriditsky E, Horowitz JM, Merchan C, Ahuja T, Brosnahan SB, McVoy L, et al. Thromboelastography profiles of critically ill patients with coronavirus disease 2019. Crit Care Med. 2020;48(9):1319–26. https://doi.org/10.1097/CCM.0000000000004471.
9. Panigada M, Bottino N, Tagliabue P, Grasselli G, Novembrino C, Chantarangkul V, et al. Hypercoagulability of COVID-19 patients in intensive care unit: a report of thromboelastography findings and other parameters of hemostasis. J Thromb Haemost. 2020;18(7):1738–42. https://doi.org/10.1111/jth.14850.
10. Wright FL, Vogler TO, Moore EE, Moore HB, Wohlauer MV, Urban S, et al. Fibrinolysis shutdown correlation with thromboembolic events in severe COVID-19 infection. J Am Coll Surg. 2020;231(2):193–203. https://doi.org/10.1016/j.jamcollsurg.2020.05.007.
11. Mortus JR, Manek SE, Brubaker LS, Loor M, Cruz MA, Trautner BW, et al. Thromboelastographic results and hypercoagulability syndrome in patients with coronavirus disease 2019 who are critically ill. JAMA Netw Open. 2020; 3(6):e2011192. https://doi.org/10.1001/jamanetworkopen.2020.11192.
12. Iba T, Levy JH, Levi M, Connors JM, Thachil J. Coagulopathy of coronavirus disease 2019. Crit Care Med. 2020;48(9):1358–64. https://doi.org/10.1097/CCM.0000000000004458.
13. Chaudhary R, Kreutz RP, Bliden KP, Tantry US, Gurbel PA. Personalising antithrombotic therapy in COVID-19: role of Thromboelastography and Thromboelastomerty. J Thromb Haemost. 2020;120(11):1594–6. https://doi.org/10.1055/s-0040-1714217.
14. Harahsheh Y, Ho KM. Use of viscoelastic tests to predict clinical thromboembolic events. A systematic review and meta-analysis. Eur J Haematol. 2018;100(2):113–23. https://doi.org/10.1111/ejh.12992.
15. Luddington RJ. Thromboelastography/thromboelastometry. Clin Lab Haem. 2005;27(2):81–90. https://doi.org/10.1111/j.1365-2257.2005.00681.x.
16. Hulshof AM, Brüggemann RAG, Mulder MMG, van de Berg TW, Sels JEM, Olie RH, et al. Serial EXTEM, FIBTEM, and tPA rotational Thromboelastometry observations in the Maastricht intensive care COVID cohort—persistence of hypercoagulability and Hypofibrinolysis despite anticoagulation. Front Cardiovasc Med. 2021;8:654174. https://doi.org/10.3389/fcvm.2021.654174.
17. Bocci MG, Maviglia R, Consalvo LM, Grieco DL, Montini L, Mercurio G, et al. Thromboelastograph clot strength profiles and effect of systemic anticoagulation in COVID-19 acute respiratory distress syndrome: a prospective, observational study. Eur Rev Med Pharmacol Sci. 2020;24(23): 12466–79. https://doi.org/10.26355/eurrev_202012_24043.
18. Pavoni V, Gianesello L, Pazzi M, Stera C, Meconi T, Frigieri FC. Evaluation of coagulation function by rotation thromboelastometry in critically ill patients with severe COVID-19 pneumonia. J Thromb Thrombolysis. 2020;50(2):281–6. https://doi.org/10.1007/s11239-020-02130-7.
19. Ranucci M, Ballotta A, Di Dedda U, Baryshnikova E, Dei Poli M, Resta M, et al. The procoagulant pattern of patients with COVID-19 acute respiratory distress syndrome. J Thromb Haemost. 2020;18(7):1747–51. https://doi.org/10.1111/jth.14854.
20. Cordier P, Pierrou C, Noel A, Paris R, Gaudray E, Martin E, et al. Complex and prolonged hypercoagulability in coronavirus disease 2019 intensive care unit patients: a thromboelastographic study. Aust Crit Care. 2021;34(2):160–6. https://doi.org/10.1016/j.aucc.2020.11.007.
21. Corrêa TD, Cordioli RL, Campos Guerra JC, da Silva BC, dos Reis RR, de Souza GM, et al. Coagulation profile of COVID-19 patients admitted to the ICU: an exploratory study. PLoS One. 2020;15(12):e0243604. https://doi.org/10.1371/journal.pone.0243604.
22. Pavoni V, Gianesello L, Pazzi M, Horton A, Suardi L. Derangements of the coagulation process using subclinical markers and viscoelastic measurements in critically ill patients with coronavirus disease 2019 penumonia and non-coronavirus disease 2019 pneumonia. Blood Coagul Fibrinolysis. 2021;32(2):80–6. https://doi.org/10.1097/MBC.0000000000000971.
23. Tang N, Li D, Wang X, Sun Z. Abnormal coagulation parameters are associated with poor prognosis in patients with novel coronavirus pneumonia. J Thromb Haemost. 2020;18(4):844–7. https://doi.org/10.1111/jth.14768.
24. Zhou F, Yu T, Du R, Fan G, Liu Y, Liu Z, et al. Clinical course and risk factors for mortality of adult inpatients with COVID-19 in Wuhan, China: a retrospective cohort study. Lancet. 2020;395(10229):1054–62. https://doi.org/10.1016/S0140-6736(20)30566-3.
25. World Health Organisation: Clinical management of Covid-19: Interim guidance. 2020 https://www.who.int/publications/i/item/clinical-management-of-covid-19. Accessed September 2020.
26. Mendelson M, Boloko L, Boutall A, Cairncross L, Calligaro G, Coccia C, et al. Clinical management of COVID-19: experiences of the COVID-19 epidemic from Groote Schuur hospital, Cape Town, South Africa. S Afr Med. 2020; 110(10):973–81. https://doi.org/10.7196/SAMJ.2020.v110i10.15157.
27. Ranieri M, Rubenfeld GD, Thompson BT, Ferguson ND, Caldwell E, Fan E, et al. Acute respiratory distress syndrome, the Berlin definition. JAMA. 2012; 307(23):2526–33. https://doi.org/10.1001/jama.2012.5669.
28. Vincent JL. In: Gullo A, editor. SOFA Score: A Keystone for Grading Multiple Organ Dysfunction. Milano: Anaesthesia, Pain, Intensive Care and Emergency A.P.I.C.E, Springer; 2008. p. 255–60.
29. Bakhtiari K, Meijers JC, de Jonge E, Levi M. Prospective validation of the International Society of Thrombosis and Haemostasis scoring system for disseminated intravascular coagulation. Crit Care Med. 2004;32(12):2416–21. https://doi.org/10.1097/01.CCM.0000147769.07699.E3.
30. Schulman S, Kearon C. Definition of major bleeding in clinical investigations of antihemostatic medicinal products in non-surgical patients. J Thromb Haemost. 2004;3(4):692–4. https://doi.org/10.1111/j.1538-7836.2005.01204.x.
31. Whiting D, DiNardo JA. TEG and ROTEM: technology and clinical applications. Am J Hematol. 2014;89(2):228–32. https://doi.org/10.1002/ajh.23599.
32. McCrath DJ, Cerboni E, Frumento RJ, Hirsh AL, Bennett-Guerrero E. Thromboelastography maximum amplitude predicts postoperative thrombotic complications including myocardial infarction. Anesth Analg. 2005;100(6):1576–83. https://doi.org/10.1213/01.ANE.0000155290.86795.12.
33. Weir CB, Jan A. BMI Classification Percentile and Cut Off Points. In: StatPearls. Treasure Island: StatPearls Publishing; 2020.
34. Becker RC. COVID-19 update: Covid-19-associated coagulopathy. J Thromb Thrombolysis. 2020;50(1):54–67. https://doi.org/10.1007/s11239-020-02134-3.
35. Carsana L, Sonzogni A, Nasr A, Rossi RS, Pellegrinelli A, Zerbi P, et al. Pulmonary post-mortem findings in a series of COVID-19 cases from northern Italy: a two-Centre descriptive study. Lancet. 2020;20(10):1135–40. https://doi.org/10.1016/S1473-3099(20)30434-5.
36. Ibañez C, Perdomo J, Calvo A, Ferrando C, Reverter JC, Tassies D, et al. High D-dimers and low global fibrinolysis coexist in COVID-19 patients: what is going on here? J Thromb Thrombolysis. 2020;51(2):308–12. https://doi.org/10.1007/s11239-020-02226-0.
37. Horby P, Lim WS, Emberson JR, Mafham M, Bell JL, Linsell L, et al. Dexamethasone in hospitalized patients with Covid-19. N Engl J Med. 2021; 384(8):693–704. https://doi.org/10.1056/NEJMoa2021436.
38. Thachil J. The versatile heparin in COVID-19. J Thromb Haemost. 2020;18(5): 1020–2. https://doi.org/10.1111/jth.14821.
39. Schlimp CJ, Solomon C, Ranucci M, Hochleitner G, Redl H, Schochl H. The effectiveness of different functional fibrinogen polymerization assays in eliminating platelet contribution to clot strength in Thromboelastometry. Anesth Analg. 2014;118(2):269–76. https://doi.org/10.1213/ANE.0000000000000058.

40. Manne BK, Denorme F, Middleton EA, Portier I, Rowley JW, Stubben C, et al. Platelet gene expression and function in patients with COVID-19. Blood. 2020;136(11):1317–29. https://doi.org/10.1182/blood.2020007214.
41. Ranucci M, Di Dedda U, Baryshnikova E. Trials and tribulations of viscoelastic-based determination of fibrinogen concentration. Anesth Analg. 2020;130(3):644–53. https://doi.org/10.1213/ANE.0000000000004522.

3

Thromboembolic and hemorrhagic risks after vaccination against SARS-CoV-2

Noppacharn Uaprasert[1,2*], Krissana Panrong[1,2], Ponlapat Rojnuckarin[1,2] and Thita Chiasakul[1,2]

Abstract

Background: Thromboembolic and bleeding events after vaccination against severe acute respiratory syndrome coronavirus 2 (SARS-CoV-2) are major public concerns leading to vaccine hesitancy. Due to low incidence, an individual randomized controlled trial (RCT) is underpowered to determine whether SARS-CoV-2 vaccines increase the risks of thromboembolism and hemorrhage.

Methods: We performed a literature search using PubMed, EMBASE, Cochrane, medRxiv databases, and reference lists of relevant articles to identify RCTs that reported thromboembolic, hemorrhagic events, and thromboembolism/hemorrhage-related death after SARS-CoV-2 vaccination. The primary aim of this systematic review and meta-analysis was to estimate the pooled thromboembolic risk related to SARS-CoV-2 vaccines compared to placebo. The secondary outcomes included estimating the risks of arterial thromboembolism (ATE), venous thromboembolisms (VTE), hemorrhage, thrombocytopenia, and thromboembolism/hemorrhage-related death.

Results: Eight RCTs of 4 vaccine platforms comprised of 195,196 participants were retrieved. SARS-CoV-2 vaccines were not associated with an increased risk of overall thromboembolism (risk ratio [RR], 1.14; 95% CI [confidence interval], 0.61–2.14; $I^2 = 35\%$), ATE (RR, 0.97; 95% CI, 0.46–2.06; $I^2 = 21\%$), VTE (RR, 1.47; 95% CI, 0.72–2.99; $I^2 = 0\%$), hemorrhage (RR, 0.97; 95% CI, 0.35–2.68; $I^2 = 0$), and thromboembolism/hemorrhage-related death (RR, 0.53; 95% CI, 0.16–1.79; $I^2 = 0$). Compared to the baseline estimated risk of these outcomes in participants administered placebos, the risk differences with vaccines were very small and not statistically significant. These findings were consistent in the subgroup analysis across 4 vaccine platforms.

Conclusion: Vaccines against SARS-CoV-2 are not associated with an increased risk of thromboembolism, hemorrhage, and thromboembolism/hemorrhage-related death.

Keywords: Thromboembolism, Hemorrhage, Vaccine, SARS-CoV-2

* Correspondence: drnoppacharn@yahoo.com
[1]Division of Hematology, Department of Medicine, Faculty of Medicine, Chulalongkorn University and King Chulalongkorn Memorial Hospital, Thai Red Cross Society, Bangkok, Thailand
[2]Research Unit in Translational Hematology, Faculty of Medicine, Chulalongkorn University and King Chulalongkorn Memorial Hospital, Thai Red Cross Society, Bangkok, Thailand

Introduction

Severe acute respiratory syndrome coronavirus 2 (SARS-CoV-2) has been identified as a causative agent of an emerging cluster of pneumonia in China in December 2019. Its outbreak has been declared as a pandemic leading to a global health crisis since March 11, 2020 [1]. As of August 2021, SARS-CoV-2 has infected more than 200 million individuals and caused over 4 million deaths worldwide [2]. Vaccines against SARS-CoV-2 were developed at unparalleled speeds to end the coronavirus disease 2019 (COVID-19) pandemic by controlling the viral spread.

To date, there are at least 4 vaccine platforms including mRNA, adenoviral vector, inactivated, and protein subunit vaccines that have demonstrated effectiveness in the prevention of symptomatic infection and reduction in hospitalization and mortality from COVID-19 [3–10]. Although these SARS-CoV-2 vaccines had acceptable safety profiles in phase 3 randomized controlled trials (RCTs), concerns regarding potential rare side effects including the risk of thromboembolism remain a reason for vaccine hesitancy [11]. A distinctive syndrome of vaccine-induced immune thrombotic thrombocytopenia (VITT) associated with pathogenic anti-platelet factor 4 antibodies (anti-PF4 Abs) has been reported after two adenoviral vector vaccines against SARS-CoV-2, ChAdOx1 nCoV-19 and Ad26.COV2.S [12–15]. However, this thrombotic complication linked to SARS-CoV-2 vaccines is extremely rare with an estimated incidence of 0.73 per 100,000 doses of the ChAdOx1 vaccine [16]. Most thromboembolic and hemorrhagic events after vaccination against SARS-CoV-2 are independent of anti-PF4 Abs. The risks of thromboembolism and hemorrhage after vaccination against SARS-CoV-2 remain largely unknown and have never been comprehensively evaluated in phase 3 RCTs.

Due to the rarity of thrombotic and hemorrhagic events reported in individual studies, a single RCT is underpowered to determine whether SARS-CoV-2 vaccines increase the risks of thromboembolism and hemorrhage. We conducted a systematic review and meta-analysis of phase 3 RCTs to estimate the risks of thromboembolism, hemorrhage, and death related to thrombosis or hemorrhage after vaccination against SARS-CoV-2.

Methods

The protocol for this review was pre-specified and registered in PROSPERO (CRD42021253193). The study was subsequently conducted following Preferred Reporting Items for Systematic reviews and Meta-Analyses (PRISMA) guidelines [17]. The primary objective of this study was to estimate the risk of overall thromboembolism including arterial and venous thromboembolism of SARS-CoV-2 vaccines compared to placebo.

Data source, search strategy and study selection

A systematic search of electronic databases was performed using PubMed, EMBASE, and Cochrane Library Database from inception to the last update on June 30, 2021 to identify RCTs reporting thromboembolic and hemorrhagic events or death related to thromboembolic and hemorrhagic events after SARS-CoV-2 vaccination. The following search terms were used: vaccine, vaccination, immunization, thromboembolism, thromboembolic, thrombosis, infarct, stroke, ischemia, ischemic, bleeding, hemorrhage, hemorrhagic, platelet, thrombocytopenia, thrombocytopenic, coagulation, coagulopathy, safety, novel coronavirus 2019, COVID-19, SARS-CoV-2, and 2019-nCoV. Additionally, studies published on the preprint server (medRxiv) and reference lists of relevant articles were manually reviewed. The inclusion criteria for eligible studies were as follows: (1) RCTs with at least 100 participants in both the vaccine and control arms, (2) reported safety outcomes which specified thromboembolic and hemorrhagic events and/or death related to thromboembolism and hemorrhage. Non-original articles (such as reviews, commentaries, or guidelines) and duplicate studies were excluded. There were no language restrictions. Two authors (N.U. and K.P.) independently searched the literature, screened titles and abstracts, and reviewed full texts to identify potentially eligible studies. Disagreements were resolved by consensus or a third reviewer (T.C.) when necessary. The selection result was reported according to the PRISMA flowchart.

Data extraction

Two authors (N.U. and K.P.) independently reviewed data from selected studies including supplementary materials and independently extracted pre-specified data. Disagreements of extracted data were resolved by consensus or a third reviewer (T.C.) when necessary. The primary outcome was the risk of arterial and/or venous thromboembolism after vaccination against SARS-CoV-2 compared to controls. The secondary outcomes included the risks of arterial thromboembolism (ATE), venous thromboembolisms (VTE), bleeding, thrombocytopenia, and death related to thromboembolism and hemorrhage after vaccination against SARS-CoV-2.

For each study, the following data were extracted: study design, phase of clinical trials, vaccine platform (mRNA, viral vector, inactivated, or protein subunit), treatment allocation, study population, number of participants, baseline characteristics of participants (age, sex, and ethnicity), thromboembolic events, hemorrhagic events, and death related to thromboembolism or hemorrhage. Corresponding authors of the BNT162b2 study were contacted twice to request additional outcome data that were not reported. However, we were unable to obtain data from the BNT162b study.

Quality assessment

An assessment of the methodological quality of included studies for meta-analysis was performed independently by two authors (N.U. and K.P.) using the revised version of the Cochrane risk-of-bias tool in RCTs [18]. Bias was assessed in the domains of randomization process, deviations from the intended interventions, missing outcome data, measurement of the outcomes, and selection of the reported results. Data on study characteristics and outcomes were extracted by using a standardized form. The risk of bias was graded as low, some concerns, or high. Discrepancies were resolved by consensus or contact with a third reviewer (T.C.).

Data analysis

The meta-analysis was performed using Comprehensive Meta-Analysis software (Version 3; Biostat, Englewood, NJ, USA). The risk ratio (RR) and the risk difference of each outcome were calculated using the Mantel-Haenszel method with random-effects model and were reported as RR and risk difference (per 100,000 persons) with 95% confidence interval (95% CI) [19]. The pre-specified subgroup analyses including the risks of thromboembolism and hemorrhage across vaccine platforms (mRNA, virus vector, inactivated, or protein subunit vaccines), age groups, sex, and races would be performed if there were sufficient data. Statistical heterogeneity was assessed using I^2 statistic which measures the inconsistency across study results. Inter-study heterogeneity was assigned as insignificant ($I^2 = 0–25\%$), low ($I^2 = 26–50\%$), moderate ($I^2 = 51–75\%$), or high ($I^2 > 75\%$) [20]. Publication bias was explored by visual inspection of the funnel plots. No formal tests for publication bias were performed as they lacked statistical power due to the low number of studies included in the meta-analysis (less than 10 studies).

Results

The study report was prepared in accordance with the Preferred Reporting Items for Systematic Reviews and Meta-Analyses guidance (Supplementary Table S1) [17]. The PRISMA flow diagram is shown in Supplementary Fig. S1. The literature search yielded 4999 articles. After 1568 duplicates removed, a total of 3847 unique studies were screened by titles and abstracts. Of these, 3816 were excluded, and 31 full texts were screened for eligibility. Eventually 8 studies [3–10] met the eligibility criteria and were included in the qualitative and quantitative synthesis. The risk of bias in each study was individually assessed. All studies [3–10] were assigned as low risk of bias (Supplementary Fig. S2).

Study characteristics

The main characteristics of the 8 included studies (7 published full-texts and 1 full-preprint report) are summarized in Table 1 [3–10]. The 8 studies contained 195,196 participants. A total of 104,779 participants were administered SARS-CoV-2 vaccines, and a total of 90,417 were administered placebos. There were 4 vaccine platforms including 2 mRNA vaccines (BNT162b2 and mRNA-1273) [3, 4], 3 adenoviral vector vaccines (Ad26.COV.2S, ChAdOx1 and rAD26/rAD5) [5–7], 1 inactivated vaccine (2 studies of CoronaVac) [8, 9], and 1 protein subunit vaccine (NVX-CoV23) [10]. All vaccines except the NVX-CoV23 vaccine were widely available under emergency use authorization. The majority of participants were younger than 60 years and predominantly Caucasian. Baseline characteristics including age groups, sex, races, and coexisting conditions among participants in the vaccine and the placebo groups were similar. The BNT162b2 study reported only death related to thromboembolism and hemorrhage, while the primary and other secondary outcomes were not reported. Detailed thromboembolic and hemorrhagic events of each study are summarized in Supplementary Table S2.

The risk of thromboembolism after vaccination against SARS-CoV-2

The estimated risk of thromboembolism including arterial and/or venous thrombosis was estimated from 7 of the 8 studies, while omitting the BNT162b study [4–10]. A total of 85,915 and 71,571 participants received either a vaccine or placebo, respectively. The pooled RR of thromboembolism after vaccination was 1.14 (95% CI, 0.61 to 2.14; $I^2 = 35\%$) (Fig. 1). With a baseline estimated risk of thromboembolism in the placebo group of 52 events per 100,000 persons (95% CI, 33 to 83; $I^2 = 37\%$), the risk difference with the vaccine group was 7.8 events per 100,000 persons (95% CI, − 20 to 36; $I^2 = 33\%$). The subgroup analysis did not demonstrate an increased risk of thromboembolism in any vaccine platform ($P = 0.80$) (Supplementary Fig. S3).

The risks of arterial thromboembolism and venous thromboembolism after vaccination against SARS-CoV-2

The risks of ATE and VTE after SARS-CoV-2 vaccination were estimated from the same 7 studies, again excluding the BNT162b2 study [4–10]. No VTE events occurred in one inactivated vaccine study (Tanriover) [8]. The pooled RR of ATE after SARS-CoV-2 vaccination was 0.97 (95% CI, 0.46 to 2.06; $I^2 = 21\%$) (Fig. 2). With an estimated risk of ATE from 7 studies [4–10] in the placebo group of 38 events per 100,000 persons (95% CI, 23 to 63; $I^2 = 20\%$), the risk difference with the vaccine group was − 1.8 events per 100,000 persons (95% CI, − 20 to 17; $I^2 = 27\%$).

Table 1 Baseline characteristics of included randomized controlled trials

Study name	Vaccine platform	Study characteristics	Treatment allocation	Number of participants (safety data)	Age (years)	Sex (male)	Race (white, black, Asian)	Countries	Comorbidities
Polack, 2020 [3]	mRNA	Primary analysis of safety and efficacy from the phase 2/3 part of BNT162b2 in preventing symptomatic COVID-19 in persons ≥16 years Median follow-up: 2 months	BNT162b2 (30 μg), 2 doses 21 days apart	18,860 (21621)	52[a] (Range; 16–89)	51.1%	82.9, 9.2, 4.2%	US 76.7%, Argentina 15.3%, Brazil 6.1%	Diabetes 8.3%, chronic lung disease 7.8%, cancers 3.9%
			Saline	18,846 (21631)	52[a] (Range; 16–91)	50.1%	82.9, 9.4, 4.3%	US 76.7%, Argentina 15.3%, Brazil 6.0%	Diabetes 8.4%, chronic lung disease 7.7%, cancers 3/5%
Baden, 2020 [4]	mRNA	Primary analysis of safety and efficacy of phase 3 RCT in preventing COVID-19 in persons ≥18 years Median follow-up: 63 days	mRNA-1273 (100 μg), 2 doses 28 days apart	15,170 (15166)	51.3[b] (Range; 18–95)	52.2%	79.2, 10.3, 4.3%	US 100%	Diabetes 9.5%, severe obesity 6.8%, cardiac disease 5%, chronic lung disease 4.7%
			Saline	15,181 (15185)	51.4[b] (Range; 18–95)	53.1%	79.1, 10.1, 4.8%	US 100%	Diabetes 9.5%, severe obesity 6.7%, cardiac disease 4.9%, chronic lung disease 4.9%
Sadoff, 2021 [5]	Adenoviral vector	Primary analysis of safety and efficacy of phase 3 RCT in preventing COVID-19 in persons ≥18 years Median follow-up: 58 days	Ad26.COV2.S (A single dose of 5×10^{10} viral particles)	21,895	52[a] (Range; 19–100)	55.1%	58.7, 19.4, 3.4%	US 44.1%, Latin America 40.9%, South Africa 15.0%	Obesity 28.7%, hypertension 10.2%, diabetes 7.8%
			Saline	21,888	52[a] (Range; 18–94)	54.7%	58.7, 19.5, 3.1%	US 44.1%, Latin America 40.9%, South Africa 15.0%	Obesity 28.4%, hypertension 10.5%, diabetes 7.7%
Voysey, 2021 [6]	Adenoviral vector	Interim analysis of 4 cohorts of phase 1/2/3 RCT parts in preventing COVID-19 in persons ≥18 years Median follow-up: 3.4 months	ChAdOx1 nCoV-19 ($2.2–6.5 \times 10^{10}$ viral particles, 2 doses 4- ≥12 weeks apart)	12,021	Age (18–55 years) 81.5%	44.2%	75.1, 10.0, 3.7%	UK 50.0%, Brazil 41.6%, South Africa 8.4%	Cardiovascular disease 12.6%, respiratory disease 9.9%, diabetes 2.8%
			Meningococcal group A, C, W, and Y conjugate vaccine or saline	11,724	Age (18–55 years) 83.5%	44.1%	75.4, 10.2, 3.3%	UK 48.8%, Brazil 42.7%, South Africa 8.5%	Cardiovascular disease 12.0%, respiratory disease 10.0%, diabetes 2.5%
Logunov, 2021 [7]	Adenoviral vector	Preliminary efficacy and safety analysis of phase 3 RCT in preventing COVID-19 in persons ≥18 years Median follow-up: 48 days	rAd26 (1st dose) and rAd5 (2nd dose) containing 1×10^{11} viral particles, 2 doses 21 days apart	14,964 (16427)	45.3[b] (SD 12.0)	61.1%	98.5%, NA, 1.5%	Russia 100%	Diabetes, hypertension, ischemic heart disease, obesity 24.7%
			Excipients	4902 (5435)	45.3[b] (SD 11.9)	61.5%	98.5%, NA, 1.5%	Russia 100%	Diabetes, hypertension, ischemic heart disease, obesity 25.2%
Tanriover, 2021 [8]	Inactivated	Interim analysis of efficacy and safety of phase 3 RCT in preventing COVID-19 in persons aged 18–59 years Median follow-up: 43 days	CoronaVac (3 μg of SARS-CoV-2 virions), 2 doses 14 days apart	6646 (6648)	45[a] (IQR; 35–51)	57.4%	NA	Turkey 100%	Hypertension 11.8%, diabetes 4.9%, chronic lung disease 2.9%
			Aluminium hydroxide diluent	3568 (3568)	45[a] (IQR; 37–51)	58.65	NA	Turkey 100%	Hypertension, 11.6%, diabetes 4.5%, chronic lung disease 2.9%
Palacios, 2021 [9] (preprint)	Inactivated	Interim analysis of efficacy and safety of phase 3 RCT in preventing COVID-19 in healthcare workers ≥18 years	CoronaVac (3 μg of SARS-CoV-2 virions), 2 doses 14 days apart	6195 (6202)	39.4[b] (SD 10.7)	36.6%	75.8, 5.3, 2.4%	Brazil 100%	Obesity 22.4%, cardiovascular disease 12.8%, diabetes 3.5%

Table 1 Baseline characteristics of included randomized controlled trials *(Continued)*

Study name	Vaccine platform	Study characteristics	Treatment allocation	Number of participants (safety data)	Age (years)	Sex (male)	Race (white, black, Asian)	Countries	Comorbidities
		Median follow-up: 2 months after the second dose	Aluminium hydroxide diluent	6201 (6194)	39.6[b] (SD 10.8)	35.0%	74.8, 5.2, 2.6%	Brazil 100%	Obesity 22.6%, cardiovascular disease 12.5%, diabetes 3.2%
Heath, 2021 [10]	Protein subunit	Interim analysis of efficacy and safety of phase 3 RCT in preventing COVID-19 in persons ≥18 years Median follow-up: 66 days after the first dose and 45 days after the second dose	NVX-CoV2373 (5 μg), 2 doses 21 days apart	7020 (7569)	56[a] (18–84)	51.4%	94.4, 0.4, 2.9%	UK 100%	Chronic lung, cardiac, renal, neurologic, hepatic, immunocompromising conditions, and obesity 44.4%
			Saline	7019 (7570)	56[a] (18–64)	51.7%	94.5, 0.4, 3.0%	UK 100%	Chronic lung, cardiac, renal, neurologic, hepatic, immunocompromising conditions, and obesity 44.8%

[a]Median; [b]Mean; COVID-19, coronavirus disease 2019; *RCT* randomized controlled trial; *US* United States; *UK* United Kingdom

The RR of VTE after SARS-CoV-2 vaccination (6 studies [4–7, 9, 10]; $N = 79{,}273$ in the vaccine group and $N = 68{,}003$ in the placebo group) was 1.47 (95% CI, 0.72 to 2.99; $I^2 = 0\%$) (Fig. 3). The risk of VTE after SARS-CoV-2 vaccination was increased only in the Ad26.COV2.S study (RR = 3.67; 95% CI, 1.02 to 13.14). With an estimated risk of VTE from 7 studies [4–10] in the placebo group of 21 events per 100,000 persons (95% CI, 13 to 36; $I^2 = 0$), the risk difference with the vaccine group was 6.3 events per 100,000 persons (95% CI, −8.5 to 21; $I^2 = 0$). The subgroup analysis did not demonstrate an increased risk of either ATE or VTE in any vaccine platform, including the adenoviral vector subtype ($P = 0.23$ and $P = 0.81$, respectively) (Supplementary Fig. S4 and Fig. S5).

The risks of hemorrhage and thrombocytopenia after vaccination against SARS-CoV-2

The risk of hemorrhage was estimated from 7 studies while excluding the BNT162b2 study ($N = 85{,}919$ in the vaccine group and $N = 71{,}751$ in the placebo group) [4–10]. No bleeding events occurred in one inactivated vaccine study (Palacios) [9]. The RR of hemorrhage after SARS-CoV-2 vaccination (6 studies [4–8, 10] included 79,724 participants in the vaccine group and 65,370 participants in the placebo group) was 0.97 (95% CI, 0.35 to 2.68, $I^2 = 0\%$) (Fig. 4). With an estimated risk of bleeding from 7 studies [4–10] in the placebo group of 18 events per 100,000 persons (95% CI, 8 to 35; $I^2 = 0$), the risk difference with the

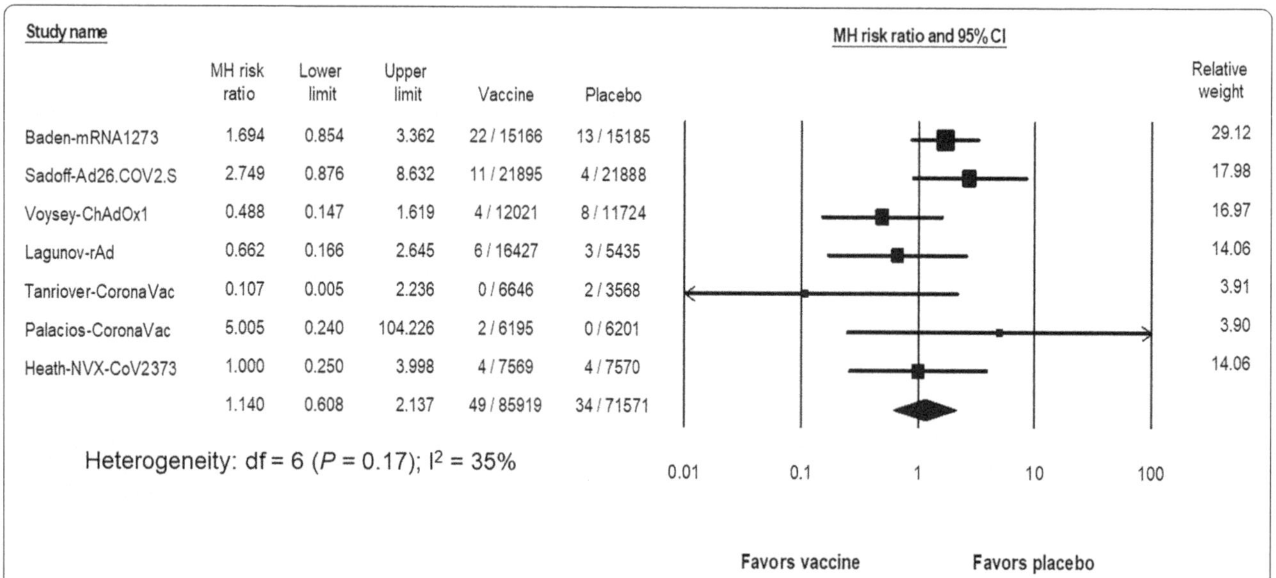

Fig. 1 The pooled risk ratio of overall thromboembolism between the SARS-CoV-2 vaccine and the placebo groups

Study name	MH risk ratio	Lower limit	Upper limit	Vaccine	Placebo	Relative weight
Baden-mRNA1273	2.003	0.857	4.678	16 / 15166	8 / 15185	36.88
Sadoff-Ad26.COV2.S	0.333	0.014	8.179	0 / 21895	1 / 21888	5.14
Voysey-ChAdOx1	0.325	0.066	1.610	2 / 12021	6 / 11724	16.82
Logunov-rAd	0.827	0.161	4.262	5 / 16427	2 / 5435	16.21
Tanriover-CoronaVac	0.107	0.005	2.236	0 / 6646	2 / 3568	5.67
Palacios-CoronaVac	3.003	0.122	73.699	1 / 6195	0 / 6201	5.14
Heath-NVX-CoV2373	1.500	0.251	8.976	3 / 7569	2 / 7570	14.14
	0.968	0.455	2.058	27 / 85919	21 / 71571	

Heterogeneity: df = 6 (P = 0.27); I^2 = 21%

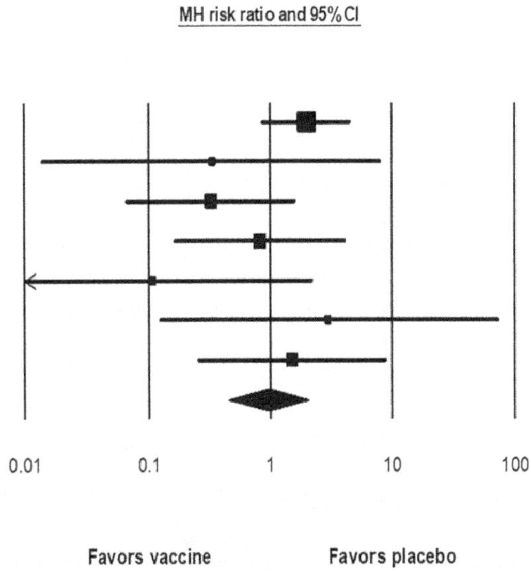

Fig. 2 The pooled risk ratio of arterial thromboembolism between the SARS-CoV-2 vaccine and the placebo groups

vaccine group was 4.1 events per 100,000 persons (95% CI, – 5.3 to 13.5; $I^2 = 0$). The subgroup analysis did not demonstrate an increased risk of bleeding in any vaccine platform ($P = 0.68$) (Supplementary Fig. S6).

The risk of thrombocytopenia after SARS-CoV-2 vaccination was not analyzed because no events were reported in the included studies.

The risk of death related to thromboembolic and hemorrhagic events after vaccination against SARS-CoV-2

The risk of death related to thromboembolism and hemorrhage was estimated from all 8 studies [3–10] ($N = 104{,}779$ in the vaccine group and $N = 90{,}417$ in the placebo group). No deaths related to thromboembolism or bleeding occurred in the ChAdOx1 study, one CoronaVac study (Tanriover) and the NVX-CoV23 study 6, 8, 10]. The RR of death from thromboembolism or hemorrhage after SARS-CoV-2 vaccination (5 studies [3–5, 7, 9] included 78,543 participants in the vaccine group and 67,555 participants in the placebo group) was 0.53 (95% CI, 0.16 to 1.79; $I^2 = 0\%$) (Fig. 5). With an estimated risk of thromboembolism/hemorrhage-related death from 8 studies [3–10] in the placebo group of 9 events per 100,000 persons (95% CI, 5 to 19; $I^2 = 0$), the risk difference with the vaccine group was – 3.7 events per 100,000 persons (95% CI, – 12.2 to 4.8; $I^2 = 0$). The

Study name	MH risk ratio	Lower limit	Upper limit	Vaccine	Placebo	Relative weight
Baden-mRNA1273	1.202	0.367	3.936	6 / 15166	5 / 15185	35.77
Sadoff-Ad26.COV2.S	3.665	1.023	13.137	11 / 21895	3 / 21888	30.91
Voysey-ChAdOx1	0.975	0.137	6.923	2 / 12021	2 / 11724	13.11
Logunov-rAd	0.331	0.021	5.289	1 / 16427	1 / 5435	6.56
Palacios-CoronaVac	3.003	0.122	73.699	1 / 6195	0 / 6201	4.92
Heath-NVX-CoV2373	0.500	0.045	5.514	1 / 7569	2 / 7570	8.74
	1.469	0.723	2.988	22 / 79273	13 / 68003	

Heterogeneity: df = 5 (P = 0.50); I^2 = 0%

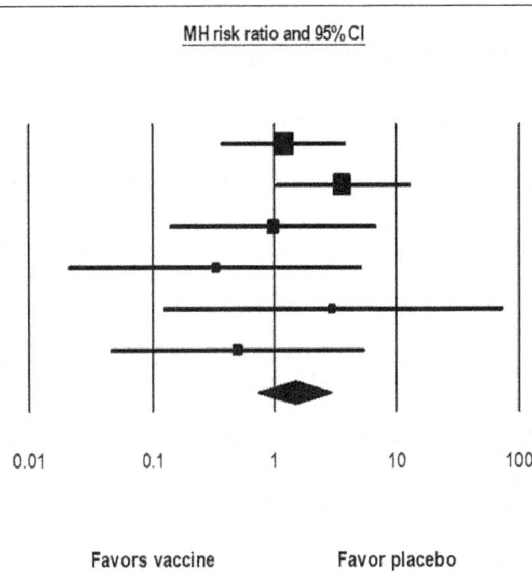

Fig. 3 The pooled risk ratio of venous thromboembolism between the SARS-CoV-2 vaccine and the placebo groups

Study name	MH risk ratio	Lower limit	Upper limit	Vaccine	Placebo	Relative weight
Baden-mRNA1273	5.006	0.240	104.269	2 / 15166	0 / 15185	11.09
Sadoff-Ad26.COV2.S	2.999	0.122	73.615	1 / 21895	0 / 21888	9.98
Voysey-ChAdOx1	0.731	0.164	3.268	3 / 12021	4 / 11724	45.65
Logunov-rAd	0.110	0.004	2.707	0 / 16427	1 / 5435	9.98
Tanriover-CoronaVac	1.611	0.066	39.531	1 / 6646	0 / 3568	9.98
Heath-NVX-CoV2373	1.000	0.063	15.987	1 / 7569	1 / 7570	13.31
	0.973	0.354	2.676	8 / 79724	6 / 65370	

Heterogeneity: df = 5 (P = 0.61); I^2 = 0%

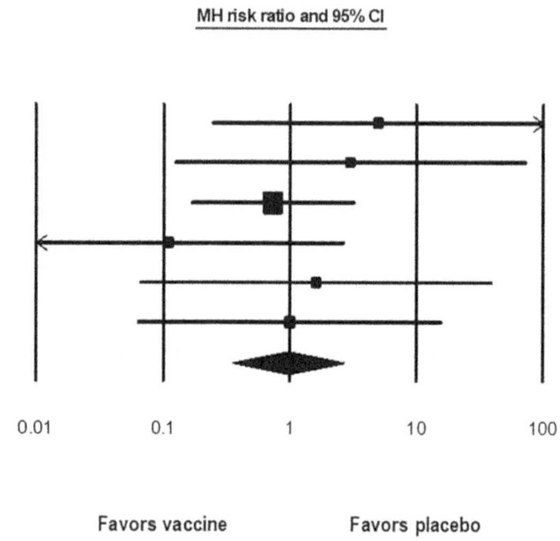

Fig. 4 The pooled risk ratio of hemorrhage between the SARS-CoV-2 vaccine and the placebo groups

subgroup analysis did not demonstrate an increased risk of death related to thromboembolism and hemorrhage in any vaccine platform (P = 0.48) (Supplementary Fig. S7).

Discussion

In this systematic review and meta-analysis of 8 RCTs involving nearly 200,000 participants, the risks of overall thromboembolism, ATE, VTE, hemorrhage, and death related to thromboembolism and hemorrhage were not significantly increased with vaccination against SARS-CoV-2. An increased risk of VTE was observed only with the Ad26.COV2.S vaccine. The absolute risk differences of all outcomes were less than 0.01% or less than 10 per 100,000 persons. This meta-analysis confirmed the rarity of thromboembolic and hemorrhagic events after SARS-CoV-2 vaccines observed in phase 3 RCTs across all vaccine platforms.

In our systematic review, there were no thrombocytopenia events reported in the included studies suggesting the rarity of significant thrombocytopenia after SARS-CoV-2 vaccination. Of note, mild asymptomatic thrombocytopenia may be undetected and underreported in clinical trials. According to population-based studies, the risk of unspecified thrombocytopenia after ChAdOx1 vaccination was increased in Denmark and Norway [21] and in England [22], while the risk of immune thrombocytopenia after ChAdOx1 vaccination was increased in Scotland and Thailand [23, 24]. Due to very low prevalence, this meta-analysis remained underpowered to detect the risk of thrombocytopenia after SARS-CoV-2 vaccination.

Study name	MH risk ratio	Lower limit	Upper limit	Vaccine	Placebo	Relative weight
Baden-mRNA1273	1.001	0.063	16.006	1 / 15166	1 / 15185	12.11
Polak-BNT162b2	0.999	0.141	7.093	2 / 18860	2 / 18846	24.24
Sadoff-Ad26.COV2.S	0.333	0.014	8.179	0 / 21895	1 / 21888	18.18
Logunov-rAd	0.110	0.004	2.707	0 / 16427	1 / 5435	27.31
Palacios-CoronaVac	0.334	0.014	8.189	0 / 6195	1 / 6201	18.16
	0.515	0.168	1.581	3 / 78543	6 / 67555	

Heterogeneity: df = 4 (P = 0.79); I^2 = 0%

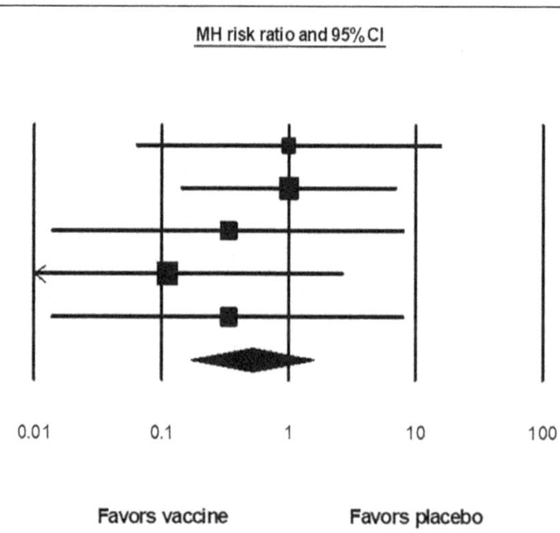

Fig. 5 The pooled risk ratio of death related to thromboembolism and hemorrhage between the SARS-CoV-2 vaccine and the placebo groups

The subgroup analysis to determine the risks of thromboembolism and hemorrhage across vaccine platforms was performed. Compared to placebo, each vaccine platform did not show an increase in the risks of thromboembolism and hemorrhage in all analyses. These findings support the general safety among different SARS-CoV-2 vaccine platforms. There were insufficient data to perform other pre-specified subgroup analysis including age, gender and race.

COVID-19 is associated with the risks of systemic coagulopathy, thrombosis, and bleeding, especially in critically ill patients [22, 25–29]. Since SARS-CoV-2 vaccines can effectively prevent symptomatic infection, hospitalization, and mortality [3–10], the risks of thromboembolism, hemorrhage, and death related to thromboembolism and hemorrhage from COVID-19 may also be reduced in vaccinated participants. However, in most studies, the SARS-CoV-2 infection status was not specified in participants who experienced thromboembolic or hemorrhagic events. A contributing risk of COVID-19 associated thromboembolism and hemorrhage could not be totally excluded.

The risks of thromboembolism and hemorrhage were also assessed in large national cohort studies. Although there was no association between the ChAdOx1 vaccine and thromboembolism in the phase 3 RCT, some national cohorts have observed an increased risk of thromboembolism after ChAdOx1 vaccination. The population-based studies from Denmark and Norway, which included 281,264 people vaccinated with the ChAdOx1 vaccine, demonstrated an increased rate of VTE and cerebral vein thrombosis, but not for ATE, and a small increased risk of unspecified thrombocytopenia among recipients of the ChAdOx1 vaccine [21]. The larger cohort from England, which included 19,608,008 people vaccinated with the ChAdOx1 vaccine, also demonstrated an increased risk of unspecified thrombocytopenia, VTE, cerebral vein thrombosis, and rare arterial thromboembolic events, but not for overall ATE, stroke, and myocardial infarction, within 28 days after ChAdOx1 vaccination [22]. However, both cohorts did not specify the numbers of VITT cases, which might have been included in both cohorts [12–16]. It remains uncertain whether the risks of VTE and thrombocytopenia after ChAdOx1 vaccination would be different from these reports if VITT cases were excluded. In contrast, the Scottish population-based study, which included 1.71 million people vaccinated with the ChAdOx1 vaccine, demonstrated an increased risk of immune thrombocytopenia and a minimally increased risk of ATE among recipients of the ChAdOx1 vaccine. Notably, there was no association between ChAdOx1 vaccination and VTE including cerebral vein thrombosis [23]. The reasons underlying different thromboembolic risks observed among these national cohorts remained unclear. Since the young age group is at higher risk for VITT, while the elderly age group is at higher risk for thromboembolism, asymmetrical age distribution of vaccine recipients among cohorts may be an important confounder. In the Scandinavian cohort, the ChAdOx1 vaccine was administered to people aged between 18 to 65 years [21]. Similarly, the ChAdOx1 vaccine was vaccinated in a higher proportion of people aged younger than 60 years in England during the study period [22]. In contrast, the highest uptake for the ChAdOx1 vaccine was found in people aged older than 65 years in Scotland [30]. Additionally, there is the potential of an overestimation of vaccine-associated adverse events with the low incidence in most study designs to assess vaccine safety [31].

Although a minimally increased risk of VTE was observed in the Ad26.COV2.S vaccine arm in the phase 3 RCT, there were very few thromboembolic events observed among 288,368 recipients of the Ad26.COV2.S vaccine in South Africa [32]. No VITT or thrombocytopenia were documented in the South African cohort.

Thromboembolic events were not specified in the BNT162b study. The Scottish population-based study, which included 0.82 million people vaccinated with the BNT162b vaccine, demonstrated no increased risks of thrombocytopenia, VTE and ATE among recipients of the BNT162b vaccine [23]. Similarly, the population-based study from Israel demonstrated no increased risks of thromboembolism, hemorrhage, and thrombocytopenia after BNT162b2 vaccination [25]. In contrast, the cohort from England, which included 9,513,625 people vaccinated with the BNT162b vaccine, demonstrated an increased risk of ATE, ischemic stroke and cerebral vein thrombosis, but not for thrombocytopenia and VTE [22]. Whether the risks of thromboembolism and thrombocytopenia might be increased after BNT162b vaccination remains undetermined due to the conflicting findings among national cohort studies. One should also be cautious to generalize the risks of thromboembolism, hemorrhage, and thrombocytopenia after SARS-CoV-2 vaccination due to different genetic and thromboembolic risks among populations.

The strength of a meta-analysis of large multinational phase 3 RCTs is its inherent advantage to have even distribution of demographic characteristics, comorbidities, especially thrombotic and bleeding risk factors, and other unmeasured covariates. All RCTs included in this meta-analysis were assessed to have low risk of bias. The included studies had insignificant or low statistical heterogeneity suggesting that the effects can reasonably be combined in a meta-analysis.

There are some limitations of this study. Although it aggregated approximately 100,000 vaccinated participants, it may be insufficient to document extremely rare events such as significant thrombocytopenia. Additionally, despite our attempts to contact the authors, we were not able to obtain the data from the BNT162b2 study, and therefore this study was not included in most analyses. Consequently, there was only one type of vaccine in the mRNA, inactivated, and protein subunit platform in subgroup analysis. The lack of detailed descriptions of participants who experienced thromboembolic or hemorrhagic events also precluded evaluation of several other important subgroups analysis such as age, sex, race, coexisting comorbidities, and COVID-19 status. Asymmetrical age distribution of vaccine recipients and potentially incomplete adjustment for covariates, especially cardiovascular comorbidities and genetic factors, may result in different estimated thromboembolic risks among population-based studies. It may require the pooled analysis of large national cohorts to have sufficient power to determine the risks of thromboembolism and hemorrhages after vaccination against SARS-CoV-2 and risks among different vaccine platforms. Incomplete data entry and a lack of adequate adjustment for baseline confounders would potentially make such analysis very challenging.

Conclusions

This meta-analysis demonstrated no increased risks of thromboembolism, hemorrhage, and death from thromboembolism and hemorrhage after vaccination against SARS-CoV-2 across all vaccine platforms. These findings provide information that may assist global vaccination campaigns in order to reduce vaccine hesitancy. Although marginal risks of thromboembolism and hemorrhage in some subgroup populations may not be excluded, the estimated incidence of these events was very low. The absolute risks of thromboembolism and hemorrhage of SARS-CoV-2 vaccines were very small in the context of the proven benefits of vaccination against SARS-CoV-2 and the globally high incidence of severe and fatal cases of SARS-CoV-2 infection.

Abbreviations

ATE: arterial thromboembolism; CI: confidence interval; COVID-19: coronavirus disease 2019; PRISMA: Preferred Reporting Items for Systematic reviews and Meta-Analyses; RCT: randomized controlled trial; RR: risk ratio; SARS-CoV-2: severe acute respiratory syndrome coronavirus 2; VITT: vaccine-induced immune thrombotic thrombocytopenia; VTE: venous thromboembolism

Acknowledgements

Not applicable.

Authors' contributions

Contribution: N.U. was involved in conceptualization, database search, screening of abstracts and full texts, data extraction and analysis, quality appraisal, and writing the manuscript; K.P. was involved in conceptualization, database search, screening of abstracts and full texts, and editing of the manuscript; P.R. was involved in data analysis, appraisal and editing of the manuscript; and T.C. was involved in conceptualization, adjudication, data analysis and editing of the manuscript. The authors read and approved the final manuscript.

References

1. Wiersinga WJ, Rhodes A, Cheng AC, Peacock SJ, Prescott HC. Pathophysiology, transmission, diagnosis, and treatment of coronavirus disease 2019 (COVID-19): a review. JAMA. 2020;324(8):782–93. https://doi.org/10.1001/jama.2020.12839.
2. Worldometer. COVID-19 coronavirus pandemic. 2020. https://www.worldometers.info/coronavirus/ (accessed August 12, 2021).
3. Polack FP, Thomas SJ, Kitchin N, Absalon J, Gurtman A, Lockhart S, et al. Safety and efficacy of the BNT162b2 mRNA Covid-19 vaccine. N Engl J Med. 2020;383(27):2603–15. https://doi.org/10.1056/NEJMoa2034577.
4. Baden LR, El Sahly HM, Essink B, Kotloff K, Frey S, Novak R, et al. Efficacy and safety of the mRNA-1273 SARS-CoV-2 vaccine. N Engl J Med. 2021;384(5):403–16. https://doi.org/10.1056/NEJMoa2035389.
5. Sadoff J, Gray G, Vandebosch A, Cardenas V, Shukarev G, Grinsztejn B, et al. Safety and efficacy of single-dose Ad26.COV2.S vaccine against Covid-19. N Engl J Med. 2021;384(23):2187–201. https://doi.org/10.1056/NEJMoa2101544.
6. Voysey M, Clemens SAC, Madhi SA, Weckx LY, Folegatti PM, Aley PK, et al. Safety and efficacy of the ChAdOx1 nCoV-19 vaccine (AZD1222) against SARS-CoV-2: an interim analysis of four randomised controlled trials in Brazil, South Africa, and the UK. Lancet. 2021;397(10269):99–111. https://doi.org/10.1016/S0140-6736(20)32661-1.
7. Logunov DY, Dolzhikova IV, Shcheblyakov DV, Tukhvatulin AI, Zubkova OV, Dzharullaeva AS, et al. Safety and efficacy of an rAd26 and rAd5 vector-based heterologous prime-boost COVID-19 vaccine: an interim analysis of a randomised controlled phase 3 trial in Russia. Lancet. 2021;397(10275):671–81. https://doi.org/10.1016/S0140-6736(21)00234-8.
8. Tanriover MD, Doğanay HL, Akova M, Güner HR, Azap A, Akhan S, et al. Efficacy and safety of an inactivated whole-virion SARS-CoV-2 vaccine (CoronaVac): interim results of a double-blind, randomised, placebo-controlled, phase 3 trial in Turkey. Lancet. 2021;398(10296):213–22. https://doi.org/10.1016/S0140-6736(21)01429-X.
9. Palacios R, Batista AP, Albuquerque CSN, Patino EG, Santos JDP, Conde MTRP, et al. Efficacy and safety of a COVID-19 inactivated vaccine in healthcare 3 professionals in Brazil: The PROFISCOV study. 2021). Available at SSRN: https://ssrn.com/abstract=3822780 or. https://doi.org/10.2139/ssrn.3822780.
10. Heath PT, Galiza EP, Baxter DN, Boffito M, Browne D, Burns F, et al. Safety and efficacy of NVX-CoV2373 Covid-19 vaccine. N Engl J Med. 2021;385(13):1172–83. https://doi.org/10.1056/NEJMoa2107659.
11. Razai MS, Chaudhry UAR, Doerholt K, Bauld L, Majeed A. Covid-19 vaccination hesitancy. BMJ. 2021;373:n1138. https://doi.org/10.1136/bmj.n1138.
12. See I, Su JR, Lale A, Woo EJ, Guh AY, Shimabukuro TT, et al. US case reports of cerebral venous sinus thrombosis with thrombocytopenia after Ad26.COV2.S vaccination, march 2 to April 21, 2021. JAMA. 2021;325(24):2448–56. https://doi.org/10.1001/jama.2021.7517.
13. Greinacher A, Thiele T, Warkentin TE, Weisser K, Kyrle PA, Eichinger S. Thrombotic thrombocytopenia after ChAdOx1 nCov-19 vaccination. N Engl J Med. 2021;384(22):2092–101. https://doi.org/10.1056/NEJMoa2104840.
14. Schultz NH, Sørvoll IH, Michelsen AE, Munthe LA, Lund-Johansen F, Ahlen MT, et al. Thrombosis and thrombocytopenia after ChAdOx1 nCoV-19 vaccination. N Engl J Med. 2021;384(22):2124–30. https://doi.org/10.1056/NEJMoa2104882.
15. Scully M, Singh D, Lown R, Poles A, Solomon T, Levi M, et al. Pathologic antibodies to platelet factor 4 after ChAdOx1 nCoV-19 vaccination. N Engl J Med. 2021;384(23):2202–11. https://doi.org/10.1056/NEJMoa2105385.
16. Chan BTB, Bobos P, Odutayo A, Pai M. Meta-Analysis of Risk of Vaccine-Induced Immune Thrombotic Thrombocytopenia Following ChAdOx1-S Recombinant Vaccine. https://www.medrxiv.org/content/10.1101/2021.05.04.21256613v1.
17. Moher D, Liberati A, Tetzlaff J, Altman DG. Preferred reporting items for systematic reviews and meta-analyses: the PRISMA statement. PLoS Med. 2009;6(7):e1000097. https://doi.org/10.1371/journal.pmed.1000097.
18. Sterne JAC, Savović J, Page MJ, Elbers RG, Blencowe NS, Boutron I, et al. RoB 2: a revised tool for assessing risk of bias in randomised trials. BMJ. 2019;366:l4898. https://doi.org/10.1136/bmj.l4898.

19. Xu C, Furuya-Kanamori L, Zorzela L, Lin L, Vohra S. A proposed framework to guide evidence synthesis practice for meta-analysis with zero-events studies. J Clin Epidemiol. 2021;135:70–8. https://doi.org/10.1016/j.jclinepi.2021.02.012.
20. Higgins JP, Thompson SG, Deeks JJ, Altman DG. Measuring in consistency in meta-analyses. BMJ. 2003;327(7414):557–60. https://doi.org/10.1136/bmj.327.7414.557.
21. Pottegård A, Lund LC, Karlstad Ø, Dahl J, Andersen M, Hallas J, et al. Arterial events, venous thromboembolism, thrombocytopenia, and bleeding after vaccination with Oxford-AstraZeneca ChAdOx1-S in Denmark and Norway: population based cohort study. BMJ. 2021;373:n1114. https://doi.org/10.1136/bmj.n1114.
22. Hippisley-Cox J, Patone M, Mei XW, Saatci D, Dixon S, Khunti K, et al. Risk of thrombocytopenia and thromboembolism after covid-19 vaccination and SARS-CoV-2 positive testing: self-controlled case series study. BMJ. 2021;374:n1931. https://doi.org/10.1136/bmj.n1931.
23. Simpson CR, Shi T, Vasileiou E, Katikireddi SV, Kerr S, Moore E, et al. First-dose ChAdOx1 and BNT162b2 COVID-19 vaccines and thrombocytopenic, thromboembolic and hemorrhagic events in Scotland. Nat Med. 2021;27(7):1290–7. https://doi.org/10.1038/s41591-021-01408-4.
24. Uaprasert N, Panrong K, Tungjitviboonkun S, Dussadee K, Decharatanachart P, Kaveevorayan P, et al. ChAdOx1 nCoV-19 vaccine-associated thrombocytopenia: three cases of immune thrombocytopenia after 107 720 doses of ChAdOx1 vaccination in Thailand. Blood Coagul Fibrinolysis. 2021. https://doi.org/10.1097/MBC.0000000000001082 Online ahead of print.
25. Barda N, Dagan N, Ben-Shlomo Y, Kepten E, Waxman J, Ohana R, et al. Safety of the BNT162b2 mRNA Covid-19 vaccine in a Nationwide setting. N Engl J Med. 2021;385(12):1078–90. https://doi.org/10.1056/NEJMoa2110475.
26. Uaprasert N, Moonla C, Sosothikul D, Rojnuckarin P, Chiasakul T. Systemic coagulopathy in hospitalized patients with coronavirus disease 2019: a systematic review and meta-analysis. Clin Appl Thromb Hemost Jan-Dec. 2021;27:1076029620987629.
27. Al-Samkari H, Karp Leaf RS, Dzik WH, Carlson JCT, Fogerty AE, Waheed A, et al. COVID-19 and coagulation: bleeding and thrombotic manifestations of SARS-CoV-2 infection. Blood. 2020;136(4):489–500. https://doi.org/10.1182/blood.2020006520.
28. Jiménez D, García-Sanchez A, Rali P, Muriel A, Bikdeli B, Ruiz-Artacho P, et al. Incidence of VTE and bleeding among hospitalized patients with coronavirus disease 2019: a systematic review and meta-analysis. Chest. 2021;159(3):1182–96. https://doi.org/10.1016/j.chest.2020.11.005.
29. Tan BK, Mainbourg S, Friggeri A, Bertoletti L, Douplat M, Dargaud Y, et al. Arterial and venous thromboembolism in COVID-19: a study-level meta-analysis. Thorax. 2021;76(10):970–9. https://doi.org/10.1136/thoraxjnl-2020-215383.
30. Vasileiou E, Simpson CR, Shi T, Kerr S, Agrawal U, Akbari A, et al. Interim findings from first-dose mass COVID-19 vaccination roll-out and COVID-19 hospital admissions in Scotland: a national prospective cohort study. Lancet. 2021;397(10285):1646–57. https://doi.org/10.1016/S0140-6736(21)00677-2.
31. Glanz JM, McClure DL, Xu S, Hambidge SJ, Lee M, Kolczak MS, et al. Four different study designs to evaluate vaccine safety were equally validated with contrasting limitations. J Clin Epidemiol. 2006;59(8):808–18. https://doi.org/10.1016/j.jclinepi.2005.11.012.
32. Takuva S, Takalani A, Garrett N, Goga A, Peter J, Louw V, et al. Thromboembolic events in the south African Ad26.COV2.S vaccine study. N Engl J Med. 2021;385(6):570–1. https://doi.org/10.1056/NEJMc2107920.

4

Cardiovascular risk factors are associated with augmented thrombogenicity in healthy individuals: Analysis using the Total Thrombus-formation Analysis System

Yuu Oda[1], Takashi Ito[1,2*], Yoichiro Yamada[3], Tadashi Koga[4], Tomoka Nagasato[1,5], Tomoko Ohnishi-Wada[5], Kazuya Hosokawa[1,5], Hiroyuki Fukase[6], Teruto Hashiguchi[7] and Ikuro Maruyama[1]

Abstract

Background: Rupture of an atherosclerotic plaque and subsequent exposure of the subendothelial prothrombotic matrix to blood cause arterial thrombosis. Circulating platelets play an indispensable role in the growth of arterial thrombi partially owing to their unique ability to adhere to the subendothelial matrix and to aggregate to each other under flow conditions. Recently, the Total Thrombus-formation Analysis System (T-TAS) was developed for ex vivo analysis of the thrombogenic potential of whole blood samples under flow conditions. Despite the potential clinical utility of the T-TAS in assessing the risk for thrombosis and bleeding, reference intervals for T-TAS analysis in healthy individuals have not been determined.

Methods: In total, 122 whole blood samples were collected from healthy volunteers ranging in age from 25 to 45 years. T-TAS analysis and hematological, physiological, and lifestyle assessments were conducted in these subjects. Whole blood samples anticoagulated with hirudin were perfused into a collagen-coated microchip (PL chip). The time to 10 kPa and the area under the flow pressure curve up to 10 min (AUC_{10}) were analyzed as representative variables for thrombogenic potential. Reference intervals, which were defined as 2.5–97.5 percentiles, were determined. Additionally, univariate and multivariate analyses were performed to identify factors associated with the AUC_{10} in the T-TAS.

Results: The time to 10 kPa and the AUC_{10} widely varied, even in healthy volunteers. The reference intervals were 1.50–4.02 min and 223.4–456.8, respectively, at a shear rate of 1500 s^{-1}. Univariate and multivariate analyses showed that platelet counts were most significantly associated with the AUC_{10} of the T-TAS. The presence of one or more cardiovascular risk factors of a high body mass index, a high pulse pressure, high fasting serum glucose levels, high low-density lipoprotein-cholesterol levels, a history of smoking, and no habitual exercise, had the second largest effect on the AUC_{10} of the T-TAS.

* Correspondence: tito@kumamoto-u.ac.jp
[1]Department of Systems Biology in Thromboregulation, Kagoshima University Graduate School of Medical and Dental Sciences, Kagoshima, Japan
[2]Department of Biomedical Laboratory Sciences, Faculty of Life Sciences, Kumamoto University, 4-24-1 Kuhonji, Kumamoto 862-0976, Japan

Conclusions: Healthy volunteers who had any cardiovascular risk factors showed augmented thrombogenicity, even in artificial uniform capillaries, compared with those without any risk factors in the T-TAS.

Background

Arterial thrombosis is a major healthcare problem not only in industrialized countries, but also in low- and middle-income countries [1]. The development of occlusive thrombi in coronary or cerebral arteries results in acute myocardial infarction or ischemic stroke, respectively, and is currently the most common cause of morbidity and mortality globally. The essential triggers for arterial thrombosis include rupture of an atherosclerotic plaque and subsequent exposure of the subendothelial prothrombotic matrix [2]. Circulating platelets play an indispensable role in the growth of arterial thrombi in part owing to their unique ability to adhere to the subendothelial matrix and to aggregate to each other under rapid flow conditions [3].

The Total Thrombus-formation Analysis System (T-TAS®, Fujimori Kogyo Co., Ltd., Yokohama, Japan) was developed for ex vivo analysis of the thrombogenic potential of whole blood under rapid flow conditions [4]. In this system, whole blood samples are perfused into artificial capillaries coated with collagen, a major subendothelial matrix protein. The thrombogenic potential is then quantified by measuring an elevation in internal flow pressure caused by growth of obstructive thrombi. Recent studies have shown that this system may be useful in evaluating the therapeutic efficacy of antiplatelet drugs [5, 6], risk of bleeding in patients undergoing percutaneous coronary intervention [7], and risk of thrombotic complications in hypoglycemic patients [8].

Despite the potential clinical utility, reference intervals for T-TAS analysis in healthy individuals have not been determined. Furthermore, blood components, other than platelets, contributing to the growth of obstructive thrombi in T-TAS have not been well defined. Therefore, this study aimed to collect whole blood samples from a sufficient number of qualified reference individuals to yield a minimum of 120 samples for establishing reference intervals for T-TAS analysis [9, 10]. This study shows that the thrombogenic potential widely varies among healthy individuals and that cardiovascular risk factors are associated with augmented thrombogenicity, even in artificial uniform capillaries.

Methods

Study subjects

This study was conducted in accordance with the Declaration of Helsinki. This study was approved by the Institutional Review Boards of CPC Clinical Trial Hospital and Kagoshima University Graduate School of Medical and Dental Sciences, both in Kagoshima, Japan. Written informed consent was obtained from all subjects prior to their participation in the study. Healthy volunteers ranging in age from 25 to 45 years were recruited in CPC Clinical Trial Hospital. Subjects participating in other clinical trials or receiving drugs and/or nutritional supplements were excluded. One hundred twenty-five volunteers were enrolled, among whom 122 (88 men and 34 women) were eligible for further analysis as healthy individuals. Daily habits of smoking, exercise, drinking, and eating were assessed by self-report questionnaires. Height, weight, blood pressure, and pulse rate were assessed in all healthy volunteers. None of them had a bleeding tendency.

Hematological examination

Blood was collected from the forearm using a 21-G needle and vacuum blood collection tubes after fasting for at least 6 h. Blood samples were anticoagulated with hirudin (Roche Diagnostics GmbH, Mannheim, Germany), ethylenediaminetetraacetic acid, or sodium citrate, which were used for T-TAS assays, complete blood cell counts, or coagulation assays, respectively. Serum samples were obtained from blood without anticoagulation, and were used for measuring levels of bilirubin, aspartate aminotransferase, alanine aminotransferase, lactate dehydrogenase, γ-glutamyl transpeptidase, albumin, globulin, creatine phosphokinase, amylase, glucose, low-density lipoprotein (LDL)-cholesterol, high-density lipoprotein (HDL)-cholesterol, triglycerides, urea nitrogen, creatinine, uric acid, sodium, potassium, and chloride.

Analysis of ex vivo thrombogenic potential using the T-TAS

The process of platelet thrombus formation was evaluated using the T-TAS, as described previously [4, 5]. Briefly, whole blood specimens (350 μL) anticoagulated with hirudin were perfused into a collagen-coated microchip (PL chip, Fujimori Kogyo Co., Ltd.) at a constant flow rate of 12, 18, or 24 μL/min, which corresponded to an initial wall shear rate of 1000, 1500, or 2000 s^{-1}. The growth of thrombus inside the microchip was quantitatively evaluated by monitoring flow pressure over time. The time to 10 kPa and the area under the flow pressure curve up to 10 min (AUC_{10}) were analyzed as representative variables for the thrombogenic potential.

Definition of cardiovascular risk factors in this study

A body mass index (BMI) ≥ 25 kg/m^2, a pulse pressure ≥ 60 mmHg, fasting serum glucose levels ≥110 mg/dL, LDL-cholesterol levels ≥120 mg/dL, a history of smoking, and no habitual exercise were defined as cardiovascular risk factors, according to previous studies [11, 12].

Statistical analysis

Statistical analyses were performed using IBM SPSS v26 (IBM Corp., Armonk NY, USA) and GraphPad Prism v8 (GraphPad Software, San Diego, CA, USA). Data are presented as the median (lower quartile–upper quartile), means ± standard deviations, or 2.5–97.5 percentiles. The relationships between the AUC_{10} (at a shear rate of 1500 s^{-1}) in the T-TAS and other explanatory variables were analyzed by Spearman's rank correlation test, the Mann–Whitney U test, or multiple regression analysis with the stepwise method. A P value of < 0.05 was considered significant.

Results

To establish reference intervals for the T-TAS, we analyzed 122 whole blood samples collected from healthy volunteers. The AUC_{10} widely varied, even in healthy volunteers (Fig. 1a). The reference interval, which was defined as 2.5–97.5 percentiles, was 223.4–456.8 at the shear rates of 1500 s^{-1} (Table 1). The AUC_{10} increased as the setting of the shear rate in the assay increased, and the reference intervals were 186.6–411.9 and 248.0–465.6 at the shear rates of 1000 and 2000 s^{-1}, respectively.

We then analyzed what determined the heterogeneity of the AUC_{10} in the T-TAS. Among 50 variables in hematological, physiological, and lifestyle parameters (Supplementary Table 1), platelet counts showed the most significant association (rho = 0.479, $P < 0.001$) with the AUC_{10} of the T-TAS at the shear rates of 1500 s^{-1} (Fig. 1b). Additionally, the hematocrit and the number of leukocytes, especially that of a monocyte fraction, showed significant associations with the AUC_{10} of the T-TAS (Fig. 1c, d). In more detailed analysis, the hematocrit and leukocyte counts were associated with the initial rise in flow pressure and platelet counts were associated with the following phase of thrombus growth (data not shown).

We then analyzed factors, other than blood cells, that might be associated with augmented thrombogenicity in the T-TAS. Serum potassium levels were unexpectedly correlated with the AUC_{10} of the T-TAS (Table 2). Among cardiovascular risk factors, BMI and pulse pressure were weakly, but significantly, associated with the AUC_{10} of the T-TAS (Fig. 2). LDL-cholesterol and fasting serum glucose levels were not associated with the AUC_{10} of the T-TAS. A positive smoking history and negative habitual exercise were associated with a higher AUC_{10} of the T-TAS. Subjects who had any of the above-mentioned cardiovascular risk factors showed augmented thrombogenicity in the T-TAS compared with those without any risk factors (Fig. 3a). The number of risks was significantly associated with the AUC_{10} of the T-TAS (Fig. 3b).

We then performed multivariate analysis to estimate the degree of the contribution of each factor to thrombogenicity in the T-TAS. Multiple regression analysis showed five main factors that had a significant effect on thrombogenicity in the T-TAS (Table 2). These factors were platelet counts (t = 4.30, $P < 0.001$), the presence of one or more cardiovascular risk factors (t = 3.17, $P = 0.002$), serum potassium levels (t = 3.02, $P = 0.003$), monocyte counts (t = 2.62, $P = 0.010$), and the hematocrit (t = 2.61, $P = 0.010$), which collectively accounted for as much as 40.6% of the variance in thrombogenicity in the T-TAS. The presence of cardiovascular risk factors had the second largest effect on thrombogenicity in the T-TAS following platelet counts.

Discussion

In this study, we analyzed 122 whole blood samples collected from healthy volunteers and clarified reference intervals for the T-TAS. Substantial heterogeneity was observed even in healthy individuals, and some of them showed unexpectedly low AUC_{10} values. The low AUC_{10} values were unlikely due to random technical errors because the AUC_{10} values were consistently low in the same individual in the different experimental conditions (three different flow rates with different microchips). Healthy subjects with low AUC_{10} values (less than 200) were also found in previous reports [13]. Although they had no bleeding tendency, few, if any, abnormalities in other clinical chemistry tests, or no drugs interfering the process of thrombus formation, they may pose a potential risk for bleeding events. Longitudinal follow-up studies will be required.

Reference intervals defined in this study were consistent with a previous report, where 31 healthy subjects (11 men and 20 women) were examined [13]. However, AUC_{10} values were slightly higher in our study. This may be due to a different composition of participants in terms of their age and gender. Participants in our study include a larger number of young men, who typically show higher AUC_{10} values. Gender-specific and age-specific reference intervals may be required in the future.

In this study, we identified factors for determining the heterogeneity of thrombogenicity in the T-TAS. These factors included the platelet number, the leukocyte number, the hematocrit, serum potassium levels, and the

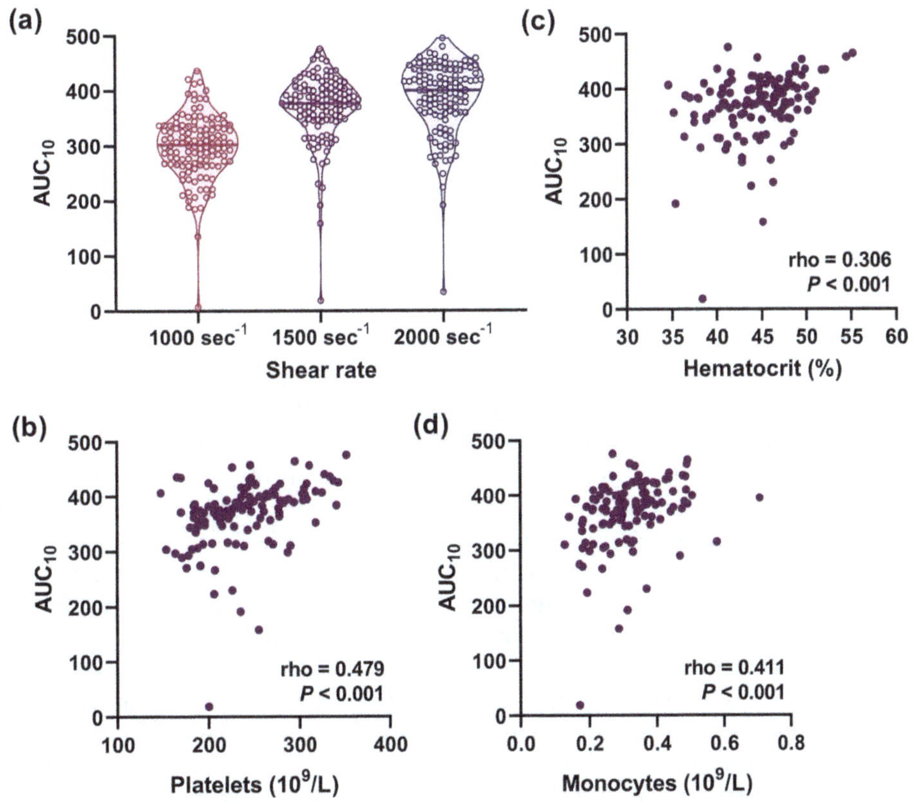

Fig. 1 Quantitative analysis of the thrombogenic potential in 122 healthy individuals. (a) The area under the flow pressure curve in T-TAS PL chips up to 10 min (AUC_{10}) was assessed as a representative variable for thrombogenic potential. The initial wall shear rates were set at 1000, 1500, or 2000 s^{-1}. The distribution of the AUC_{10} in 122 healthy volunteers is shown as violin plots. Bold horizontal lines indicate median values. (b–d) Correlations between the AUC_{10} (at a shear rate of 1500 s^{-1}) in the T-TAS and platelet counts (b), hematocrit (c), and monocyte counts (d) were analyzed by Spearman's rank correlation test

presence of one or more cardiovascular risk factors. Although a small portion of healthy subjects in this study showed slightly elevated serum glucose, serum triglyceride (and/or low HDL-cholesterol), or blood pressure levels above the criteria for metabolic syndrome [14], they were considered to be otherwise healthy.

In this study, platelet counts showed the strongest correlation with the AUC_{10} at the shear velocity of 1500 s^{-1}. Platelet counts were more clearly associated with the time to occlusion (60 kPa) than with the time to 10 kPa. Therefore, the number of platelets might be more important in the later stage of the thrombus growth process than in the earlier stage of platelet adhesion. We previously reported that aspirin prolonged the time to 60 kPa, but not the time to 10 kPa [5]. This finding suggested that not only platelet counts but also platelet activity may play an important role in the later stage of thrombus growth.

Leukocytes are also involved in the thrombus formation process [15]. They are larger than red blood cells or platelets, and therefore, can decrease the rate of blood flow, enabling easier growth of a thrombus under flow conditions. Among leukocytes, monocytes showed the strongest correlation with thrombogenicity in the T-TAS. This finding may have occurred because monocytes and/or platelet–monocyte complexes can promote the growth of platelet-rich thrombi [16, 17] or simply because monocytes have the largest nucleus, which can generate resistance to blood flow in capillaries.

The hematocrit was more clearly associated with the time to 10 kPa than with the time to 60 kPa in this study. This finding suggested that the volume of red blood cells played a role in the initial stage of thrombus growth. Previous studies have shown experimentally and clinically that red blood cells determine blood viscosity [18, 19]. Furthermore, under blood flow conditions, red blood cells generate an axial stream, which secondarily generates near-wall excess of platelets and plasma proteins. Therefore, an increase in the hematocrit may lead to a higher platelet density around the capillary wall, which enables platelets to more readily attach to the wall [20, 21].

Table 1 Reference intervals of T-TAS values based on data from 122 healthy individuals

Shear rate	Measurement	Mean	Median	Reference interval (95%)		
1000 s^{-1}	T10 (min:s)	03:02	02:48	01:41	–	04:39
	AUC_{10}	298.0	301.9	186.6	–	411.9
1500 s^{-1}	T10 (min:s)	02:34	02:25	01:30	–	04:01
	AUC_{10}	367.6	376.6	223.4	–	456.8
2000 s^{-1}	T10 (min:s)	02:35	02:22	01:33	–	04:02
	AUC_{10}	385.1	399.8	248.0	–	465.6

T10: time to 10 kPa

Serum potassium levels varied within a relatively narrow range (3.6–4.7 mEq/L) in this study. However, a significant correlation was observed between serum potassium levels and thrombogenicity in the T-TAS. There were no correlations of potassium levels with other parameters, except for a weak correlation with a BMI > 25 kg/m^2. Potassium may directly affect thrombus formation without any effect on coagulation and fibrinolysis [22]. Potassium may also be an "innocent bystander" in hemolysis, which can be a confounding factor directly related to thrombus formation. Hemolysis results in the extracellular release of adenosine diphosphate, calcium ions, and hemoglobin, all of which activate platelets [23, 24]. Further studies are required to examine the effect of potassium and/or hemolysis on thrombus formation in the T-TAS, although completely excluding minor hemolysis during the blood sampling is difficult.

In this study, a BMI ≥ 25 kg/m2, a pulse pressure ≥ 60 mmHg, fasting blood glucose levels ≥110 mg/dL, LDL-cholesterol levels ≥120 mg/dL, a history of smoking, and a low daily physical activity level were considered as cardiovascular risk factors [25–27]. Age is another important risk factor related to cardiovascular events. However, in the present study, we did not include age as a risk factor because all of the subjects were young (25–45 years). Among cardiovascular risk factors analyzed in the present study, a history of smoking showed the strongest correlation with thrombus formation. Smoking may augment thrombogenicity by enhancing platelet agglutinability via oxidative stress or by increasing blood viscosity due to secondary polycythemia [28]. Systolic blood pressure and pulse pressure were weakly correlated with thrombus formation in the T-TAS, with a slightly stronger correlation observed in pulse pressure. In previous studies in older people, pulse pressure was a risk factor for cardiovascular events and was independent of systolic blood pressure and average blood pressure [29, 30]. In this study, although the majority of subjects were young, a correlation between pulse pressure and thrombus formation was observed.

Generally, cardiovascular risk factors are considered to increase the incidence of ischemic or hemorrhagic vascular events by accelerating atherosclerosis or vascular injury [31, 32]. However, the effect of cardiovascular risk factors on the thrombogenicity of blood components rather than vascular components has rarely been discussed. In this study, we showed that the presence of cardiovascular risk factors was associated with augmented thrombogenicity, even in the artificial uniform capillaries, in the T-TAS. This finding suggests that cardiovascular risk factors have a significant effect on the thrombogenicity of blood components.

Longitudinal follow-up studies are required in the future. Determining whether individuals who show a high AUC_{10} in the T-TAS will experience thrombotic events more frequently than those who show a low AUC_{10} is important. Determining whether individuals with a very low AUC_{10} in the T-TAS will experience bleeding events is also important. Findings from these investigations will provide confirmatory evidence and the basis of a strategy for assessing and managing cardiovascular risks.

Table 2 Univariate and multivariate analyses for identifying factors associated with the AUC_{10} of the T-TAS

Explanatory variable	Correlation analysis		Multivariate analysis		
	Spearman's rho	Significance probability	Standardization coefficient	t value	Significance probability
Platelets	0.479	< 0.001	0.319	4.30	< 0.001
Risk factor(s)	0.459	< 0.001	0.241	3.17	0.002
Monocytes	0.411	< 0.001	0.201	2.62	0.010
Potassium	0.322	< 0.001	0.225	3.02	0.003
Hematocrit	0.306	0.001	0.204	2.61	0.010

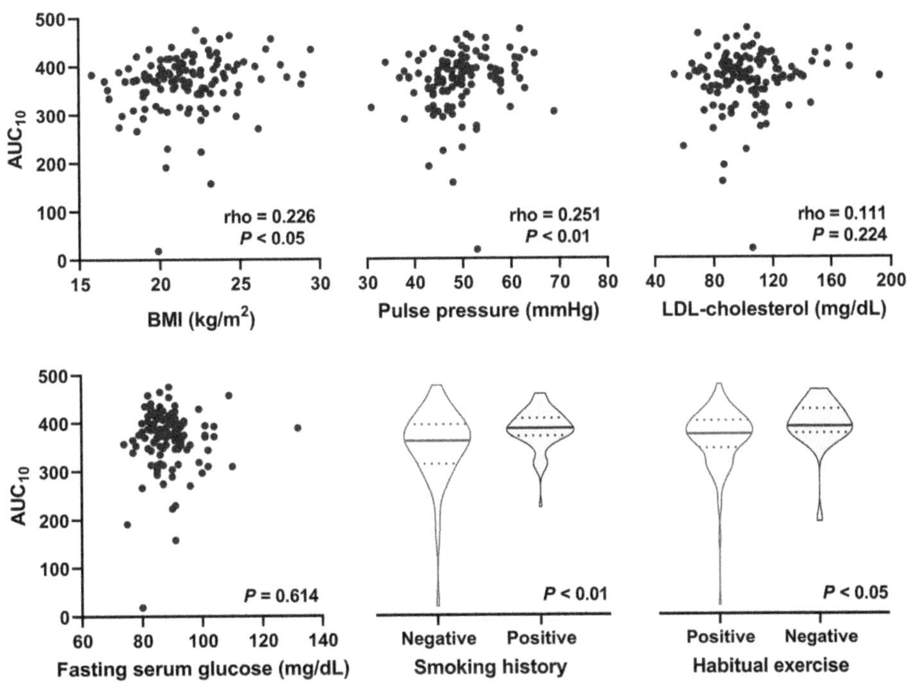

Fig. 2 Correlations between the thrombogenic potential and cardiovascular risk factors in 122 healthy individuals. Correlations between the AUC_{10} (at a shear rate of $1500\ s^{-1}$) in the T-TAS and BMI, pulse pressure, LDL-cholesterol levels, fasting serum glucose levels, smoking history, and habitual exercise were analyzed by Spearman's rank correlation test or the Mann–Whitney U test

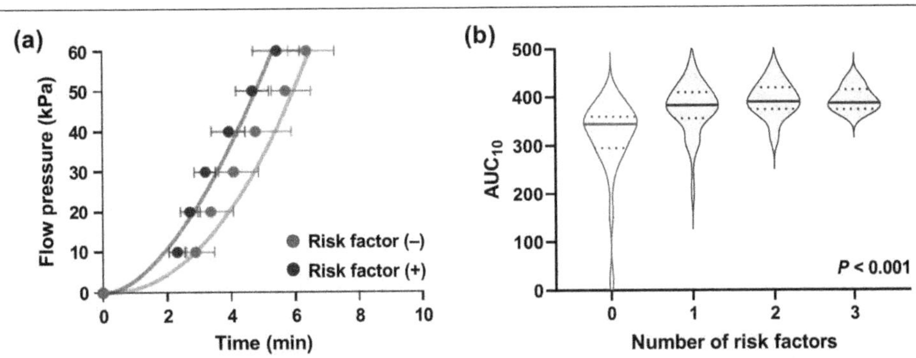

Fig. 3 Healthy individuals with one or more cardiovascular risk factors show augmented thrombogenicity. (a) The times to 10, 20, 30, 40, 50, and 60 kPa (at a shear rate of $1500\ s^{-1}$) in the T-TAS in healthy individuals with or without cardiovascular risk factor(s) are shown. Filled circles and error bars indicate medians and interquartile ranges, respectively. A nonlinear curve fit model was used for estimating theoretical flow pressure curves in individuals with or without cardiovascular risk factor(s). (b) The distribution of the AUC_{10} in the T-TAS in healthy individuals without ($n = 28$) or with one ($n = 59$), two ($n = 26$), or three ($n = 9$) cardiovascular risk factors is shown as violin plots. Bold and dotted horizontal lines indicate medians and quartiles, respectively. The correlation between the AUC_{10} (at a shear rate of $1500\ s^{-1}$) in the T-TAS and the number of cardiovascular risk factors was analyzed by Spearman's rank correlation test

Conclusions

Reference intervals for T-TAS analysis were determined by an analysis of 122 whole blood samples collected from healthy individuals. The platelet number, the leukocyte number, the hematocrit, serum potassium levels, and the presence of one or more cardiovascular risk factors determine the heterogeneity of the thrombogenic potential in the T-TAS

Abbreviations

AUC_{10}: Area under the flow pressure curve up to 10 min; BMI: Body mass index; HDL: High-density lipoprotein; LDL: Low-density lipoprotein; SD: Standard deviation; T-TAS: Total Thrombus-formation Analysis System

Acknowledgments

The authors thank Ellen Knapp, PhD, from Edanz (https://edanz.com/ac) for editing a draft of this manuscript.

Authors' contributions

YO analyzed data and wrote the manuscript. TI designed the experimental protocol and wrote the manuscript. YY, TK, and HF recruited the healthy volunteers and examined individual thrombogenic potential using the T-TAS. TN, TO, and KH analyzed the data. TH and IM critically appraised the manuscript. All authors read and approved the final manuscript.

Author details

[1]Department of Systems Biology in Thromboregulation, Kagoshima University Graduate School of Medical and Dental Sciences, Kagoshima, Japan. [2]Department of Biomedical Laboratory Sciences, Faculty of Life Sciences, Kumamoto University, 4-24-1 Kuhonji, Kumamoto 862-0976, Japan. [3]PPD-SNBL K.K., Kagoshima, Japan. [4]Clinical Study Support, Inc., Nagoya, Japan. [5]Research Institute, Fujimori Kogyo Co., Ltd., Yokohama, Japan. [6]Clinical Research Hospital, Tokyo, Japan. [7]Department of Laboratory and Vascular Medicine, Kagoshima University Graduate School of Medical and Dental Sciences, Kagoshima, Japan.

References

1. Wendelboe AM, Raskob GE. Global burden of thrombosis: epidemiologic aspects. Circ Res. 2016;118(9):1340–7.
2. Ross R. Atherosclerosis--an inflammatory disease. N Engl J Med. 1999;340(2): 115–26.
3. Jackson SP. Arterial thrombosis--insidious, unpredictable and deadly. Nat Med. 2011;17(11):1423–36.
4. Hosokawa K, Ohnishi T, Fukasawa M, Kondo T, Sameshima H, Koide T, et al. A microchip flow-chamber system for quantitative assessment of the platelet thrombus formation process. Microvasc Res. 2012;83(2):154–61.
5. Hosokawa K, Ohnishi T, Sameshima H, Miura N, Ito T, Koide T, et al. Analysing responses to aspirin and clopidogrel by measuring platelet thrombus formation under arterial flow conditions. Thromb Haemost. 2013; 109(1):102–11.
6. Arima Y, Kaikita K, Ishii M, Ito M, Sueta D, Oimatsu Y, et al. Assessment of platelet-derived thrombogenicity with the total thrombus-formation analysis system in coronary artery disease patients receiving antiplatelet therapy. J Thromb Haemost. 2016;14(4):850–9.
7. Oimatsu Y, Kaikita K, Ishii M, Mitsuse T, Ito M, Arima Y, et al. Total Thrombus-formation Analysis System Predicts Periprocedural Bleeding Events in Patients With Coronary Artery Disease Undergoing Percutaneous Coronary Intervention. J Am Heart Assoc. 2017;6(4):e005263.
8. Yamamoto K, Ito T, Nagasato T, Shinnakasu A, Kurano M, Arimura A, et al. Effects of glycemic control and hypoglycemia on Thrombus formation assessed using automated microchip flow chamber system: an exploratory observational study. Thromb J. 2019;17:17.
9. Horowitz GL, Altaie S, Boyd JC. Defining, establishing, and verifying reference intervals in the clinical laboratory; approved guideline - third edition. Wayne: CLSI; 2010.
10. Jones G, Barker A. Reference intervals. Clin Biochem Rev. 2008;29(Suppl 1(Suppl 1)):S93–7.
11. Tanaka F, Makita S, Onoda T, Tanno K, Ohsawa M, Itai K, et al. Predictive value of lipoprotein indices for residual risk of acute myocardial infarction and sudden death in men with low-density lipoprotein cholesterol levels < 120 mg/dl. Am J Cardiol. 2013;112(8):1063–8.
12. Staessen JA, Gasowski J, Wang JG, Thijs L, Den Hond E, Boissel JP, et al. Risks of untreated and treated isolated systolic hypertension in the elderly: meta-analysis of outcome trials. Lancet. 2000;355(9207):865–72.
13. Yamaguchi Y, Moriki T, Igari A, Matsubara Y, Ohnishi T, Hosokawa K, et al. Studies of a microchip flow-chamber system to characterize whole blood thrombogenicity in healthy individuals. Thromb Res. 2013;132(2):263–70.
14. World Health O. Definition, diagnosis and classification of diabetes mellitus and its complications : report of a WHO consultation. Part 1, diagnosis and classification of diabetes mellitus. In. Geneva: World Health Organization; 1999.
15. Belch J. The role of the white blood cell in arterial disease. Blood Coagul Fibrinolysis. 1990;1(2):183–91.
16. Dentan C, Lesnik P, Chapman MJ, Ninio E. Phagocytic activation induces formation of platelet-activating factor in human monocyte-derived macrophages and in macrophage-derived foam cells. Relevance to the inflammatory reaction in atherogenesis. Eur J Biochem FEBS. 1996; 236(1):48–55.
17. Sarma J, Laan CA, Alam S, Jha A, Fox KA, Dransfield I. Increased platelet binding to circulating monocytes in acute coronary syndromes. Circulation. 2002;105(18):2166–71.
18. Baskurt OK, Meiselman HJ. Blood rheology and hemodynamics. Semin Thromb Hemost. 2003;29(5):435–50.
19. Spivak JL. Polycythemia vera: myths, mechanisms, and management. Blood. 2002;100(13):4272–90.
20. Aarts P, Van Den Broek S, Prins GW, Kuiken G, Sixma JJ, Heethaar RM. Blood platelets are concentrated near the wall and red blood cells, in the center in flowing blood. Arterioscler Thromb Vasc Biol. 1988;8(6):819–24.
21. Ikeda Y, Handa M, Kawano K, Kamata T, Murata M, Araki Y, et al. The role of von Willebrand factor and fibrinogen in platelet aggregation under varying shear stress. J Clin Invest. 1991;87(4):1234–40.
22. Lin H, Young DB. Interaction between plasma potassium and epinephrine in coronary thrombosis in dogs. Circulation. 1994;89(1):331–8.
23. Helms C, Marvel M, Zhao W, Stahle M, Vest R, Kato G, et al. Mechanisms of hemolysis-associated platelet activation. J Thromb Haemost. 2013;11(12): 2148–54.
24. Takano K, Asazuma N, Satoh K, Yatomi Y, Ozaki Y. Collagen-induced generation of platelet-derived microparticles in whole blood is dependent on ADP released from red blood cells and calcium ions. Platelets. 2004;15(4): 223–9.
25. Stone NJ, Robinson JG, Lichtenstein AH, Bairey Merz CN, Blum CB, Eckel RH, et al. 2013 ACC/AHA guideline on the treatment of blood cholesterol to reduce atherosclerotic cardiovascular risk in adults: a report of the American College of Cardiology/American Heart Association task force on practice guidelines. Circulation. 2014;129(25 Suppl 2):S1–s45.
26. Kitamura A, Sato S, Kiyama M, Imano H, Iso H, Okada T, et al. Trends in the incidence of coronary heart disease and stroke and their risk factors in Japan, 1964 to 2003: the Akita-Osaka study. J Am Coll Cardiol. 2008; 52(1):71–9.
27. Inoue M, Iso H, Yamamoto S, Kurahashi N, Iwasaki M, Sasazuki S, et al. Daily total physical activity level and premature death in men and women: results from a large-scale population-based cohort study in Japan (JPHC study). Ann Epidemiol. 2008;18(7):522–30.
28. Yanbaeva DG, Dentener MA, Creutzberg EC, Wesseling G, Wouters EF. Systemic effects of smoking. Chest Journal. 2007;131(5):1557–66.
29. Franklin SS, Khan SA, Wong ND, Larson MG, Levy D. Is pulse pressure useful in predicting risk for coronary heart disease? The Framingham Heart Study. Circulation. 1999;100(4):354–60.
30. Blacher J, Staessen JA, Girerd X, Gasowski J, Thijs L, Liu L, et al. Pulse pressure not mean pressure determines cardiovascular risk in older hypertensive patients. Arch Intern Med. 2000;160(8):1085–9.
31. Kaplan NM. The deadly quartet: upper-body obesity, glucose intolerance, hypertriglyceridemia, and hypertension. Arch Intern Med. 1989;149(7):1514–20.
32. Yusuf HR, Giles WH, Croft JB, Anda RF, Casper ML. Impact of multiple risk factor profiles on determining cardiovascular disease risk. Prev Med. 1998; 27(1):1–9.

5

Endovascular revascularization strategies using catheter-based thrombectomy versus conventional catheter-directed thrombolysis for acute limb ischemia

Maofeng Gong, Xu He, Boxiang Zhao, Jie Kong, Jianping Gu and Guoping Chen*

Abstract

Background: Acute limb ischemia (ALI) is an important clinical event threatening both life and the affected limbs, but the optimal treatment for ALI remains undefined. The aim of this study was to compare the safety and effectiveness of thrombectomy approaches via either catheter-based thrombectomy (CBT) or catheter-directed thrombolysis (CDT).

Methods: A total of 98 patients (mean age 69.7 years, 60 male) who underwent endovascular intervention for ALI from January 2015 to July 2019 were included. Of these, 57 were treated with primary CBT via a large-bore catheter, an AngioJet catheter or Rotarex catheter, and/or underwent low-dose CDT, and 41 were treated with primary CDT. The safety and effectiveness of CBT compared to conventional CDT and other various endovascular techniques were evaluated.

Results: More Rutherford IIb patients were treated with primary CBT (68.4%) than CDT (26.8%; $P < .001$). Patients who underwent primary CDT achieved a higher technical success rate than those who underwent primary CBT in a shorter procedure time ($P < .001$), whereas 42.1% of patients who underwent CBT did not need adjunctive CDT. The duration and dosage of adjunctive CDT in the CBT group were significantly decreased compared with those in the primary CDT group (both $P < .001$), and the CBT group achieved a shorter in-hospital length of stay ($P < .001$). Subgroup analysis revealed that patients treated with AngioJet and Rotarex catheters achieved slightly lower dosages, shorter CDT durations and shorter in-hospital stay lengths than those treated with large-bore catheters ($P > .05$). Clinical success was estimated to be achieved in 98.2% of patients who underwent CBT, which is similar to the 97.6% estimated in those who underwent primary CDT ($P = 1.000$), and this finding was similar among the CBT subgroups. Patients who underwent CBT had a higher procedure-related distal embolization rate and economic cost than those who underwent primary CDT ($P < .05$), but it had slightly fewer complications than those who underwent primary CDT ($P = .059$), especially minor complications ($P = .036$). The freedom from amputation at 6 and 12 months for CBT and CDT was assessed (93.0% vs 90.2% respectively, $P = .625$; 89.5% vs 82.9%, respectively, $P = .34$,). Comparable limb salvage was found for different techniques of large bore catheters, AngioJet catheters and Rotarex catheters. The Kaplan-Meier table analysis also showed similar limb salvage rates between groups.

* Correspondence: chenguoping_72@163.com
Department of Interventional and Vascular Radiology, Nanjing First Hospital, Nanjing Medical University, Jiangsu 210006 Nanjing, People's Republic of China

Conclusions: Endovascular treatment of ALI with the use of catheter-based therapies is an effective modality that can reduce the requirement for thrombolysis, with expected reductions in hemorrhagic complications, but at the risk of remediable distal emboli and increased economic cost. It has a similar clinical outcome to conventional CDT alone. Different CBT techniques have comparable efficacy but different adverse event profiles.

Keywords: Acute limb ischemia, Endovascular treatment, Catheter-based thrombectomy, Percutaneous mechanical thrombectomy, Catheter-directed thrombolysis

Article highlights Type of Research: Single-center retrospective cohort study.

Key findings: CBT was successful as a stand-alone first-line endovascular technique in close to one-half of patients, with the remainder of patients requiring adjunctive CDT due to residual thrombus or emboli into distal small arteries where the CBT catheters could not safely reach. CBTs had the advantages of pronounced reduction of large volumes of thrombus in a moderate time and quicker return of blood flow and had comparable limb salvage rates, but at the risk of remediable distal emboli and increased economic cost. In contrast, primary CDT had greater technical success but was associated with more bleeding complications, including one bleeding-related death. Moreover, comparisons among CBT techniques revealed comparable outcomes in ALI patients regardless of which of the 3 modalities were used as first-line treatment but showed that the modalities had different adverse event profiles.

Take home message: Endovascular treatment of ALI with the use of catheter-based therapies is an effective modality that can reduce the requirement for thrombolysis, with expected reductions in hemorrhagic complications, but at the risk of remediable distal emboli and increased economic cost. It has a similar clinical outcome to conventional CDT alone. Regarding Rutherford IIb ischemia, CBT may have an advantage over CDT. In terms of CBT modalities, different techniques have comparable efficacy but have different adverse event profiles.

Table of contents summary: This retrospective single-center study analyzed the endovascular revascularization and outcomes of 98 acute limb ischemia patients. The study suggests that endovascular treatment of ALI with the use of catheter-based therapies is an effective modality that can reduce the requirement for thrombolysis, with expected reductions in hemorrhagic complications, but at the risk of remediable distal emboli and increased economic cost. It has a similar clinical outcome to conventional CDT alone. Regarding Rutherford IIb ischemia, CBT may have an advantage over CDT. In terms of CBT modalities, different techniques have comparable efficacy but have different adverse event profiles.

Introduction

Acute limb ischemia (ALI), referred to as ischemia symptoms that emerge within 2 weeks, is one of the most common arterial emergencies [1, 2]. The most common causes of ALI are embolism, thrombosis of native arteries or reconstructions, peripheral arterial aneurysm, dissection and traumatic arterial injury [3]. ALI manifesting as "6P syndrome" can be catastrophic, with a potential threat to limb viability due to insufficient time for new vessel growth to compensate for the sudden interruption of limb perfusion [4, 5]. Ischemia is graded clinically according to the Rutherford ALI classification system. For acute, viable or marginally threatened ALI, timely recognition and revascularization aiming at restoring perfusion is recommended (Class I) [1, 2, 5].

ALI is a potential lethal event leading to not only amputation (12–50% of cases) but also death (20–40% of cases) without prompt treatments [4]. A majority of adverse outcomes occur within the initial days after presentation, indicating that intervention time is limited. Therefore rapid and effective revascularization following an episode of ALI is pivotal, as it will most likely improve the prognosis. However, determination of the optimal option for revascularization remains particularly challenging [1]. Surgical and endovascular approaches have been a longstanding topic of debate; both appear equally effective in the ALI patient population [6, 7] but have different adverse event profiles. Two recent guidelines, the European Society of Cardiology (ESC) and the European Society for Vascular Surgery (ESVS) guidelines [1, 8], have put a spotlight on ALI, and an evolution towards less invasive interventions has taken place, which may be an opportunity to encourage endovascular interventions in addition to surgery [9].

For endovascular approaches, conventional catheter-directed thrombolysis (CDT) is one of the most well established and employed techniques [10, 11]. Recently, a variety of new endovascular modalities aimed at mechanical disruption of the thrombus have emerged, and catheter-based thrombectomy (CBT) techniques, including thromboaspiration, microfragmentation, pharmacomechanical thrombectomy and ultrasound-accelerated CDT, have emerged and been made more available [12]. Even if all of the above techniques have been widely applied in clinical practice, relatively little is known about critical points such as safety and competitive device performance. Thus, the primary objective of this study was to compare the safety and effectiveness of CBT to conventional CDT in the management of ALI, as well as to evaluate various endovascular techniques with large bore catheters, Rotarex catheters and AngioJet catheters.

Methods

Patients and study design

This was a retrospective cohort study which included confirmed ALI patients who underwent endovascular revascularization as first-line treatment at a single academic center from January 2015 to July 2019. All patients underwent treatment via the CBT and/or CDT approach, and data were retrospectively derived from the medical database system and paper records. This data collection protocol was approved by the institutional review board, and the need for informed consent was waived owing to the retrospective nature of this study. A study flow-chart is shown in Fig. 1.

Management strategies details

ALI was initially assessed in the majority of patients with urgent duplex ultrasound and CT arteriography (CTA). Then, the therapeutic approach was left to the discretion of the treatment group, consisting of 3 interventional radiologists with at least 15 years of experience. The decision to proceed with either CBT or CDT as the first-line treatment was determined by the interventional radiologist operators based mainly on the degree of ischemia, experience and devices available. Although the procedural details varied slightly in different cases depending on individuality therapy, procedures were largely similar, and the exact CBT reperfusion details are shown in Supplementary Table 1. If residual in situ thrombus or distal embolization was found after embolectomy, further widely used alternative conjunction with CDT was considered.

Patients who underwent conventional CDT as first-line treatment were infused a bolus dose of 5 mg of recombinant tissue-type plasminogen activator (rt-PA) (Actilyse; Boehringer Ingelheim; Ingelheim, Germany) via a multiple-side hole thrombolytic catheter (Uni*Fuse; Angio-Dynamic; Latham, NY). Both CDT techniques subsequently received a continuous infusion of reduced-dose rt-PA for further treatment. Thrombolytic therapy with rt-PA was administered as follows: 20 mg of actilyse in 500 ml of 0.9% saline was administered through the reserved thrombolysis catheter at an infusion rate of 0.01 mg/kg/h; the maximum rate was no more than 1.0 mg/h. Thrombolysis with actilyse was only administered when the fibrinogen level, which was monitored at 12–24 hourly intervals, was greater than 1.0 g/L. Follow-up angiography was performed to assess efficacy every 24 h. In the absence of any contraindications, CDT was continued if the thrombus load remained and discontinued when treatment was complete or in the event of an adverse event.

If more than the indicated minimum of 50% stenosis remained after thrombus removal, balloon angioplasty and/or stenting was performed. During each thrombolysis therapy or at the end of CDT, low molecular weight heparin (Hebei Changshan Biochemical Pharmaceutical; Shijiazhuang, China) therapy at a dose of 100 IU/kg per 12 h was started immediately. In the absence of local hemorrhagic complications, dual antiplatelet therapy (aspirin 100 mg/d and clopidogrel 75 mg/d) and statin therapy (atorvastatin, 20 mg/d) were prescribed after discharge. Outpatient follow-ups were conducted by our center at 1, 3, 6, and 12 months postprocedure via ankle-brachial index (ABI), duplex ultrasound and/or CTA; additional procedures and complications were recorded during follow-up.

Definitions of outcome and safety measures

The clinical severity of ALI was classified by the Rutherford classification system details are listed in Supplementary Table 2 [5]. Technical success of the primary procedure was defined as complete in situ thrombus clearance of CBT or CDT alone, and adjunctive treatment of CDT to achieve thrombus clearance for CBT was considered to indicate assistant technical success. Clinical success (improvement in clinical status) was defined as the absence and/or relief of symptoms related to ALI according to accepted guidelines [5, 11], or an improvement in the Rutherford grade of at least one category with objective evidence of hemodynamic change (at least 0.1 increase in ABI). Limb salvage was defined as freedom from major amputation (performed above the ankle), and maintained functional autonomy (walking or standing) was determined in accordance to accepted guidelines [5]. The need for necessary additional techniques (such as balloon angioplasty and/or stenting) to treat underlying chronic disease to obtain sufficient distal perfusion within the same hospital stay was recorded but not considered clinical failure. Safety was classified as major or minor complications in accordance with the criteria of the Society of Interventional Radiology (SIR) classification scale [13].

Statistical analysis

The *SPSS* statistical software package (version 23.0; *SPSS* statistical software, Chicago, Illinois, USA) was used to perform all statistical analyses in this study. Continuous variables are expressed as the mean ± standard deviation. Qualitative variables are presented as numbers and

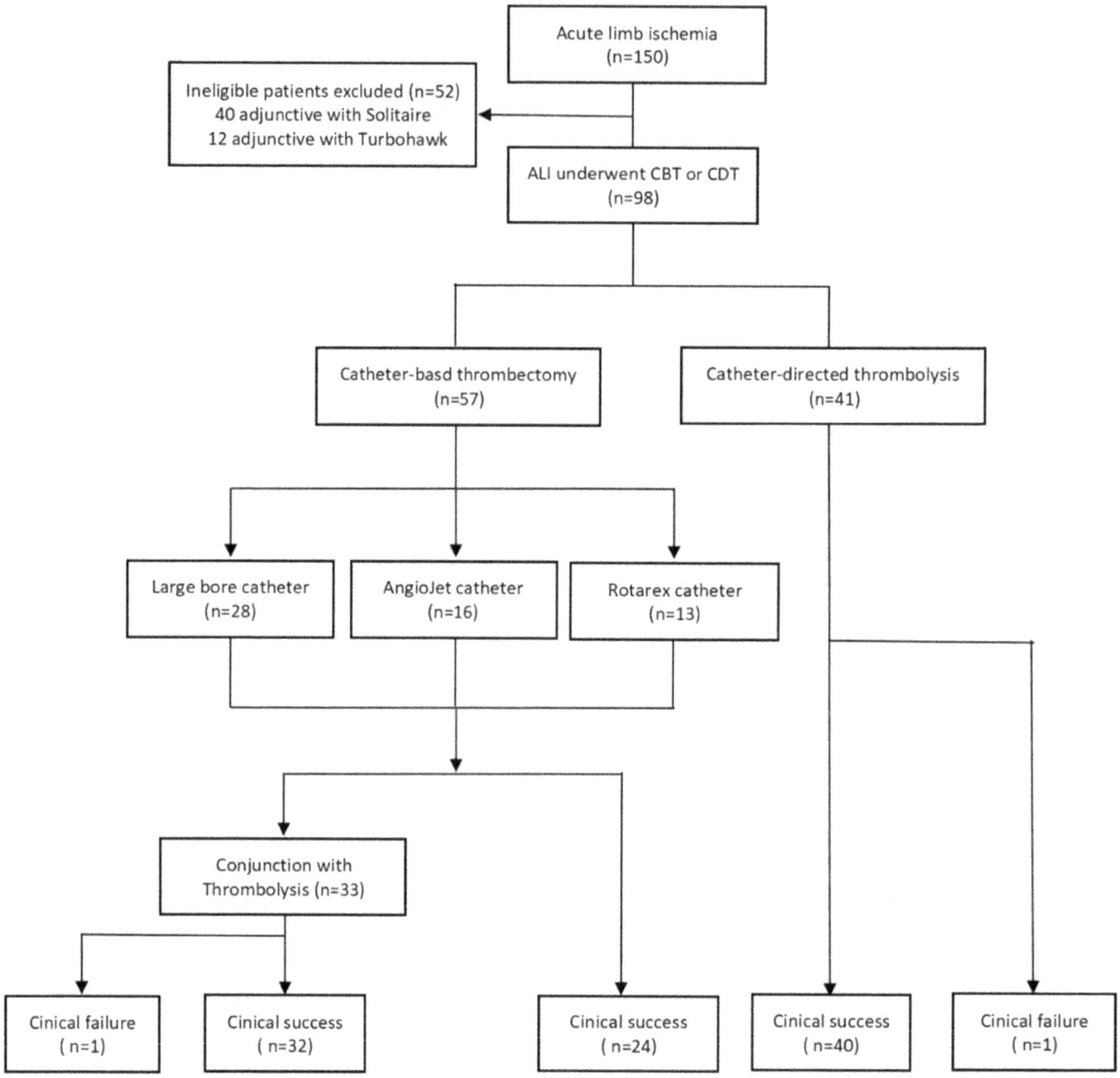

Fig. 1 Study Flowchart. CBT = catheter-based thrombectomy; CDT = catheter-directed thrombolysis

percentages. When assessing the correlation between pre- and postprocedural variables, a paired *t*-test was used. The significance of qualitative variables was tested with a *chi-square* test or *Fisher's* exact test. Findings with a *P* value less than 0.05 were deemed statistically significant.

Results

Baseline characteristics and ischemia classification of patients

A total of 98 patients [mean age 69.7 years, 61.2% male ($n = 60$)] with ALI who underwent endovascular revascularization with either CBT or CDT were included. Of those patients who underwent CBT as first-line treatment, 28 were treated with large-bore catheters, 16 with AngioJet catheters, and 13 with Rotarex catheters, and 41 underwent conventional CDT solely as the first-line treatment. The demographics, comorbidities, presentation and lesion characteristics of 98 patients are summarized in Table 1. Procedure characteristics and outcomes are outlined in Tables 2, and 3 summarizes outcomes by subgroups of interest.

The mean duration of ischemia symptoms before presentation was slightly longer in the CBT group of than that in the CDT group (37.2 ± 32.8 h vs 31.0 ± 28.2 h, respectively; $P = .332$). Within the CBT group, the Rotarex

Table 1 Demographics, Comorbidities, Presentation and Lesion Characteristics of ALI Patients

Characteristic	Primary CBT ($n = 57$)	Primary CDT ($n = 41$)	p value
Age, y, mean ± SD (range)	68.89 ± 11.88	70.63 ± 10.87	.461
Male sex	35 (61.4%)	25 (61.0%)	.966
Duration of symptoms at presentation, h, mean ± SD (range)	37.2 ± 32.8	31.0 ± 28.2	.332
Risk factors			
Diabetes mellitus	20 (35.1)	12 (29.3)	.545
Coronary artery disease	19 (33.3)	13 (31.7)	.886
Rheumatic heart disease	9 (15.8)	5 (12.2)	.616
Previous cerebrovascular accident	7 (12.3)	3 (7.3)	.644
Renal insufficiency	5 (8.8)	3 (7.3)	1.00
Hypertension	38 (66.7)	31 (75.6)	.339
Hyperlipidemia	18 (31.6)	13 (31.7)	.989
Diagnosed atrial fibrillation	35 (61.4)	27 (65.9)	.652
Current diagnosis of cancer	3 (5.3)	1 (2.4)	.858
History of smoking	17 (29.8)	13 (31.7)	.842
History of peripheral artery disease	20 (35.1)	12 (29.3)	.545
Thrombosed segment			
Iliac	7 (12.3)	3(7.3)	.644
Iliofemoral (including iliofemoral stents)	42 (73.7)[a]	24 (58.5)	.115
Femoropopliteal	8 (14.0)	12 (29.3)	.065
Crural and Tibial	0 (0)	2 (4.9)	.173**
Ischemia level (Rutherford category)			
I (viable limb)	1 (1.8)	4 (9.8)	.076
II a (marginally threatened limb)	17 (29.8)	26 (63.4)	.001*
II b (immediately threatened limb)	39 (68.4)	11 (26.8)	.000*

ALI Acute limb ischemia, *CBT* Catheter-based thrombectomy, *CDT* Catheter-directed thrombolysis
Continuous data are presented as the means ± standard deviations; categorical data are given as the counts (percentage)
*$P < .05$; ** Fisher exact
[a]Includes two patients of thrombus in stents

subgroup had a longer duration of ischemia (50.8 ± 30.0 h, $P = .208$). With regard to etiology, the major risk factors for the development of ALI were hypertension (70.4%), diagnosed atrial fibrillation (63.3%) and coronary artery disease (32.7%). In the majority of cases, the thrombosed segment primarily resided in the iliac, iliofemoral arteries for the CBT group, and iliofemoral or femoropopliteal arteries for the CDT group; two cases in the CBT group had iliofemoral thrombus of existing stents, and two cases in the CDT group had distal artery thrombus. There were no statistically significant differences in baseline characteristics between the two groups or among the subgroups of large-bore catheters, AngioJet catheters and Rotarex catheters ($P > .05$). With regard to the ischemia classification of patients, the primary CDT group had a slightly higher proportion of patients with Rutherford grade I ischemia ($P = .076$); there were fewer Rutherford grade IIa patients treated with primary CBT ($n = 17$, 29.8%) than those treated with CDT ($n = 26$, 63.4%; $P = .001$), and more Rutherford grade IIb patients were treated with the use of primary CBT ($n = 39$, 68.4%) than those treated with CDT ($n = 11$, 26.8%; $P < .001$).

Outcomes of technical and clinical success

Procedure characteristics and outcomes are outlined in Tables 2 and 3. Patients who underwent primary CDT achieved a higher technical success rate ($n = 39$, 95.1%) than those who underwent primary CBT ($n = 24$, 42.1%) in a shorter time [1.32 ± .44 h versus 1.89 ± .52 h; $P < .001$)]. In the subgroup analysis, large-bore catheters had slightly shorter procedure lengths than AngioJet or Rotarex catheters. In the 57 patients who underwent primary CBT and experienced technical failure, 33 patients required adjunctive CDT due to either residual in situ thrombus ($n = 19$) or dislodged distal thrombus ($n = 14$). At completion, additional balloon angioplasty and/or secondary stenting for underlying chronic disease to obtain sufficient distal reperfusion was performed in 81.6%

Table 2 Procedure Characteristics by Treatment Approach and Outcomes

Characteristics	Primary CBT ($n = 57$)	Primary CDT ($n = 41$)	p value
Technical success of thrombus/embolus removal			
With primary intervention only	24 (42.1)	39 (95.1)	.000
Including adjuvant thrombolysis	57 (100)	41 (100)	1.000
Adjunctive angioplasty/stenting after thrombus/embolus removal	47 (82.5)	33 (80.5)	.804
Duration of operation procedure, h	1.89 ± .52	1.32 ± .44	.000
Total duration of thrombolysis, d	1.74 ± .98	3.07 ± 1.38	.000
Rt-PA dose, mg	14.14 ± 5.75	29.27 ± 11.70	.000
ABI scores			
Pretreatment	.29 ± .09	.31 ± .08	.747
Treatment completion	.72 ± .16	.66 ± .13	.101
Clinical success	56 (98.2)	40 (97.6)	1.000
Limb salvage at 6 months	53 (93.0)	37(90.2)	.625
Limb salvage at 12 months	51 (89.5)	34 (82.9)	.346
30-day complications	10 (17.5)	14 (34.1)	.059
Minor (SIR A, B: nominal or no therapy, no consequence)	6 (10.5)	11(26.8)	.036
Major (SIR C, D, E: requires therapy or permanent sequelae)	3 (5.3)	2 (4.9)	1.000
Major-death (SIR F: death)	1 (1.8)	1 (2.4)	1.000
Procedure- related distal embolization	14 (24.6)	2 (4.9)	.009
In-hospital length of stay, d	4.97 ± .13	6.04 ± .95	.000

CBT Catheter-based thrombectomy, *CDT* Catheter-directed thrombolysis
Continuous data are presented as the means ± standard deviations; categorical data are given as the counts (percentages)

of patients ($n = 80$), without a significant difference between the two groups ($P = .804$).

The duration and dosage of adjunctive CDT were significantly lower when compared to those for primary CDT (duration was 1.74 ± .98 days vs 3.07 ± 1.38 days, mean dosage rt-PA 14.14 ± 5.75 mg vs 29.27 ± 11.70 mg, both $P < .001$). The CBT group also demonstrated a shorter in-hospital length of stay ($P < .001$). In the subgroup analysis, AngioJet and Rotarex catheters achieved slightly lower dosages, shorter CDT durations and shorter length of in-hospital stay than large-bore catheters. Clinical success estimates were achieved in 98.2% of patients ($n = 56$) who underwent primary CBT, which was similar to the 97.6% ($n = 40$) success in those who underwent primary CDT ($P = 1.000$). These were similar among the subgroups of CBT, despite differences in the proportions of patients with Rutherford IIa and Rutherford IIb ischemia treated with each modality. Of these, the clinical success rates of patients in Rutherford IIa and IIb were 100% and 97.4%, respectively ($P = 1.000$). In both groups, ABI was significantly improved from preprocedure measurements to those after treatment completion ($P < .001$); however, the difference was not statistically significant between each other or among the subgroups ($P > .05$).

The average procedural costs including devices and thrombolytic agents and total cost of hospitalization were CNY ¥ 46,522.1 ± 14,724.8 and CNY ¥ 69,633.4 ± 27,460.6 per patient for patients who underwent primary CBT, which were higher than CNY ¥ 35,249.9 ± 8177.2 and CNY ¥ 49,734.3 ± 10,710.8 in those who underwent primary CDT ($P < .05$).

Complications and treatment therapy

The 30-day complications recorded are listed in Tables 2 and 3. Patients who underwent primary CBT had slightly fewer complications than those who underwent primary CDT ($P = .059$), especially for minor complications ($P = .036$). Minor complications for the CBT group included vessel spasm ($n = 3$), dissection of the superficial femoral artery ($n = 1$), hematuria ($n = 1$) and hematoma of the puncture site ($n = 1$); the rate of complications was significantly lower than that for CDT. Minor complications in the CDT group were presented mainly as hemorrhage events, including hematoma of the puncture site (diameter 3–5 cm, $n = 6$), pseudoaneurysm ($n = 2$), hematuria ($n = 2$) and calf hematoma ($n = 1$). Local pressure dressing was applied for observation and treatment of minor hemorrhage, and minor complications experienced less serious adverse consequences. The major complication except for distal embolization of the CBT group was compartment syndrome ($n = 3$) requiring surgery for calf fasciotomy. Two patients in

Table 3 Comparisons of Outcomes by Treatment Approach (large bore catheter and Rotarex and AngioJet devices)

Characteristic	Large bore catheter	Rotarex catheter	AngioJet catheter	*p* value
Age, y, mean ± SD (range)	69.7 ± 13.2	67.6 ± 9.9	68.8 ± 11.7	.862
Sex, male	17 (60.7)	9 (56.3)	9 (69.2)	.768
Duration of symptoms at presentation, h, mean ± SD (range)	31.2 ± 36.5	50.8 ± 30.0	36.7 ± 25.8	.208
Ischemia level (Rutherford category)				
I (viable limb)	1 (3.6)	0 (0)	0 (0)	.590
II a (marginally threatened limb)	11 (39.3)	3 (18.8)	3 (23.1)	.292
II b (immediately threatened limb)	16 (57.1)	13 (81.3)	10 (76.9)	.186
Procedure length (h, mean ± SD)	1.74 ± .54	2.03 ± .53	2.04 ± .38	.103
Technical and clinical success with initial endovascular procedure only	13 (46.4)	5 (31.3)	6 (46.2)	.584
Total duration of thrombolysis, d	.775 ± .20	.56 ± .16	.61 ± .22	.092
rt-PA dosage, mg	16.67 ± 5.56	12.31 ± 5.63	12.1 ± 4.88	.076
In-hospital length of stay, d	5.21 ± .92	4.78 ± .71	4.69 ± 1.18	.165
ABI scores				
Pre procedure	.30 ± .11	.29 ± .09	.28 ± .04	.743
Treatment completion	.68 ± .15	.75 ± .17	.75 ± .16	.179
Limb salvage at 6 months	26 (92.9)	15 (93.8)	12 (92.3)	.988
Limb salvage at 12 months	25 (89.3)	14 (87.5)	12 (92.3)	.915
Procedure-related complications				
Minor (SIR A, B: nominal or no therapy, no consequence)	3 (10.7)	2 (12.5)	1 (7.7)	.912
Major (SIR C, D, E: requires therapy or permanent sequelae)	1 (3.6)	1(6.3)	1 (7.7)	.841
Major-death (SIR F: death)	1 (3.6)	0 (0)	0 (0)	–
Procedure- related distal embolization	6 (21.4)	5 (31.3)	3 (23.1)	.765

Data are presented as the mean ± standard deviation or number (percentage)

the CDT group required transfusion of two units of red blood cell suspension due to major gastrointestinal hemorrhage. Fortunately, all these events resolved without permanent sequelae. One death in each group was recorded: one subject in the CBT group died from cardiac failure after amputation, which was unrelated to the procedure, and the one subject in the CDT group died from intracranial hemorrhage after CDT despite surgical decompression. CBT had a higher procedure-related distal embolization rate than those who underwent primary CDT ($P = .009$), in the subgroup analysis, Rotarex catheters had more procedure-related distal emboli than large-bore catheters and AngioJet catheters, yet the difference was not statistically significant among the 3 groups ($P = .765$). Owing to the small size of these vessels and underlying chronic disease, adjunctive CDTs were performed, the dislodged thrombus was well treated without permanent sequelae.

Follow-up and limb freedom from amputation

No patients were lost to follow-up, and 98.0% (96/98) of patients were alive when discharged from the hospital. The reintervention rates at 6 months and 12 months were 9.2% ($n = 9$) and 17.3% ($n = 17$), respectively. A total of four patients in each group suffered major amputations at 6 months for the CBT and CDT groups and six and seven at 12 months, which were primarily attribute to intractable infection caused by diabetes, osteomyelitis or repeat embolism event. The freedom from amputation at 6 months in the CBT and CDT groups was 93.0 and 90.2%, respectively, and at 12 months was 89.5 and 82.9%, respectively ($P > .05$). The Kaplan-Meier analysis also showed similar limb salvage rates between groups (Fig. 2). Similarly, no significant differences were seen among groups ($P > .05$).

Discussion

Present study demonstrated that CBT is successful as a stand-alone first-line endovascular technique in close to one-half of patients with ALI, with the remainder requiring adjunctive CDT due to residual thrombus or emboli into distal small arteries where the CBT catheters could not safely reach. CBTs had the advantages of pronounced reduction of large volumes of thrombus in a moderate time, speedy recanalization of blood flow and comparable limb salvage, but at the risk of remediable distal emboli and increased economic cost. In contrast, primary CDT had greater technical success but with

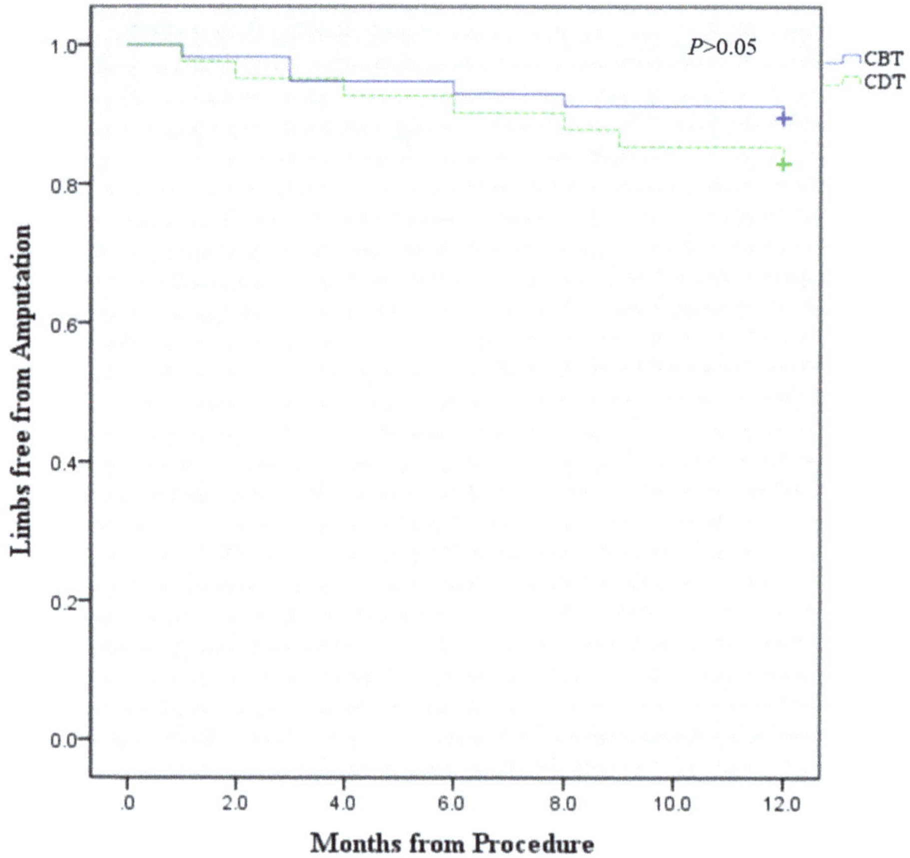

Fig. 2 Kaplan-Meier estimates of limbs salvage for the CBT and CDT cohort at 12 months. CBT = catheter-based thrombectomy; CDT = catheter-directed thrombolysis

more bleeding complications (statistically significant for minor bleeds), including one bleeding-related death. Moreover, the comparison among CBTs revealed comparable outcomes in ALI patients regardless of which of the 3 modalities were used as first-line treatment, but had different adverse event profiles. Because ALI might threaten limbs and life, especially quality of life, shared decision making between clinicians, patients and families based on the best available option for ALI patients seems to be important.

The strategy options for ALI treatment in our study depended mainly on the severity of ischemia. CDT for revascularization often takes time, and ischemia may progress during treatment if the thrombus is not removed in a timely manner [1, 2, 6]. In this study, 73.2% of CDT therapy was applied in patients with Rutherford grade I and IIa ischemia considering its inherent defects of slow opening of the lumen. In 68.4% of patients with Rutherford grade IIb, more emergency revascularization techniques, including large-bore catheters, Rotarex catheters and AngioJet catheters, were used as the preferred first-line methods to restore perfusion. Although clinical success and freedom from amputation in the Grip et al. [7] study were inferior in patients with Rutherford grade IIb than IIa ischemia, the present study demonstrates that outcomes were no worse for patients with Rutherford grade IIb ischemia. CBT was empirically performed for iliac and iliofemoral thrombosed segment and CDT was used primarily for iliofemoral and femoropopliteal segment. Patients who underwent CBT achieved similar outcomes, removing emboli/thrombus and opening the lumen with shorter procedure times than CDT. The strategy of CBT for Rutherford grade IIb ischemia seems to be a suitable alternative when initiated promptly.

In the present cohort study of patients treated by CDT and CBT, both techniques were shown to be useful. We compared CBT and CDT as the primary endovascular procedures, and the results indicated that technical success rates of CBT were 42.1%, which was lower than that of CDT as 57.9% of CBT patients underwent conjunctive CDT. This number was lower than that reported by Zehnder et al. [14], which may be attributed to a more stringent definition (not including adjunctive CDT) of technical success in the present study. A matched analysis comparing clinical success and limb salvage between the two groups showed slightly better outcomes and comparable limb salvage in the CBT group. The patients who were free from amputation at 6 months and 12 months was approximately 93.0% versus 90.2% and 89.5% versus 82.9% in both groups, which was similar to those of other published studies [15, 16]. While more patients with Rutherford grade IIb ischemia were considered, CBT attained a better outcome. These results indicated that it might be better to perform CBT initially than CDT. A limitation of CBTs was the inability to use the devices in the small-caliber arteries of the lower limbs; however, it was managed by conjunctive low-dose CDT. Even if adjuvant therapy was possible, and the procedure time tended to be shorter in CDT, CBT seemed to have the advantages of a lower CDT duration and rt-PA dosages than conventional CDT. Several studies have examined whether the risk factors for bleeding risk during CDT are related to the duration and dosages of CDT used [17, 18]. Approximately one-half of patients with ALI did not require adjunctive CDT, and the present study supported the major potential advantage of CBT, which, if successful as a stand-alone treatment, obviates the requirement for CDT with a concomitant reduction in the risk of hemorrhagic complications.

One study that compared CDT with or without pharmacomechanical thrombolysis using the AngioJet device showed that CBT increased technical success rates but at the cost of more distal emboli, causing embolization of both large and small particles. Notably, patients treated with CBT in our study also encountered distal emboli events, similar to a published study [16]. The dislodged thrombus was successful treated by adjunctive CDT, without permanent sequelae, which seems remediable. It should be noted that a variety of distal embolic protection devices have been developed for carotid artery stenosis and deep vein thrombosis, a situation of minor embolization and less serious consequences [19]. The use of distal embolic protection devices has been considered suitable but not yet advocated in ALI treatments. The mean rt-PA dosage was lower in CBT than in CDT. Although there was no significant difference in the frequency of major complications between the two groups, two cases of major hemorrhage and one death complication were noted in CDT, while no such cases were recorded in CBT. Furthermore, three patients who underwent CBT required calf compartment decompression due to compartment syndrome after reperfusion, which was not recorded in CDT. A possible explanation for this may lie in the differences in ischemia grade at presentation for each group; more patients with Rutherford grade IIb ischemia were present in the primary CBT group, and more ALI patients with Rutherford IIa ischemia were present in the primary CDT group. In addition to the severity of ischemia, another possible explanation may be related to the shorter time taken to achieve reperfusion with CBT compared with CDT, which may result in massive blood perfusion and exudation [20, 21]. The risks of CBT may lead to hyperkalemia, myoglobinuria, and renal damage [15], but these risks were not recorded in the present study.

Subgroup analysis evaluated within distinct patients showed that three techniques exhibited comparable outcomes but had different adverse event profiles. The PEARL registry study showed AngioJet catheter as a modality for treating ALI, with a technical success rate of 52%, and adjuvant CDT improved this success rate to 83% [15]. Rotarex devices were described with a technical success rate of 68.7% as a stand-alone technique but with additional thrombolysis in 90.5% [22]. Patients with ALI assigned to an initial large-bore catheter and AngioJet catheter tended to have improved technique success rates in the present study and had less need for adjunctive intervention. The Rotarex device revealed a lower technical success rate and a greater need for additional CDT due to distal artery emboli. A physiological circulation model study [23] revealed that the Rotarex system had slight advantages, but significantly more thromboemboli and vascular injuries; however, the AngioJet was more tissue preserving. Similar to our subgroup analysis, AngioJet and large bore catheter had slightly first pass recanalization and lower distal emboli when compared to Rotarex catheter in a "real-world" contemporary clinical setting.

Some limitations of the present study should be mentioned. Due to the aim of present study was to investigate the endovascular revascularization strategies, patients who underwent surgical revascularization were not included. The strategy employed mainly depended on the severity of ischemia and the expertise and facilities of the treating team, and the study was not randomized, which could have resulted in potential selection biases and confounding variables. Although the outcome in the subgroup analysis of PAT with a large-bore catheter and PMT with an AngioJet/Rotarex catheter was conducted, the conclusion was limited to a small subgroup of cases, which may need to be confirmed, and there is a need for future research in this field. Meanwhile, devices such as Penumbra/Indigo had not been utilized in the present study. Therefore, the thromboaspiration device used in the present study was limited to a simple large-bore catheter. Nevertheless, this study hopes to help clinicians choose between approaches for individual patients, but is inevitably hampered by a lack of robust data. The conclusions of the present study are limited due to the small, retrospective and nonrandomized analysis from a single center. These data may help prompt the design of RCTs that may differ from the guidelines.

Conclusion

This study demonstrates that endovascular treatment of ALI with the use of catheter-based therapies is an effective modality that can reduce the requirement for thrombolysis, with expected reductions in hemorrhagic complications, but at the risk of remediable distal emboli and increased economic cost. It has a similar clinical outcome to conventional CDT alone, CBT was empirically performed for iliac and iliofemoral thrombosed segment and CDT was used primarily for iliofemoral and femoropopliteal segment. Regarding Rutherford IIb ischemia, CBT may have an advantage over CDT. In terms of CBT modalities, different techniques have comparable efficacy, but have different adverse event profiles. Insufficient data are available to determine a preference for a specific technique among CBTs. Future trials regarding ALI need to be designed carefully, ensuring comparable study groups, and should follow standardized practices of outcome reporting.

Abbreviations

ABI: Ankle-brachial index; ALI: Acute limb ischemia; ESC: European Society of Cardiology; ESVS: European Society for Vascular Surgery; LMWH: Low molecular weight heparin; MALE: Major adverse limb events; PTA: Percutaneous transluminal angioplasty; PAT: Percutaneous aspiration thrombectomy; RCT: Randomized controlled trial; rt-PA: Recombinant tissue plasminogen activator; SFA: Superficial femoral artery

Supplementary Information

Additional file 1 Supplementary Table 1. Techniques and devices for catheter-based therapy and catheter-directed thrombolysis of Acute Ischemia Patients. **Supplementary Table 2.** Rutherford categories of Acute Ischemia Patients.

Authors' contributions

MF Gong: contributed to data collection, manuscript writing/editing. X He and BX Zhao: contributed to project development, data collection, data analysis. J Kong: contributed to project development, data collection, data analysis, manuscript editing. JP Gu: contributed to project development. GP Chen: contributed to project development. The authors read and approved the final manuscript.

References

1. Björck M, Earnshaw JJ, Acosta S, Bastos Gonçalves F, Cochennec F, Debus ES, et al. Editor's choice-European Society for Vascular Surgery (ESVS) 2020 clinical practice guidelines on the management of acute limb ischaemia. Eur J Vasc Endovasc Surg. 2020;59(2):173–218. https://doi.org/10.1016/j.ejvs.2019.09.006.
2. Hess CN, Huang Z, Patel MR, Baumgartner I, Berger JS, Blomster JI, et al. Acute limb ischemia in peripheral artery disease: insights from EUCLID. Circulation. 2019;140(7):556–65. https://doi.org/10.1161/CIRCULATIONAHA.119.039773.
3. Howard DP, Banerjee A, Fairhead JF, Hands L, Silver LE, Rothwell PM. Population-based study of incidence, risk factors, outcome, and prognosis of ischemic peripheral arterial events: implications for prevention. Circulation. 2015;132(19):1805–15. https://doi.org/10.1161/CIRCULATIONAHA.115.016424.
4. Korabathina R, Weintraub AR, Price LL, Kapur NK, Kimmelstiel CD, Iafrati MD, et al. Twenty-year analysis of trends in the incidence and in-hospital mortality for lower-extremity arterial thromboembolism. Circulation. 2013;128(2):115–21. https://doi.org/10.1161/CIRCULATIONAHA.113.003543
5. Rutherford RB, Baker JD, Ernst C, Johnston KW, Porter JM, Ahn S, et al. Recommended standards for reports dealing with lower extremity ischemia: revised version. J Vasc Surg. 1997;26(3):517–38. https://doi.org/10.1016/S0741-5214(97)70045-4.
6. Kolte D, Kennedy KF, Shishehbor MH, Mamdani ST, Stangenberg L, Hyder ON, et al. Endovascular versus surgical revascularization for acute limb ischemia: a propensity-score matched analysis. Circ Cardiovasc Interv. 2020;13(1):e008150.
7. Grip O, Wanhainen A, Michaelsson K, Lindhagen L, Bjorck M. Open or endovascular revascularization in the treatment of acute lower limb ischaemia. Br J Surg. 2018;105(12):1598–606. https://doi.org/10.1002/bjs.10954.
8. Aboyans V, Ricco JB, Bartelink MEL, Bjorck M, Brodmann M, Cohnert T, et al. Editor's choice e-2017 ESC guidelines on the diagnosis and treatment of peripheral arterial diseases, in collaboration with the European Society for Vascular Surgery (ESVS). Eur J Vasc Endovasc Surg. 2018;55(3):305–68. https://doi.org/10.1016/j.ejvs.2017.07.018.
9. Davis FM, Albright J, Gallagher KA, Gurm HS, Koenig GC, Schreiber T, et al. Early outcomes following endovascular, open surgical, and hybrid revascularization for lower extremity acute limb ischemia. Ann Vasc Surg. 2018;51:106–12. https://doi.org/10.1016/j.avsg.2017.12.025.
10. Ebben HP, Jongkind V, Wisselink W, Hoksbergen AWJ, Yeung KK. Catheter directed thrombolysis protocols for peripheral arterial occlusions: a systematic review. Eur J Vasc Endovasc Surg. 2019;57(5):667–75. https://doi.org/10.1016/j.ejvs.2018.11.018.
11. Lian WS, Das SK, Hu XX, Zhang XJ, Xie XY, Li MQ. Efficacy of intra-arterial catheter-directed thrombolysis for popliteal and infrapopliteal acute limb ischemia. J Vasc Surg. 2020;71(1):141–8. https://doi.org/10.1016/j.jvs.2019.03.081.
12. Byrne RM, Taha AG, Avgerinos E, Marone LK, Makaroun MS, Chaer RA. Contemporary outcomes of endovascular interventions for acute limb ischemia. J Vasc Surg. 2014;59(4):988–95. https://doi.org/10.1016/j.jvs.2013.10.054.
13. Rajan DK, Patel NH, Valji K, Cardella JF, Brown DB, Brountzos EN, et al. Quality improvement guidelines for percutaneous management of acute limb ischemia. J Vasc Intervent Radiol. 2009;20(7):S208–18. https://doi.org/10.1016/j.jvir.2009.04.010.
14. Zehnder T, Birrer M, Do DD, Baumgartner I, Triller J, Nachbur B, et al. Percutaneous catheter thrombus aspiration for acute or subacute arterial occlusion of the legs: how much thrombolysis is needed? Eur J Vasc Endovasc Surg. 2000;20(1):41–6. https://doi.org/10.1053/ejvs.2000.1117.
15. Leung DA, Blitz LR, Nelson T, Amin A, Soukas PA, Nanjundappa A, et al. Rheolytic pharmacomechanical thrombectomy for the management of acute limb ischemia: results from the PEARL registry. J Endovasc Ther. 2015;22(4):546–57. https://doi.org/10.1177/1526602815592849.
16. Kwok CHR, Fleming S, Chan KKC, Tibballs J, Samuelson S, Ferguson J, et al. Aspiration thrombectomy versus conventional catheter-directed thrombolysis as first-line treatment for non-iatrogenic acute lower limb ischemia. J Vasc Interv Radiol. 2018;29(5):607–13. https://doi.org/10.1016/j.jvir.2017.11.030.
17. Kuoppala M, Akeson J, Svensson P, Lindblad B, Franzen S, Acosta S. Risk factors for haemorrhage during local intra-arterial thrombolysis for lower limb ischaemia. J Thromb Thrombolysis. 2011;31(2):226–32. https://doi.org/10.1007/s11239-010-0520-2.
18. Lee K, Istl A, Dubois L, DeRose G, Forbes TL, Wiseman D, et al. Fibrinogen level and bleeding risk during catheter-directed thrombolysis using tissue plasminogen activator. Vasc Endovasc Surg. 2015;49(7):175–9. https://doi.org/10.1177/1538574415611234.
19. Harada K, Morioka J, Higa T, Saito T, Fukuyama K. Significance of combining distal filter protection and a guiding catheter with temporary balloon occlusion for carotid artery stenting: clinical results and evaluation of debris capture. Ann Vasc Surg. 2012;26(7):929–36. https://doi.org/10.1016/j.avsg.2012.04.022.
20. Funke C, Pfiffner R, Husmann M, Pfammatter T. The use of the "preclosure" technique for antegrade aspiration thrombectomy with large catheters in acute limb ischemia. Cardiovasc Interv Radiol. 2013;36(2):377–84. https://doi.org/10.1007/s00270-012-0455-4.
21. von Keudell AG, Weaver MJ, Appleton PT, Bae DS, Dyer GSM, Heng M, et al. Diagnosis and treatment of acute extremity compartment syndrome. Lancet. 2015;386(10000):1299–310. https://doi.org/10.1016/S0140-6736(15)00277-9.
22. Heller S, Lubanda JC, Varejka P, Chochola M, Prochazka P, Rucka D, et al.

Percutaneous mechanical thrombectomy using Rotarex S device in acute limb ischemia in infrainguinal occlusions. Biomed Res Int. 2017;2017: 2362769–8. https://doi.org/10.1155/2017/2362769.

23. Rusch R, Trentmann J, Hummitzsch L, Rusch M, Aludin S, Haneya A, et al. Effectiveness and safety of percutaneous thrombectomy devices: comparison of Rotarex and Angiojet in a physiological circulation model. Eur J Vasc Endovasc Surg. 2020;59(6):983–9. https://doi.org/10.1016/j.ejvs.2020.01.016.

6

Morphologic change in deep venous thrombosis in the lower extremity after therapeutic anticoagulation

Tanapong Panpikoon*, Wisanu Phattharaprueksa, Tharintorn Treesit, Chinnarat Bua-ngam, Kaewpitcha Pichitpichatkul and Apichaya Sriprachyakul

Abstract

Background: To evaluate the anticoagulant treatment response in venous thrombi with different morphologies (size, shape, and echogenicity) by measuring the change in thrombus thickness.

Materials and methods: This was a retrospective cohort study of 97 lower extremity DVT patients diagnosed by venous ultrasound between March 2014 and February 2018. The demographics, clinical risk factors, anticoagulant treatment, and ultrasound findings at the first diagnosis and 2–6 months after treatment were evaluated.

Results: The anticoagulant treatment with LMWH followed by VKAs showed a significant decrease in the mean maximum difference in lower extremity DVT thrombus thickness compared with VKAs alone (*P*-value < 0.001). After adjustment by treatment, the thrombi found in dilated veins showed a significant decrease in the thickness of such thrombi compared with those found in small veins: 4 mm vs. 0 mm (Coef. = 3, 95% CI: 1.9, 4.1 and *P*-value < 0.001). Anechoic and hypoechoic thrombi showed a significant decrease in the thickness compared with hyperechoic thrombi: 5 mm vs. 0 mm (Coef. = 4, 95% CI: 3.25, 4.74 and *P*-value < 0.001) and 3 mm vs. 0 mm (Coef. = 2, 95% CI: 1.34, 42.66 and *P*-value < 0.001), respectively. Concentric thrombi showed a significant decrease in thickness compared with eccentric thrombi: 4 mm vs. 0 mm (Coef. = 2, 95% CI: 1.45, 2.55 and *P*-value < 0.001).

Conclusion: The anticoagulant treatment with LMWH followed by VKAs shows a significant decrease in lower extremity DVT thrombus thickness compared with VKAs alone. After adjustment by treatment, the morphologic finding of acute thrombi shows a significantly decreased thickness compared with the morphologic finding of chronic thrombi.

Keywords: Deep vein thrombosis, Venous duplex ultrasound, Thrombus resolution, Anticoagulant treatment

Introduction

Deep venous thrombosis (DVT), which commonly occurs in the lower extremities and is associated with pulmonary embolism (PE) and referred to together as venous thromboembolism (VTE), is a significant global health burden [1]. Accurate VTE diagnosis is essential due to the morbidity and mortality associated with missed diagnoses and the potential side effects, patient inconvenience, and resource implications of anticoagulant treatment [2].

The diagnosis of VTE based on clinical manifestations alone is unreliable [3]. The D-dimer test for exclusion of DVT, followed by proximal lower extremity ultrasound, is recommended in a population with low pretest probability (PTP) of lower extremity DVT. Initial proximal lower extremity ultrasound followed by whole leg

* Correspondence: tanapong.pai@mahidol.ac.th
Department of Diagnostic and Therapeutic Radiology, Faculty of Medicine Ramathibodi Hospital, Mahidol University, 270 Rama VI Rd. Phyathai, Ratchathewi, 10400 Bangkok, Thailand

ultrasound is recommended in a population with intermediate and high PTPs of lower extremity DVT [2].

The diagnostic criteria of DVT are lack of complete cross-sectional vein compressibility or direct visualization of an intraluminal thrombus in B-mode, combined or not combined with colour-Doppler ultrasound. Initial (5–21 days following diagnosis) and long-term (3–6 months following diagnosis) treatment are mandatory for all patients with positive ultrasound for DVT. Extended treatment (beyond the first 3–6 months) is based on the risk/benefit balance of continued anticoagulation, patient compliance and preference [4]. Follow-up venous ultrasound at 3–6 months after coagulation treatment has a role in evaluating recurrent DVT. A 2- or 4-mm increase in venous diameter between two measurements of the common femoral and popliteal veins is the most validated criterion for the diagnosis of recurrent DVT [5].

In addition to thrombus visualization, ultrasound also provides morphological information on the thrombus related to the progression of the thrombus-forming process, namely, fibrin deposition in the first few days, thrombolysis within a week, and fibroblast invasion and capillary development within several weeks [6]. The varied staging of thrombi results in different responses to anticoagulant treatment. Morphological information, such as the size, shape and echogenicity of the thrombus, may be another concerning factor for initial and extended anticoagulation treatment unless the patient's factors. However, there is no study to support this hypothesis.

The purpose of this study was to evaluate the response of anticoagulation treatment in venous thrombi with different morphologies (size, shape and echogenicity) by measuring the thrombus thickness change between the maximum thickness at the first diagnosis and that at 3–6 months after long-term treatment.

Materials and methods

A retrospective cohort study was conducted on lower extremity DVT patients diagnosed by venous ultrasound between March 2014 and February 2018. The demographics, clinical risk factors, anticoagulation treatment, and ultrasound findings at the first diagnosis and 2–6 months after treatment were evaluated. The Institutional Review Board approved the study, and informed consent was waived.

According to the standard protocol, four consultant radiologists with a minimum of 5 years of postqualification experience performed whole leg ultrasound (proximal and distal lower extremity veins). A similar protocol was used in the first diagnosis and follow-up study after anticoagulant treatment.

The protocol of lower extremity venous ultrasound begins with cross-sectional greyscale compression of the common femoral vein (CFV), femoral vein (FV) and popliteal vein (Pop V) at 2-cm intervals. Dual images before and during compression were recorded at CFV, proximal FV, mid-FV, distal FV and the popliteal vein.

The criteria from DVT diagnosis are as follows:

1. Lack of complete compressibility
2. Visualization of an intraluminal thrombus

Suppose the intraluminal thrombus or incomplete compressibility is presented. The anterior-posterior thickness of the thrombus or the incomplete compressed vein will be measured in millimetres (mm). A colour flow image is an option for confirmation of suspicious intraluminal thrombus and complete haemodynamic information. An equivalent technical examination was performed on the calf veins. No video recording was made. A Toshiba Aplio 500 ultrasound scanner equipped (Canon Medical Systems Corporation, Japan) with a 14-MHz linear-array transducer (PLT-705BT) was used in the study.

The different thicknesses of venous thrombi between the first diagnosis and 3–6 months after the long-term treatment were remeasured by three radiologists. The mean value of the three measurements was used. The thrombus, which showed the maximum difference in thickness from one of five locations (CFV, prox-FV, mid-FV, dis-FV and the popliteal vein) and one side per patient, was selected for the statistical analysis.

The consensus from three experienced radiologists was used for the morphological classification according to the following criteria:

1. Size (Fig. 1)

- Increased size; the affected vein is more than two times larger than the adjacent artery.
- Normal size: the affected vein is equal to or not more than two times larger than the adjacent artery.
- Decreased size; the affected vein is smaller than the adjacent artery.

2. Echogenicity (Fig. 2)

- Anechoic; the thrombus appears black on the screen.
- Hypoechoic; the thrombus appears grey on the screen.
- Hyperechoic; the thrombus appears white on the screen

3. Shape (Fig. 3)

- Concentric: the presence of an acute angle between the thrombus and venous wall or total occlusion
- Eccentric: the presence of an obtuse angle between the thrombus and venous wall.

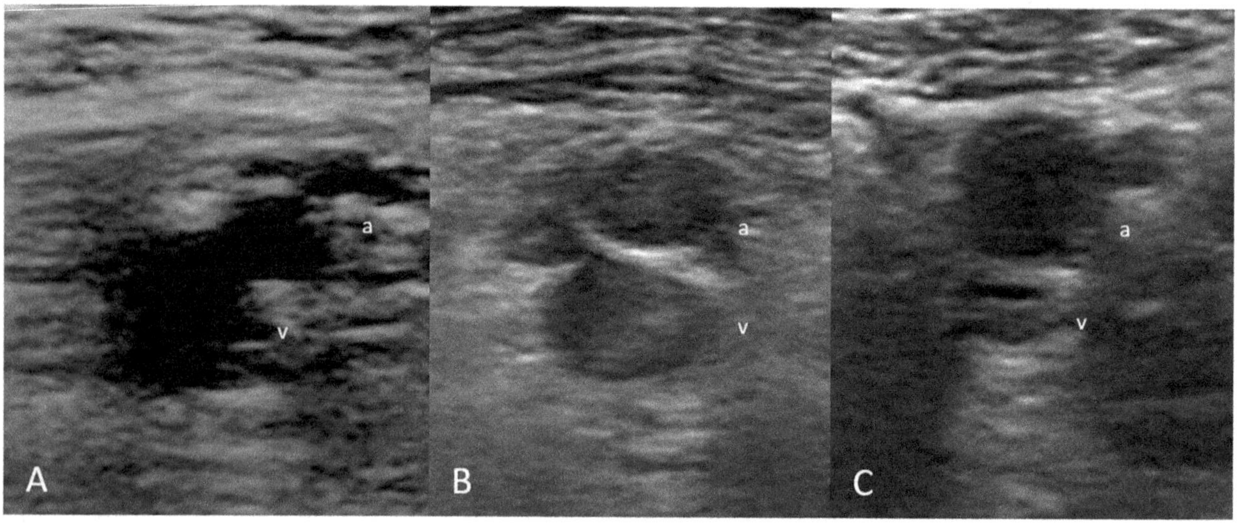

Fig. 1 Size of the affected vein: **A** Increased size; The thrombus in the femoral vein (FV) is larger than that in the adjacent superficial femoral artery (SFA). **B** Normal vein size. The thrombus in the FV is equal to the adjacent SFA. **C** Decreased vein size; The thrombus in the FV is smaller than the adjacent SFA. a = superficial femoral artery, v = femoral vein.

Patient selection

Inclusion criteria

- Lower extremity DVT patients were diagnosed, treated and followed by the venous ultrasound from March 2014 to February 2019.

Exclusion criteria

- Patients whose sonographic image were inadequate for interpretation.
- Patients with isolated DVT in the calf vein.
- Patients younger than 18 years old.

Statistical analysis

Categorical variables and clinical and sonographic characteristics were evaluated. Normally distributed data are presented as the mean and standard deviation. Nonnormally distributed data are presented as the median and range. The comparison was performed by median regression analysis between morphologic findings and the maximum difference in thrombus thickness. Multiple median regression analyses were applied to individual variables (treatment and the timing of the repeat ultrasound). Analytical results are presented as a coefficient and 95% confidence intervals (CI). A *p*-value of < 0.05 was considered statistically significant. STATA version 15.1 (Stata Corp, College Drive, Texas) statistical software was used to analyse the data.

Results

Between March 2014 and February 2019, 106 lower extremity DVT patients were diagnosed and followed by venous ultrasound. Four patients were excluded from the study due to inadequate sonographic imaging for interpretation, and five patients were excluded due to isolated DVT in the calf vein. Ninety-seven patients were enrolled in the study population.

Out of the 97 patients, 57 (58.8%) patients were male. The age of the patients ranged from 20 to 85 years, with a mean age of 60.4 years. A history of malignancy was the most common risk factor (25.8%), followed by immobility (15.5%), sepsis (2.1%) and trauma (2.1%).

All patients were treated with anticoagulants based on the clinical signs and symptoms before the ultrasound examination. Thirty-seven (38.1%) patients had a history of malignancy, or the clinical signs and symptoms of extensive DVT were treated by low molecular weight heparin (LMWH) 1 mg/kg subcutaneous q 12 h in the initial phase followed by long-term oral vitamin K antagonists (VKAs). Sixty (61.9%) patients were treated with VKAs alone (maintaining INR at 2.0–3.0) (Table 1). The timing of the repeat ultrasound in both groups ranged from 74 to 192 days (the median was 141 days). In the multiple median regression analysis, anticoagulation treatment was significantly associated with the maximum difference in lower extremity DVT thrombus thickness ($P < 0.001$). The adjusted coefficient (95% CI) of LMWH followed by VKAs compared with VKAs alone was − 4 (95% CI: − 4.6, − 3.4). In contrast, the timing of the repeat ultrasound was not significantly associated (P value = 0.217) (Table 2).

Venous thrombi were predominantly located in the left lower extremities compared with the right lower extremities (62.9 vs 37.1%). The most common location was the popliteal vein (81.4%). However, the

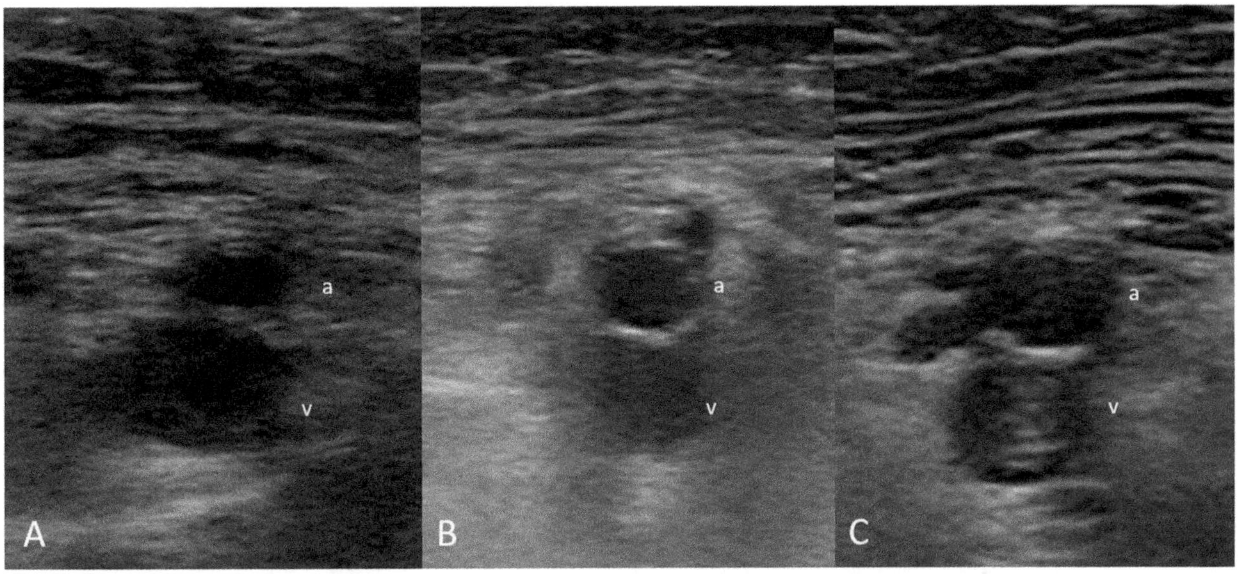

Fig. 2 Echogenicity of the thrombus: **A** Anechoic thrombus; The thrombus appears black on the screen. **B** Hypoechoic thrombus; The thrombus appears grey on the screen. **C** Hyperechoic thrombus; The thrombus appears white on the screen. a = superficial femoral artery, v = femoral vein.

maximum thrombus thickness change was found commonly in the proximal femoral vein (32.0%), followed by the common femoral vein (30.9%) and popliteal vein (18.6%). At the first diagnosis, 46.4% of thrombi were found in small veins; 63.9% were hyperechoic thrombi, and 61.9% were eccentric thrombi (Table 3).

The thrombi found in dilated veins showed a significant decrease in the mean maximum difference in thickness of the thrombus compared with that of thrombi found in small veins: 4 mm vs. 0 mm (Coef. = 3, 95% CI: 1.9, 4.1 and *P*-value < 0.001). Anechoic and hypoechoic thrombi showed a significant decrease in the mean maximum difference in thickness of the thrombus compared with that of hyperechoic thrombi, 5 mm vs 0 mm (Coef. = 4, 95% CI: 3.25, 4.74 and *P*-value < 0.001) and 3 mm vs 0 mm (Coef. = 2, 95% CI: 1.34, 42.66 and *P*-value < 0.001), respectively. Concentric thrombi showed a significant decrease in the mean maximum difference in thickness compared with that of eccentric thrombi: 4 mm vs. 0 mm (Coef. = 2, 95% CI: 1.45, 2.55 and *P*-value < 0.001). Results

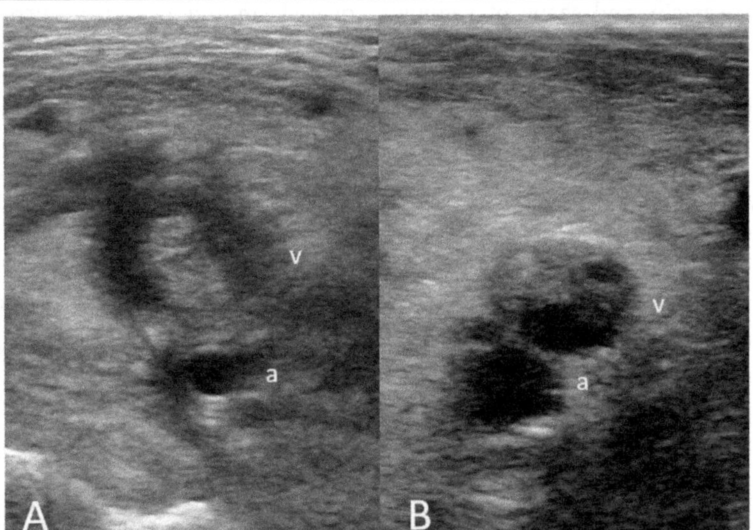

Fig. 3 Shape of the thrombus: **A** Concentric thrombus; the thrombus causes total occlusion of the popliteal vein. **B** Eccentric thrombus: the thrombus causes partial occlusion and forms an obtuse angle with the venous wall. a = popliteal artery, v = popliteal vein.

Table 1 Clinical characteristics data of the study population

Characteristics	Sample (*n* = 97)
Gender, n (%)	
Male	57 (58.8)
Female	40 (41.2)
Age, mean (SD)	60.4 (46.6)
Risk factor, n (%)	
Malignancy	25 (25.8)
Immobility	15 (15.5)
Sepsis	2 (2.1)
Trauma	2 (2.1)
Cardiac arrythmia	1 (1)
Hormonal treatment	1 (1)
Obesity	1 (1)
Pregnancy	0 (0)
Follow-up time, median (min-max) days	141 (74–192)
Treatment, n (%)	
LMWH followed by VKAs	37 (38.1)
VKAs alone	60 (61.9)

DVT Deep vein thrombosis, *LMWH* Low molecular weight heparin, *LMWH* Low molecular weight heparin, *VKAs* Vitamin K antagonists

of median regression analysis between morphologic findings and the maximum difference in thickness of the thrombus after adjustment by the anticoagulant treatment are shown in Table 4.

Discussion

The results of this study advocate the benefit of venous thrombus morphology classification by ultrasound apart from the first imaging modality for DVT diagnosis. Differences in the size, echogenicity and shape of venous thrombi show different responses to anticoagulant treatment. A concentric anechoic or hypoechoic thrombus, which causes dilatation of the affected vein, shows a statistically significant decrease in thrombus thickness compared with that of eccentric hyperechoic thrombi in retracted veins, which offers minimal to no change in thickness after anticoagulant treatment. No previous clinical studies have reported this issue. Most reviews of venous ultrasound after anticoagulation treatment have focused on the risk of recurrent VTE when residual thrombus occurs [6–8].

Table 3 Characteristic data of the venous thrombus

Characteristics	Sample (*n* = 97)
Side of cases showing DVT involvement, n (%)	
Right	36 (37.1)
Left	61 (62.9)
Anatomic distribution of thrombi, n (%)	
Common femoral vein (CFV)	62 (63.9)
Proximal femoral vein (prox FV)	72 (74.2)
Mid femoral vein (mid FV)	71 (73.2)
Distal femoral vein (dis FV)	74 (76.3)
Popliteal vein (Pop)	79 (81.4)
Location at maximum thrombus thickness change, n (%)	
Common femoral vein (CFV)	30 (30.9)
Proximal femoral vein (prox FV)	31 (32.0)
Mid femoral vein (mid FV)	8 (8.3)
Distal femoral vein (dis FV)	10 (10.3)
Popliteal vein (Pop)	18 (18.6)
Size of affected vein (relative to adjacent artery), n (%)	
Increased size	23 (23.7)
Normal size	29 (29.9)
Decreased size	45 (46.4)
Echogenicity of thrombus, n (%)	
Anechoic	17 (17.5)
Iso/hypoechoic	18 (18.6)
Hyperechoic	62 (63.9)
Shape of thrombus, n (%)	
Concentric	37 (38.1)
Eccentric	60 (61.9)

DVT Deep vein thrombosis

With knowledge of the natural history of thrombus formation, ultrasound may specify the age of the thrombus by the difference in morphology. Fibrinogen is converted to fibrin in 1 day, forming a mesh that traps platelets and red blood cells and produces a thrombus. The cross-linking of fibrin and the development of internal zones of haemolysis are responsible for the anechoic-hypoechogenicity of the thrombus. The newly

Table 2 Factor associated with maximum difference thickness of the thrombus

Factor	Coef. (95% CI)	*P* value
Follow up time	0.009 (−0.006, 0.025)	0.217
Treatment		
Maximum difference thickness in LMWH followed by VKAs	−4 (−4.6, −3.4)	< 0.001*
Maximum difference thickness in VKAs alone	0	

LMWH Low molecular weight heparin, *VKAs* Vitamin K antagonists
* *P*-value <0.05 was considered statistically significant

Table 4 Correlation of morphologic sonographic findings and maximum difference in thrombus thickness after adjustment by treatment

Morphologic findings	Maximum difference thickness (min-max) mm	Coef. (95% CI)	*P* Value
Size of the affected vein (relative to adjacent artery)			
Increased size	4 (0–12)	3 (1.90, 4.10)	< 0.001*
Normal size	1 (1–6)	0 (0.00, 0.82)	1.00
Decreased size	0 (0–2)	0	
Echogenicity of the thrombus			
Anechoic	5 (0–8)	4 (3.25, 4.74)	< 0.001*
Iso/hypoechoic	3 (0–12)	2 (1.34, 2.66)	< 0.001*
Hyperechoic	0 (0–2)	0	
Shape of the thrombus			
Concentric	4 (1–12)	2 (1.45, 2.55)	< 0.001*
Eccentric	0 (0–2)	0	

* P-value <0.05 was considered statistically significant

formed thrombus tends to obstruct the vein lumen and expand the venous diameter entirely. The thrombin net squeezes red blood cells and fluid components out of the thrombi during thrombus ageing [9–11]. The proportion of red blood cells in the thrombus decreases with time, and the ultrasound signal intensity is affected by the number of red blood cells in the thrombus. This accounts for the increased echogenic appearance of the aged thrombus [12]. In the following 2–8 weeks, the thrombus organizes or dissolves from balancing clot formation and degradation. A mixture of the hyperplastic response of the endothelium at the site of thrombus deposition and residual thrombus incorporated into the wall during the scarring or fibrotic response causes asymmetrical wall thickening or an eccentric thrombus. The affected vein is often retracted [9–11]. Therefore, an acute obstructing DVT is typically hypoechogenic-concentric shaped, and the vein lumen is dilated. In contrast, the residual thrombus in chronic DVT is often hyperechogenic-eccentric shaped and adheres to one side of the vein wall, and the vein lumen is small.

The thrombus is transformed from being composed predominantly of platelets to having a fibrin composition with replacement by dense connective tissue [13]. Therefore, anticoagulation cannot break apart the chronic thrombus. The results of this study show minimal to no change in thickness (0–2 mm) of eccentric, hyperechoic thrombi in retracted veins. This supports the conclusion that the presence of a chronic thrombus in a symptomatic patient without a new acute thrombus does not require anticoagulant therapy [14].

Although this study shows the different responses to anticoagulants in cases with different venous sizes and echogenicities of thrombi, neither venous size nor thrombi echogenicity reliably distinguishes acute from chronic thrombi [15]. An acute nonobstructing thrombus does not often cause dilatation of the affected vein. Chronic thrombi can be found in dilated veins, especially after the development of venous reflux. The concentric shape of the thrombus remains in the small vein when there is no recanalization. Furthermore, the differentiation of acute and chronic thrombi by morphology remains mainly qualitative and nonstandardized. The ageing of the thrombus and the treatment decision may be purely based on patient reporting of symptoms.

Ultrasound elastography for assessing thrombus stiffness is a quantitative method for determining thrombus age. Few clinical studies involving lower extremity ultrasound have reported the difference between acute and chronic thrombi's median normalized strain magnitude [16]. The strain ratio of the chronic and subacute thrombosis groups was found to be higher than that of the acute thrombosis group ($P < 0.001$, < 0.05) [17]. Combining thrombus morphology and ultrasound elastography may enhance ultrasound accuracy in thrombus age determination and require further study.

In addition, the limitation of this investigation is that it was a single-centre, retrospective cohort study with a small study population. Approximately 60% of the study population was diagnosed by the clinical manifestation and received LMWH before the ultrasound examination. No recurrent DVT or increase in thrombus thickness was found in our study population. Therefore, the value of differentiating thrombus morphology in follow-up ultrasound after anticoagulant treatment was not discovered.

Conclusion

The anticoagulant treatment with LMWH followed by VKAs shows a significant decrease in lower extremity

DVT thrombus thickness compared with VKAs alone. After adjustment by treatment, the morphologic finding of acute thrombi (concentric, anechoic/hypoechoic and dilated vein) shows a significantly decreased thickness than the morphologic finding of chronic thrombi (eccentric, hyperechoic and retracted vein). Although the chronic thrombi show minimal to no change in thickness, the increase in thickness or recurrent DVT did not occur after anticoagulant treatment.

Abbreviations

VTE: Venous thromboembolism; DVT: Deep venous thrombosis; PE: Pulmonary embolism; PTP: Pretest probability; CFV: Common femoral vein; FV: Femoral vein; Pop V: Popliteal vein; LMWH: Low molecular weight heparin; VKAs: Vitamin K antagonists

Acknowledgements

We would like to thank the following doctors for taking part in treating patients with DVT: Dr. Gorawee Tepsamrithporn and Dr. Nutsiri Kitritirapong from the Department of Surgery, Faculty of Medicine, Ramathibodi Hospital, Mahidol University, Thailand.

Authors' contributions

Dr.Tanapong Panpikoon, Dr. Wisanu Phattharaprueksa, Dr. Tharintorn Treesit, Dr. Chinnarat Bua-ngam, Dr. Kaewpitcha Pichitpichatkul and Dr. Apichaya Sriprachyakul designed and conducted this study, including patient recruitment, data collection and data analysis. Dr. Wisanu Phattharaprueksa, Dr. Kaewpitcha Pichitpichatkul and Dr. Apichaya Sriprachyakul prepared the manuscript draft with important intellectual input from Dr. Tanapong Panpikoon, Dr. Tharintorn Treesit and Dr. Chinnarat Bua-ngam. All authors approved the final manuscript. The department of Clinical Epidemiology and Biostatistics, Faculty of Medicine, Ramathibodi Hospital, Mahidol University, Thailand, provided statistical support in analyzing the data.

References

1. Nisio MD, Es NV, Buller HR. Deep vein thrombosis and pulmonary embolism. Lancet. 2016;388:3060–73.
2. Lim W, Le Gal G, Bates HM, Righini M, Haramati LB, et al. American Society of Hematology 2018 guidelines for management of venous thromboembolism: diagnosis of venous thromboembolism. Blood advances. 2018;2:3226–56.
3. Pollack CV, Schreiber D, Goldhaber SZ, Slattery D, Fanikos J, O'Neil BJ, et al. Clinical characteristics, management, and outcomes of patients diagnosed with acute pulmonary embolism in the emergency department: initial report of EMPEROR (multicenter emergency medicine pulmonary embolism in the RealWorld registry). J Am Coll Cardiol. 2011;57(6):700–6.
4. Mazzolai L, Aboyans V, Ageno W, Agnelli G, Alatri A, Bauersachs R, et al. Diagnosis and management of acute deep vein thrombosis: a joint consencus document from the European society of cardiology working groups of aorta and peripheral vascular diseases and pulmonary circulation and right ventricular function. Eur Heart J. 2017;00:1–14.
5. Le Gal G, Kovacs MJ, Carrier M, Do K, Kahn SR, Wells PS, et al. Validation of a diagnostic approach to exclude recurrent venous thromboembolism. J Thromb Haemost. 2009;7:752–9.
6. Prandoni P, Lensing AW, Prins MH, Bernardi E, Marchiori A, Bagatella P, et al. Residual venous thrombosis as a predictive factor of recurrent venous thromboembolism. Ann Intern Med. 2002;137:955–60.
7. Piovella F, Crippa L, Barone M, Vigano D'Angelo S, Serafini S, Galli L, et al. Normalization rates of compression ultrasonography in patients with first episode of deep vein thrombosis of the lower limbs: association with recurrence and new thrombosis. Haematologica. 2002;87:515–22.
8. Young L, Ockelford P, Miline D, Rolfe-vyson V, Mckelvie S, Harper P. Post-treatment residual thrombus increases the risk of recurrent deep vein thrombosis and mortality. J Thromb Haemost. 2006;4:1919–24.
9. Karande GY, Hedgire SS, Sanchez Y, Baliyan V, Mishra V, et al. Advanced imaging in acute and chronic deep vein thrombosis. Cardiovascular diagnosis and therapy. 2016;6:493–507.
10. Dupuy DE. Venous US of lower extremity deep venous thrombosis. Radiographics. 2000;20:1195–200.
11. Leslie MS, Joshua C, Ulrike MH. Ultrasound diagnosis of lower extremity venous thrombosis. In: John SP, Joseph FP, editors. Introduction to vascular Sonography. 6th ed. Philadephia: Elsevier Saunders; 2012. p. 377–95.
12. Fang J, Wa YL, Chen CK, Tsui PH. Discrimination between newly formed and aged thrombi using empirical mode decomposition of ultrasound B-scan image. Biomed Res Int. 2015;2015:403293 Epub 2015 Jan 28.
13. Peter H, Alex W, Mark S, Andrew F, Yash P, Nirvikar D, et al. Elastography techniques in the evaluation of deep vein thrombosis. Cardiovasc Diagn Ther. 2017;7(Suppl 3):S238–45.
14. Büller HR, Agnelli G, Hull RD, Myers TM, Prins MH, Raskob GE. Antithrombotic therapy for venous thromboembolic dis- ease: the seventh ACCP conference on antithrombotic and thrombolytic therapy. Chest. 2004; 126(suppl):401S–28S.
15. Murphy TP, Cronan JJ. Evolution of deep venous thrombosis: a prospective evaluation with US. Radiology. 1990;177:543–8.
16. Rubin JM, Xie H, Kim K, et al. Sonographic elasticity imaging of acute and chronic deep venous thrombosis in humans. J Ultrasound Med. 2006;25: 1179–86.
17. Yi X, Wei X, Wang Y, et al. Role of real-time elastography in assessing the stage of thrombus. Int Angiol. 2017;36:59–63.

7

D-dimer for risk stratification and antithrombotic treatment management in acute coronary syndrome patients

Flavio Giuseppe Biccirè[1,2], Alessio Farcomeni[3], Carlo Gaudio[1], Pasquale Pignatelli[1], Gaetano Tanzilli[1] and Daniele Pastori[1*]

Abstract

Background: Data on the prognostic role of D-dimer in patients with acute coronary syndrome (ACS) are controversial. Our aim was to summarize current evidence on the association between D-dimer levels and short/long-term poor prognosis of ACS patients. We also investigated the association between D-dimer and no-reflow phenomenon.

Methods: Systematic review and metanalysis of observational studies including ACS patients and reporting data on D-dimer levels. PubMed and SCOPUS databases were searched. Data were combined with hazard ratio (HR) and metanalysed. The principal endpoint was a composite of cardiovascular events (CVEs) including myocardial infarction, all-cause and cardiovascular mortality.

Results: Overall, 32 studies included in the systematic review with 28,869 patients. Of them, 6 studies investigated in-hospital and 26 studies long-term outcomes. Overall, 23 studies showed positive association of high D-dimer levels with CVEs. D-dimer levels predicted poor prognosis in all studies reporting in-hospital outcomes. Five studies satisfied inclusion criteria and were included in the metanalysis, with a total of 8616 patients. Median follow-up was 13.2 months with 626 CVEs. The pooled HR for D-dimer levels and CVEs was 1.264 (95% CI 1.134–1.409). Five out of 7 studies (4195 STEMI patients) investigating the association between D-dimer levels and no-reflow showed a positive correlation of D-dimer levels with no-reflow.

Conclusions: In patients with ACS, D-dimer was associated with higher in-hospital and short/long-term complications. D-dimer was also higher in patients with no-reflow phenomenon. The use of D-dimer may help to identify patients with residual thrombotic risk after ACS.

* Correspondence: daniele.pastori@uniroma1.it
[1]Department of Clinical Internal, Anesthesiological, and Cardiovascular Sciences, Sapienza University of Rome, Viale del Policlinico 155, 00161 Rome, Italy

Keywords: D-dimer, Myocardial infarction, No-reflow phenomenon, Prognosis, Acute coronary syndrome

Introduction

Coronary artery disease (CAD) is the leading cause of death worldwide with acute myocardial infarction (MI) representing the clinical condition associated with the greatest morbidity and mortality, up to 30% of in-hospital deaths [1, 2]. Prompt reperfusion with percutaneous coronary intervention (PCI), advances in acute cardiovascular care and more effective medical therapy have improved the prognosis of patients with MI in the last years [3].

This increased survival revealed a previously unrecognized long-term risk of recurrent thrombotic events despite optimal medical therapy [2]. Indeed, almost one fifth of MI patients suffer from re-hospitalization within 1 year and 10% from recurrent MI [3, 4].

There is therefore a growing need of a more accurate risk stratification of MI patients to identify those at higher risk for adverse events and worse prognosis [5].

Current guidelines of the American Heart Association and the European Society of Cardiology highlighted the lack of useful biomarkers to predict in-hospital complications and short/long term prognosis of patients with MI, recommending for this purpose only to measure troponin and brain natriuretic peptide (BNP) serum levels, with the latter associated with a low level of evidence [6, 7].

During last decades, several studies, mostly conducted in the 90's before the routine use of dual antiplatelet therapy, described the pivotal and prognostic role of coronary thrombosis and hypercoagulable state in the pathophysiology of MI, correlating increased coagulation activity with recurrent event and poor outcome after MI [8–10].

As a marker of rapid fibrin turnover and high thrombotic activation in both arterial and venous system, interest in D-dimer has grown over time, and its predictive role has been investigated in several acute and chronic cardiovascular care, [11]. In patients with MI, high circulating D-dimer levels have been correlated with recurrent MI and poor prognosis [12, 13] and early reduction in plasma concentration of D-dimer by Ximelagatran administration was associated with decreased risk of new cardiovascular events [14].

In addition, there are some data indicating that D-dimer may be higher in MI patients experiencing no-reflow phenomenon [15], a severe condition in which high thrombotic burden interfere with complete restoration of myocardial blood supply after PCI, known to be correlated with adverse outcomes and poor prognosis [16].

Despite many studies published, conclusive data on the real usefulness and additional value of D-dimer in the management of patients with MI are lacking.

The aim of this systematic review and meta-analysis is to summarize current evidence on the potential prognostic role of D-dimer levels in CAD patients and its association with no-reflow phenomenon.

Materials and methods

Strategy search

We conducted a systematic review of literature searching MEDLINE via PubMed and Scopus databases using a combination of the following keywords: "D-dimer" and "myocardial infarction" and "coronary artery disease" and "acute coronary syndrome". There was no time restriction and the last search was run on May 1, 2021. We included only journal articles in English language with full text available. We excluded case-control studies, case reports, editorials/comments, letters, review and meta-analysis, and experimental studies. Supplementary Fig. 1 report strategy searches which were performed according to the PRISMA guidelines.

Study selection and quality assessment

Two physicians (FGB, DP) independently screened the titles and abstracts of manuscripts identified through the database searches to identify studies potentially eligible for further assessment. A third physician (GT) reviewed eligible studies for appropriateness and completeness. The study selection was performed in multiple phases. In the first phase, potentially relevant studies were obtained by combined searches of electronic databases using the selected above-mentioned keywords and exclusion criteria. In the second phase, potentially eligible studies were reviewed to assess the appropriateness with the study question. Finally, the quality of pertinent studies included in the metanalysis was assessed by the Newcastle–Ottawa scale. Studies with a score ≥ 7 were considered of good quality. Quality assessment is reported in Supplementary Table 1.

Endpoints

The principal endpoint was a composite of cardiovascular events (CVEs) including MI, all-cause and cardiovascular mortality. The type of endpoint reported in each study is given in Table 1. Given the lack of high-quality studies, the association between D-dimer and no-reflow was not formally analysed but only systematically reviewed. Ethical approval was not required given the study type.

Statistical analysis

When available, hazard ratios (HRs) and odds ratios (ORs) were recorded from each study.

A separate meta-analysis was conducted for each endpoint, using a hierarchical Bayesian model which therefore would take into account heterogeneity among studies. This technique was chosen due to the limited number of studies included. Formally, each study-specific effect was assumed to be distributed according to a log-Gaussian random variable, centered on a pooled effect. The variance on the log-scale was assumed to correspond to 1.25 times the squared standard error, as evaluated through confidence intervals reported in each study.

All analyses were conducted with R version 3.5.1, using the 'metafor and 'adaptMCMC' packages.

Results

Characteristics of studies

The association between D-dimer levels and clinical outcomes has been investigated in populations enrolled using different definitions of ischemic heart disease, such as CAD, ST segment elevation myocardial (STEMI), non-ST segment elevation myocardial infarction (NSTE MI), acute MI and acute coronary syndrome (ACS). Characteristics of these studies have been separately described according to each definition (Table 1). Supplementary Table 2 and Supplementary Table 3 display the method used to dose D-dimer, cut-off levels and antithrombotic therapy across included studies.

Cardiovascular events

PRISMA flow diagram showing study search strategy about cardiovascular events is reported in Supplementary Fig. 1. After screening, 42 potentially eligible studies were identified and were considered for detailed analysis (Supplementary Fig. 1); 32 studies were included in the systematic review with 28,869 patients. Of these, 9 were retrospective, 20 prospective, 1 ambispective, 1 cross sectional study and 1 post-hoc analysis of a randomized clinical trial.

According to different inclusion criteria, 13 studies included STEMI, 3 NSTEMI, 7 MI, 9 CAD patients.

ST segment elevation myocardial (STEMI)

Overall, a sample of 7729 patients was analysed. The mean age ranged from 41 to 70.2 years and the proportion of women ranged from 8.45 to 54.7%. Four studies investigated outcomes occurred during hospital stay, while 7 studies investigated long-term outcomes (Table 1).

Overall, 11 studies showed an association between high plasma D-dimer levels and CVEs in STEMI patients. In particular, D-dimer predicted worse prognosis in all studies considering in-hospital outcomes, and in 5 out of 7 studies with long-term follow-up (Table 1).

Non-ST segment elevation myocardial infarction (NSTEMI)

A total of 1949 NSTEMI patients, with a mean age that ranged from 57.2 to 67.4 years was included. The proportion of female patients ranged from 24.8 to 35.8%. All studies investigated long-term prognosis. Overall, 1 out of 3 studies showed a positive association between high plasma D-dimer levels and CVEs incidence. However, one study showing no association between D-dimer and outcomes showed an association between D-dimer and NSTEMI severity, as assessed by Global Registry of Acute Coronary Events (GRACE) and thrombolysis in myocardial infarction (TIMI) risk scores, and included only mortality as endpoint; the other study had a short follow-up (6 months) and included also heart failure among cardiovascular outcomes (Table 1).

Myocardial infarction

Seven studies included a total of 12,320 patients with MI, with a mean age ranging from 62.8 to 74.2 years. The proportion of women ranged from 20 to 33.6% and 2 studies investigated in-hospital outcomes. Overall, 4 out of 7 studies consistently showed that D-dimer associated with CVEs (Table 1). Two studies also investigated the existence of a sex-based difference in the prognostic role of D-dimer providing conflicting evidence. Indeed, the study by Wang et al. found that D-dimer predicted all-cause mortality in women but not men. In this study, women were significantly older than men (74 vs 61 years). The opposite was found in the THROMBO study, in which however the mean age was lower and the endpoint included a composited of non-fatal events and cardiovascular death (Table 1).

Acute coronary syndrome (ACS) or CAD

Nine studies included 6871 ACS/CAD patients with a mean age ranging from 57.2 to 71.1 years. The proportion of female patients ranged from 11.1 to 54.1%. Overall, 8 out of 9 studies found that D-dimer was a predictive risk factor for CVEs in patients with ACS or CAD. In one study [45], the association between D-dimer and mortality was not confirmed at multivariable analysis; however, this study included a very

Table 1 Clinical characteristics of studies investigating major adverse cardiac events and all-cause mortality included in the systematic review

Author/ year	Setting	N	Age (years)	Women (%)	Study Design	FU (months)	Endpoints	D-dimer	Main findings
STEMI									
Biccirè 2021 [17]	STEMI	132	64	19.1	R	In-hospital	Adverse events (cardiogenic shock, resuscitated cardiac arrest and death).	Events vs control group: log-transformed D-dimer 6.8 ± 1.1 vs 6.3 ± 0.8, $p = 0.019$	Patients experiencing in-hospital adverse events had higher values of D-dimer compared to those free from events.
Huang 2020 [18]	STEMI	1165	63.5	17	R	In-hospital	CVEs including cardiac death, non-fatal AMI, revascularization, and stroke.	≥ 800 vs < 800 ng/mL	Increased D-dimer level predicted CVEs (OR 8.408, 95% CI 4.065–17.392, $P = 0.001$). D-dimer AUC was 0.840 (95% CI 0.769–0.911). The best cut-off value was 640 ng/mL. In the subgroup with no-reflow phenomenon, increased D-dimer predicted CVEs (OR 8.114, 95%CI 1.598–41.196, $p = 0.012$)
Luo 2020 [19]	STEMI	400	62.5	21	R	12	CVEs (all-cause death, TVR, MI, UA, HF, stroke or TIA)	Groups (μg/L) 1: 74.0; 2: 146.0; 3: 256.5; 4: 576.0.	The incidence of CVEs and all-cause mortality within 30 days ($p < 0.001$), 6 months ($p = 0.001$), and 1 year ($p = 0.001$) after PCI in the highest quartile of the D-dimer groups were higher than those in the other 3 groups.
Qi Zhou 2020 [20]	STEMI	872	63.7	19.8	R	29	All-cause mortality	Groups (μg/mL) 1: ≤0.33; 2: 0.33–0.64; 3: 0.64–1.33; 4: ≥1.33.	Higher in-hospital HF (40.2 vs 10.2%, $p < 0.0001$), malignant arrhythmia (14.2 vs 2.3%, $p < 0.0001$), and all-cause mortality (5.9 vs 0%, $p < 0.0001$) rates were observed in Group 4. 84 patients died. Group 4 was a predictor of all-cause mortality (HR: 2.53, 95%CI 1.02–6.26, $p = 0.045$).
Lin 2020 [21]	STEMI	550	63.5	12.2	P	16	CI-AKI, in-hospital outcomes and long-term mortality and CVEs §	D-dimer quartiles (μg/mL): 1: < 0.38; 2: 0.38–0.67; 3: 0.68–1.03; 4: > 1.03 .	D-dimer > 0.69 μg/mL was an independent risk factor for long-term mortality (HR: 3.41 [95% CI, 1.4–8.03], $p = 0.005$) and CVEs
Zhang 2018 [22]	STEMI	926	52.6	54.7	P	In-hospital	Mortality	383.1 ng/mL ± 264.2	Patients without pre-infarction angina with high D-dimer level on admission had significantly increased in-hospital mortality compared to the other patients ($p = 0.041$).
Gao 2018	STEMI	822	62.5	46.1	P	100	Mortality	D-dimer 430.0	Patients with high

Table 1 Clinical characteristics of studies investigating major adverse cardiac events and all-cause mortality included in the systematic review *(Continued)*

Author/ year	Setting	N	Age (years)	Women (%)	Study Design	FU (months)	Endpoints	D-dimer	Main findings
[23]	with T2DM							ng/mL ± 256.8	plasma D-dimer level on admission showed a significantly shorter survival time (*p* < 0.001 in the log-rank test).
Hansen 2018 [24]	STEMI	971	61	20	cross-sectional cohort study	55	Composite of all-cause mortality, reinfarction, stroke, unscheduled revascularization, HF rehospitalization Secondary outcome was total mortality	Median D-dimer 456 ng/mL (IQR 286–801).	Adjusted OR for composite endpoints for D-dimer above 456 ng/mL: 1.179 (95% CI, 0.814–1.706 *p* = 0.384) Adjusted OR for total mortality for D-dimer above 456 ng/mL: 2.01 (95% CI, 1.06–3.83; *p* = 0.034)
Sarli 2015 [25]	STEMI	266	64	38	P	in-hospital	CVEs: nonfatal MI, in-stent thrombosis, and in-hospital mortality during hospitalization.	D-dimer (µg/l): 686 (±236) vs 418 (±164), *p* < 0.001.	D-dimer level predicted CVEs (OR: 1.002; 95% CI: 1.000–1.004; *p* = 0.029). Optimal cut-off value was 544 µg/mL for CVEs.
Erkol 2014 [15]	STEMI	569	56	16	A	38	Mortality and CVEs (death, non-fatal MI, stroke, revascularization, and advanced HF at long-term follow-up)	D-dimer overall 0.40 mg/L (0.20–0.87).	Univariable HR for long-term mortality 1.56 (95%CI, 1.24–1.95, p < 0.001) and CVEs 1.60 (95%CI, 1.37–1.83, *p* < 0.001); not significant association at multivariable analysis.
HORIZONS-AMI substudy 2014 [26]	STEMI	461	1st: 55.8 2nd: 61.0 3rd: 70.2	20.61	R	36	CVEs (composite of all-cause death, recurrent MI, stroke, or TVR for ischemia.)	Tertiles (µg/mL): 1: < 0.30 (*n* = 215) 2: 0.30–0.71 (*n* = 161) 3: ≥0.71 (*n* = 85)	D-dimer levels ≥0.71 µg/mL on admission predicted CVEs (HR 2.58 [95% CI, 1.44–4.63], *p* = 0.0014), compared to the lowest group.
Ozgur Akgul 2013 [27]	STEMI	453	55.6	19.65	P	6	Mortality	High D-dimer group: > 0.72 µg/mL; Low D-dimer group: lowest two tertiles (≤0.72 µg/mL).	Highest tertile of D-dimer associated with in-hospital CV mortality and 6-month all-cause mortality (7.2 vs. 0.6%, *p* < 0.001 and 13.9 vs. 2%, p < 0.001, respectively). Fatal reinfarction, advanced HF, and CVEs were more frequent in high D-dimer group (p < 0.001).
Pineda 2010 [28]	AMI STEMI (85.9%)	142	41	8.45	P	36	Adverse CV events included stroke, ACS, CABG/PCI, hospitalisation due to congestive HF, CV and global mortality.	Event 360.0 ng/mL vs no event 297.5 ng/mL, *p* = 0.314	No significant differences in D-dimer levels in the event group.
NSTEMI									
Lu 2021 [29]	NSTEMI	1357	65	31.4	P	12	Mortality and CVEs including all-cause death, hospital admission for UA and/or HF, nonfatal recurrent MI	0.380 µg/mL (0.27–0.65) Event group (mortality at 1 year): 0.95	HR for D-dimer for 1-year death and CVEs: 2.12 (95%CI, 1.50–2.99, p < 0.0001).

Table 1 Clinical characteristics of studies investigating major adverse cardiac events and all-cause mortality included in the systematic review *(Continued)*

Author/ year	Setting	N	Age (years)	Women (%)	Study Design	FU (months)	Endpoints	D-dimer	Main findings
							and stroke)	(0.50, 2.00) Control group: 0.37 (0.26, 0.60)	
Hulusi Satilmisoglu 2017 [30]	NSTEMI	234	57.2	24.8	R	14	Mortality	Non-survivors: 1568 ± 1489 ng/mL Survivors: 632 ± 995 ng/mL	D-dimer correlated with GRACE ($r = 0.215$, $p = 0.01$) and TIMI scores ($r = 0.253$, $p < 0.001$). Higher levels recorded for D-dimer assay ($p = 0.003$) in non-survivors. At multivariate analysis, D-dimer assay no significant predictor of increased mortality risk.
Tello-Montoliu 2007 [31]	NSTEMI	358	67.4	35.8	R	6	Death, new ACS, revascularization, and HF	Overall D-dimer level: 340 (211–615) ng/mL	Admission D-dimer levels did not predict events [HR: 1.26 (0.79–2.02), $p = 0.337$).
AMI									
Fu 2020 [32]	AMI with ESRD	113	69.2	33.6	R	In-hospital	Mortality	Mortality: 3.2 mg/L Survival: 1.1 mg/L $p = 0.023$	D-dimer ≥2.4 mg/L predicted in-hospital mortality (OR 2.771 [95% CI, 1.017–8.947], $p < 0.001$).
Wang 2020 [33]	AMI	197	Male 61.8 Female 74.2	20	P	6	All-cause mortality (in- and out-of-hospital deaths) or readmission.	Male D-dimer (mg/L) 0.4 vs 1.0 $P < 0.001$ Female D-dimer (mg/L) 0.4 vs 0.6 $p = 0.015$.	HR for continuous D-dimer in women 2.029 (95%CI, 1.403–2.933; $p < 0.001$). D-dimer ≥0.43 mg/L as an independent predictor of poor prognosis in female AMI patients.
Zhang 2020 [34]	AMI	4495	62	31.03	P	24	All-cause mortality	< 145 ng/mL ≥145 ng/mL	Elevated D-dimer was associated with mortality (univariable HR 1.20, 95%CI, 1.04–1.37, $p = 0.01$) and in the patients in different groups (HFpEF, HFrEF, non-HF).
Yu 2019 [35]	AMI	5923	62.2	30.5	P	In-hospital	Mortality	D-dimer tertiles (ng/mL): Low: ≤88; Intermediate: 89–179; High: > 179.	After multivariable adjustment, D-dimer significantly predicted in-hospital mortality (OR 1.060 [95% CI, 1.026–1.094], $p < 0.001$). D-dimer levels significantly improved the prognostic performance of GRACE score (C-statistic: $p = 2.269$, $p = 0.023$; IDI: 0.016, $p = 0.032$; no-reflowl: 0.291, $p = 0.035$).
REBUS study 2017 [36]	AMI	412	67	22.3	P	24	Composite endpoint (all-cause death, MI, congestive HF, or all-cause stroke)	Median D-dimer was 677 μg/L at inclusion	D-dimer was not associated with the composite endpoint (HR 1.22 [95% CI 0.99–1.51], $p = 0.06$, for one SD increase).
Smid 2011	AMI	135	61	26	P	12	CV death, recurrent MI,	On admission	D-dimer on admission

Table 1 Clinical characteristics of studies investigating major adverse cardiac events and all-cause mortality included in the systematic review *(Continued)*

Author/ year	Setting	N	Age (years)	Women (%)	Study Design	FU (months)	Endpoints	D-dimer	Main findings
[37]							a second PCI or CABG and ischemic stroke.	D-dimer: 370 (260–718) ng/mL	was higher in patients with recurrent thrombotic CV event (medians 550 vs. 365 ng/mL, p = 0.06) OR for D-dimer against endpoints: 2.9 (95%CI 0.9–8.8)
THROMBO study 2000 [38]	AMI	1045	Male 58 Female 62	24.3	P	26	Recurrent cardiac events (nonfatal reinfarction or cardiac death)	D-dimer mean in men 508 ± 690 ng/mL vs women 564 ± 430 ng/mL	D-dimer had prognostic value in men (HR 2.35, 95%CI 1.27–4.35], *p* = 0.006) but not in women (HR 1.58, 95%CI 0.59–4.22, *p* = 0.360).
ACS/CAD									
Chen 2018 [39]	CAD (76.9% AMI)	238	64.4	21.1	P	24	All-cause mortality and CVEs (cardiac death and nonfatal outcomes: recurrent MI, TVR or re-admission due to advanced HF).	Mean D-dimer: 0.7 ± 1.1 mg/L.	OR for long-term CVEs: 1.526 (95% CI, 1.174–1.983), *p* = 0.002. D-dimer in multivariate Cox regression of CVEs: 1.420 (1.069–3.014), *p* = 0.046
Kosaki 2018 [40]	ACS (76.3% AMI)	400	71.1	27.2	P	27	CVEs (all-cause mortality, recurrent MI, unplanned repeat revascularization, surgical revascularization, fatal arrhythmia, admission for HF, and stroke.	Patients without CVEs: 1.67 mg/mL ± 2.49 Patients with CVEs: 2.11 mg/mL ±2.72 *p* = 0.0003	Univariate analysis for D-dimer ≥0.84 mg/mL predicting CVEs: OR 2.49 (95%CI 1.54–4.11), *p* = 0.0001
ATLAS ACS-TIMI46 Trial Substudy 2018 [41]	ACS (73.9% AMI)	1834	Placebo 57.9 Rivaroxaban 57.2	23.2	Post-hoc RCT	6	Composite endpoint of CV death, myocardial infarction, or stroke	Baseline D-dimer (μg/mL) Placebo 0.39 (0.24–0.73) vs Rivaroxaban 0.42 (0.24–0.78) *p* = 0.370	Continuous D-dimer prognostic factor for composite outcome: univariate OR 1.15 (1.03–1.29) *p* = 0.015, multivariate OR 1.13 (1.0–1.28) *p* = 0.048
Mjelva, 2016 [42]	CAD (44.3% AMI)	871	69.5	38.7	P	84	All-cause mortality; a combined endpoint consisting of death or recurrent non-fatal MI; recurrent non-fatal MI alone.	194 (106–437) μg/L Median D-dimer in survivors vs non-survivors were for 153 vs 346 μg/L (*p* < 0.001)	D-dimer above 436 μg/L independently predicted mortality (4th vs 1st quartile HR 1.83 [95% CI 1.20–2.78], *p* = 0.005) Death or MI (4th vs 1st quartile HR 1.38 [95% CI 0.96–1.98], *p* = 0.08) Recurrent MI (4th vs 1st quartile HR 0.70 [95% CI 0.43–1.15], *p* = 0.16)
Gong 2016 [43]	CAD (29.2% AMI)	2209	58.58	25.9	P	18	Cardiac death, nonfatal MI, recurrence of MI, and stroke	Tertiles (μg/mL) 1: < 0.23, *n* = 816; 2: 0.23–0.36, *n* = 629; 3: > 0.36, *n* = 764.	D-dimer was linked to the severity of CAD (95% CI: 1.20–6.84, p = 0.005) Continuous D-dimer predictor of total outcome (HR = 1.22, 95% CI: 1.09–1.37, *p* = 0.001).
Charoensri 2011 [44]	ACS (61% AMI)	74	66	54.1	R	In-hospital	CHF, arrhythmias and death	D-dimer levels (μg/L) CHF: 1475 vs No CHF 385; Arrhythmia	D-dimer levels correlated with complication of ACS (CHF; p < 0.001, arrhythmia; *p* = 0.007

Table 1 Clinical characteristics of studies investigating major adverse cardiac events and all-cause mortality included in the systematic review *(Continued)*

Author/ year	Setting	N	Age (years)	Women (%)	Study Design	FU (months)	Endpoints	D-dimer	Main findings
								5422 vs No arrhythmia 550; Death 5118 vs No death 2550	and death; $p = 0.009$). D-dimer was significantly increased with the number of coronary arteries affected ($p = 0.03$).
Brugger-Andersen 2008 [45]	STEMI (15%), NSTEMI (29,3%), UA (9,4%), No ACS (46,3%)	871	69.6	39	P	24	All-cause mortality, CVEs (cardiac death or recurrent positive troponin T)	Quartiles of D-dimer (μg/l): Q1 < 106, Q2 ≥ 106–191, Q3 ≥ 191–438, Q4 ≥ 438.	In the univariate analysis highest D-dimer quartile predicted all-cause mortality compared with the lowest quartile (Q1) (OR 7.78 [95%IC, 3.95–15.33], $p < 0.001$), but not confirmed at multivariable logistic regression analysis (OR 1.80 [95%IC, 0.81 to 3.97]; $p = 0.148$).
Prisco 2001 [46]	CAD (52,9% AMI)	54	60 (44–75) 65 (38–81)	11.1	P	18	Restenosis	D-dimer before PCI: AMI (group 1) 55 ng/mL vs elective PCI (group 2) 29.0 ng/mL, $p < 0.001$	In group 1, D-dimer levels at the end of the procedure were higher in patients with restenosis than in those without ($p < 0.005$). Increased D-dimer in patients with restenosis (61%) than those without (25%, $p < 0.05$).
Oldgren 2001 [12]	ACS	320	66	–	P	29	Death, MI, and refractory angina during and after anticoagulant treatment in unstable CAD	< 82 μg/L ($N = 105$); 82–149 μg/L ($N = 106$); > 149 μg/L ($N = 103$)	No difference in clinical outcome at 72 h, 7 days and 30 days. During long-term follow-up, there was a relation between higher baseline levels of D-dimer and increased mortality ($p = 0.003$).

Study design: *A* ambispective, *P* prospective, *R* retrospective

§including recurrent MI, required renal replacement therapy, stent thrombosis, bleeding and length of hospital stay, hospital costs, and mortality and long-term CVEs (mortality, stent restenosis, non-fatal MI and TVR)

ACS acute coronary syndrome, *AMI* acute myocardial infarction, *AUC* area under curve, *CABG* coronary artery bypass grafting, *CAD* coronary artery disease, *CHF* congestive heart failure, *CI-AKI* Contrast-induced acute kidney injury, *CV* cardiovascular, CVEs cardiovascular events, *ESRD* end-stage renal disease, *HF* heart failure, *HFpEF* heart failure with preserved ejection fraction, *HFrEF* heart failure with reduced ejection fraction, *HR* hazard ratio, *NSTEMI* non-ST segment elevation myocardial infarction, *NT-proBNP* N-terminal pro-B-type natriuretic peptide, *OR* odds ratio, *PCI* percutaneous coronary intervention, *STEMI* ST segment elevation myocardial infarction, *TIA* transient ischemic attack, *TIMI* Thrombolysis in Myocardial Infarction, *TVR* target vessel revascularization, *UA* unstable angina

heterogeneous population mixing STEMI, NSTEMI, unstable angina and no ACS patients.

Results of meta-analysis

Five studies satisfied inclusion criteria and were included in the metanalysis: 4 prospective and 1 retrospective studies (Table 1) with a total of 8616 patients. Only studies reporting HR for continuous values were formally analysed. Median follow-up was 13.2 months with a total of 626 CVEs. The weighted mean age was 61.9 years. The percentage of women ranged from 25.9 to 100% (in one study). The pooled HR for D-dimer levels and CVEs was 1.264 (95% CI 1.134–1.409) (Fig. 1).

No-reflow phenomenon in STEMI patients

We also performed a systematic search using "D-dimer" and "no-reflow". After screening, 7 potentially eligible studies were identified (3 prospective, 3 retrospective and 1 ambispective) (Supplementary Fig. 2). A total of 4195 STEMI patients were included, with mean age ranged from 52.6 to 64.0 mean years (female patients from 16 to 53.7%). Overall, 1327 patients (31.6%) had no-reflow phenomenon (Table 2). Five out of 7 studies showed a positive correlation of D-dimer levels with no-reflow phenomenon. Given the high variability in the methods of each study (cut-off of D-dimer used, measures of association) a formal analysis was not performed.

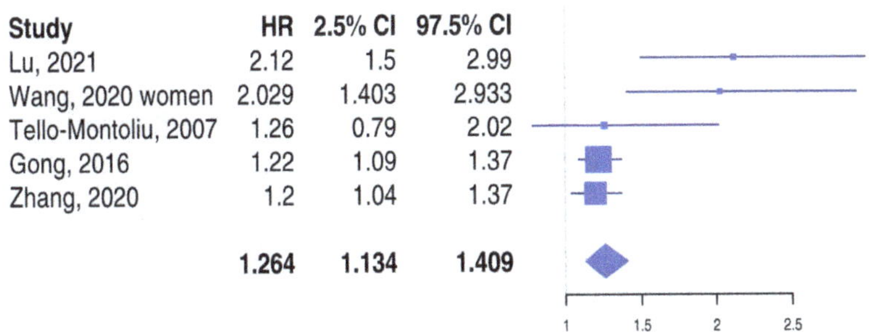

Fig. 1 Forest plot of the hazard ratio for the risk of composite endpoints according to D-dimer values in patients with acute MI. HR: hazard ratio; CI: confidence interval

Discussion

Our study shows that most studies including patients with ischemic heart disease showed a consistent association between D-dimer levels and worse clinical outcomes. This association was particularly evident in studies investigating in-hospital adverse events.

The rationale of investigating D-dimer levels in CAD patients relies on the persistent hypercoagulable state described in MI patients, which may lead to worse clinical outcomes in these patients through several mechanisms [14]. Clotting activation may contribute to thrombus growth and no-reflow phenomenon, along with impaired thrombolysis which has been frequently described in CAD patients [49], all factors contributing to an increased CAD severity and myocardial injury (Fig. 2).

Reperfusion fails to occur after thrombolytic therapy in approximate 40% of patients, as shown by a study including 427 STEMI patients undergo rescue PCI [50]. Indeed, high D-dimer levels have been shown to be significantly higher in lysis-resistant thrombi from STEMI patients [51].

Table 2 Clinical characteristics of studies investigating no-reflow phenomenon included in the systematic review

Author/ year	N[a]	Age (years)	Women (%)	Study design	Events	D-dimer levels		Odds Ratio	Low CI	High CI	Main findings
						No-reflow group	Control group				
Gong 2020 [47]	229	63.7	17	R	28	1600 ± 1400 ng/mL	500 ± 600 ng/mL	2.520	1.160	5.470	D-dimer level can independently predict no-reflow after PCI. D-dimer value of 530 ng/mL was an effective cut-off point for postprocedural no-reflow with 85.7% of sensitivity and 67.7% of specificity (AUC = 0.78; $p = 0.049$).
Huang 2020 [18]	1165	63.5	17	R	165	≥ 800 ng/mL	< 800 ng/mL	1.399	0.929	2.106	D-dimer group had more frequently no-reflow (13.1% vs. 18.8%. $p = 0.028$).
Cheng 2019 [48]	218	58.7	17.5	R	39	410.3 ± 237.2 ng/mL	536.9 ± 291.7 ng/mL	1.001	1.000	1.003	No-reflow patients were older, diabetics, with longer pain-to balloon time, lower blood pressure, higher platelet count and higher levels of D-dimer and Cystatin C.
Zhang 2018 [22]	926	52.6	53.7	P	435	508.5 ± 254.7 ng/mL	272.0 ± 218.9 ng/mL	2.563	1.910	3.439	Multivariate OR for predicting no-reflow for D-dimer above mean (383.1 ng/mL).
Gao 2018 [23]	822	62.5	46.1	P	418	533.0 ± 244.0 ng/mL	323.4 ± 224.4 ng/mL	4.212	2.973	5.967	Diabetic patients with high D-dimer levels showed higher risk of no-reflow. Sensitivity of high plasma D-dimer levels in predicting no-reflow was 0.766.
Sarli 2015 [25]	266	64	38	P	63	686 ± 236 µg/l	418 ± 164 µg/l	1.005	1.003	1.007	D-dimer levels predicted no-reflow (OR: 1.005; 95% CI: 1.003–1.007; $p < 0.001$). Optimal cut-off for no-reflow was 549 µg/l.
Erkol 2014 [15]	569	56	16	A	179	720 (280–1490) mg/L	350 (170–620) mg/L	1.640	1.260	2.140	D-dimer (per each 1 mg/L increase) predictor of angiographic no-reflow ($p < 0.001$).

[a]all STEMI patients. Study design: *A* ambispective, *P* prospective, *R* retrospective. *PCI* percutaneous coronary intervention. *CVEs* cardiovascular ev

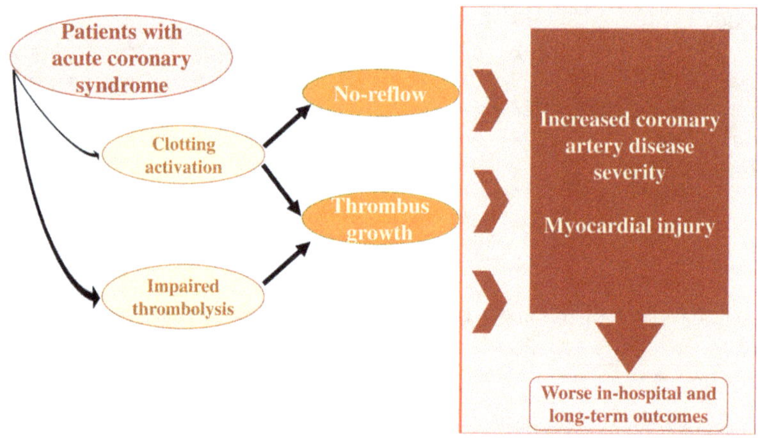

Fig. 2 Pathophysiological mechanisms linking clotting activation and impairment of thrombolysis with the severity of acute coronary syndrome presentation and clinical outcomes

The pathogenesis of no-reflow remains unclear, but it is likely to be multifactorial, including endothelial damage platelet and clotting activation leading to thrombus formation at the level of small vessels [52]. Few studies investigated the occurrence of no-reflow in STEMI patients undergoing PCI and its relationship with D-dimer [15, 22, 23, 25, 47, 48]. In 229 consecutive STEMI patients, X. Gong et al. [47] found that a D-dimer value of 530 ng/mL (FEU) was associated with postprocedural no-reflow, with 85.7% of sensitivity and 67.7% of specificity (area under the curve [AUC] = 0.78; $p = 0.049$). Similarly, Sarli et al. found that optimal D-dimer cut-off value for predicting no-reflow was 549 µg/l (FEU) [25]. In 218 STEMI patients, Cheng et al. [48] found that no-reflow patients were older, diabetics, with longer pain-to balloon time, lower blood pressure, higher platelet counts and higher levels of D-dimer and Cystatin C than patients without no-reflow.

Risk stratification using D-dimer

In the past decades, an increasing number of biomarkers have been tested to improve cardiovascular risk stratification in patients with ACS [6, 53]. In particular, some studies suggested that the use of a combination of multiple biomarkers may improve risk stratification. This is the case of D-dimer, which if used alone is currently recommended to only exclude acute venous thromboembolism, but its addition to other biomarkers/risk scores gave promising results.

Indeed, the addition of D-dimer has been investigated to some biomarkers such as C-reactive protein (CRP), NT-proBNP and clinical scores, such as the Global Registry of Acute Coronary Events (GRACE) risk score has been investigated. Fu et al. included D-dimer levels ≥2.4 mg/L FEU in a risk score model together with CRP, left ventricular ejection fraction, age ≥ 65 years old and heart rate [32]. In ROC curve analysis, this model demonstrated a good power in predicting in-hospital mortality (AUC = 0.895, 95% CI 0.814–0.96; $p < 0.001$), better than the predictive power of the GRACE risk score alone (AUC = 0.754, 95% CI 0.641–0.868; p < 0.001). D-dimer has been tested combined to GRACE score also in the study by Lin et al. who found that the combination of NT-pro-BNP and D-dimer improved the predictive accuracy of GRACE score for all-cause death [29]. In 5923 ACS patients undergoing PCI, GRACE score combined with D-dimer achieved a better prognostic performance than GRACE score, and D-dimer could significantly improve the prognostic performance of GRACE score [35]. This result is in keeping with that described by Yu et al., in which [35] D-dimer levels significantly improved the prognostic performance of GRACE score.

Management and therapeutic implications

Altogether, current evidence suggest that D-dimer may identify patients at higher risk for a more severe CAD and worse prognosis. Of note, clotting activation is not lowered by antiplatelet therapy [54], as shown by previous studies reporting no effect of aspirin and DAPT in reducing D-dimer levels [55]. Conversely, oral and parenteral anticoagulation, in addition or not to DAPT, has been demonstrated to decrease D-dimer levels in patients with MI [41, 56, 57]. Thus, ATLAS ACS 2-TIMI 51 and COMPASS trials have recently proved the utility of adding low-dose anticoagulation to antiplatelet medications. In ATLAS ACS 2-TIMI 51, introduction of low-dose rivaroxaban therapy (2.5 mg or 5 mg twice daily, with 93% of patients on DAPT) has shown to be effective in reducing the risk of death from cardiovascular causes, myocardial infarction, or stroke [58], even if the use of rivaroxaban increased the risk of major bleeding and intracranial haemorrhages. Similarly, the COMPASS trial demonstrated that rivaroxaban plus aspirin was effective in decreasing the primary outcome of cardiovascular death, stroke or MI with a 22% reduction in the net clinical benefit endpoint (defined as the composite of primary outcome, fatal bleeding and symptomatic bleeding into a critical organ/area) [59]. Moreover, a subanalysis of the COMPASS trial has shown that patients with high thrombotic profile (i.e., peripheral arterial disease) may benefit more from adding anticoagulation therapy to reduce residual thrombotic risk.

However, these studies did not stratified patients according to D-dimer levels. Data from the literature let to hypothesize that the benefit conferred by an association therapy of oral anticoagulation and antiplatelet therapy may be even more evident in patients with the features of clotting activation (i.e. high D-dimer). This aspect would deserve a specific investigation.

Another group of patients who deserve particular attention is represented by patients presenting with no-reflow. Preliminary data from the literature suggest an association between high-D-dimer levels and no-reflow. Moreover, in MI patients who cannot undergo cardiac catheterization, D-dimer concentrations may also be helpful to predict severity of coronary disease [60].

Finally, D-dimer levels might be helpful in identifying MI patients at high risk of complications and worse outcome. In Fig. 3, we propose a D-dimer guided strategy to tailored therapy in patients at higher thrombotic risk such as those with MI undergoing PCI. Firstly, MI patients with high D-dimer levels may benefit from specific pharmacological management and technical procedures to reduce the probability of no-reflow phenomenon. These include the use of glycoprotein IIb/IIIa inhibitors, higher heparin dose and direct stenting without predilation [61–64]. Those high-risk patients might also take advantage from prolonged parenteral anticoagulation after PCI during in-hospital staying to reduce early complications. At discharge, patients presenting with high-risk features, including presence of comorbidities, multivessel disease, age > 65 years, recurrent MI, multiple stent insertion, may benefit from adding a low dose of oral anticoagulant agent to conventional antiplatelet therapy to reduce the residual thrombotic risk (i.e., rivaroxaban 2.5 mg twice daily).

Study limitations. A formal analysis for D-dimer against no-reflow phenomenon was not performed given the high variability in the methods of each study (cut-off of D-dimer used, measures of association) was not performed.

Conclusions

In conclusion, given its association with CVEs, the use of D-dimer may help physicians to improve outcome and manage residual thrombotic risk in MI

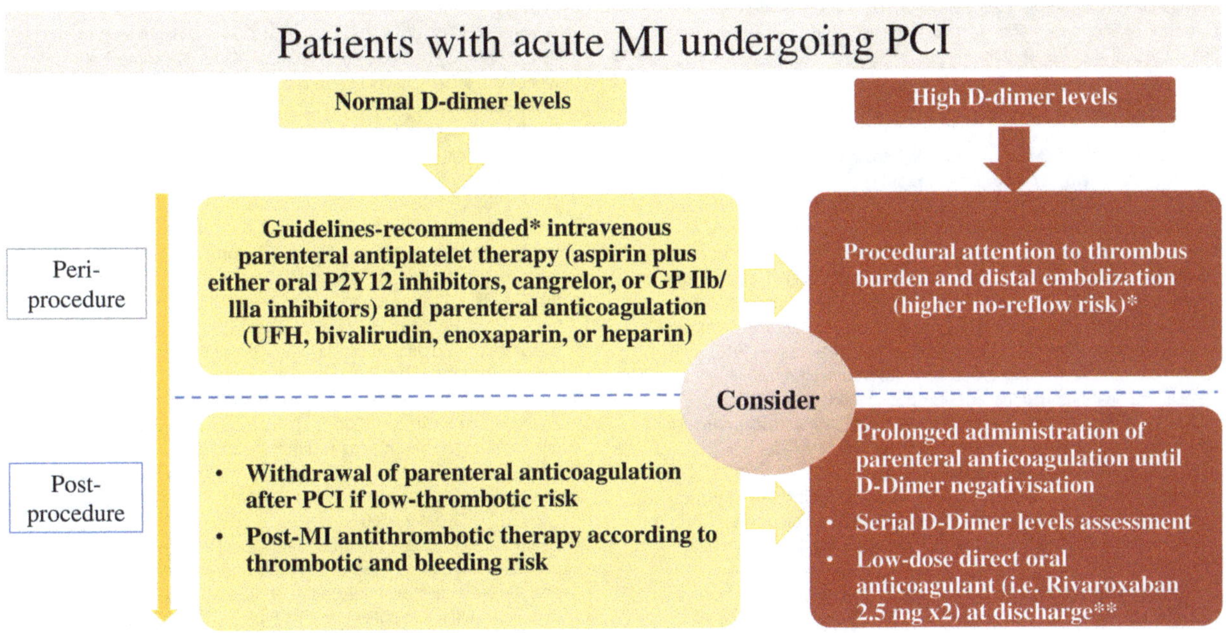

*2020 ESC Guidelines

** especially in patients with high-risk features (age ≥ 50 years with one or more of the following criteria: age ≥ 65 years, diabetes mellitus in pharmacological treatment, previous MI, multivessel disease, chronic kidney disease with <60 ml/min eGFR).

Fig. 3 Proposed flow-chart for the management of patients with acute MI according to D-dimer values. MI: myocardial infarction; PCI: percutaneous coronary intervention; UFH: unfractionated Heparin patients. D-dimer may therefore represent a valuable guide in the difficult decision-making process on the use of oral anticoagulation in addition to currently recommended antithrombotic therapy in patients with ACS.

Abbreviations

CAD: Coronary artery disease; MI: Myocardial infarction; PCI: Percutaneous coronary intervention; CVEs: Cardiovascular events; STEMI: ST segment elevation myocardial; NSTEMI: Non-ST segment elevation myocardial infarction; ACS: Acute coronary syndrome; CRP: C-reactive protein; GRACE: Global registry of acute coronary events; TIMI: Thrombolysis in myocardial infarction

Supplementary Information

Additional file 1. Supplementary data.

Acknowledgements

this research did not receive any specific grant from funding agencies in the public, commercial, or not-for-profit sectors.

Authors' contributions

F.G.B. and D.P. are the guarantors of the manuscript and responsible for project administration, study concept, design and literature search. Data collection/interpretation/analysis: F.G.B, D.P., A.F. and G.T. Manuscript writing/revisions, validation, visualization and drafting of figures: F.G.B., D.P., A.F., C.G., F.V., P.P. and G.T. The authors read and approved the final manuscript.

Author details

[1]Department of Clinical Internal, Anesthesiological, and Cardiovascular Sciences, Sapienza University of Rome, Viale del Policlinico 155, 00161 Rome, Italy. [2]Department of General and Specialized Surgery "Paride Stefanini", Sapienza University of Rome, Viale del Policlinico 155, 00161 Rome, Italy. [3]Department of Economics and Finance, University of Rome "Tor Vergata", Via Columbia 2, 00133 Rome, Italy.

References

1. Roth GA, Huffman MD, Moran AE, Feigin V, Mensah GA, Naghavi M, et al. Global and regional patterns in cardiovascular mortality from 1990 to 2013. Circulation. 2015;132(17):1667–78. https://doi.org/10.1161/CIRCULATIONAHA.114.008720.
2. Jernberg T, Hasvold P, Henriksson M, Hjelm H, Thuresson M, Janzon M. Cardiovascular risk in post-myocardial infarction patients: nationwide real world data demonstrate the importance of a long-term perspective. Eur Heart J. 2015;36(19):1163–70. https://doi.org/10.1093/eurheartj/ehu505.
3. Townsend N, Wilson L, Bhatnagar P, Wickramasinghe K, Rayner M, Nichols M. Cardiovascular disease in Europe: epidemiological update 2016. Eur Heart J. 2016;37(42):3232–45. https://doi.org/10.1093/eurheartj/ehw334.
4. Global, regional, and national age-sex-specific mortality for 282 causes of death in 195 countries and territories, 1980–2017: a systematic analysis for the Global Burden of Disease Study 2017. Lancet. 2018;392(10159):1736–88. https://doi.org/10.1016/S0140-6736(18)32203-7.
5. Dhingra R, Vasan RS. Biomarkers in cardiovascular disease: statistical assessment and section on key novel heart failure biomarkers. Trends Cardiovasc Med. 2017;27(2):123–33. https://doi.org/10.1016/j.tcm.2016.07.005.
6. Collet JP, Thiele H, Barbato E, Barthélémy O, Bauersachs J, Bhatt DL, et al. ESC guidelines for the management of acute coronary syndromes in patients presenting without persistent ST-segment elevation. Eur Heart J. 2020;2020(3):4418. https://doi.org/10.15829/1560-4071-2021-4418.
7. Amsterdam EA, Wenger NK, Brindis RG, Casey DE Jr, Ganiats TG, Holmes DR Jr, et al. AHA/ACC guideline for the Management of Patients with non-ST-elevation acute coronary syndromes: a report of the American College of Cardiology/American Heart Association task force on practice guidelines. J Am Coll Cardiol. 2014;64:e139–228. https://doi.org/10.1016/j.jacc.2014.09.017.
8. Galvani M, Ferrini D, Ottani F, Eisenberg PR. Early risk stratification of unstable angina/non-Q myocardial infarction: biochemical markers of coronary thrombosis. Int J Cardiol. 1999;68(Suppl 1):S55–61. https://doi.org/10.1016/S0167-5273(98)00292-7.
9. Ardissino D, Merlini PA, Gamba G, Barberis P, Demicheli G, Testa S, et al. Thrombin activity and early outcome in unstable angina pectoris. Circulation. 1996;93(9):1634–9. https://doi.org/10.1161/01.CIR.93.9.1634.
10. Merlini PA, Bauer KA, Oltrona L, Ardissino D, Cattaneo M, Belli C, et al. Persistent activation of coagulation mechanism in unstable angina and myocardial infarction. Circulation. 1994;90(1):61–8. https://doi.org/10.1161/01.CIR.90.1.61.
11. Giannitsis E, Mair J, Christersson C, Siegbahn A, Huber K, Jaffe AS, et al. How to use D-dimer in acute cardiovascular care. Eur Heart J Acute Cardiovasc Care. 2017;6(1):69–80. https://doi.org/10.1177/2048872615610870.
12. Oldgren J, Linder R, Grip L, Siegbahn A, Wallentin L. Coagulation activity and clinical outcome in unstable coronary artery disease. Arterioscler Thromb Vasc Biol. 2001;21(6):1059–64. https://doi.org/10.1161/01.ATV.21.6.1059.
13. Soomro AY, Guerchicoff A, Nichols DJ, Suleman J, Dangas GD. The current role and future prospects of D-dimer biomarker. Eur Heart J Cardiovasc Pharmacother. 2016;2(3):175–84. https://doi.org/10.1093/ehjcvp/pvv039.
14. Christersson C, Oldgren J, Bylock A, Siegbahn A, Wallentin L. Early decrease in coagulation activity after myocardial infarction is associated with lower risk of new ischaemic events: observations from the ESTEEM trial. Eur Heart J. 2007;28(6):692–8. https://doi.org/10.1093/eurheartj/ehl564.
15. Erkol A, Oduncu V, Turan B, Kılıçgedik A, Sırma D, Gözübüyük G, et al. The value of plasma D-dimer level on admission in predicting no-reflow after primary percutaneous coronary intervention and long-term prognosis in patients with acute ST segment elevation myocardial infarction. J Thromb Thrombolysis. 2014;38(3):339–47. https://doi.org/10.1007/s11239-013-1044-3.
16. Rezkalla SH, Dharmashankar KC, Abdalrahman IB, Kloner RA. No-reflow phenomenon following percutaneous coronary intervention for acute myocardial infarction: incidence, outcome, and effect of pharmacologic therapy. J Interv Cardiol. 2010;23(5):429–36. https://doi.org/10.1111/j.1540-8183.2010.00561.x.
17. Biccirè FG, Pastori D, Tanzilli A, Pignatelli P, Viceconte N, Barillà F, et al. Low serum albumin levels and in-hospital outcomes in patients with ST segment elevation myocardial infarction. Nutr Metab Cardiovasc Dis. 2021;31(10):2904–11.
18. Huang D, Gao W, Wu R, Zhong X, Qian J, Ge J. D-dimer level predicts in-hospital adverse outcomes after primary PCI for ST-segment elevation myocardial infarction. Int J Cardiol. 2020;305:1–4. https://doi.org/10.1016/j.ijcard.2020.02.010.
19. Luo E, Wang D, Liu B, Hou J, Yan G, Tang C. The value of d-dimer level in predicting contrast-induced acute kidney injury in patients with acute ST-segment elevation myocardial infarction after PCI. Clin Appl Thromb Hemost. 2020;26:1076029620944492. https://doi.org/10.1177/1076029620944492.
20. Zhou Q, Xue Y, Shen J, Zhou W, Wen Y, Luo S. Predictive values of D-dimer for the long-term prognosis of acute ST-segment elevation infarction: a retrospective study in southwestern China. Medicine (Baltimore). 2020;99(16):e19724. https://doi.org/10.1097/MD.0000000000019724.
21. Lin KY, Chen HC, Jiang H, Wang SY, Chen HM, Wu ZY, et al. Predictive value of admission D-dimer for contrast-induced acute kidney injury and poor outcomes after primary percutaneous coronary intervention. BMC Nephrol. 2020;21(1):90. https://doi.org/10.1186/s12882-020-01743-7.
22. Zhang H, Qiu B, Zhang Y, Cao Y, Zhang X, Wu Z, et al. The value of pre-infarction angina and plasma D-dimer in predicting no-reflow after primary percutaneous coronary intervention in ST-segment elevation acute myocardial infarction patients. Med Sci Monit. 2018;24:4528–35. https://doi.org/10.12659/MSM.909360.
23. Gao R, Wang J, Zhang S, Yang G, Gao Z, Chen X. The value of combining plasma D-dimer and Endothelin-1 levels to predict no-reflow after percutaneous coronary intervention of ST-segment elevation in acute myocardial infarction patients with a type 2 diabetes mellitus history. Med Sci Monit. 2018;24:3549–56. https://doi.org/10.12659/MSM.908980.
24. Hansen CH, Ritschel V, Andersen G, Halvorsen S, Eritsland J, Arnesen H, et al. Markers of thrombin generation are associated with long-term clinical outcome in patients with ST-segment elevation myocardial infarction. Clin Appl Thromb Hemost. 2018;24(7):1088–94. https://doi.org/10.1177/1076029618764847.
25. Sarli B, Akpek M, Baktir AO, Sahin O, Saglam H, Arinc H, et al. Impact of D-

dimer level on postinterventional coronary flow and in-hospital MACE in ST-segment elevation myocardial infarction. Herz. 2015;40(3):507–13. https://doi.org/10.1007/s00059-013-4029-2.
26. Kikkert WJ, Claessen BE, Stone GW, Mehran R, Witzenbichler B, Brodie BR, et al. D-dimer levels predict ischemic and hemorrhagic outcomes after acute myocardial infarction: a HORIZONS-AMI biomarker substudy. J Thromb Thrombolysis. 2014;37(2):155–64. https://doi.org/10.1007/s11239-013-0953-5.
27. Akgul O, Uyarel H, Pusuroglu H, Gul M, Isiksacan N, Turen S, et al. Predictive value of elevated D-dimer in patients undergoing primary angioplasty for ST elevation myocardial infarction. Blood Coagul Fibrinolysis. 2013;24(7):704–10. https://doi.org/10.1097/MBC.0b013e3283610396.
28. Pineda J, Marín F, Marco P, Roldán V, Valencia J, Ruiz-Nodar JM, et al. The prognostic value of biomarkers after a premature myocardial infarction. Int J Cardiol. 2010;143(3):249–54. https://doi.org/10.1016/j.ijcard.2009.02.019.
29. Lu PJ, Gong XW, Liu Y, Tian FS, Zhang WJ, Liu YW, et al. Optimization of GRACE risk stratification by N-terminal pro-B-type natriuretic peptide combined with D-dimer in patients with non-ST-elevation myocardial infarction. Am J Cardiol. 2021;140:13–9. https://doi.org/10.1016/j.amjcard.2020.10.050.
30. Satilmisoglu MH, Ozyilmaz SO, Gul M, Ak Yildirim H, Kayapinar O, Gokturk K, et al. Predictive values of D-dimer assay, GRACE scores and TIMI scores for adverse outcome in patients with non-ST-segment elevation myocardial infarction. Ther Clin Risk Manag. 2017;13:393–400. https://doi.org/10.2147/TCRM.S124794.
31. Tello-Montoliu A, Marín F, Roldán V, Mainar L, López MT, Sogorb F, et al. A multimarker risk stratification approach to non-ST elevation acute coronary syndrome: implications of troponin T, CRP, NT pro-BNP and fibrin D-dimer levels. J Intern Med. 2007;262(6):651–8. https://doi.org/10.1111/j.1365-2796.2007.01871.x.
32. Fu Y, Sun H, Guo Z, Xu L, Yang X, Wang L, et al. A risk score model to predict in-hospital mortality of patients with end-stage renal disease and acute myocardial infarction. Intern Emerg Med. 2020;16(4):905–12. https://doi.org/10.1007/s11739-020-02529-3.
33. Wang P, Yao J, Xie Y, Luo M. Gender-specific predictive markers of poor prognosis for patients with acute myocardial infarction during a 6-month follow-up. J Cardiovasc Transl Res. 2020;13(1):27–38. https://doi.org/10.1007/s12265-019-09946-6.
34. Zhang X, Wang S, Sun L, Fang S, Yu B. Prognostic value of D-dimer in acute myocardial infarction complicated by heart failure with preserved ejection fraction. ESC Heart Fail. 2020;7(6):4118–25. https://doi.org/10.1002/ehf2.13027.
35. Yu T, Jiao Y, Song J, He D, Wu J, Sun Z, et al. Hospital mortality in acute coronary syndrome: adjustment of GRACE score by D-dimer enables a more accurate prediction in a prospective cohort study. BMC Cardiovasc Disord. 2019;19(1):252. https://doi.org/10.1186/s12872-019-1239-4.
36. Christersson C, Lindahl B, Berglund L, Siegbahn A, Oldgren J. The utility of coagulation activity for prediction of risk of mortality and cardiovascular events in guideline-treated myocardial infarction patients. Ups J Med Sci. 2017;122(4):224–33. https://doi.org/10.1080/03009734.2017.1407849.
37. Smid M, Dielis AW, Winkens M, Spronk HM, van Oerle R, Hamulyák K, et al. Thrombin generation in patients with a first acute myocardial infarction. J Thromb Haemost. 2011;9(3):450–6. https://doi.org/10.1111/j.1538-7836.2010.04162.x.
38. Kalaria VG, Zareba W, Moss AJ, Pancio G, Marder VJ, Morrissey JH, et al. Gender-related differences in thrombogenic factors predicting recurrent cardiac events in patients after acute myocardial infarction. The THROMBO Investigators. Am J Cardiol. 2000;85(12):1401–8. https://doi.org/10.1016/S0002-9149(00)00785-2.
39. Chen H, Lu N, Zheng M. A high circulating FGF21 level as a prognostic marker in patients with acute myocardial infarction. Am J Transl Res. 2018;10(9):2958–66.
40. Kosaki R, Minoura Y, Ogura K, Oishi Y, Tanaka L, Arai K, et al. Thrombomodulin can predict the incidence of second events in patients with acute coronary syndrome: single-center, retrospective cohort study. J Cardiol. 2018;72(6):494–500. https://doi.org/10.1016/j.jjcc.2018.05.006.
41. AlKhalfan F, Kerneis M, Nafee T, Yee MK, Chi G, Plotnikov A, et al. D-dimer levels and effect of rivaroxaban on those levels and outcomes in patients with acute coronary syndrome (an ATLAS ACS-TIMI 46 trial substudy). Am J Cardiol. 2018;122(9):1459–64. https://doi.org/10.1016/j.amjcard.2018.07.032.
42. Mjelva ØR, Pönitz V, Brügger-Andersen T, Grundt H, Staines H, Nilsen DW. Long-term prognostic utility of pentraxin 3 and D-dimer as compared to high-sensitivity C-reactive protein and B-type natriuretic peptide in suspected acute coronary syndrome. Eur J Prev Cardiol. 2016;23(11):1130–40. https://doi.org/10.1177/2047487315619733.
43. Gong P, Yang SH, Li S, Luo SH, Zeng RX, Zhang Y, et al. Plasma d-dimer as a useful marker predicts severity of atherosclerotic lesion and short-term outcome in patients with coronary artery disease. Clin Appl Thromb Hemost. 2016;22(7):633–40. https://doi.org/10.1177/1076029616634885.
44. Charoensri N, Pornratanarangsi S. D-dimer plasma levels in NSTE-ACS patient. J Med Assoc Thail. 2011;94(Suppl 1):S39–45.
45. Brügger-Andersen T, Pönitz V, Staines H, Grundt H, Hetland Ø, Nilsen DW. The prognostic utility of D-dimer and fibrin monomer at long-term follow-up after hospitalization with coronary chest pain. Blood Coagul Fibrinolysis. 2008;19(7):701–7. https://doi.org/10.1097/MBC.0b013e32830b1512.
46. Prisco D, Antonucci E, Fedi S, Margheri M, Giglioli C, Comeglio M, et al. D-dimer increase after percutaneous transluminal angioplasty and clinical recurrence after primary revascularization in acute myocardial infarction? A pilot study. Clin Exp Med. 2001;1(4):219–24. https://doi.org/10.1007/s102380100006.
47. Gong X, Lei X, Huang Z, Song Y, Wang Q, Qian J, et al. D-dimer level predicts angiographic no-reflow phenomenon after percutaneous coronary intervention within 2-7 days of symptom onset in patients with ST-segment elevation myocardial infarction. J Cardiovasc Transl Res. 2020;14(4):728–34. https://doi.org/10.1007/s12265-020-09991-6.
48. Cheng C, Liu X-B, Bi S-J, Lu Q-H, Zhang J. Serum cystatin C levels relate to no-reflow phenomenon in percutaneous coronary interventions in ST-segment elevation myocardial infarction. PLoS One. 2019;14(8):e0220654. https://doi.org/10.1371/journal.pone.0220654.
49. Okafor ON, Gorog DA. Endogenous fibrinolysis: an important mediator of Thrombus formation and cardiovascular risk. J Am Coll Cardiol. 2015;65(16):1683–99. https://doi.org/10.1016/j.jacc.2015.02.040.
50. Gershlick AH, Stephens-Lloyd A, Hughes S, Abrams KR, Stevens SE, Uren NG, et al. Rescue angioplasty after failed thrombolytic therapy for acute myocardial infarction. N Engl J Med. 2005;353(26):2758–68. https://doi.org/10.1056/NEJMoa050849.
51. Sambola A, García Del Blanco B, Ruiz-Meana M, Francisco J, Barrabés JA, Figueras J, et al. Increased von Willebrand factor, P-selectin and fibrin content in occlusive thrombus resistant to lytic therapy. Thromb Haemost. 2016;115(6):1129–37. https://doi.org/10.1160/TH15-12-0985.
52. Kloner RA, Ganote CE, Jennings RB. The "no-reflow" phenomenon after temporary coronary occlusion in the dog. J Clin Invest. 1974;54(6):1496–508. https://doi.org/10.1172/JCI107898.
53. Thygesen K, Mair J, Mueller C, Huber K, Weber M, Plebani M, et al. Recommendations for the use of natriuretic peptides in acute cardiac care†: a position statement from the study group on biomarkers in cardiology of the ESC working group on acute cardiac care. Eur Heart J. 2011;33(16):2001–6. https://doi.org/10.1093/eurheartj/ehq509.
54. Ardissino D, Merlini PA, Bauer KA, Galvani M, Ottani F, Franchi F, et al. Coagulation activation and long-term outcome in acute coronary syndromes. Blood. 2003;102(8):2731–5. https://doi.org/10.1182/blood-2002-03-0954.
55. Morelli F, Schol-Gelok S, Arends LR, Boersma E, Kruip M, Versmissen J, et al. Effect of antiplatelet drugs on D-dimer levels: a systematic review and Meta-analysis. J Cardiovasc Pharmacol. 2019;73(6):343–51. https://doi.org/10.1097/FJC.0000000000000670.
56. Ding S, Xu S, Chen X, Wu S. Effects of atorvastatin combined with bivalirudin on coagulation function, cardiac function, and inflammatory factors of percutaneous coronary intervention in elderly patients with acute myocardial infarction. Ann Palliat Med. 2020;9(4):1905–11. https://doi.org/10.21037/apm-20-925.
57. Oldgren J, Budaj A, Granger CB, Khder Y, Roberts J, Siegbahn A, et al. Dabigatran vs. placebo in patients with acute coronary syndromes on dual antiplatelet therapy: a randomized, double-blind, phase II trial. Eur Heart J. 2011;32(22):2781–9. https://doi.org/10.1093/eurheartj/ehr113.
58. Mega JL, Braunwald E, Wiviott SD, Bassand J-P, Bhatt DL, Bode C, et al. Rivaroxaban in patients with a recent acute coronary syndrome. N Engl J Med. 2011;366(1):9–19. https://doi.org/10.1056/NEJMoa1112277.
59. Eikelboom JW, Connolly SJ, Bosch J, Dagenais GR, Hart RG, Shestakovska O, et al. Rivaroxaban with or without aspirin in stable cardiovascular disease. N Engl J Med. 2017;377(14):1319–30. https://doi.org/10.1056/NEJMoa1709118.
60. Carvalho JF, Belo A, Congo K, Neves D, Santos AR, Piçarra B, et al. Left main

and/or three-vessel disease in patients with non-ST-segment elevation myocardial infarction and low-risk GRACE score: prevalence, clinical outcomes and predictors. Rev Port Cardiol. 2018;37(11):911–9. https://doi.org/10.1016/j.repc.2018.03.016.

61. Antoniucci D, Valenti R, Migliorini A, Moschi G, Bolognese L, Cerisano G, et al. Direct infarct artery stenting without predilation and no-reflow in patients with acute myocardial infarction. Am Heart J. 2001;142(4):684–90. https://doi.org/10.1067/mhj.2001.117778.
62. Qin T, Xie L, Chen MH. Meta-analysis of randomized controlled trials on the efficacy and safety of intracoronary administration of tirofiban for no-reflow phenomenon. BMC Cardiovasc Disord. 2013;13(1):68. https://doi.org/10.1186/1471-2261-13-68.
63. Zeng Q, Zhang LD, Wang W. A meta-analysis of randomized controlled trials investigating tirofiban combined with conventional drugs by intracoronary administration for no-reflow prevention. Anatol J Cardiol. 2021;25(1):7–16. https://doi.org/10.14744/AnatolJCardiol.2020.99469.
64. Rossington JA, Sol E, Masoura K, Aznaouridis K, Chelliah R, Cunnington M, et al. No-reflow phenomenon and comparison to the normal-flow population postprimary percutaneous coronary intervention for ST elevation myocardial infarction: case-control study (NORM PPCI). Open Heart. 2020; 7(2):e001215. https://doi.org/10.1136/openhrt-2019-001215.

8

Coexistence of antithrombin deficiency and suspected inferior vena cava atresia in an adolescent and his mother

M. Müller-Knapp[1], C. F. Classen[2], R. Knöfler[3], C. Spang[1,4], C. Hauenstein[5], T. Heinrich[6], F. L. P. Gabriel[7], J. Däbritz[8], D. A. Reuter[4] and J. Ehler[1,4*]

Abstract

Background: Antithrombin deficiency (ATD) is an autosomal dominant thrombophilia presenting with varying phenotypes. In pediatric patients with ATD, thrombosis typically develops during the neonatal period or adolescence. However, to date there are no consistent recommendations on the therapeutic management of children with ATD. Inferior vena cava atresia (IVCA) belongs to a range of congenital or acquired vena cava malformations and is described as an independent risk factor for thrombosis.
The present case report explores two cases of combined ATD and IVCA in an adolescent and his mother.

Case presentation: A 14-year-old male presented with extensive deep venous thromboses (DVTs) of both lower extremities as well as an IVCA. The patient had previously been diagnosed with an asymptomatic ATD without therapeutic consequences at that time. His mother was suffering from an ATD and had herself just been diagnosed with IVCA, too.
The DVTs in the adolescent were treated by systemic anticoagulation and catheter-directed local thrombolysis causing favourable results. Yet, despite adequate oral anticoagulation the DVTs in both lower extremities reoccurred within 1 week after the patient was discharged from hospital. This time, thrombolysis could not be fully achieved. Surprisingly, probing and stenting of the IVCA was achieved, indicating an acquired IVCA which could have occurred after undetected thrombosis in early childhood.
Genetic analyses showed the same mutation causing ATD in both son and mother: heterozygote missense mutation c.248 T > C, p.(Leu83Pro), within the heparin binding domain of antithrombin. This mutation was never reported in mutation databases before.

* Correspondence: johannes.ehler@med.uni-rostock.de
[1]Department of Pediatrics, Interdisciplinary Pediatric Intensive Care Medicine, University Medical Center Rostock, Rostock, Germany
[4]Department of Anesthesiology and Intensive Care Medicine, Interdisciplinary Pediatric Intensive Care Medicine, University Medical Center Rostock, Rostock, Germany

Conclusions: To our knowledge this is the first case report discussing combined ATD and IVCA in two family members. Since ATDs present with clinical heterogeneity, taking a thorough family history is crucial for the anticipation of possible complications in affected children and decisions on targeted diagnostics and therapeutic interventions. Affected families must be educated on risk factors and clinical signs of thrombosis and need an immediate diagnostic workup in case of clinical symptoms. IVCA in patients with ATD could occur due to thrombotic occlusion at a very early age. Therefore, in case of family members with IVCA and ATD ultrasound screening in newborns should be considered.

Keywords: Pediatric hematology, Pediatric thrombophilia, Antithrombin deficiency, Inferior vena cava atresia, Thrombosis, Genetic analysis, Gene mutation

Background

Antithrombin deficiency (ATD) is an autosomal dominant thrombophilia caused by mutations in the *SERPINC1* gene [1, 2]. ATD has a prevalence of 1:2000–5000 [1, 2] and more than 300 different defects with varying phenotypes are currently listed in common mutation databases (ClinVar, HGMD, gnomAD). There are two different types of ATD: patients with quantitative type 1 ATD generally have a higher risk for thrombosis than patients with qualitative type 2 ATD [2, 3]. In pediatric patients with ATD, thrombosis typically develops during the neonatal period or adolescence. Thrombosis tends to be provoked by additional risk factors such as immobilization, and is associated with severe morbidity and mortality [4, 5]. Inferior vena cava atresia (IVCA) belongs to a range of congenital or acquired vena cava malformations and has been observed as a risk factor for thrombosis [6, 7].

Here, we explore two cases of combined ATD and IVCA in an adolescent and his mother and report on new etiologic and therapeutic perspectives concerning this relevant condition.

Case presentation

A 14-year-old male adolescent presented to the emergency department with subfebrile temperatures for 1 week and localized pain in his right popliteal fossa for 3 days. Prior to the onset of these symptoms, he had been immobilized for several days following a minor sports injury.

The adolescent had no permanent medication and no prior medical history except for an asymptomatic ATD diagnosed at the age of six by functional antithrombin assay (antithrombin activity of 57%, age adapted reference: 77–125%). Since at that time, there were no clinical signs of thrombosis, the diagnosis of ATD did not lead to any therapeutic consequences. Screening for ATD at this early age had been carried out on parental request, as his mother was diagnosed with ATD in her early adulthood. Interestingly, his mother now reported that she had very recently been diagnosed with IVCA (preexisting chromogenic test results showed an antithrombin activity of 50% for the mother, the age adjusted reference range being 80 to 130%).

The coexistence of other hereditary thrombophilic disorders in our patient and his mother (protein S deficiency, protein C deficiency, factor V Leiden mutation, prothrombin-mutation, antiphospholipid syndrome) was ruled out by respective laboratory analyses.

Laboratory blood analysis in the emergency department showed markedly elevated D-dimers of 25 mg/l FEU (reference: < 0.5 mg/l FEU) and of C-reactive protein (CrP) of 184 mg/l (reference < 5 mg/l). Antithrombin activity on admission was reduced to 61% (age adjusted reference 83–118%).

A vascular ultrasound examination upon admission confirmed the clinically suspected thrombosis of the right lower extremity involving the external iliac, common and superficial femoral as well as the popliteal vein. The ultrasound examination of the left lower extremity veins did not give evidence of thromboses upon admission. The patient was treated with continuous infusion of unfractionated heparin at a therapeutical dose including several bolus administrations and antithrombin (4000 IE within the first 36 h) was substituted reaching levels in the target range between 80 and 100%. Subsequent monitoring of the activated partial thromboplastin time (aPTT) showed an insufficient response to heparin treatment (aPTT was 29 s before the administration of heparin and did not exceed a maximum value of 33.6 s during heparin treatment). The anticoagulative therapy was therefore switched to direct thrombin inhibition by argatroban at a dose of 1.5–2.0 µg/kg/min, which led to target aPTT values of 50–60s.

Due to the elevated CrP levels and subfebrile temperatures, empirical antibiotic treatment with intravenous cefuroxim was initiated.

A magnetic resonance imaging (MRI) scan on day three confirmed a complete DVT of the right lower extremity, and now additionally extended thromboses of the left lower extremity and thrombosis of both iliac vessels. Furthermore, it revealed an occlusion of the inferior vena cava (IVC) with prominent venous lumbar collaterals, suggestive of IVCA. Surrounding the lumbar vertebrae, several of these collaterals appeared to be fully thrombotic, which was confirmed by angiography (Fig. 1A).

The following day, a catheter-directed local thrombolysis using recombinant tissue plasminogen activator (rt-PA) at a daily dose of 0.25 mg/kg was initiated in both extremities and carried out for a total of 48 h. For the right leg, an additional ultrasound-accelerated thrombolysis using the EKOS® system was performed.

During hospitalization, the anticoagulative therapy was switched from argatroban to the vitamin K antagonist phenprocoumon with a target International Normalized Ratio (INR) of 2.0–2.5. Oral anticoagulation will most likely be continued lifelong due to the combination of extended multilocal thromboses with underlying ATD, as well as IVCA, which in itself is a risk factor for thrombosis.

The patient was discharged on day eight after hospital admission. An ultrasound examination upon discharge showed full recanalization of the femoral and iliac veins of both legs.

During a routine follow-up 1 week later, the patient presented free of any clinical complaints. However, despite continued oral anticoagulation since hospital discharge, vascular ultrasound now revealed extended re-thrombosis of both the right and left pelvic axis and the right lower extremity, thus leading to a second hospital admission and re-induction of therapy with both intravenous antithrombin and catheter-directed thrombolysis.

Recanalization of the right lower extremity and pelvic axis was subsequently achieved, whereby IVC occlusion was confirmed (Fig. 1B). However, the left pelvic vessels remained thrombotic even after 5 days of catheter-directed thrombolysis.

Surprisingly, one of the angiographies allowed for location of the occluded area of the IVC by rendezvous-technique between the superior and inferior vena cava, which prior to this had been thought to be atretic

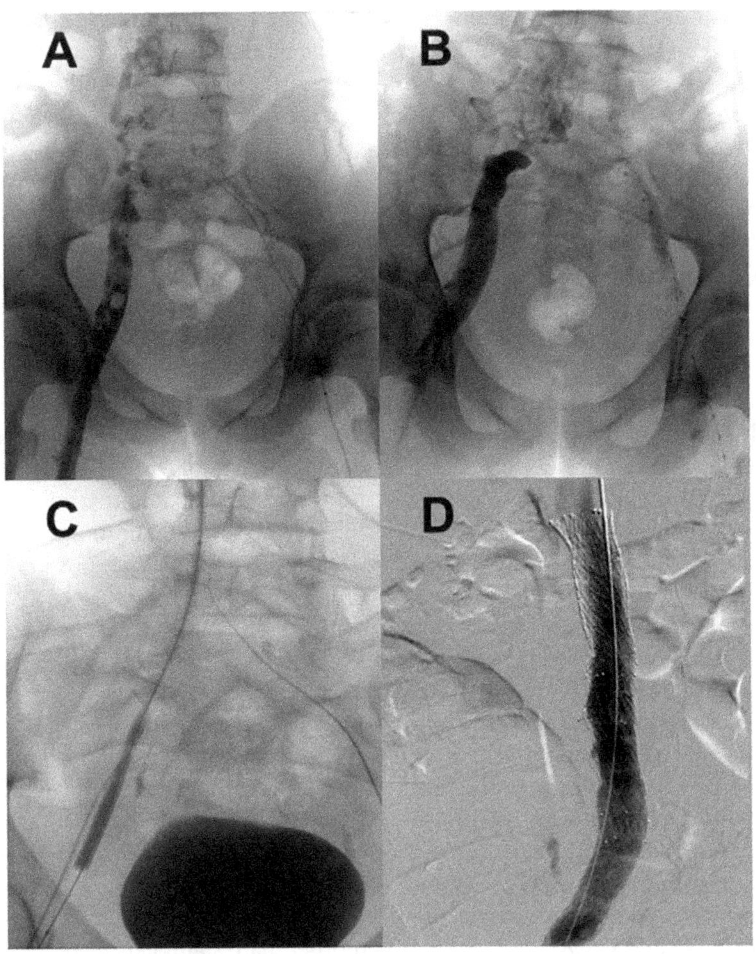

Fig. 1 Angiography images in our 14-year-old patient. **A** Angiography shows a thrombotic right pelvic axis with suspected inferior vena cava atresia and prominent paravertebral collaterals; **B** Angiography confirms inferior vena cava atresia; **C** Location of the occluded inferior vena cava by rendezvous-technique between superior and inferior vena cava; **D** Recanalized inferior vena cava after successful stenting

(Fig. 1C). The vessel was successfully recanalized using balloon dilation and subsequent stenting (Fig. 1D).

Throughout the clinical stay, the patient's oral anticoagulation with phenprocoumon was intensified to a new target INR of 2.5–3.0 in order to prevent re-thrombosis.

The patient was discharged from hospital on day seven after admission. Regular follow-up examinations at our outpatient clinic did not give evidence for any new thrombotic events to date (time since first occurrence of thrombosis was 9 months).

Concerning the thrombotic left iliac vessels, a follow-up angiographic intervention relying on special equipment was performed, but recanalization could not be achieved.

Fortunately, the IVC of the patient's mother could also be recanalized by angiographic intervention.

Discussion and conclusions

In pediatric patients ATD increases the risk for thrombotic events by factor 300, and morbidity and mortality of these thromboses tend to be high [4, 5, 8]. Yet, to date there is a lack of consistent recommendations for the therapeutic management of children affected by ATD [2, 9].

Here, wepresent an impressive case of hereditary ATD in a patient who did not only suffer from extensive thromboses, but also presented with IVCA, which in itself is a known risk factor for thrombosis [6, 7].

During the course of treatment, angiographic recanalization of the patient's IVC was achieved, thus pointing towards an acquired and not congenital IVCA. Retrospectively, an obliteration of the IVC, maybe at an early age and most likely due to thrombosis, has to be discussed. This is supported by the presence of extensive lumbar collaterals which were thrombotic upon admission, thus possibly promoting the recent development of thromboses in the patient's lower extremities.

On this issue, Mabud et al. recently described an association between hereditary thrombophilias and IVCAs, hypothesizing that in many of these combined cases, IVCAs might not represent primary agenesis, but instead arise secondarily due to thrombotic events [10]. This is consistent with previous case reports referring to the rare KILT (kidney and inferior vena cava anomaly with leg thrombosis) syndrome [6]. Most importantly, a recent and large study by de la Morena-Barrio et al. found a high penetrance of IVCAs in patients with the homozygous antithrombin Budapest 3 variant, a form of ATD with generally high risk for thrombosis [11]. To our knowledge, this is the first study showing an association between a specific form of ATD and IVCA.

Thrombotic events that could cause IVCA are most likely to develop during early childhood or the neonatal period, when the risk of thrombosis in patients with ATD is known to be particularly high. These early thrombotic events resulting in subsequent IVCA might not present with typical clinical signs such as bilateral leg swelling due to the relative immobility of the young patients. Thrombosis may therefore be undetected and untreated [10].

During the clinical stay of our patient, intensified reviewing of the family history revealed that the mother of our patient had herself been diagnosed with ATD at the age of 24 years and had suffered multiple extensive thromboses from the age of 12 years onwards. Additionally, she was diagnosed with IVCA just 5 months prior to her son and was awaiting angiography herself.

Genetic analysis in our patient confirmed the same mutation in the *SERPINC1*-gene that had already been detected in his mother (heterozygous missense mutation c.248 T > C, p.(Leu83Pro), within the heparin binding domain of antithrombin; reference transcript: NM_000488.3). To date, this variant has not been reported in mutation databases (ClinVar, HGMD, gnomAD). Following guidelines of the American College of Medical Genetics and Genomics [12] and considering (a) in silico predictions of pathogenicity, (b) functional consequences (antithrombin assay), and (c) familial segregation the variant was classified as "likely pathogenic" (class 4 mutation). One might speculate that initially insufficient therapeutic response to heparin in our patient was influenced by this particular mutation type affecting the heparin binding site.

As mentioned above, antithrombin activity had been reduced to 61% on admission (analysis performed with the INNOVANCE® Anti-Xa assay, age adapted reference 83–118%). To further classify the ATD, a blood sample was sent off for combined analyses of functional antithrombin assay and antithrombin antigen. This sample revealed an antithrombin activity of 40% and antithrombin antigen of 33% (quantified by radial immunodiffusion, age adjusted cutoff 77–125%) thus indicating a type 1 ATD. Concerning the difference in antithrombin activity between the different samples (61% upon admission and 40% during repeat analysis) it is known that antithrombin analyses can be influenced by various factors such as pre-analytical variables or circadian variations [13]. Most importantly antithrombin measurements are not reliable in the acute phase of a thrombotic event and should thus be re-evaluated 3 months after the event (which holds true for the second measurement of antithrombin activity of 40%) [14].

Regarding the preexisting laboratory test results, the mother had significantly reduced antithrombin activity of 50% (via chromogenic assay, age adjusted cutoff 80–130%), too. Antithrombin antigen values were not available.

It is known that hereditary ATDs present with great clinical heterogeneity [1]. Mutations affecting the heparin binding site are generally classified as type II mutations and expected to be associated with medium thrombogenic risk [1], except for antithrombin Budapest 3 *homo*zygotes, where the risk for thrombosis is extremely high. However, this particular mutation shows reduced antithrombin functional activity and reduced antigen levels and is therefore characterized as type I mutation. The substitution of leucine by proline at position 83 affects a relatively conserved residue in the serpin superfamily. This change probably disturbs the folding of the native conformation of antithrombin (due to the conformational rigidity exerted by the proline ring structure) thereby leading to the type I deficiency.

In our adolescent patient, the mutation led to multiple extensive thromboses at the age of 14, which occurred after a short period of immobilization. He later developed re-thrombosis despite adequate anticoagulation and without further risk factors present. We speculate that he possibly suffered from an undetected thrombosis at an early age, resulting in a secondary obliteration of the IVC. Notably, the family history finally revealed a strikingly similar clinical course in his mother, which led us to speculate that she too might have suffered from an undetected early childhood thrombosis leading to obliteration of the IVC.

It has been observed previously that clinical severity for antithrombin heparin binding site mutations significantly depends on the individual pathogenic variant [15] illustrating the complex genotype-phenotype relationship of *SERPINC1* genetic alterations. The missense mutation c.248 T > C, p.(Leu83Pro) identified in the two members of our family (mother and son) was detected in heterozygote state. It is known that homozygosity for *SERPINC1* mutations in type I deficiency and in most type II deficiencies is incompatible with life, whereas homozygosity for specific type II mutations, namely AT Budapest 3 (p.Leu131Phe), is often found in the background of pediatric thrombosis cases, due to the high frequency of this mutation and due to its very severe behavior [16].

To date, there are no guidelines for the therapeutic management of pediatric patients with ATD [2, 9]. However, after carefully reviewing both our clinical case and the related literature, we would like to propose the following cornerstones for the care of (potentially) affected children:

1.) Family history as a base for diagnostic deliberations
ATDs present with great clinical heterogeneity, thus conducting a thorough family history is crucial for anticipation of possible complications in affected children. In case of adults with early and extensive thromboses associated with a proven ATD, the indication for targeted thrombophilia diagnostics in their children should be considered and discussed on an individual basis with respect to potential legal restrictions regarding testing of asymptomatic minors.

2.) Education of affected families and regular clinical monitoring
In case of positive ATD diagnostics in a child, the family should be advised about risk factors for and clinical symptoms of thrombosis. Medical attention should be sought immediately if risk factors or symptoms become present. In case of high risk thrombophilic situations such as complete immobilization for several days after surgical procedures primary prophylactic anticoagulation should be performed.
Thromboses in young children with ATD tend to occur in otherwise uncommon locations (e.g. the renal/ cerebral veins or upper extremities) [3] and this should be taken into account for any symptom constellation in the child.

3.) Prophylactic and therapeutic anticoagulation
Long-term prophylactic anticoagulation in children with asymptomatic ATD is generally not recommended but may be discussed in cases with extensive risk (e.g. uncommon homozygous ATD and elder sibling with catastrophic thrombosis at an early age) [17].
After the first occurrence of thromboses, long-term and possibly lifelong anticoagulation has to be considered.

4.) IVCA as an indicator for highly thrombogenic ATD
To our knowledge, there are only two other case reports describing singular patients with ATD and IVCA to date. Both reports regard the occurrence of ATD and IVCA as unrelated events [7, 18]. However, recent data [10] as well as our clinical case with a suspected IVCA that could be recanalized support the hypothesis that IVCA in thrombophilic patients may not necessarily be due to primary agenesis but instead arise following thrombotic occlusion with subsequent obliteration at an early age.
If parents or other family members with ATD are known to suffer from IVCA, ultrasound screening of newborns should be considered immediately after birth and – in case of asymptomatic ATD – possibly be repeated until the child is fully mobile. This could help to diagnose asymptomatic thromboses of the IVC and enable early treatment in order to prevent significant complications.
In conclusion, the diagnostic and therapeutic management of pediatric patients with ATD should

encompass a multidimensional and multidisciplinary approach.
According to recent publications and our clinical experience, IVCA in patients with ATD should also strongly be considered as a possible residue of a previous thrombotic event.
The specialized diagnostic and therapeutic management including decisions on possible long-term anticoagulation in children should be performed in experienced pediatric centers.

Abbreviations

aPTT: Activated partial thromboplastin time; ATD: Antithrombin deficiency; CrP: C-reactive protein; DVT: Deep venous thrombosis; INR: International Normalized Ratio; IVC: Inferior vena cava; IVCA: Inferior vena cava atresia; MRI: Magnetic resonance imaging; rt-PA: Recombinant tissue plasminogen activator

Acknowledgements

The authors gratefully thank Dr. B. Krammer-Steiner for providing details on the past medical history of the patient's mother.

Authors' contributions

MKM is the main author auf the manuscript and compiled the patient data, did the literature research, collected all data from relevant specialists/ co-authors in the field. She wrote the first draft of the case report and revised the draft according to the co-authors input. *EJ* was supervising MKM at all stages in writing the case report. He provided extensive input on the clinical proceedings regarding the patient. EJ was involved in all communications with other co-authors regarding this manuscript as well as multiple revisions of the manuscript. *CCF* provided hematological input regarding the case report and substantially revised the manuscript. *KR* provided hematological input regarding the case/ ATDs in general, he has been especially involved in the Discussions/Conclusions section of this manuscript and substantially revised the manuscript. *SC* provided input on the clinical care of the patient. He was in close touch with the patient family and was responsible for obtaining the family's consent. *HC* provided detailed input regarding the radiological/angiological aspects and proceedings of the case. She was in charge of the selection of appropriate images regarding the case. *HT* provided detailed input regarding the genetical diagnostics of the patient, possible clinical implications of the genetic diagnostics as well as current deliberations concerning mutations in SERPINC1. *GFLP* provided haematological input regarding coagulation diagnostics performed in our patient. *DJ* substantially revised the manuscript. *RDA* substantially revised the manuscript. All authors read and approved the final manuscript.

Author details

[1]Department of Pediatrics, Interdisciplinary Pediatric Intensive Care Medicine, University Medical Center Rostock, Rostock, Germany. [2]Department of Pediatrics, Oncology and Hematology Unit, University Medical Center Rostock, Rostock, Germany. [3]Department of Pediatrics, Division of Pediatric Hemostaseology, University Hospital Carl Gustav Carus, Technical University Dresden, Dresden, Germany. [4]Department of Anesthesiology and Intensive Care Medicine, Interdisciplinary Pediatric Intensive Care Medicine, University Medical Center Rostock, Rostock, Germany. [5]Institute of Diagnostic and Interventional Radiology, Paediatric Radiology and Neuroradiology, University Medical Center Rostock, Rostock, Germany. [6]MVZ für Humangenetik und Molekularpathologie GmbH, Rostock, Germany. [7]Institute for Clinical Chemistry and Laboratory Medicine, University Medical Center Rostock, Rostock, Germany. [8]Department of Pediatrics, University Medical Center Rostock, Rostock, Germany.

References

1. Corral J, de la Morena-Barrio ME, Vicente V. The genetics of antithrombin. Thromb Res. 2018;169(July):23–9.
2. Kumar R, Chan AKC, Dawson JE, Forman-Kay JD, Kahr WHA, Williams S. Clinical presentation and molecular basis of congenital antithrombin deficiency in children: a cohort study. Br J Haematol. 2014;166(1):130–9.
3. Patnaik MM, Moll S. Inherited antithrombin deficiency: a review. Haemophilia. 2008;14(6):1229–39.
4. de la Morena-Barrio B, Orlando C, de la Morena-Barrio ME, Vicente V, Jochmans K, Corral J. Incidence and features of thrombosis in children with inherited antithrombin deficiency. Haematologica. 2019;104(12):2512–8.
5. Ishiguro A, Ezinne CC, Michihata N, Nakadate H, Manabe A, Taki M, et al. Pediatric thromboembolism: a national survey in Japan. Int J Hematol. 2017; 105(1):52–8.
6. Lauener S, Bütikofer A, Eigenheer S, Escher R. Thrombophlebitis hiding under a KILT - case report on 40 years long-term follow-up of neonatal renal vein thrombosis. BMC Pediatr. 2019;19(1):1–7.
7. Muscianese L, Seese RR, Graham W, Williams JH. Congenital atresia of the inferior vena cava and antithrombin III deficiency in a young adult: compounding risk factors for deep vein thrombosis. BMJ Case Rep. 2015; 2015:bcr2014205729.
8. Bergmann F, Knöfler R. Hereditäre Thrombophilie bei Kindern und Jugendlichen. In: Hoffmann GF, Lentze MJ, Spranger J, Zepp F, Berner R, editors. Pädiatrie: Grundlagen und Praxis. Berlin: Springer Berlin Heidelberg; 2020. p. 1–10.
9. Young G, Albisetti M, Bonduel M, Brandao L, Chan A, Friedrichs F, et al. Impact of inherited thrombophilia on venous thromboembolism in children: a systematic review and meta-analysis of observational studies. Circulation. 2008;118(13):1373–82.
10. Mabud TS, Sailer AM, Swee JKY, Tamboli M, Arendt VA, Jeon GS, et al. Inferior vena cava atresia: characterisation of risk factors, treatment, and outcomes. Cardiovasc Intervent Radiol. 2020;43(1):37–45.
11. de la Morena-Barrio ME, Gindele R, Bravo-Pérez C, Ilonczai P, Zuazu I, Speker M, et al. High penetrance of inferior vena cava system atresia in severe thrombophilia caused by homozygous antithrombin Budapest 3 variant: description of a new syndrome. Am J Hematol. 2021;96(11):1363–73.
12. Richards S, Aziz N, Bale S, Bick D, Das S, Gastier-Foster J, et al. Standards and guidelines for the interpretation of sequence variants: a joint consensus recommendation of the American College of Medical Genetics and Genomics and the Association for Molecular Pathology. Genet Med. 2015; 17(5):405–24.
13. Undar L, Ertuğrul C, Altunbaş H, Akça S. Circadian variations in natural coagulation inhibitors protein C, protein S and antithrombin in healthy men: a possible association with interleukin-6. Thromb Haemost. 1999;81(4): 571–5.
14. Kottke-Marchant K, Duncan A. Antithrombin deficiency: issues in laboratory diagnosis. Arch Pathol Lab Med. 2002;126(11):1326–36.
15. Orlando C, Heylen O, Lissens W, Jochmans K. Antithrombin heparin binding site deficiency: a challenging diagnosis of a not so benign thrombophilia. Thromb Res. 2015;135(6):1179–85.
16. Gindele R, Oláh Z, Ilonczai P, Speker M, Udvari A, Selmeczi A, et al. Founder effect is responsible for the p.Leu131Phe heparin-binding-site antithrombin mutation common in Hungary: phenotype analysis in a large cohort. J Thromb Haemost. 2016;14(4):704–15.
17. Limperger V, Klostermeier UC, Kenet G, Holzhauer S, Alhenc Gelas M, Finckh U, et al. Clinical and laboratory characteristics of paediatric and adolescent index cases with venous thromboembolism and antithrombin deficiency. An observational multicenter cohort study. Thromb Heamostasis. 2014; 112(3):478–85.
18. Bianchi M, Giannini D, Balbarini A, Castiglioni MG. Congenital hypoplasia of the inferior vena cava and inherited thrombophilia: rare associated risk factors for idiopathic deep vein thrombosis. A case report. J Cardiovasc Med. 2008;9(1):101–4.

9

Incidence and characteristics of arterial thromboemboli in patients with COVID-19

Nancy Glober[1†], Lauren Stewart[1†], JangDong Seo[1], Christopher Kabrhel[2], Kristen Nordenholz[3], Carlos Camargo[2] and Jeffrey Kline[4*]

Abstract

Background: Studies have reported COVID-19 as an independent risk factor for arterial thromboemboli.

Methods: From a cross-sectional sample, we determined the incidence and location of arterial thromboemboli (myocardial infarction, ischemic stroke, peripheral artery), stratified by COVID-19 status, in the RECOVER database, which included data on patients at 45 United States medical centers in 22 states. Epidemiological factors, clinical characteristics and outcomes were collected through a combination of individual chart review and automatic electronic query and recorded in REDCap®. We investigated the association of baseline comorbidities on the development of arterial thromboemboli and analyzed results based on the presence or absence of concomitant COVID-19 infection, testing this association with Chi-squared. We also described use of anticoagulants and statins.

Results: Data were collected on 26,974 patients, of which 13,803 (51.17%) tested positive for COVID-19. Incidence of arterial thromboemboli during hospitalization was 0.13% in patients who tested positive for COVID-19 and 0.19% in patients who tested negative. Arterial thromboemboli tended to be more common in extremities than in core organs (heart, kidney, lung, liver) in patients with COVID-19, odds ratio 2.04 (95% CI 0.707 – 5.85). Patients with COVID-19 were less likely to develop an arterial thrombus when on baseline statin medication (p=0.014). Presence of metabolic syndrome predicted presence of core arterial thrombus (p=0.001) and extremity arterial thrombus (p=0.010) in those with COVID-19. Arterial thromboemboli were less common in patients with COVID-19 than in those who tested negative for COVID-19.

Conclusions: Presence of a composite metabolic syndrome profile may be associated with arterial clot formation in patients with COVID-19 infection.

Introduction

Since the beginning of the coronavirus disease 2019 (COVID-19) pandemic, studies have reported increased incidence of arterial thromboemboli, prognosticating poor outcomes in patients infected with COVID-19.[1–5] Researchers speculated that SARS-CoV-2 infects endothelial cells through the angiotensin-converting enzyme 2 receptor leading to arterial thromboemboli.[6, 7] However, reports describing the incidence of arterial thromboemboli vary, [2, 7, 8], and the mechanisms leading to occurrence of arterial thromboemboli in those patients remain unclear.

Many studies investigating arterial thromboemboli are small retrospective studies or case series.[2, 9] As arterial thromboemboli are uncommon,[2] small studies are extremely limited in their ability to describe patterns in those patients. However, though the overall incidence is low, arterial thromboemboli remain a critical complication of infection with COVID-19. Thus, understanding factors contributing to arterial thromboemboli in patients with COVID-19 remains of great importance.

The purpose of this study was to query a large nationwide sample, the REgistry of suspected COVID-19 in EmeRgency care (RECOVER) database, in an effort to

* Correspondence: jkline@wayne.edu
[4]Department of Emergency Medicine, Wayne State University School of Medicine, 4201 St. Antoine, 48201 Detroit, Michigan, United States

describe the incidence and location of arterial thromboemboli. We further described factors associated with the development of arterial thromboemboli and the effect of treatment with anticoagulants and statins. Specifically, we observed the incidence of comorbid metabolic syndrome as well as its associated risk for the development of arterial thromboemboli in COVID-19 infected patients.

Methods

The RECOVER network collected data on Emergency Department (ED) patients at 45 United States medical centers who received diagnostic testing for SARS-CoV-2. Clinical factors and outcomes were documented for all patients with a positive swab molecular test or antibody testing within 30 days. A patient was considered positive for SARs-CoV-2 infection if either a molecular diagnostic test from a swab or serological IgM or IgG antibody test within 30 days was positive. A patient was considered negative for SARs-CoV-2 if in the absence of positive test results or clinical diagnosis of COVID-19 within 30 days. Patients were excluded if the test was done for automated or administrative purposes. Patients were only included in the database once, not multiple times in cases of multiple tests. The institutional review boards (IRBs) at all sites reviewed and approved the RECOVER registry protocol. A more detailed description of overall study methodology has been previously described.[10].

Each site collected data on at least 500 patients through a combination of automated electronic query and individual chart review by emergency medicine clinician-investigators using previously described methods.[10] Data were collected in REDCap®.

We recorded the incidence and location of arterial thromboemboli, stratified by COVID-19 status, and analyzed results using descriptive statistics. We investigated the association of various baseline comorbidities on the development of arterial thrombus and analyzed results based on the presence or absence of concomitant COVID-19 infection, testing this association with the Pearson's Chi-squared. We also described patterns of use of different anticoagulants and statins. Analyses were done with SAS software 9.4 (SAS Institute, Cary, NC).

Results

Data were collected on 26,974 patients, of which 13,803 (51.2%) tested positive for COVID-19. Of those included, 2,743 (10.2%) died, including 2,044 (74.5%) who tested positive and 699 (25.5%) who tested negative. We found significantly higher rates of positive COVID-19 testing among men (54.4% vs. 48.0%, $p<0.001$). Caucasian and African American patients were most commonly tested (Table 1). Patients who tested positive for COVID-19 were older and less likely to be of White race than those who tested negative ($P<0.001$, unpaired t-test and Chi-square, respectively). Of those with a positive COVID-19 test result, 265 (1.9%) were admitted to an observation unit, 2,581 (18.7%) were admitted to a regular or monitored floor, 4,278 (31.0%) were admitted to stepdown or progressive care, and 865 (6.3%) were admitted to an intensive care unit.

As noted in prior studies, we found an increased risk for new venous thromboembolism within 30 days in patients with severe COVID-19 infection, requiring hospitalization ($p<0.001$) (Table 2).

Table 1 Distribution of patient epidemiology and COVID-19 test results

	COVID-19 Test Results					
	Negative		**Positive**		**Total**	
Patient Characteristics	N (n=13,166)	% (48.8)	N (n=13,803)	% (51.2)	N (n=26,974)	% (100)
Gender						
Male	6098	45.6	7289	54.4	13,387	49.6
Female	7073	52.1	6514	48.0	13,587	51.2
Age (mean)	49.63 (SD 20.89)		56.51 (SD 19.46)			
Race						
Asian	392	1.5	414	1.5	806	3.0
Black	2923	10.9	4816	17.9	7739	28.7
Native Hawaiian or Other Pacific Islander	62	0.2	37	0.1	99	0.4
American Indian or Alaskan Native	84	0.3	62	0.2	146	0.5
Multiple Races	31	0.1	11	0.1	42	0.2
Unknown	1701	6.3	4504	16.7	6205	23.0
White	7959	29.5	3948	14.7	11,907	44.2

Table 2 Incidence of acute venous thromboemboli by hospitalization status in patients with or without COVID-19

COVID-19 Status	Venous Thromboemboli	Observation Admission *n*=1028 (%)	Regular or monitored floor admission *n*=9347 (%)	Stepdown or progressive care admission *n*=9018 (%)	Intensive care unit admission *n*=2623 (%)
Negative	**Yes**	7 (0.92)	168 (2.48)	79 (1.67)	85 (4.83)
	No	757 (99.08)	6599 (97.52)	4661 (98.33)	1674 (95.17)
Positive	**Yes**	3 (1.14)	66 (2.56)	64 (1.50)	45 (5.21)
	No	261 (98.86)	2514 (97.44)	4214 (98.50)	819 (94.79)

The incidence of arterial thromboemboli was 0.13% in patients who tested positive for COVID-19 and 0.19% in patients who tested negative. Patients with COVID-19 experienced a greater proportion of arterial thromboemboli in extremities (rather than core organs) as compared to those without COVID-19, although this did not reach statistical significance (Odds Ratio 2.04, 95% CI 0.71 – 5.85) (Table 3). Two patients had two extremity arterial thrombi, whereas the others had one each. Only one patient had two core arterial thrombi, and the others had one each. All arterial clots were found in patients who were hospitalized within 30 days of COVID-19 testing.

Significantly more patients who tested positive for COVID-19 were started on some type of thromboprophylaxis. Of those who tested positive for COVID-19, 4,959 (36.1%) were started on thromboprophylaxis. Of those who tested negative for COVID-19, only 1,143 (8.7%%) were started on thromboprophylaxis ($p<0.001$). Aspirin use was documented in 4261 (15.9%) of patients. Arterial thromboemboli were documented in 25 (0.59%) of patients who were taking aspirin and 41 (0.22%) of patients not taking aspirin ($p<0.001$).

Disseminated Intravascular Coagulation (DIC) was diagnosed in a total of 29 (0.11%) patients, and incidence was not significantly different based on whether or not patients had a positive COVID-19 test (15 vs. 14, $p=0.950$). Ischemic stroke was diagnosed in 164 (0.61%) of all patients, 70 (0.53%) of whom had a negative COVID-19 test, and 94 (0.68%) of whom tested positive ($p=0.115$).

We investigated the association of various baseline comorbidities on the development of arterial thrombus and analyzed results based on the presence or absence of concomitant COVID-19 infection. We found a history of hypertension to be significantly associated with arterial thrombus, with patients with underlying hypertension having a significantly higher risk of developing core thrombi than patients without a history of hypertension, regardless of COVID-19 status (Chi-square, $p=0.001$ in COVID-19 positive and $p=0.001$ in COVID-19 negative). In COVID-19 positive patients, we also noted an association between hypertension and extremity thrombi ($p=0.0174$). The presence of baseline diagnosis of diabetes also was associated with arterial thrombi, although thrombus location depended on COVID-19 status. In COVID-19 positive patients, there was a significant association between diabetes and extremity thrombi ($p=0.003$), while COVID-19 negative patients were found to have an associated between diabetes and core thrombi ($p=0.011$). Hyperlipidemia was positively associated with both core and extremity thrombi, regardless of COVID-19 status. We found no association between obesity and arterial thrombi (Table 4).

Table 3 Incidence of arterial thromboemboli by type in patients with or without COVID-19

	COVID-19 Test Negative *n*= 38 (%)	COVID-19 Test Positive *n*= 25 (%)
Arterial Extremity Thromboemboli	**5**	**11**
Left arm	1 (2.6)	2 (8.0)
Left leg	1 (2.6)	3 (12.0)
Right arm	0 (0.0)	3 (12.0)
Right leg	3 (7.9)	3 (12.0)
Arterial Core Thromboemboli	**33**	**14**
Heart	13 (3.4)	6 (24.0)
Brain	19 (50.0)	6 (24.0)
Kidney	2 (5.3)	0 (0.0)
Intestine	0 (0.0)	2 (8.0)

Table 4 Association of comorbidities with arterial thrombi and COVID status

	Core arterial thrombus present		Extremity arterial thrombus present	
	COVID-19 Test Positive	COVID-19 Test Negative	COVID-19 Test Positive	COVID-19 Test Negative
Hypertension				
Yes	12	24	7	3
No	2	9	2	2
p-value	0.001	0.001	0.017	0.383
Diabetes				
Yes	6	13	6	1
No	8	20	3	4
p-value	0.100	0.011	0.003	0.944
Hyperlipidemia				
Yes	8	17	5	1
No	6	16	4	4
p-value	0.002	0.002	0.020	0.009
Obesity				
Yes	4	6	1	4
No	10	27	7	1
p-value	0.460	0.445	0.572	0.211

We created an additional composite parameter for metabolic syndrome, defined as patients with a documented diagnosis of at least three of the following four conditions: obesity (BMI >30 kg/m^2), hypertension, hyperlipidemia, and diabetes, and examined the effect of metabolic syndrome in patients with arterial thromboemboli. Of the n= 61 patients with arterial thromboemboli, a total of 23 (37.70%) met criteria for composite metabolic syndrome diagnosis. Comparatively, 15.14% of the total population met criteria for metabolic syndrome.

The presence of metabolic syndrome was associated with the development of core arterial thrombus (p= 0.001) and extremity arterial thrombus (p=0.010) in those with COVID-19. Conversely, the absence of metabolic syndrome was associated with core arterial thrombus in those without COVID-19 (p=0.001), but there was no difference in presence of extremity arterial thrombus in those without COVID-19 based on presence or absence of metabolic syndrome (p=0.330) (Table 5).

Table 5 Incidence of extremity or core arterial thromboemboli stratified by COVID-19 status and metabolic syndrome

	COVID-19 Test Negative N (%)	COVID-19 Test Positive N (%)
Extremity Thromboemboli	5	9*
With metabolic syndrome	0 (0.00)	4 (0.20)
Without metabolic syndrome	5 (0.05)	5 (0.04)
Core Thromboemboli	33	14
With metabolic syndrome	12 (0.57)	7 (0.35)
Without metabolic syndrome	21 (0.19)	7 (0.06)

**Two patients had incomplete history leading to inability to conclude whether or not the patients had metabolic syndrome*

Finally, we examined the effect of statin therapy on arterial clots in those patients with metabolic syndrome. We excluded all patients for whom statin therapy status was undocumented (n=1,116, 4.15%). Of all patients included in the study, 5,880 (22.8%) were on statins and 19,830 (77.2%) were not. Of all patients with metabolic syndrome, n= 3,912 (71.14%) were on statins. Of all patients with metabolic syndrome who also had arterial thromboemboli, four were taking statins and one was not.

In patients who were COVID-19 positive, preexisting use of statins was associated with a lower incidence of arterial thromboemboli (p=0.014) (Table 6).

Discussion

This study represents the largest investigation to date of arterial thromboemboli in patients with COVID-19. As such, it adds to existing literature and better characterizes the extent of arterial thromboemboli complicating COVID-19 infection. Overall, we found that arterial thromboemboli were uncommon, precluding a more extensive analysis. However, we were able to describe common features of these patients. Interestingly, COVID-19

Table 6 Incidence of arterial clots in patients with and without COVID-19 as modified by use of statins

		Statin Use		Total
COVID-19 Status	Arterial Thrombus	Yes	No	
Negative	Yes	14 (0.24%)	21 (0.11%)	35
	No	3,042 (51.73%)	9,190 (46.34%)	12,232
	Sub total	3,056 (51.97%)	9,211 (46.45%)	12,267
Positive	Yes	9 (0.15%)	12 (0.06%)	21
	No	2,815 (47.87%)	10,607 (53.49%)	13,422
	Sub total	2,824 (48.03%)	10,619 (53.55%)	13,443
		5,880 (100%)	19,830 (100%)	25,710

positive patients were more likely to sustain a limb arterial thrombosis than those who did not have COVID-19. While the mechanism behind this finding is unclear, this finding could inform understanding of comorbid conditions which predispose patients with SARS-CoV-2 to arterial thromboemboli.

In examination of patients' baseline comorbidities, we found that three of the four components of metabolic syndrome (hypertension, diabetes and hyperlipidemia) likely mediated arterial clots, perhaps more significantly than COVID-19 infection status. This is a critical finding as metabolic syndrome is common [11] and is known to lead to an inflammatory and hypercoagulable state, causing endothelial dysfunction, and subsequent vascular remodeling and thrombosis.[11–13] We did not appreciate additive effects of metabolic syndrome and concurrent COVID-19 infection.

Interestingly, we did not find an association between obesity (the fourth component of metabolic syndrome) and arterial clots. Many studies have shown a paradoxical association of cardiovascular disease and obesity, in which obese patients with strokes or other cardiovascular disease have a better prognosis, including reduced mortality.[14–17] This paradox remains controversial and requires a higher quality of evidence to further clarify, but our results add to prior findings suggesting the need for distinction between obesity alone and a more complete metabolic syndrome profile.

Results of this large nationwide study indicate that baseline use of statins to control metabolic syndrome risk factors may lead to reduced risk of arterial thromboembolism in patients with new COVID-19 diagnosis, although overall numbers are small and need to be further studied.

Limitations

This represents a retrospective secondary analysis of a prospective registry study. Not all patients were tested for arterial thromboemboli, as testing occurred at physician discretion. Therefore, it is possible that some arterial thromboemboli were not detected. Further, because the overall numbers of patients with arterial thromboemboli were so small, we were unable to perform a statistically meaningful multiple regression analysis, thus limiting our analysis to describing trends with Chi-squared tests. Potential bias exists in testing patients for COVID-19 because they required admission to the hospital. Patients admitted for ischemic stroke or myocardial infarction, for example, but with relatively few risk factors for COVID-19 infection could disproportionately fall into the COVID-19 negative cohort, inflating the incidence of arterial thromboemboli in that cohort.

Conclusions

In a patient with newly diagnosed COVID-19 infection, there does not appear to be an increased risk of arterial thromboemboli. Presence of a composite metabolic syndrome profile may be associated with arterial clot formation.

Acknowledgements
none.

Authors' contributions
NG and LS wrote the manuscript and performed data analysis. JDS performed data analysis. CK, KN, and CC collected the data and edited the manuscript. JK conceived of the idea, supervised the project including data collection, cleaned the data as noted in the RECOVERY database, and edited the manuscript. The author(s) read and approved the final manuscript.

Author details
[1]Indiana University, Indianapolis, Indiana, United States. [2]Harvard Medical School, Boston, Massachusetts, United States. [3]University of Colorado Anschutz Medical Campus, Colorado, Aurora, United States. [4]Department of Emergency Medicine, Wayne State University School of Medicine, 4201 St. Antoine, 48201 Detroit, Michigan, United States.

References

1. Tang N, Li D, Wang X, Sun Z. Abnormal coagulation parameters are associated with poor prognosis in patients with novel coronavirus pneumonia. J Thromb Haemost. 2020;18(4):844–7.
2. Indes JE, Koleilat I, Hatch AN, Choinski K, Jones DB, Aldailami H, et al. Early experience with arterial thromboembolic complications in patents with COVID-19. J Vasc Surg. 2020.

3. Zhou F, Yu T, Du R, Fan G, Liu Y, Liu Z, et al. Clinical course and risk factors for mortality of adult inpatients with COVID-19 in Wuhan, China: a retrospective cohort study. Lancet. 2020;395(10229):1054–62.
4. Guan WJ, Ni ZY, Hu Y, Liang WH, Ou CQ, He JX, et al. Clinical Characteristics of Coronavirus Disease 2019 in China. N Engl J Med. 2020;382(18):1708–20.
5. Huang C, Wang Y, Li X, Ren L, Zhao J, Hu Y, et al. Clinical features of patients infected with 2019 novel coronavirus in Wuhan, China. Lancet. 2020;395(10223):497–506.
6. Obi AT, Tignanelli CJ, Jacobs BN, Arya S, Park PK, Wakefield TW, et al. Empirical systemic anticoagulation is associated with decreased venous thromboembolism in critically ill influenza A H1N1 acute respiratory distress syndrome patients. J Vasc Surg Venous Lymphat Disord. 2019;7(3):317–24.
7. Bellosta R, Luzzani L, Natalini G, Pegorer MA, Attisani L, Cossu LG, et al. Acute limb ischemia in patients with COVID-19 pneumonia. J Vasc Surg. 2020;72(6):1864–72.
8. Lameijer JRC, van Houte J, van Berckel MMG, Canta LR, Yo LSF, Nijziel MR, et al. Severe arterial thromboembolism in patients with Covid-19. J Crit Care. 2020;60:106–10.
9. Abou-Ismail MY, Diamond A, Kapoor S, Arafah Y, Nayak L. Corrigendum to "The hypercoagulable state in COVID-19: Incidence, pathophysiology, and management" [Thromb. Res., 194, October 2020, Pages 101-115]. Thromb Res. 2020.
10. Kline J, Pettit K, Kabrhel C, Courtney D, Nordenholz K, Camargo C. Multicenter registry of United States emergency department patients tested for SARS-CoV-2. Journal of the American College of Emergency Physicians2020.
11. Franchini M, Targher G, Montagnana M, Lippi G. The metabolic syndrome and the risk of arterial and venous thrombosis. Thromb Res. 2008;122(6): 727–35.
12. Dentali F, Squizzato A, Ageno W. The metabolic syndrome as a risk factor for venous and arterial thrombosis. Semin Thromb Hemost. 2009;35(5):451–7.
13. Prandoni P. Venous and Arterial Thrombosis: Is There a Link? Adv Exp Med Biol. 2017;906:273–83.
14. Lavie CJ, Milani RV, Patel D, Artham SM, Ventura HO. Disparate effects of obesity and left ventricular geometry on mortality in 8088 elderly patients with preserved systolic function. Postgrad Med. 2009;121(3):119–25.
15. Lavie CJ, Milani RV, Ventura HO. Obesity and cardiovascular disease: risk factor, paradox, and impact of weight loss. J Am Coll Cardiol. 2009;53(21): 1925–32.
16. Forlivesi S, Cappellari M, Bonetti B. Obesity paradox and stroke: a narrative review. Eat Weight Disord. 2021;26(2):417–23.
17. Quiñones-Ossa GA, Lobo C, Garcia-Ballestas E, Florez WA, Moscote-Salazar LR, Agrawal A. Obesity and Stroke: Does the Paradox Apply for Stroke? Neurointervention. 2021;16(1):9–19.

10

Replacement of traditional prothrombin time monitoring with the new Fiix prothrombin time increases the efficacy of warfarin without increasing bleeding

Pall T. Onundarson[1*], Ragnar Palsson[2], Daniel M. Witt[3] and Brynja R. Gudmundsdottir[4]

Abstract

The antithrombotic effect of vitamin K antagonists (VKA) depends on controlled lowering of the activity of factors (F) II and X whereas reductions in FVII and FIX play little role. PT-INR based monitoring, however, is highly influenced by FVII, which has the shortest half-life of vitamin K-dependent coagulation factors. Hence, variability in the anticoagulant effect of VKA may be partly secondary to an inherent flaw of the traditional monitoring test itself. The Fiix prothrombin time (Fiix-PT) is a novel test that is only sensitive to reductions in FII and FX and is intended to stabilize the VKA effect. Two clinical studies have now demonstrated that when warfarin is monitored with the Fiix-PT based normalized ratio (Fiix-NR) instead of PT-INR, anticoagulation is stabilized and less testing and fewer dose adjustments are needed. Furthermore, the relative risk of thromboembolism was reduced by 50–56% in these studies without an increase in major bleeding.

Keywords: Warfarin, Oral anticoagulation, Monitoring, Fiix, Prothrombin time

Introduction

From their advent, 70 years ago, the effect of vitamin K antagonists (VKAs) has been monitored by measuring the prothrombin time (PT), either Quick or Owren type [1, 2], that equally reflect reductions in vitamin K-dependent (VKD) coagulation factors (F) II, VII or X but not FIX [3, 4] to effectively prevent and treat thromboembolism (TE) [5, 6]. However, the pharmacodynamic effect of PT-monitored warfarin (hereafter referred to as PT-warfarin) is quite variable in many patients. International standardization of PT ratios for the purpose of VKA monitoring, leading to the international normalized ratio (INR, hereafter referred to as PT-INR) [7], has not reduced intra-individual anticoagulation variability that is mainly blamed on food and drug interactions and patient non-adherence.

In this article, we argue that the reasons for using the PT to monitor VKAs are primarily historical. Based on knowledge that accumulated after the development of the PT, it can be questioned whether the most relevant anticoagulant effect of VKAs has been monitored throughout the decades of their use. This article reviews recent data suggesting that the PT-INR suboptimally reflects the anticoagulant effect of warfarin and that anticoagulation outcomes can be improved considerably by monitoring a different effect, namely only the influence of FII and FX [3, 8, 9] while ignoring FVII and FIX.

* Correspondence: pallt@landspitali.is
[1]Central Laboratory/Hematology, Landspitali National University Hospital of Iceland and University of Iceland Faculty of Medicine, Hringbraut, 101 Reykjavik, Reykjavik, Iceland

Efficacy and safety of current oral anticoagulants

In accordance with recent clinical guidelines [10, 11], the unmonitored newer direct oral anticoagulants (DOACs) have increasingly replaced warfarin as first-line anticoagulants in non-valvular atrial fibrillation (AF) and venous thromboembolism (VTE). In addition to convenience, this practice-shift is mainly based on pharmaceutical industry initiated clinical trials that have concluded that DOACs are at least similarly effective as warfarin that is dosed based on traditional PT-warfarin monitoring and that DOACs carry lower risk of intracranial hemorrhage [12, 13]. However, PT-warfarin has been found to be more effective and safer than DOACs in high thrombogenic-risk patients with mechanical heart valves [14] or triple-positive antiphospholipid antibody syndrome [15–17] and possibly as well following anterior wall myocardial infarction [18]. If PT-warfarin has advantages over DOACs in high-risk patients, why not also in patients that are at lower risk? Poor warfarin management, i.e. low time within target INR range (TTR), associates with high risk of TE, bleeding and mortality [5, 19–21]. Is it possible that poor PT-warfarin management or other quality issues in the control groups of the DOAC trials (e.g. low TTR) influenced the study outcomes? Some published data suggest so [22–24]. Furthermore, two real-world practice studies involving 130,911 and 196,061 patients have suggested that PT-warfarin may actually be more effective in clinical practice than are the DOACs. The authors of those studies suggest that the benefit of reduced intracranial bleeding with DOACs has been overemphasized as it may be at the cost of more thromboembolism due to lower anticoagulation level [25, 26].

There is little argument that DOACs have the major advantage of not needing to be routinely monitored. However, warfarin patients with very stable INR control can safely go up to 12-weeks between PT-INR tests [27]. Therefore, if the effectiveness and stability of warfarin could be further improved then further comparative effectiveness studies would at least seem warranted.

Prothrombin time based VKA monitoring; history

The Quick-PT, invented in 1935 [1], in its original form mixed undiluted thromboplastin of rabbit brain origin and calcium chloride into citrated patient plasma and the ensuing clotting ("prothrombin") time was measured. At the time, it was only known to be affected by a reduction in either of two then known coagulation factors, i.e., fibrinogen (FI) or prothrombin (FII), only the latter being a VKD factor. PT monitoring made VKA use possible in humans around 1950. Two new factors influencing the PT had then just been discovered, the non-VKD FV [28] and proconvertin (FVII) [2, 29]. For the purpose of VKA monitoring, Owren modified the PT in order to eliminate the influence of reduced non-VKD factors (fibrinogen or FV) on the PT [2]. Two further VKD coagulation factors, FIX and FX, only the latter of which influences Quick PT and Owren PT, were described in the 1950s [30, 31]. Over the ensuing decades the common wisdom was that an equal reduction in all VKD factors was necessary for full VKA anticoagulation, although it was considered sufficient to monitor only reductions in three out of the four, namely FII, FVII and FX.

Thromboplastins from different sources have different "strengths"; a strong thromboplastin has a short clotting time and does not detect the VKA effect as accurately as the more "sensitive thromboplastins" that have longer clotting times. Due to major differences observed in PT ratios, obtained from the same test plasmas from patients managed with VKAs with different thromboplastins, PT-ratios were later standardized as international normalized ratios (INR, PT-INR) [7]. This finally made the anticoagulation level comparable between clinical laboratories despite use of different thromboplastins and instruments [7]. Nevertheless, the use of a sensitive thromboplastin is generally recommended for VKA monitoring. The implementation of PT-INR worldwide improved the efficacy, safety and comparability of VKA management but did not solve the problem of high intra-individual variability.

Target ranges and the therapeutic window

VKAs need monitoring of their anticoagulant effect. Although inconvenient, monitoring has benefits such as improving drug adherence [32] and providing the ability to identify food and drug interactions that remain obscure for the DOACs. Measuring a biological effect in blood has also led to an understanding of the relationship between PT-INR variability, TE and bleeding and it is universally accepted that VKAs have a narrow therapeutic window [5]. Over the decades, a consensus has been reached empirically on standard (2.0–3.0) and high intensity (2.5–3.5) PT-INR target ranges, the latter being used mainly for those with mechanical heart valves [5]. A low and in the authors' opinion too narrow target range of 1.5–2.0 was shown to be less effective than a range of 2.0–3.0 in VTE [33]. Although a target range is a different concept from a therapeutic range, calculating the time that the PT-INR stays within specified target ranges (TTR) has turned out to be a useful surrogate measure of likely efficacy and safety during VKA therapy [19, 21]. Other informative variability measures include variance growth rate (VGR) [34–36], monitoring testing frequency, and dose change frequency [36, 37].

VKA dose

The daily dose of warfarin varies from 0.5 to 20 mg daily between patients and this causes problems during initiation [38]. The dose is influenced by hereditary metabolic differences in sensitivity to VKA action but the daily dose requirement is also influenced by vitamin K supply from food and colonic bacteria [5, 6, 38]. However, the likely dose range needed for each patient becomes evident during the first treatment weeks. Once the dose range is established the main difficulty becomes variable PT-INR that influences the TTR.

Factors adversely influencing the ability to maintain stable warfarin dosing include geographical and cultural differences (e.g. distance from clinical laboratories, health insurance issues, dietary practices) and patient factors such as drug interactions, genetic factors, female gender, age, presence of chronic disorders such as heart failure, variable vitamin K intake, high PT-INR target (≥3), sudden change in lifestyle and poor adherence. Factors that associate with high TTR and favorable clinical outcome include dosing by specialized staff, self-management using portable INR monitors, formal dosing algorithms, and use of dosing software [5, 6]. Finally, studies on the value of genotyping cytochrome P450 2C9 or the VKOR genes at the initiation of VKA therapy have yielded conflicting results and continue to be debated [38, 39]. Although predictive of dose, the usefulness of genotyping during long-term anticoagulation is unknown.

PT-INR variability

The variable anticoagulant effect of VKAs as indicated by the PT-INR may be the single most problematic feature of VKA management following the initiation phase. PT-INR variability is assumed to correctly reflect antithrombotic effect variability and, therefore, leads to dose adjustments, repeat testing and further dose adjustments. Furthermore, variable PT-INR associates with occurrence of both TE and bleeding [34, 35, 37]. PT-INR variability is usually blamed on food and drug interactions or patient non-adherence [5, 6, 40]. The question has, however, been raised whether the perceived variability in the antithrombic effect when measured as PT-INR could be partly due to the PT-test being affected by a factor that confounds anticoagulation assessment and dosing, namely FVII.

The PT-INR is similarly affected by reduced concentrations of FII, FVII or FX (Fig. 1A) [3]. The very short half-life of FVII (4–6 h) leads to this particular factor having a major influence on the PT-INR in the short term, e.g. during initiation, after dose changes, and when dose changes are made repeatedly within short time intervals. As further discussed later, it should be noted that during stable PT-warfarin management the percent normal activity levels of FII, FVII, FIX and FX differ considerably, i.e. FII 27 (95% range 15–40), FVII 48 (18–79), FIX 61 (32–89) and FX 15 [11–19] [41]. The activity range variation is higher for FVII and FIX which may reflect their shorter half-lives, 4–6 h and 21–30 h, respectively, than those of factors and II and X, 42–72 h and 27–48 h, respectively.

The antithrombotic effect of warfarin

The assumed need to reduce all VKD coagulation factors similarly to obtain a full anticoagulant effect of VKAs has been questioned for decades. First, in the 1980's Furie and Furie published studies suggesting that monitoring the native prothrombin antigen was a more

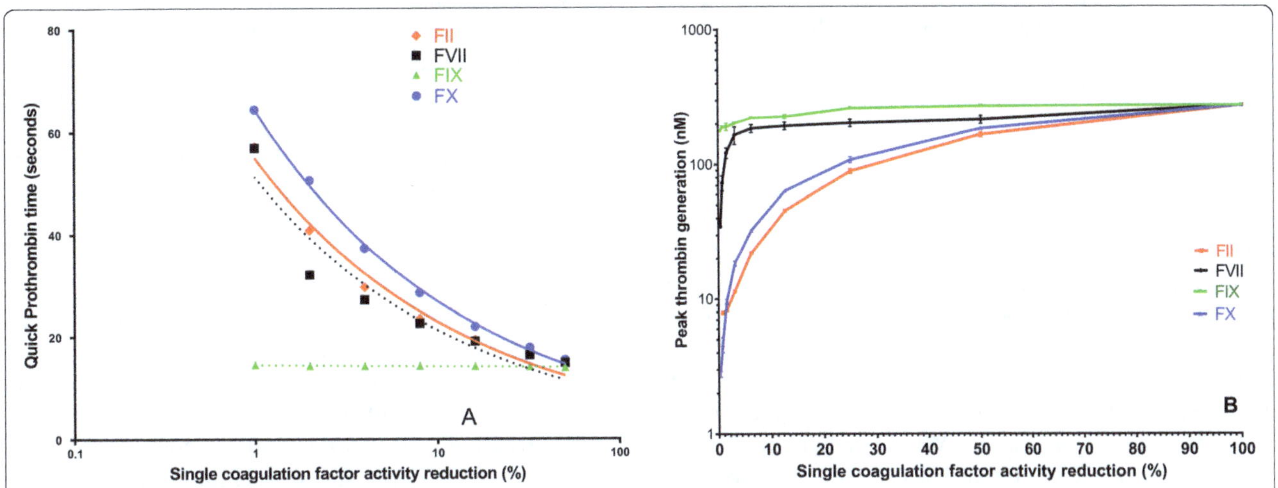

Fig. 1 Influence of selective reduction in vitamin K dependent factors, a single factor at a time while others remain within normal range, on the undiluted Quick prothrombin time (Neoplastin with ISI 1.3, Stago, Asnieres, France: panel A) and and automated peak thrombin generation with clotting activated with a diluted thromboplastin (Neoplastin diluted 1:17,000: panel B) The figures are reproduced with permission from Thrombosis Research 2012;130:674–81 [3] and Journal of Thrombosis and Haemostasis 2016;15:131–9, respectively [41].

effective monitoring method of warfarin than the PT ratio which was, however, poorly standardized at the time [42, 43]. Second, in vitro experiments demonstrated that thrombin generation was linearly dependent on the prothrombin concentration at any activity level and also dependent on FX concentration at activity levels < 25–30% but almost independent of the activity of FVII and FIX unless their activity was markedly reduced to << 5% [8]. Third, animal experiments demonstrated that the antithrombotic effect of warfarin depends on reductions in FII and FX and that reductions in FVII and FIX have little role at concentrations expected during therapeutic VKA anticoagulation [9]. Finally, these conclusions were confirmed by in vitro experiments suggesting a similar effect of reductions in FII and FX but not of FVII or FIX on automated thrombin generation and ROTEM clot formation [3, 41]. Based on those experiments, at the activity levels of VKD factors present during maintenance phase warfarin anticoagulation [41] only FII (15–40 u/dL) and FX (11–19 u/dL) would be expected to significantly reduce thrombin generation in vitro (Fig. 1B).

Is the PT-INR partly to blame for PT-warfarin anticoagulation instability?

Based on the discussion in the previous sections the following issue emerges: The PT-INR that has been the basis of all therapeutic VKA use for seven decades is highly sensitive to reductions of a VKD coagulation factor (FVII) that has little role in bringing about the required antithrombotic effect. Furthermore, due to FVII's much shorter half-life than that of VKD factors II and X, it is a major cause of short-term variability in the measured PT-INR effect, even within a day. If only FII and X reductions matter, monitoring FVII has little meaningful role but confounds assessment as it exaggerates food and drug interactions and day to day variations in the drug effect.

The Fiix prothrombin time and Fiix normalized ratio (Fiix-NR)

Experimental basis

Our group (PTO, BRG) hypothesized that by ignoring FVII in addition to FIX and measuring only the influence of FII and FX reductions during warfarin monitoring, anticoagulation variability could be decreased, potentially to a degree favorably affecting the efficacy and/or safety of VKA management. In turn a new modified PT was designed that is only sensitive to reductions in FII or FX, called Fiix-PT (pronounced "fix PT") [3]. The new Fiix-test is not affected by reduced fibrinogen, FV or FVII but only by reductions in factors FII or FX as FIIX-deficient plasma is mixed into diluted test plasma, thereby normalizing all factor levels except those of FII and FX [3, 41]. Other coagulation activators can also be used but when thromboplastin is used to initiate clotting, the Fiix test principle can also be achieved by adding FII, FIX and FX deficient plasma to the test sample and bioequivalent results will be obtained, namely measuring only the influence of FII and FX. A Fiix normalized ratio (Fiix-NR) can then be calculated based on the Fiix-PT ratio in a manner identical to the traditional PT based international normalized ratio (INR, PT-INR) using standards traceable to the WHO international sensitivity index (ISI) standards [7, 44].

The Quick-PT and the Owren's PT have previously been shown to correlate excellently with each other [4]. In samples drawn during stable warfarin management, the Fiix-NR has been shown to correlate well with both the Quick-PT based INR (R^2 0.91x; y = 0,91 + 0,20; 49 samples) and the Owren's PT based INR (R^2 = 0.92; y = 0.95x + 0.05; 60 samples These previously unpublished data from the study of Gudmundsdottir BR et al. 2012 [3] are shown in Fig. 2 A and B. On the other hand, during warfarin initiation and when factor VII is low for any reason the PT-INR and the Fiix-NR may diverge as illustrated in Fig. 3 [3]..

Fiixing warfarin management

The Fiix trial

To test the hypothesis, in an investigator initiated single-center double-blind randomized non-inferiority clinical trial, named the Fiix-trial [35] mostly warfarin-experienced patients with typical mixed indications for anticoagulation were randomized to either Fiix-NR monitoring (Neoplastin and Fiix-deficient plasma, *n* = 573) or standard Quick PT-INR monitoring (Neoplastin, *n* = 575). Fiix-NR or PT-INR (depending on blinded assignment) measured in the central laboratory was reported as a blinded "research INR" to patients, dosing staff and event adjudicators. After a median follow-up of 1.7 years, Fiix-NR anticoagulation variability (variance growth rate) [34], was reduced, TTR was higher (84 vs 80%), and testing and dose adjustments were reduced. Furthermore, a 48% statistically non-inferior reduction was observed in thromboembolic events in Fiix-warfarin patients compared to the PT-warfarin controls (Fig. 4A). As reduced TE became evident only 180 days after the laboratory switched to Fiix-NR monitoring, a post-hoc analysis was performed after excluding the first 180 days and then a statistically superior 59% reduction in TE was observed ($P_{superiority}$ = 0.0307). Despite improved efficacy, major bleeding (MB) was not increased (2.3% per person year in both study arms). With Fiix monitoring, dose change frequency and INR variability were reduced and TTR increased as well, all statistically significantly so. Overall, the Fiix-trial confirmed the hypothesis that the PT-INR is a source of warfarin anticoagulation variability. Further analysis confirmed that higher variability associated with adverse outcomes [37]. One interpretation of these results is that Fiix-warfarin patients have a more consistent anticoagulation level than PT-warfarin patients leading

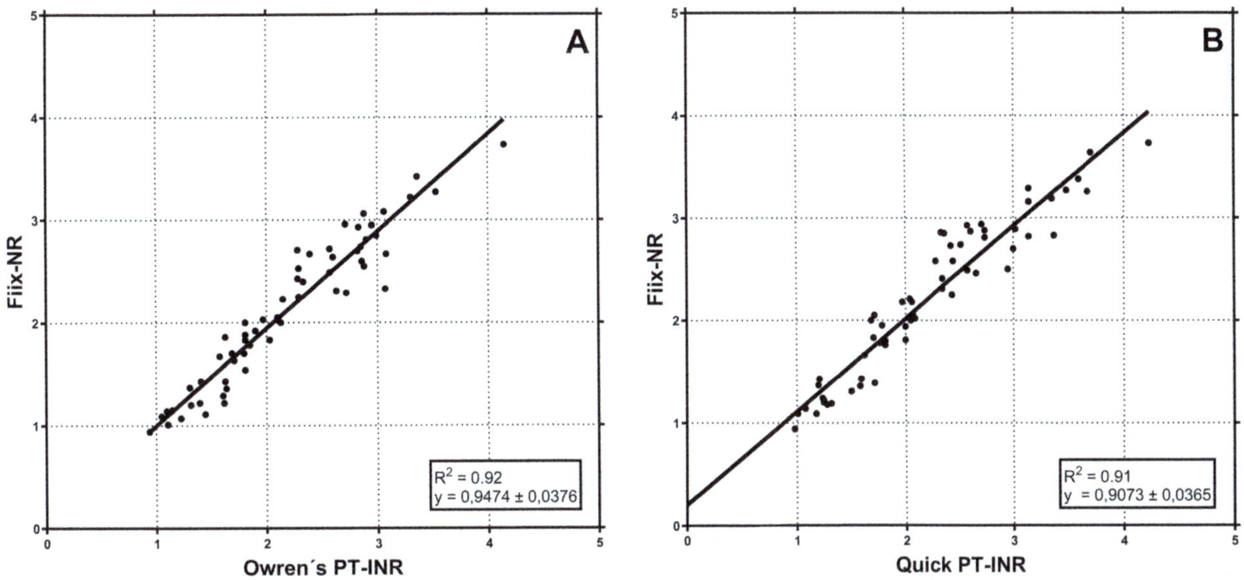

Fig. 2 Correlation of Fiix-normalized ratio with undiluted Owren's PT-INR (SPA, Stago, Asnieres, France: upper panel) or undiluted Quick PT-INR (Neoplastin, Stago, Asnieres, France: lower panel) in samples from patients on stable warfarin therapy. Previously unpublished data from the study described in Thrombosis Research 2012;130:674–81 [3].

to reduced TE but that reduced variability at the same time may prevent a simultaneous increased bleeding risk.

Meta-analysis comparing Fiix-warfarin to PT-warfarin and DOACs in non-valvular atrial fibrillation

Using meta-analytic methods [45], outcomes of Fiix-trial patients with non-valvular AF monitored with PT-warfarin ($n = 427$) or Fiix-warfarin ($n = 406$) were compared to the outcomes of patients with non-valvular AF on PT-warfarin ($n = 29{,}272$) or on rivaroxaban, apixaban, edoxaban, or dabigatran (n = 42,411) in the pivotal pharmaceutical company initiated RCTs [46–49]. The reported adverse events´ incidence of PT-warfarin control groups in all included trials was similar. This analysis found a statistically significant 49% reduction in composite stroke, systemic embolism or myocardial

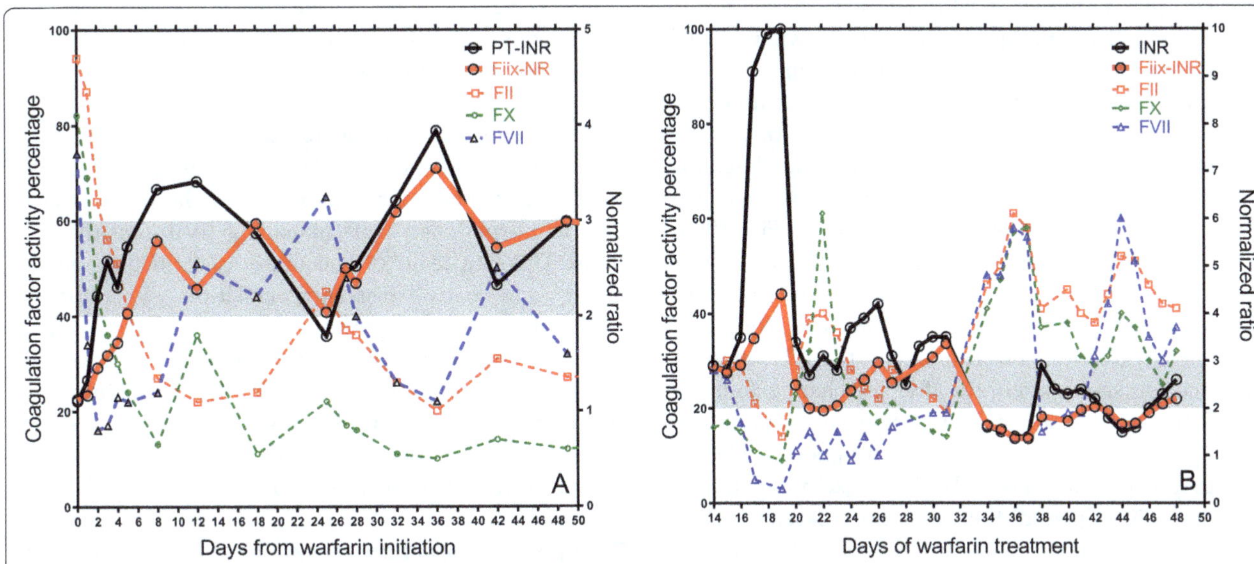

Fig. 3 Examples of differences in PT-INR and Fiix-NR during warfarin initiation when factor VII is fluctuating due to dose changes. Both the PT-INR and Fiix-NR were measured using undiluted Neoplastin CI Plus with ISI 1.3 (Diagnostica Stago, Asnieres, France) but in the Fiix-NR measurement factor II and X deficient plasma is added to diluted test plasma prior to addition of Neoplastin. Reproduced with permission from Thrombosis Research 2012;130:674–81 [3]

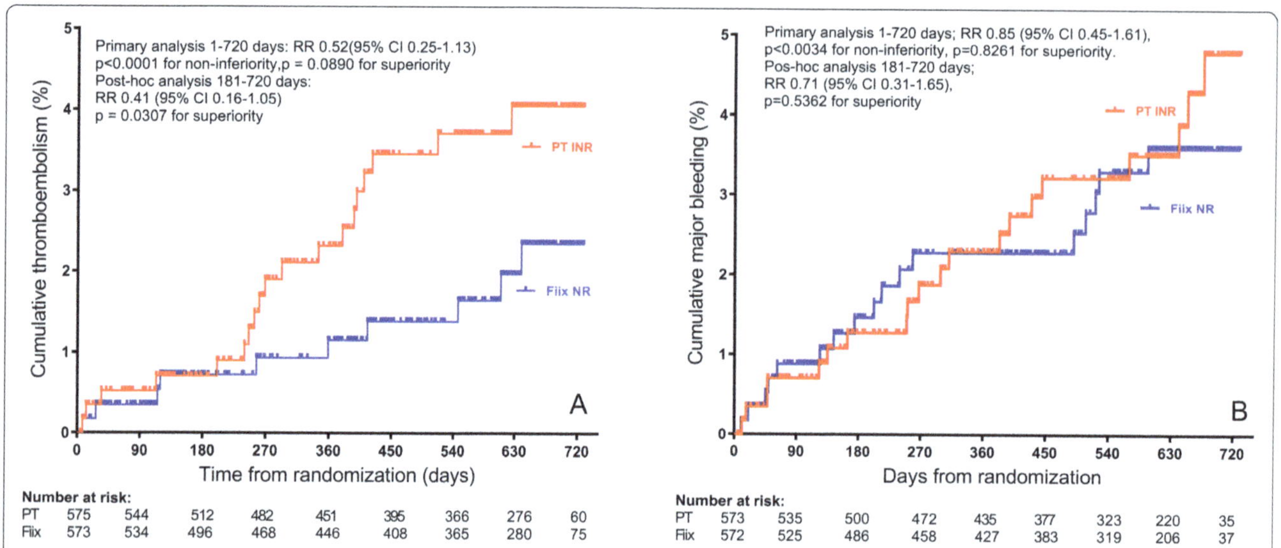

Fig. 4 Cumulative non-fatal and fatal thromboembolic events (panel A) and major bleeding (panel B) during treatment days 1–720 of the randomized double blind Fiix trial in patients monitored either with Fiix-warfarin (blue) or PT-warfarin (red). Reproduced with permission from The Lancet Haematology 2015;2:e231-e40 [35].

infarction (MI) in Fiix-warfarin patients when compared to outcome with PT-warfarin control patients in these trials. MB was numerically 37% lower but this finding was non-significant. Point estimates suggested that Fiix-warfarin might also compare favorably to the pooled clinical outcome with the combined DOAC drugs with a 39% reduction in composite stroke or systemic embolism (SSE) or MI and 24% fewer major bleeds but due to limited power these findings were non-significant.

Fiix in real world practice

After completing the Fiix-trial in February 2014, all warfarin patients at the Reykjavik center were switched back to the prior Owren's type PT-INR monitoring. All were then transitioned to Fiix-NR monitoring beginning on July 1st 2016. The effect of the transition was then retrospectively assessed [36]. This real-world single-cohort interrupted time series study assessed the incidence of TE and MB in 2667 patients and compared Fiix-NR to Owren's PT-INR. Incidence was assessed at monthly intervals during 12 months prior to and 18 months after laboratory switching to Fiix-NR monitoring. Using two-segmented regression, a breakpoint in total TE monthly incidence was seen six months after the change, followed by a 56% reduction in total TE incidence (from 2.82 to 1.23% per patient year, $P = 0.019$; number needed to treat to prevent one TE = 63). After excluding this 6-month transition period, there was no difference in MB between the 12-month Fiix-period (2.3%) and the 12-month PT-period (2.7%, $p = 0.25$). A separate analysis showed that Fiix-monitoring significantly reduced testing, dose adjustments and normalized ratio variability by about one third and increased TTR as well albeit to a minor degree ($P = 0.0157$). A further analysis shown in Fig. 5 demonstrated that the relative risk of suffering any TE, was reduced to 0.45 (0.27–0.75) during Fiix-NR compared to PT-INR monitoring and even more in patients treated long-term. The relative risk of suffering major bleeding was not significantly reduced in that analysis (0.80 (0.53–1.21).

The results of this pre-post study were similar to the Fiix-trial results. Together the two clinical studies suggest that Fiix-NR monitoring is an improvement over monitoring with two standard but different thromboplastin reagents, namely Neoplastin (Quick PT-INR, rabbit brain, ISI 1.3) and the SPA reagent (Owren's PT-INR, rabbit brain, ISI 1.1).

Fiix-warfarin initiation dose protocol

During warfarin initiation, Fiix-NR changes will be observed later than most physicians might predict based on their experience with managing FVII sensitive PT-INRs. This can lead to inaccurate warfarin dose adjustments and early over-anticoagulation. Therefore, a modified initiation algorithm must be used (Table 1) that prevents early over-anticoagulation during Fiix-warfarin initiation [44]. However, during maintenance Fiix-warfarin treatment, the dosing algorithm designed for PT-warfarin patients is appropriate as this did associate with favorable outcomes in our studies [35, 36].

Other possible uses of the Fiix test: the dilute Fiix-PT (dFiix-PT)

Measuring DOAC anticoagulant effect may have useful applications [50] but no single test can be used for this purpose [50]. A test using highly diluted thromboplastin,

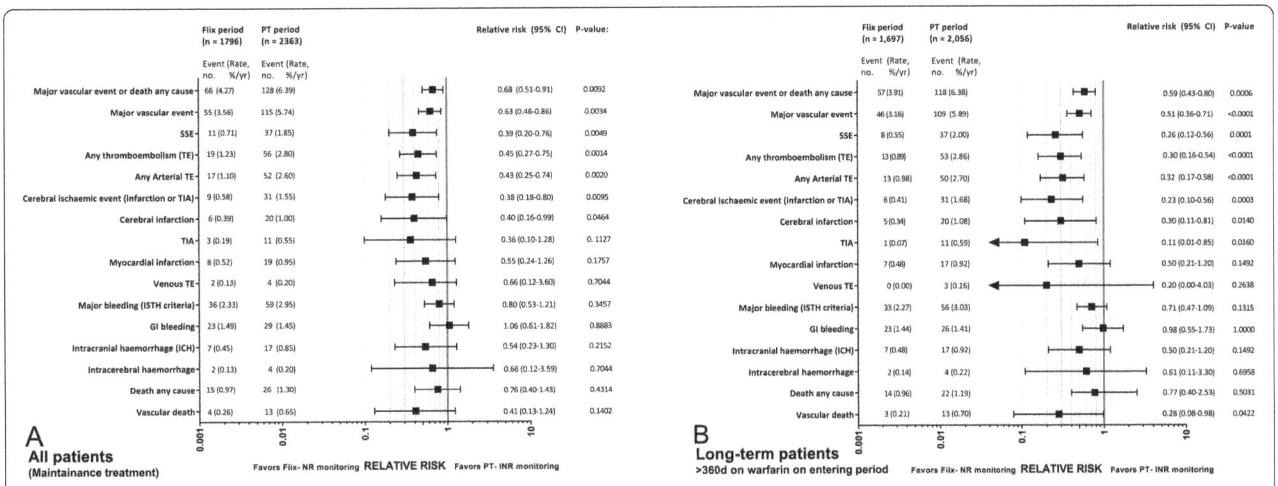

Fig. 5 Relative risk plots showing major vascular event rates and relative risk plots comparing clinical outcome during Fiix-NR or traditional PT-INR. Reproduced with permission from Blood 2021;137 [20]:2745–55 [36].

the tissue thromboplastin inhibition test (a dilute PT (dPT) assay) used in the past for lupus anticoagulant detection was known to be sensitive to heparin, thrombin and anti-Xa inhibitors but not to pentasaccharide [51]. The sensitivity of both dPT and dilute Fiix-PT clotting times for the detection of different anticoagulants were tested using high dilutions of thromboplastin hypothesizing that the dFiix-PT might be less influenced by confounders. In short, the dFiix-PT at a single thromboplastin dilution could determine warfarin normalized ratios and quantitative concentrations of dabigatran, rivaroxaban, apixaban, unfractionated heparin and enoxaparin but not of fondaparinux. The PT was less effective as two dilutions had to be used and the dPT ratio did not correlate well with the INR in warfarin patient samples [52].

Adoption of Fiix-PT into clinical practice

The Fiix test is already available as a CE marked product from a single manufacturer in Europe and can be easily

Table 1 Old PT-INR based initiation protocol and new initiation protocol modified for the slower responding Fiix prothrombin time (Fiix-NR). Modified from Journal of Thrombosis and Thrombolysis 2019;48:685–9 [44].

Starting daily dose on day 1	Normalized ratio on day 4	Warfarin dose; Old PT-INR initiation protocol (mg/day)	Warfarin dose; New adapted Fiix-NR initiation protocol (mg/day)*
< 65 year old; 4 mg daily			
	< 1.3	6	5
	1.3	4	4
	1.4–1.5	4	3
	1.6–1.7	4	2
	1.8–2.5	2	1.0–1.3
	> 2.5	1.3	Dose skipped and adapted**
≥65 year old; 6 mg daily			
	< 1.3	9	8
	1.3	6	6
	1.4–1.5	6	4.5
	1.6–1.7	6	3
	1.8–2.5	3	1.5–2.0
	> 2.5	2	Dose skipped and adapted**

*The Fiix normalized ratio (Fiix-NR) responds slower than the PT-INR due to insensitivity to factor VII reductions. ** Dose usually skipped for 1–2 days and dose then reduced based on rate of rise of the normalized ratio automated. The additional Fiix-reagent (Fiix deficient plasma) adds somewhat to the cost of the reagent compared to traditional PT tests and this may initially be seen as an issue by laboratory directors. However, it must be considered that the benefit of Fiix-NR monitoring is to the patient, health insurance and society due to fewer serious events that have long-term consequences. A cost-benefit study will therefore be important along the way of introducing the Fiix concept to different stakeholders in health care.

Conclusion

The new Fiix test was based on the hypothesis that monitoring VKAs should focus on the two factors responsible for the antithrombotic effect, namely FII and FX, and that ignoring FVII (in addition to already traditionally ignoring FIX) is reasonable as VKA therapy rarely produces reduction in FVII and FIX activity sufficiently low to be associated with spontaneous bleeding. Two clinical studies now suggest that the hypothesis has merits but further study by independent investigators would be welcomed. As the Fiix-NR is insensitive to factor VII, the measured effect is more stable than was previously achievable and this leads to fewer dose-adjustments and, therefore, less variable warfarin anticoagulation. The TTR was improved as well in the high TTR populations studied, albeit less notable than the variability reduction. In future studies it will be important to assess how Fiix-monitored warfarin compares to clinical outcomes with DOAC drugs. Future studies could also investigate if a lower Fiix-NR target range could improve safety without much loss of efficacy. However, although these findings remain to be externally validated, Fiix-NR monitored warfarin appears to be an improved potentially practice-changing anticoagulant-monitoring test combination compared traditional PT-INR monitored warfarin.

Nomenclature

Fiix = factors II and X only (pronounced "fix").

Fiix prothrombin time (Fiix-PT).

Fiix-NR = Fiix normalized ratio.

PT-warfarin = warfarin monitored with traditional PT-INR.

Fiix-warfarin = warfarin monitored with the new Fiix-NR.

VKA = vitamin K antagonists.

VKD = vitamin K dependent.

TTR = time within target INR range by Rosendaal method.

Authors' contributions

PTO wrote the first manuscript draft that was then critically edited by RP, DMW and BRG.

Author details

[1]Central Laboratory/Hematology, Landspitali National University Hospital of Iceland and University of Iceland Faculty of Medicine, Hringbraut, 101 Reykjavik, Reykjavik, Iceland. [2]Nephrology Division, Department of Medicine, Massachusetts General Hospital, Boston, MA, USA. [3]Department of Pharmacotherapy, University of Utah College of Pharmacy, Salt Lake City, UT, USA. [4]Central Laboratory/Hematology, Landspitali National University Hospital of Iceland , Reykjavik, Iceland.

References

1. Quick AJ, Stanley-Brown M, Bancroft FW. A study of the coagulation defect in hemophilia and in jaundice. Am J Med Sci. 1935;190(4):501–11. https://doi.org/10.1097/00000441-193510000-00009.
2. Owren PA, Aas K. The control of dicumarol therapy and the quantitative determination of prothrombin and proconvertin. Scand J Clin Lab Invest. 1951;3(3):201–8. https://doi.org/10.3109/00365515109060600.
3. Gudmundsdottir BR, Francis CW, Bjornsdottir AM, Nellbring M, Onundarson PT. Critical role of factors II and X during coumarin anticoagulation and their combined measurement with a new Fiix-prothrombin time. Thromb Res. 2012;130(4):674–81. https://doi.org/10.1016/j.thromres.2011.12.013.
4. Haraldsson HM, Onundarson PT, Einarsdottir KA, Gudmundsdottir BR, Petursson MK, Palsson K, et al. Performance of prothrombin-proconvertin time as a monitoring test of oral anticoagulation therapy. Am J Clin Pathol. 1997;107(6):672–80. https://doi.org/10.1093/ajcp/107.6.672.
5. Ageno W, Gallus AS, Wittkowsky A, Crowther M, Hylek EM, Palareti G, et al. Oral anticoagulant therapy: antithrombotic therapy and prevention of thrombosis, 9th ed: American College of Chest Physicians Evidence-Based Clinical Practice Guidelines. Chest. 2012;141(2 Suppl):e44S–88S. https://doi.org/10.1378/chest.11-2292.
6. Ansell J, Hirsh J, Hylek E, Jacobson A, Crowther M, Palareti G. Pharmacology and management of the vitamin K antagonists: American College of Chest Physicians Evidence-Based Clinical Practice Guidelines (8th edition). Chest. 2008;133(6):160S–98S. https://doi.org/10.1378/chest.08-0670.
7. Kirkwood TB. Calibration of reference thromboplastins and standardisation of the prothrombin time ratio. Thromb Haemost. 1983;49(3):238–44. https://doi.org/10.1055/s-0038-1657371.
8. Xi M, Beguin S, Hemker HC. The relative importance of the factors II, VII, IX and X for the prothrombinase activity in plasma of orally anticoagulated patients. Thromb Haemost. 1989;62(2):788–91. https://doi.org/10.1055/s-0038-1646904.
9. Zivelin A, Rao LV, Rapaport SI. Mechanism of the anticoagulant effect of warfarin as evaluated in rabbits by selective depression of individual procoagulant vitamin K-dependent clotting factors. J Clin Invest. 1993;92(5):2131–40. https://doi.org/10.1172/JCI116814.
10. January CT, Wann LS, Alpert JS, Calkins H, Cigarroa JE, Cleveland JC Jr, et al. 2014 AHA/ACC/HRS guideline for the management of patients with atrial fibrillation: a report of the American College of Cardiology/American Heart Association task force on practice guidelines and the Heart Rhythm Society. J Am Coll Cardiol. 2014;64(21):e1–76. https://doi.org/10.1016/j.jacc.2014.03.022.
11. Kearon C, Akl EA, Ornelas J, Blaivas A, Jimenez D, Bounameaux H, et al. Antithrombotic therapy for VTE disease: CHEST guideline and expert panel report. Chest. 2016;149(2):315–52. https://doi.org/10.1016/j.chest.2015.11.026.
12. Ruff CT, Giugliano RP, Braunwald E, Hoffman EB, Deenadayalu N, Ezekowitz MD, et al. Comparison of the efficacy and safety of new oral anticoagulants with warfarin in patients with atrial fibrillation: a meta-analysis of randomised trials. Lancet. 2014;383(9921):955–62. https://doi.org/10.1016/S0140-6736(13)62343-0.
13. van der Hulle T, den Exter PL, Kooiman J, van der Hoeven JJ, Huisman MV, Klok FA. Meta-analysis of the efficacy and safety of new oral anticoagulants in patients with cancer-associated acute venous thromboembolism. J Thromb Haemost. 2014;12(7):1116–20. https://doi.org/10.1111/jth.12605.
14. Eikelboom JW, Connolly SJ, Brueckmann M, Granger CB, Kappetein AP, Mack MJ, et al. Dabigatran versus warfarin in patients with mechanical heart valves. N Engl J Med. 2013;369(13):1206–14. https://doi.org/10.1056/NEJMoa1300615.
15. Pengo V, Denas G, Zoppellaro G, Jose SP, Hoxha A, Ruffatti A, et al. Rivaroxaban vs warfarin in high-risk patients with antiphospholipid syndrome. Blood. 2018;132(13):1365–71. https://doi.org/10.1182/blood-2018-04-848333.

16. Ordi-Ros J, Saez-Comet L, Perez-Conesa M, Vidal X, Riera-Mestre A, Castro-Salomo A, et al. Rivaroxaban versus vitamin K antagonist in Antiphospholipid syndrome: a randomized noninferiority trial. Ann Intern Med. 2019;171(10):685–94. https://doi.org/10.7326/M19-0291.
17. Pengo V, Hoxha A, Andreoli L, Tincani A, Silvestri E, Prisco D, et al. Trial of rivaroxaban in AntiPhospholipid syndrome (TRAPS): two-year outcomes after the study closure. J Thromb Haemost. 2021;19(2):531–5. https://doi.org/10.1111/jth.15158.
18. Robinson AA, Trankle CR, Eubanks G, Schumann C, Thompson P, Wallace RL, et al. Off-label Use of Direct Oral Anticoagulants Compared With Warfarin for Left Ventricular Thrombi. JAMA Cardiol. 2020. https://doi.org/10.1001/jamacardio.2020.0652.
19. Rosendaal FR, Cannegieter SC, van der Meer FJ, Briet E. A method to determine the optimal intensity of oral anticoagulant therapy. Thromb Haemost. 1993;69(3):236–9. https://doi.org/10.1055/s-0038-1651587.
20. Wan Y, Heneghan C, Perera R, Roberts N, Hollowell J, Glasziou P, et al. Anticoagulation control and prediction of adverse events in patients with atrial fibrillation: a systematic review. Circulation Cardiovascular quality and outcomes. 2008;1(2):84–91. https://doi.org/10.1161/CIRCOUTCOMES.108.796185.
21. Björck F, Renlund H, Lip GYH, Wester P, Svensson PJ, Själander A. Outcomes in a warfarin-treated population with atrial fibrillation. JAMA Cardiol. 2016;1(2):172–80. https://doi.org/10.1001/jamacardio.2016.0199.
22. Wallentin L, Yusuf S, Ezekowitz MD, Alings M, Flather M, Franzosi MG, et al. Efficacy and safety of dabigatran compared with warfarin at different levels of international normalised ratio control for stroke prevention in atrial fibrillation: an analysis of the RE-LY trial. Lancet. 2010;376(9745):975–83. https://doi.org/10.1016/S0140-6736(10)61194-4.
23. Wallentin L, Lopes RD, Hanna M, Thomas L, Hellkamp A, Nepal S, et al. Efficacy and safety of apixaban compared with warfarin at different levels of predicted international normalized ratio control for stroke prevention in atrial fibrillation. Circulation. 2013;127(22):2166–76. https://doi.org/10.1161/CIRCULATIONAHA.112.142158.
24. Garmendia CA, Nassar Gorra L, Rodriguez AL, Trepka MJ, Veledar E, Madhivanan P. Evaluation of the inclusion of studies identified by the FDA as having falsified data in the results of Meta-analyses: the example of the Apixaban trials. JAMA Intern Med. 2019;179(4):582–4. https://doi.org/10.1001/jamainternmed.2018.7661.
25. Shpak M, Ramakrishnan A, Nadasdy Z, Cowperthwaite M, Fanale C. Higher incidence of ischemic stroke in patients taking novel Oral anticoagulants. Stroke. 2018;49(12):2851–6. https://doi.org/10.1161/STROKEAHA.118.022636.
26. Vinogradova Y, Coupland C, Hill T, Hippisley-Cox J. Risks and benefits of direct oral anticoagulants versus warfarin in a real world setting: cohort study in primary care. Bmj. 2018;362:k2505. https://doi.org/10.1136/bmj.k2505.
27. Holbrook A, Schulman S, Witt DM, Vandvik PO, Fish J, Kovacs MJ, et al. Evidence-based management of anticoagulant therapy: antithrombotic therapy and prevention of thrombosis, 9th ed: American College of Chest Physicians Evidence-Based Clinical Practice Guidelines. Chest. 2012;141(2 Suppl):e152S–e84S. https://doi.org/10.1378/chest.11-2295.
28. Owren PA. Parahaemophilia; haemorrhagic diathesis due to absence of a previously unknown clotting factor. Lancet. 1947;1(6449):446–8. https://doi.org/10.1016/S0140-6736(47)91941-7.
29. Owen CA, Bollman JL. Prothrombin conversion factor of dicumarol plasma. Proceedings of the Society for Experimental Biology and Medicine Society for Experimental Biology and Medicine. 1948;67(2):231–4. https://doi.org/10.3181/00379727-67-16262.
30. Biggs R, Douglas AS, Macfarlane RG, Dacie JV, Pitney WR. Merskey. Christmas disease: a condition previously mistaken for haemophilia. Br Med J. 1952;2(4799):1378–82. https://doi.org/10.1136/bmj.2.4799.1378.
31. Duckert F, Fluckiger P, Matter M, Koller F. Clotting factor X; physiologic and physico-chemical properties. Proceedings of the Society for Experimental Biology and Medicine Society for Experimental Biology and Medicine. 1955;90(1):17–22. https://doi.org/10.3181/00379727-90-21927.
32. Burn J, Pirmohamed M. Direct oral anticoagulants versus warfarin: is new always better than the old? Open heart. 2018;5(1):e000712. https://doi.org/10.1136/openhrt-2017-000712.
33. Kearon C, Ginsberg JS, Kovacs MJ, Anderson DR, Wells P, Julian JA, et al. Comparison of low-intensity warfarin therapy with conventional-intensity warfarin therapy for long-term prevention of recurrent venous thromboembolism. N Engl J Med. 2003;349(7):631–9. https://doi.org/10.1056/NEJMoa035422.
34. Ibrahim S, Jespersen J, Poller L. European, action, on, et al. the clinical evaluation of international normalized ratio variability and control in conventional oral anticoagulant administration by use of the variance growth rate. J Thromb Haemost. 2013;11(8):1540–6. https://doi.org/10.1111/jth.12322.
35. Onundarson PT, Francis CW, Indridason OS, Arnar DO, Bjornsson ES, Magnusson MK, et al. Fiix-prothrombin time versus standard prothrombin time for monitoring of warfarin anticoagulation: a single Centre, double-blind, randomised, non-inferiority trial. The Lancet Haematology. 2015;2(6):e231–e40. https://doi.org/10.1016/S2352-3026(15)00073-3.
36. Oskarsdottir AR, Gudmundsdottir BR, Jensdottir HM, Flygenring B, Palsson R, Onundarson PT. Ignoring instead of chasing after coagulation factor VII during warfarin management: an interrupted time series study. Blood. 2021;137(20):2745–55. https://doi.org/10.1182/blood.2020008698.
37. Oskarsdottir AR, Gudmundsdottir BR, Indridason OS, Lund SH, Arnar DO, Bjornsson ES, et al. Reduced anticoagulation variability in patients on warfarin monitored with Fiix-prothrombin time associates with reduced thromboembolism: the Fiix-trial. J Thromb Thrombolysis. 2017;43(4):550–61. https://doi.org/10.1007/s11239-017-1482-4.
38. Pirmohamed M. Warfarin: The End or the End of One Size Fits All Therapy? J Pers Med. 2018;8(3).
39. Furie B. Do pharmacogenetics have a role in the dosing of vitamin K antagonists? N Engl J Med. 2013;369(24):2345–6. https://doi.org/10.1056/NEJMe1313682.
40. Witt DM, Delate T, Clark NP, Martell C, Tran T, Crowther MA, et al. Twelve-month outcomes and predictors of very stable INR control in prevalent warfarin users. J Thromb Haemost. 2010;8(4):744–9. https://doi.org/10.1111/j.1538-7836.2010.03756.x.
41. Jonsson PI, Letertre L, Juliusson SJ, Gudmundsdottir BR, Francis CW, Onundarson PT. During warfarin induction, the Fiix-prothrombin time reflects the anticoagulation level better than the standard prothrombin time. J Thromb Haemost. 2017;15(1):131–9. https://doi.org/10.1111/jth.13549.
42. Furie B, Diuguid CF, Jacobs M, Diuguid DL, Furie BC. Randomized prospective trial comparing the native prothrombin antigen with the prothrombin time for monitoring oral anticoagulant therapy. Blood. 1990;75(2):344–9. https://doi.org/10.1182/blood.V75.2.344.344.
43. Furie B, Liebman HA, Blanchard RA, Coleman MS, Kruger SF, Furie BC. Comparison of the native prothrombin antigen and the prothrombin time for monitoring oral anticoagulant therapy. Blood. 1984;64(2):445–51. https://doi.org/10.1182/blood.V64.2.445.445.
44. Onundarson PT, Gudmundsdottir BR. The need for an adapted initiation nomogram during Fiix prothrombin time monitoring of warfarin. J Thromb Thrombolysis. 2019;48(4):685–9. https://doi.org/10.1007/s11239-019-01928-4.
45. Onundarson PT, Arnar DO, Lund SH, Gudmundsdottir BR, Francis CW, Indridason OS. Fiix-prothrombin time monitoring improves warfarin anticoagulation outcome in atrial fibrillation: a systematic review of randomized trials comparing Fiix-warfarin or direct oral anticoagulants to standard PT-warfarin. Int J Lab Hematol. 2016;38(Suppl 1):78–90. https://doi.org/10.1111/ijlh.12537.
46. Connolly SJ, Ezekowitz MD, Yusuf S, Eikelboom J, Oldgren J, Parekh A, et al. Dabigatran versus warfarin in patients with atrial fibrillation. N Engl J Med. 2009;361(12):1139–51. https://doi.org/10.1056/NEJMoa0905561.
47. Patel MR, Mahaffey KW, Garg J, Pan G, Singer DE, Hacke W, et al. Rivaroxaban versus warfarin in nonvalvular atrial fibrillation. N Engl J Med. 2011;365(10):883–91. https://doi.org/10.1056/NEJMoa1009638.
48. Granger CB, Alexander JH, McMurray JJ, Lopes RD, Hylek EM, Hanna M, et al. Apixaban versus warfarin in patients with atrial fibrillation. N Engl J Med. 2011;365(11):981–92. https://doi.org/10.1056/NEJMoa1107039.
49. Giugliano RP, Ruff CT, Braunwald E, Murphy SA, Wiviott SD, Halperin JL, et al. Edoxaban versus warfarin in patients with atrial fibrillation. N Engl J Med. 2013;369(22):2093–104. https://doi.org/10.1056/NEJMoa1310907.
50. Onundarson PT, Flygenring B. Oral anticoagulant monitoring: are we on the right track? Int J Lab Hematol. 2019;41(Suppl 1):40–8. https://doi.org/10.1111/ijlh.13008.
51. Gerbutavicius R, Iqbal O, Messmore HL, Wehrmacher WH, Hoppensteadt DA, Gerbutaviciene R, et al. Differential effects of DX-9065a, argatroban, and synthetic pentasaccharide on tissue thromboplastin inhibition test and dilute Russell's viper venom test. Clin Appl Thromb Hemost. 2003;9(4):317–23. https://doi.org/10.1177/107602960300900407.
52. Letertre LR, Gudmundsdottir BR, Francis CW, Gosselin RC, Skeppholm M, Malmstrom RE, et al. A single test to assay warfarin, dabigatran, rivaroxaban, apixaban, unfractionated heparin, and enoxaparin in plasma. J Thromb Haemost. 2016;14(5):1043–53. https://doi.org/10.1111/jth.13300.

11

Changes of antithrombotic prescription in atrial fibrillation patients with acute coronary syndrome or percutaneous coronary intervention and the subsequent impact on long-term outcomes

Chiao-Chin Lee[1†], Chiao-Hsiang Chang[1†], Yuan Hung[1], Chin-Sheng Lin[1], Shih-Ping Yang[1], Shu-Meng Cheng[1], Fan-Han Yu[1], Wei-Shiang Lin[1] and Wen-Yu Lin[1,2*]

Abstract

Objectives: The choice of optimal antithrombotic therapy in atrial fibrillation (AF) patients with acute coronary syndrome (ACS) or percutaneous coronary intervention (PCI) remains controversial. The aim of this longitudinal cohort study is to investigate the prescribing pattern of antithrombotic regimen in different cohorts and its subsequent impact.

Setting and design: Longitudinal data from the Tri-Service General Hospital-Coronary Heart Disease (TSGH-CHD) registry, between January 2016 and August 2018 was screened.

Participants and method: Patients with prior history of nonvalvular AF, who had ACS presentation or underwent PCI were selected, and these patients were divided into cohort 1 and cohort 2, according to the index date of antithrombotic prescription before and after the PIONEER AF-PCI study.

Primary and secondary outcomes: The primary safety endpoints were composites of major bleeding and/or clinically relevant non-major bleeding. The secondary efficacy endpoints included the occurrence of all-cause mortality, stroke/systemic embolization, nonfatal myocardial infarction (MI), and >30-days coronary revascularization.

* Correspondence: salmon.lin1019@gmail.com
[1]Division of Cardiology, Department of Medicine, Tri-Service General Hospital, National Defense Medical Center, Taipei, Taiwan
[2]Division of Cardiology, Department of Internal Medicine Tri-Service General Hospital, National Defense Medical Center, No. 325, Cheng-Gong Road, Section 2, Neihu 114, Taipei, Taiwan

Results: A total of 121 patients were included into analysis (cohort 1=35; cohort 2=86). Comparing with cohort 1, the prescription rate of triple antithrombotic therapy (TAT) increased from 17.1 to 38.4%, especially the regimen with dual antiplatelet therapy (DAPT) plus low-dose non-vitamin-K dependent oral anticoagulation (NOAC). However, the prescription rate of dual antithrombotic therapy (DAT) decreased (14.3–10.5%), as well as the prescription rate of DAPT (68.6–51.2%). These changes of antithrombotic prescription across different cohorts were not associated with risk of adverse safety (HR= 0.87; 95% CI, 0.42-1.80, p=0.710) and efficacy outcomes (HR=0.96; 95% CI, 0.40-2.32, p=0.930).

Conclusions: Entering the NOAC era, the prescription of TAT increased alongside the decrease in DAT. As the prescription rate of DAPT without anticoagulation remained high, future efforts are mandatory to improve the implementation of guidelines and clinical practice.

Keywords: Antithrombotic, Prescription, Atrial fibrillation, Acute coronary syndrome, Percutaneous coronary intervention, Cohort

Introduction

Atrial fibrillation (AF) is the most common sustained cardiac arrhythmia in the world and is associated with significant symptoms, impaired quality of life, and cardiovascular morbidity and mortality. [1] Moreover, AF shares several common risk factors with coronary artery disease (CAD), such as age, obesity, hypertension, diabetes mellitus, and dyslipidemia, so that the prevalence of CAD in patients with AF is expected to be high, reported ranging from approximate 20-40%[2, 3].

However, the strategy of optimal antithrombotic therapy in patients with AF and concomitant CAD remains challenging. [4, 5] Thromboembolism as a result of AF has a stasis and fibrin drive, whereas atherothrombosis is mainly driven by endothelial plaque rupture, platelet aggregation, and even partially thrombin generation. [6] Clinically, dual antiplatelet therapy (DAPT) with a $P2Y_{12}$ inhibitor plus aspirin were recommended in patients with acute coronary syndrome (ACS) or who underwent percutaneous coronary intervention (PCI) with implantation of stent. [7, 8] Oral anticoagulation (OAC), on the other hand, has been proved to be superior to DAPT for prevention of stroke and systemic thromboembolism in patients with AF. [9] As a consequence, so-called triple antithrombotic therapy (TAT) with DAPT plus an OAC will be considered after ACS or successful PCI in AF patients. Unfortunately, but inevitably, the more aggressive of antithrombotic regimen being used, the higher risk of bleeding. [10, 11].

Entering the non-vitamin-K dependent oral anticoagulation (NOAC) era, PIONEER AF-PCI (Open-Label, Randomized, Controlled, Multicenter Study Exploring Two Treatment Strategies of Rivaroxaban and a Dose-Adjusted Oral Vitamin K Antagonist Treatment Strategy in Subjects with Atrial Fibrillation who Undergo Percutaneous Coronary Intervention) trial, published in December 2016, was one of the first attempts to try to clarify the optimal antithrombotic strategy in patients with AF undergoing PCI with placement of stents. [12] The study provided that dual antithrombotic therapy (DAT), a $P2Y_{12}$ inhibitor plus rivaroxaban 15 mg once daily was associated with a lower rate of significant bleeding related to standard TAT with DAPT plus vitamin-K antagonist (VKA), without compromising the risk of major adverse cardiovascular events and stent thrombosis. Taking advantage of safety, DAT with combination of a $P2Y_{12}$ inhibitor and a NOAC may be an alternative option; or even a favorable choice to balance the risk of ischemic event and bleeding. [13, 14] However, the contemporary real world data of antithrombotic management is limited. In this longitudinal cohort study, we did not intend to represent which antithrombotic regimen is better than others. Instead, the scope of the study is to demonstrate the cohort effects on the changes of antithrombotic prescribing habits and its impact on patients' outcomes.

Methods

Study cohorts

Tri-Service General Hospital-Coronary Heart Disease (TSGH-CHD) registry is a single-center, prospective, and longitudinal cohort database and it was established since 2014. [15] Patients were eligible for enrollment into the registry if they presented with stable angina (SA) or acute coronary syndrome (ACS), including unstable angina (UA), non-ST-segment elevation myocardial infarction (NSTEMI), or ST-segment elevation myocardial infarction (STEMI). All patients were admitted to the hospital and received coronary angiography (CAG) with or without coronary interventional therapy. All patients' clinical data have thoroughly been reviewed and recorded by a specialized research assistant. Baseline demographic characteristics, medical history, clinical presentation, laboratory parameters, echocardiographic findings, phenotype of coronary arteries, coronary angiography results, interventional procedures and discharge medication are comprehensively evaluated from medical records.

Patients with prior history of nonvalvular AF, who had ACS presentation or had underwent PCI were selected from the TSGH-CHD registry between January 2016 and August 2018. These patients were indicated clinical requirement of concomitant anticoagulation and antiplatelet therapy. In order to analyze the differences of prescribing pattern of antithrombotic regimen before and after the publication of PIONEER AF-PCI study, we divided these eligible patients into two longitudinal cohorts by the index date of antithrombotic prescription. Patients were categorized into cohort 1 if the prescribing date was before the publication of PIONEER AF-PCI study (December 31, 2016) and cohort 2 was defined as the cohort after PIONEER AF-PCI study. The study was ethically approved by the institutional review board (IRB NO. A202005128). This was an observational study that patients were not recruited to receive intervention. Informed consent was not required in the study.

Stroke and bleeding risks assessment

Stroke risk was assessed with the use of CHA_2DS_2-VASc scores, which has been proved to be correlated with the risk of stroke and systemic embolization among patients with nonvalvular AF who are not receiving anticoagulant therapy. [16] The CHA_2DS_2-VASc scores ranges from 0 to 9 and represents the sum of points for the following conditions: congestive heart failure, hypertension, diabetes mellitus, vascular diseases, age of 65-74 years (1 points for each), and age ≥75 years, prior stroke or transient ischemic attack (2 points for each). The clinical utility of HAS-BLED score has been described before and it was used for bleeding risk assessment in our cohort study. [17] The HAS-BLED score ranges from 0 to 9 and represents the sum of points for the conditions: hypertension, abnormal renal function (dialysis, kidney transplantation, or ≥creatinine 2.3 mg/dL), abnormal liver function (aspartate aminotransferase or alanine aminotransferase more than 3-fold the upper limit of normal or bilirubin more than 2-fold the upper limit of normal), previous history of stroke, bleeding history or tendency, labile international normalized ratio (INR), elderly with age >65 years, concomitant usage of drugs of antiplatelet agents or non-steroid anti-inflammatory drug (NSAID), and excess alcohol intake. The higher HAS-BLED score reflects the higher risk of bleeding.

Antithrombotic regimen

Clinical decisions regarding prescribing antithrombotic regimen were made by the attending physicians after assessing patients' characteristics, clinical thrombotic and bleeding risk. The antithrombotic regimens were categorized into three major patterns: triple antithrombotic therapy (TAT), DAPT, and dual antithrombotic therapy (DAT). The composition of TAT included DAPT plus VKA, DAPT plus full-dose NOAC, and DAPT plus low-dose NOAC. The composition of DAT included single antiplatelet therapy (SAPT) plus VKA, SAPT plus full-dose NOAC and SAPT plus low-dose NOAC. The full-dose NOAC indicated 50 mg twice daily for dabigatran; 15 mg daily for rivaroxaban; 5 mg twice daily for apixaban; and 60 mg daily for edoxaban. However, the low-dose NOAC indicated 110 mg twice daily for dabigatran; 10 mg daily for rivaroxaban; 2.5 mg twice daily for apixaban; and 30 mg daily for edoxaban.

Follow-up and study outcomes

The primary safety endpoint of the study was occurrence of major or clinically relevant non-major bleeding as defined by the International Society on Thrombosis and Hemostasis (ISTH). The definition of major bleeding in non-surgical patients was (1) fetal bleeding and/or (2) symptomatic bleeding in a critical organ (e.g. intracranial, intraspinal, intraocular, retroperitoneal, intraarticular, pericardial, or intramuscular with compartment syndrome) and/or (3) bleeding causing a fall in hemoglobin level of 2 g/dL or more, or leading to transfusion at least 2 units of whole blood or red cells. The clinically relevant non-major bleeding was defined as an acute or subacute clinically over bleed that leads to at least one of the following: (1) a hospital admission for bleeding or (2) a physician guided medical or surgical treatment for bleeding, or (3) a change in antithrombotic therapy. The secondary endpoint was efficacy endpoints which included the occurrence of all-cause mortality, stroke/systemic embolization, nonfatal myocardial infarction (MI), and coronary revascularization (>30 days after discharge). All medical records were reviewed carefully, and every patient was followed up to 1.5 years maximally if they did not meet the criteria of our endpoints.

Statistical analysis

Continuous variables are presented as mean and standard deviation. Categorical variables are presented as the number of patients and the corresponding percentage. The differences between the continuous values were assessed by using an unpaired two-tail Student t test or one-way analysis of variance post-hoc Benferroni test for normally distributed continuous variables; Mann-Whitney rank-sum test for skewed variables. Nominal variables were compared with Pearson chi-square test or Fisher exact test. Kaplan-Meier method was used to present cumulative incidence in the two longitudinal cohorts. A Cox proportional regression analysis was conducted to compare the differences of study outcomes between the two longitudinal cohorts, with the results presented as a hazard ratio (HR) with a 95% confidence internal (CI). All statistical analyses were performed with a software package (IBM SPSS Statistics Version 25.0), and differences were considered significant as p value < 0.05.

Results

Study population and clinical characteristics

Figure 1 displayed the details of selection criteria and patient deposition. Between January 2016 and August 2018, a total of 4,061 patients were selected retrospectively from the TSGH-CHD registry. After comprehensive assessment, 121 patients with prior nonvalvular AF with ACS or PCI were included into analysis. Among these, 35 patients were categorized into cohort 1 in which the index date of prescribing antithrombotic regimen was before the publication of PIONEER AF-PCI study; and 86 patients were categorized into cohort 2.

Table 1 demonstrated the characteristics of patients in the two cohorts. No differences were observed in age, gender, and underlying comorbidities. The prevalence of uremia, requiring hemodialysis was approximately 20% in both cohorts. Regarding the echocardiographic findings, there were no significant differences in left atrium size and left ventricular systolic function between the two cohorts. The proportion of paroxysmal AF was

Table 1 Comparison of clinical characteristics between two longitudinal cohorts

Characteristics	Overall population (*N*=121)		P value
	Cohort 1 (*N*=35)	Cohort 2 (*N*=86)	
Baseline characteristics			
Age (years)	71.7±11.4	73.6±12.3	0.418
Male, N (%)	25 (71.4)	60 (69.8)	0.856
Hypertension, N (%)	32 (91.4)	73 (84.9)	0.259
Diabetes mellitus, N (%)	20 (57.1)	37 (43.0)	0.158
Dyslipidemia, N (%)	12 (34.3)	32 (37.2)	0.762
Prior MI, N (%)	18 (51.4)	42 (48.8)	0.796
Prior stroke/TIA, N (%)	9 (25.7)	16 (18.6)	0.381
Prior heart failure, N (%)	17 (48.6)	34 (39.5)	0.361
Uremia, N (%)	7 (20.0)	17 (19.8)	0.977
Echocardiographic characteristics			
LAD (mm)	46.59±7.88	44.04±8.25	0.138
LVEF (%)	49.69±14.36	51.67±16.34	0.552
AF characteristics			
Paroxysmal AF, N (%)	24 (68.6)	36 (41.9)	0.008
CHA_2DS_2-VASc score	4.5±1.9	4.1±1.7	0.187
HAS-BLED score	3.5±1.1	3.2±1.1	0.182

MI, myocardial infarction; TIA, transient ischemic attack; LAD, left atrium dimension; LVEF, left ventricular ejection fraction; AF, atrial fibrillation

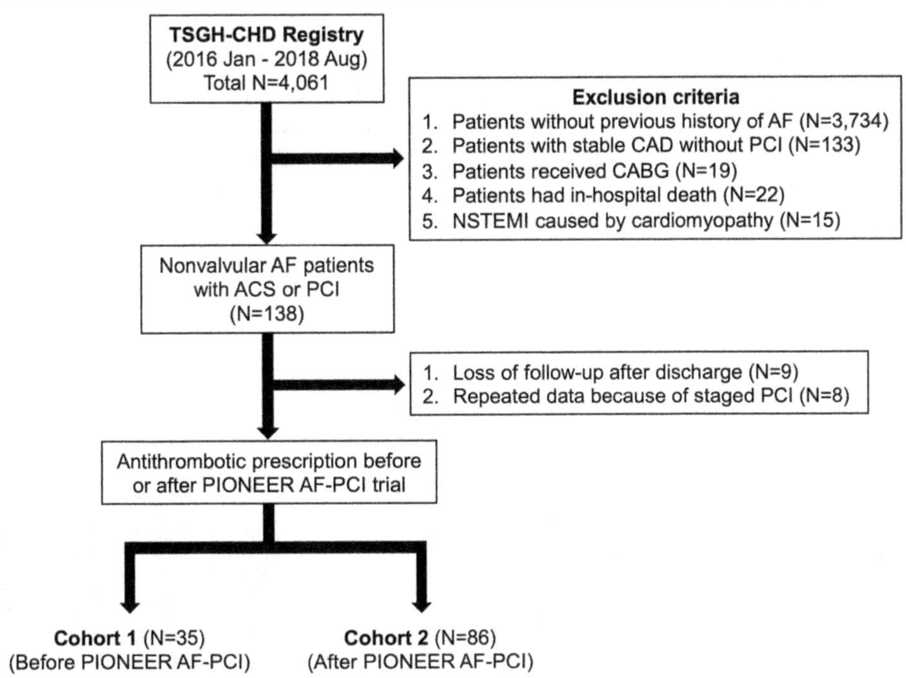

Fig. 1 Algorithm of study design. The flow chart demonstrated the selection criteria and patient deposition by the timing of PIONEER AF-PCI study. AF, atrial fibrillation; ACS, acute coronary syndrome; PCI, percutaneous coronary intervention; CAD, coronary artery disease; CABG, coronary artery bypass grafting, NSTEMI, non-ST-segment elevation myocardial infarction

significantly higher in cohort 1 compared to cohort 2 (68.6% vs. 41.9%, P=0.008). The mean CHA_2DS_2-VASc (4.5±1.9 vs. 4.1±1.7) and HAS-BLED (3.5±1.1 vs. 3.2± 1.1) scores were similar between cohort 1 and cohort 2. Figure 2 demonstrated the detailed distribution of CHA_2DS_2-VASc and HAS-BLED scores in the two cohorts. Based on the similar mean CHA_2DS_2-VASc score, patients in cohort 1 had more proportion of CHA_2DS_2-VASc score of over 5 than cohort 2. On the contrary, patients in the cohort 2 had higher proportion of CHA_2DS_2-VASc score of 4 and 5. Regarding the HAS-BLED score, patients in cohort 1 had higher proportion of HAS-BLED score of 5 than patients in cohort 2.

Table 2 showed the clinical characteristics of coronary artery disease in the two cohorts. There were nearly 40% patients presented as acute coronary syndrome (ACS) in both cohorts and almost 90% of patients had received successful stent placement. The left anterior descending (LAD) coronary artery was the most commonly stenosed coronary artery. Despite the recent practical guideline had recommended contemporary drug-eluting stent (DES) as the preferred stent type during management of PCI in AF patients treated with oral anticoagulation, [18] there was only 51.4% of patients received DES placement in cohort 1 and 61.6% in the cohort 2. No significant differences in stent type were observed between the two cohorts.

Table 2 Comparison of clinical presentation, coronary lesion characteristics, and stent types between two longitudinal cohorts

Characteristics	Overall population (N=121)		P value
	Cohort 1 (N=35)	Cohort 2 (N=86)	
Clinical presentation			
ACS presentation, N (%)	13 (37.1)	33 (38.4)	0.899
Coronary lesion characteristics			
LM lesion, N (%)	3 (2.3)	5 (5.7)	0.421
LAD lesion, N (%)	35 (100.0)	77 (89.5)	0.041
LCX lesion, N (%)	24 (68.6)	54 (62.8)	0.547
RCA, N (%)	28 (80.0)	61 (70.9)	0.305
Stent placement, N (%)	30 (85.7)	77 (89.5)	0.544
Stent types			
DES, N (%)*	18 (51.4)	53 (61.6)	0.302
BMS, N (%)	13 (37.1)	23 (26.7)	0.257
BVS, N (%)	1 (2.9)	1 (1.2)	0.497

ACS, acute coronary syndrome; LM, left main coronary artery; LAD, left anterior descending artery; LCX, left circumflex artery; RCA, right coronary artery; DES, drug-eluting stent, BMS, bare-metal stent; BVS, bioresorbable scaffold
* Two patients received both drug-eluting stent and bare-metal stent placement during the same procedure in cohort 1

Prescribing pattern of antithrombotic regimen

Figure 3 A displayed the percentages of three major prescribing patterns of antithrombotic regimen in the two longitudinal cohorts. Comparing with cohort 1, the percentage of TAT was significantly higher in cohort 2 (17.1% vs. 38.4%, p= 0.023). The prescription rate of DAT decreased from 14.3 to 10.5% even despite PIONEER AF-PCI study provided superior safety with DAT, a $P2Y_{12}$ inhibitor plus rivaroxaban (15 mg once daily) over TAT with warfarin. Although the percentage of DAPT decreased from 68.6 to 51.2%, this regimen remained the most common prescription in both cohorts. Comprehensive information regarding all compositions of antithrombotic regimen was illustrated in Fig. 3B. Among the composition of TAT, DAPT plus low-dose NOAC was the most common prescription than DAPT plus warfarin and DAPT plus full-dose NOAC in both cohort 1 and cohort 2. Regarding DAT, the percentage of prescription of SAPT plus a VKA was common (11.4%) in cohort

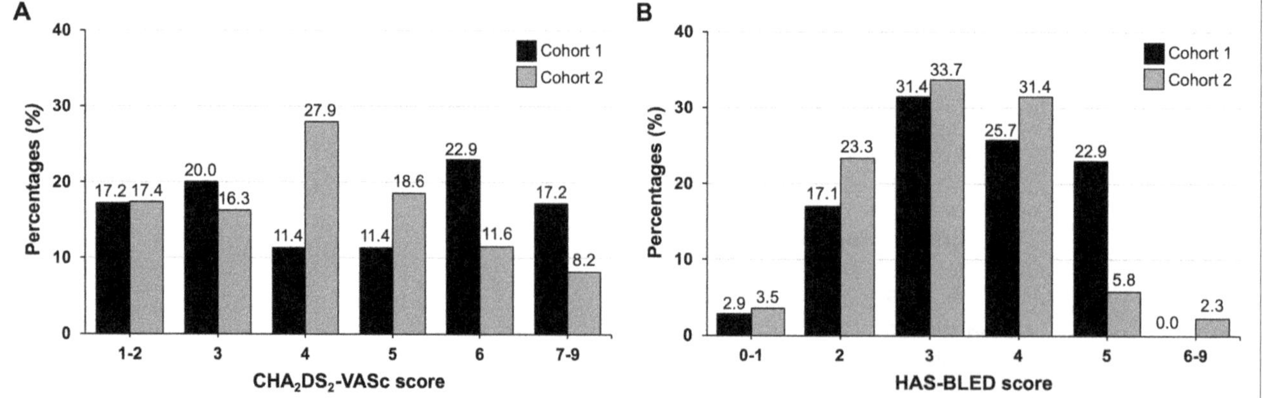

Fig. 2 The distribution of CHA_2DS_2-VASc and HAS-BLED scores in the two longitudinal cohorts. The detailed information of **(A)** CHA_2DS_2-VASc and **(B)** HAS-BLED score were presented. The mean values of CHA_2DS_2-VASc and HAS-BLED scores were similar between the two cohorts

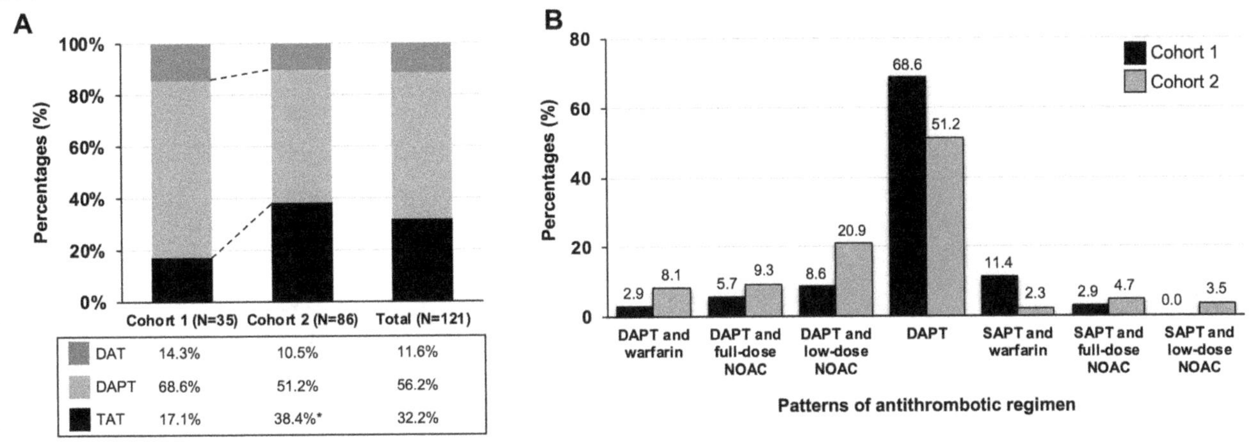

Fig. 3 Prescribing patterns of antithrombotic regimen in the two longitudinal cohorts. **A** The bar plot demonstrated the longitudinal changes of prescribing patterns of antithrombotic regimens. **B** The detailed information regarding distribution of all compositions of antithrombotic regimen in the tow cohorts. * indicated the significant difference between the two cohorts

1, and the SAPT plus a NOAC was more common (8.2%) in the cohort 2.

The prevalence of male gender was much lower in patients received DAT regimen, related to DAPT and TAT (35.7% vs. 77.9% and 69.2%, respectively) (Supplement Table). The prescription of DAT was more common in patients with prior history of stroke or transient ischemic attack. Among patients received DAPT, 32.4% had ESKD requiring hemodialysis that was significantly higher than patients received DAT and TAT. Compared with those received DAT and DAPT, patients received TAT has lower HAS-BLED score (3.5±1.2, 3.4±1.2 vs. 2.9±0.8, respectively).

Follow-up of study outcomes

Table 3 showed no differences in discharge medication between the two cohorts; including medication of renin-angiotensin system (RAS) blockade, beta-blockade, statin, and antiarrhythmic drugs. During follow-up, 11 (31.4%) patients suffered from primary safety endpoints in cohort 1 and 22 (25.6%) patients in cohort 2 (HR=0.87; 95% CI, 0.42-1.80, p=0.710) (Table 4). There were no significant differences in individual components of the safety endpoints between the two cohorts. Regarding the secondary efficacy endpoints, the incidence was 20.0% in cohort 1 as compared with 19.8% in cohort 2 (HR=0.96; 95% CI, 0.40-2.32, p=0.930). The incidence of individual components of the efficacy endpoints were also provided in Table 4. Similarly, no differences in individual components of the efficacy endpoints were observed. Figure 4 demonstrated the Kaplan-Meier curve of cumulative incidence of primary safety endpoints and secondary efficacy endpoints. Although the prescription of antithrombotic regimen changes in different cohorts, the incidence of primary safety endpoints and secondary efficacy endpoints were similar during follow up.

Table 3 Comparison of medication at discharge between two longitudinal cohorts

Characteristics	Overall population (N=121)		P value
	Cohort 1 (N=35)	Cohort 2 (N=86)	
ACEI/ARB, N (%)	13 (37.1)	48 (55.8)	0.063
Aldactone, N (%)	7 (20.0)	23 (26.7)	0.436
Beta-blocker, N (%)	29 (82.9)	65 (75.6)	0.383
Statin, N (%)	21 (60.0)	48 (55.8)	0.673
Digoxin, N (%)	4 (11.4)	9 (10.5)	1.000
Propafenone, N (%)	1 (2.9)	1 (1.2)	0.497
Cordarone, N (%)	7 (20.0)	29 (33.7)	0.134

ACEI, angiotensin converting enzyme inhibitor; ARB, angiotensin II receptor blocker

Discussion

Our study provided the real-world practice of antithrombotic management in AF patients with ACS or PCI in two longitudinal cohorts. Entering the NOAC era, the percentage of DAPT prescription decreased but it remained the most common antithrombotic regimen rather than TAT and DAT. The prescription of TAT, especially low-dose NOAC-based regimen increased, accompanied with decrease of DAT prescription. Moreover, these changes of prescribing pattern of antithrombotic regimen were not associated with long-term risks of clinical bleeding, all-cause mortality, and adverse cardiovascular events.

Table 4 Comparison of clinical outcomes between two longitudinal cohorts

Clinical Outcomes	Overall Cohort (*N*=121)		Cohort 2 vs. Cohort 1	P Value
	Cohort 1 (*N*=35)	Cohort 2 (*N*=86)	Hazard ratio (95% CI)	
Primary safety endpoint, N (%)	11 (31.4)	22 (25.6)	0.87 (0.42-1.80)	0.710
Major bleeding, N (%)	10 (28.6)	17 (19.8)	0.74 (0.34-1.62)	0.456
CRNMB, N (%)	1 (2.9)	5 (5.8)	2.16 (0.25-18.45)	0.483
Secondary efficacy endpoint, N (%)	7 (20.0)	17 (19.8)	0.96 (0.40-2.32)	0.930
All-cause death, N (%)	2 (5.7)	8 (9.3)	1.57 (0.33-7.41)	0.567
Stroke/SE, N (%)	1 (2.9)	4 (4.7)	1.60 (0.18-14.28)	0.676
Nonfatal MI, N (%)	2 (5.7)	2 (2.3)	0.39 (0.06-2.79)	0.350
Revascularization, N (%)	2 (5.7)	3 (3.5)	0.60 (0.10-3.59)	0.576

Antithrombotic strategy in the NOAC era

A major breakthrough in the antithrombotic management in AF patients requiring anticoagulation has been represented by the introduction of NOACs. [18–21] Moreover, four large clinical trials addressed on the optimal antithrombotic strategy for specific subgroup of AF patients with ACS or PCI requiring concomitant DAPT has been recently generated. [12, 22–24] The PIONEER AF-PCI study, the first one of them, compared three treatment strategies in AF patients after PCI and the study demonstrated the superiority in safety outcomes with DAT (rivaroxaban 15 mg once daily plus a $P2Y_{12}$ inhibitor, mostly clopidogrel) relative to traditional TAT with DAPT plus VKA. [12] The rates of cardiovascular death, myocardial infarction (MI), or stroke were similar between these two antithrombotic regimens. Univocally, other three trials also showed significantly reduced risk of major bleeding in prescribing DAT with a $P2Y_{12}$ inhibitor plus a NOAC when compared with TAT. A recent meta-analysis also suggested combination of a $P2Y_{12}$ inhibitor and a NOAC, without aspirin may be the most favorable treatment option as TAT with DAPT plus VKA may cause more bleeding risk without improvement in antithrombotic efficacy. [25].

However, some key issues should be emphasized. Firstly, the four clinical trials, included AF patients with ACS and/or undergoing PCI were primarily investigating the safety and had no sufficient power to provide definite robust evidence of benefit about ischemic outcome. [26] Secondly, patients with extremely high risk of stent thrombosis were largely under-represented in these trials. In the RE-DUAL PCI trial, there was a numerical trend for increased thrombotic endpoints when treating with SAPT plus dabigatran 100 mg twice daily. [22] In a subgroup analysis of 3498 AF patients underwent PCI with stenting in AUGUST trial, 57 (1.6%) patients developed stent thrombosis over 6 months. The majority of the definite or probable stent thrombosis occurred within 30 days. [27] In addition, according to a comprehensive meta-analysis, Ravi V. et al. suggested the

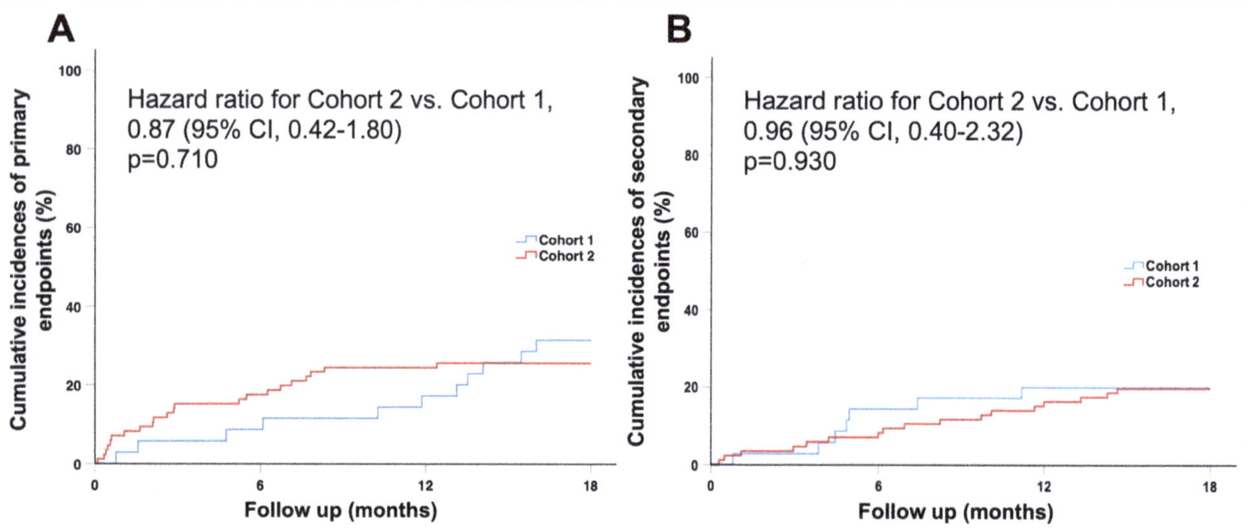

Fig. 4 Kaplan-Meier curve of cumulative incidence of study endpoints. The Kaplan-Meier curve of accumulative incidences of **(A)** primary safety endpoints and **(B)** secondary efficacy endpoints showed no significant differences in the two cohorts

potential increase in the risk of stent thrombosis when choosing DAT in patients with AF and CAD, especially for those at a higher risk of ischemic events. [28] Our longitudinal cohort study showed the prescription of DAT decreased from 14.3 to 10.5%. In cohort 2, only 4.7% of patients received DAT with SAPT plus full-dose NOAC at discharge, like the regimen recommended by clinical trials. This finding suggested that cardiovascular interventionist may hesitate to prescribe DAT at charge because of the unmet need of power in preventing ischemic events of stent thrombosis.

Current guideline/consensus recommendation

Currently, most of guidelines or consensus recommended TAT as the initial medical strategy for most AF patients with ACS and/or underwent PCI, especially those with high ischemic risk and low bleeding risk. [7, 29–31] In the four clinical trials, the duration of TAT between index PCI and study randomization varied from 1 to 14 days. [12, 22–24] That indicated a short course of TAT after coronary stenting could be desirable. In the 2020 ESC guideline for the diagnosis and management of atrial fibrillation, short course of TAT and early cessation (≤1 week) of aspirin was recommended in AF patients with ACS underwent an uncomplicated PCI. [31] The duration of TAT could be extended up to 1 month when risk of stent thrombosis outweighs the bleeding risk. In the North American expert consensus update focusing on AF patients undergoing PCI, TAT was even recommended only during index hospitalization for most patients. [32] DAT with SAPT plus an OAC should be prescribed immediately after hospital discharge and up to 12 months as a default strategy. One-month of TAT should only be recommended for those at high ischemic/thrombotic risk and low bleeding risk. Our study demonstrated the percentage of TAT prescription at discharge increased significantly from 17.1 to 38.4% in the two longitudinal cohorts, especially the increment of DAPT plus low-dose NOAC (from 8.6 to 20.9%). Nevertheless, the information regarding duration of TAT after discharge was limited in our study. Another point is that only half of our patients with coronary stenting received drug-eluting stent (DES) implantation. Despite the recent practical guideline recommended contemporary DES as the preferred stent type during management of PCI in AF patients treated with oral anticoagulation. [33].

Under prescribing of anticoagulation in real-world data

One important finding in our study is that the percentage of DAPT prescription decreased from 68.6 to 51.2% as more physicians were aware of the optimal antithrombotic management. In other words, that pointed out approximately half of AF patients with ACS or PCI who required concomitant use of antiplatelet therapy and anticoagulation were prescribed with DAPT only rather than TAT and DAT. This under prescribing of anticoagulation reflected a gap between guideline recommendation and real-world practice.

However, our result is not a unique instance, but has its counterpart. [34] Wang et al. reported 53.3% of patients were prescribed DAPT at discharge in a retrospective cohort study in Taiwan, which included AF patients with a new ACS or PCI from 2008 to 2016. [35] In a Korean nationwide study investigating the 10-year trends of antithrombotic prescription from 2006 to 2015, Park et al. reported the prescription rate of TAT increased gradually (22.7–38.3%) in patients with AF undergoing PCI. [36] However, the prescription rate of DAPT remained high with 60.3% in 2015. Mai et al. reported a retrospective data in Southern China that showed the prescription rate of OACs at discharge for patients with AF and ACS from 2013 to 2018 was only 21.7%.[37] The inadequate implementation of guidelines recommendation were more common in Asia as individuals of Asian ethnicity were considered more vulnerable to anticoagulant-related bleeding, especially using VKA. [38] Among 12,165 Danish population of AF patients hospitalized with MI or PCI between 2001 and 2009, only 3,590 (29.5%) patients received DAPT. [39] Rubboli et al. reported that DAPT was prescribed to 18% of AF patients undergoing PCI and stent implantation in a large European multicenter observational study. [40] Several factors may also contribute the inadequate anticoagulation in our study. The prevalence of baseline HAS-BLED score ≥3 were 80% and 73.2% in cohort 1 and cohort 2, which indicated a relatively higher bleeding risk in our cohort and this situation could discourage physicians to pursue more aggressive antithrombotic strategy. Moreover, the prevalence of uremia was high in both cohorts, with approximately one fifth. We believed that was because Taiwan has the highest prevalence of uremia in the world the the incidence of AF is notably high in uremic patients who requiring hemodialysis. [41] Therefore, uremia, a contraindication to NOAC, could also precipitate the under-prescription of anticoagulation. A meta-analysis suggested the use of VKA for AF may be associated with an unfavorable risk/benefit ratio in patients with ESKD. [42] Therefore, physician would rather not prescribe VKA when treating AF patients with ESKD and our study demonstrated that 92% (22/24) of ESKD patients were treated with DAPT only.

Study limitations

Some limitations were observed in this study. This is a single-center, observational and non-randomized cohort study and it provides regional data only. Some discrepancies may exist in different areas. Another major limitation is the small sample size which may affect the significance of the results. In addition, not all dosage of NOAC were available in the single medical institution (e.g. Rivaroxaban 20 mg) and this may affect the decision of antithrombotic strategy. The lack of information regarding the duration of antithrombotic treatment after hospital discharge may influenced the patients' outcome during follow-up. Finally, there was a low prescription rate of guideline-medical therapy, including RAS blockade, beta-blockade, and statin in our study which might also affect the clinical outcome during follow-up.

Conclusions

In this real-world, longitudinal cohort study, we found that the prescribing pattern of antithrombotic regimen in AF patients with ACS or PCI were changing over time. Entering the NOAC era, the prescription of TAT increased, especially the regimen of DAPT plus low-dose NOAC. Noteworthy, still half of individuals of AF with ACS and/or underwent PCI were treated with DAPT only. We need more efforts to increase the physician awareness and improve the adherence of guidelines for the optimal antithrombotic management of AF patients with ACS or PCI. Finally, our study demonstrated these changes of antithrombotic prescription were not associated with increased risk of clinical bleeding, all-cause mortality, and adverse cardiovascular events.

Abbreviations

AF: Atrial fibrillation; CAD: Coronary artery disease; ESKD: End-stage kidney disease; ACS: Acute coronary syndrome; PCI: Percutaneous coronary intervention; CAG: Coronary angiography; SA: Stable angina; UA: Unstable angina; NSTEMI: Non-ST-segment elevation myocardial infarction; STEMI: ST-segment elevation myocardial infarction; DAPT: Dual antiplatelet therapy; SAPT: Single antiplatelet therapy; OAC: Oral anticoagulation; NOAC: Non-vitamin-K dependent oral anticoagulation; VKA: Vitamin K antagonist; TAT: Triple antithrombotic therapy; DAT: Dual antithrombotic therapy; DES: Drug-eluting stent; RAS: Renin-angiotensin system

Acknowledgements

I would like to thank all participating colleagues who contributed to this study and reviewers/editor for their comments.

Authors' contributions

CH Chang, CC Lee, and WY Lin conceived and designed the study. Y Hung, CS Lin, SP Yang, SM Cheng, FH Yu, WS Lin, and WY Lin participated in the collection of patients' data and organization of manuscript writing. CH Chang, CC Lee, and WY Lin performed the statistical analysis, interpreted the data, and drafted the manuscript. WY Lin critically revised the manuscript and supervised the project. All the authors approved and agreed the final manuscript.

References

1. Colilla S, Crow A, Petkun W, Singer DE, Simon T, Liu X. Estimates of current and future incidence and prevalence of atrial fibrillation in the U.S. adult population. Am J Cardiol. 2013;112(8):1142–1147.
2. Nucifora G, Schuijf JD, Tops LF, et al. Prevalence of coronary artery disease assessed by multislice computed tomography coronary angiography in patients with paroxysmal or persistent atrial fibrillation. Circ Cardiovasc Imaging. 2009;2(2):100–106.
3. Kralev S, Schneider K, Lang S, Süselbeck T, Borggrefe M. Incidence and Severity of Coronary Artery Disease in Patients with Atrial Fibrillation Undergoing First-Time Coronary Angiography. PLoS One. 2011;6(9):e24964.
4. Capodanno D, Huber K, Mehran R, et al. Management of Antithrombotic Therapy in Atrial Fibrillation Patients Undergoing PCI: JACC State-of-the-Art Review. J Am Coll Cardiol. 2019;74(1):83–99.
5. Buccheri S, Angiolillo DJ, Capodanno D. Evolving paradigms in antithrombotic therapy for anticoagulated patients undergoing coronary stenting. Ther Adv Cardiovasc Dis. 2019;13:1753944719891688.
6. Chan NC, Weitz JI. Antithrombotic Agents. Circ Res. 2019;124(3):426–436.
7. Valgimigli M, Bueno H, Byrne RA, et al. 2017 ESC focused update on dual antiplatelet therapy in coronary artery disease developed in collaboration with EACTS. Eur Heart J. 2018;39(3):213–254.
8. Li YH, Wang YC, Wang YC, et al. 2018 Guidelines of the Taiwan Society of Cardiology, Taiwan Society of Emergency Medicine and Taiwan Society of Cardiovascular Interventions for the management of non ST-segment elevation acute coronary syndrome. J Formos Med Assoc. 2018;117(9):766–790.
9. Connolly S, Pogue J, Pfeffer M, et al. Clopidogrel plus aspirin versus oral anticoagulation for atrial fibrillation in the Atrial fibrillation Clopidogrel Trial with Irbesartan for prevention of Vascular Events (ACTIVE W): a randomised controlled trial. Lancet. 2006;367(9526):1903–1912.
10. Paikin JS, Wright DS, Crowther MA, Mehta SR, Eikelboom JW. Triple antithrombotic therapy in patients with atrial fibrillation and coronary artery stents. Circulation. 2010;121(18):2067–2070.
11. Shiroto T, Sakata Y, Nochioka K, et al. Clinical benefits and risks of antithrombotic therapy in patients with atrial fibrillation with comorbidities – A report from the CHART-2 Study. Int J Cardiol. 2020;299:160–168.
12. Gibson CM, Mehran R, Bode C, et al. Prevention of Bleeding in Patients with Atrial Fibrillation Undergoing PCI. N Engl J Med. 2016;375(25):2423–2434.
13. Golwala HB, Cannon CP, Steg PG, et al. Safety and efficacy of dual vs. triple antithrombotic therapy in patients with atrial fibrillation following percutaneous coronary intervention: a systematic review and meta-analysis of randomized clinical trials. Eur Heart J. 2018;39(19):1726-1735a.
14. Lopes R, Hong H, Harskamp R, et al. Optimal Antithrombotic Regimens for Patients With Atrial Fibrillation Undergoing Percutaneous Coronary Intervention. JAMA Cardiol. 2020;5(5):1–8.
15. Lin WY, Hung Y, Lin GN, et al. Profiles of hospitalized patients with angiographic coronary heart disease in Taiwan during 2014-2016: Report of a tertiary hospital. Acta Cardiol Sin. 2021;37(4):365–376.
16. Lip GYH, Nieuwlaat R, Pisters R, et al. Refining clinical risk stratification for predicting stroke and thromboembolism in atrial fibrillation using a novel risk factor-based approach: The Euro Heart Survey on atrial fibrillation. Chest. 2010;137(2):263–272.
17. Pisters R, Lane DA, Nieuwlaat R, et al. A novel user-friendly score (HAS-BLED) to assess 1-year risk of major bleeding in patients with atrial fibrillation: The euro heart survey. Chest. 2010;138(5):1093–1100.
18. Connolly SJ, Ezekowitz MD, Yusuf S, et al. Dabigatran versus Warfarin in Patients with Atrial Fibrillation. N Engl J Med. 2009;361(12):1139–1151.
19. Patel MR, Mahaffey KW, Garg J, et al. Rivaroxaban versus Warfarin in Nonvalvular Atrial Fibrillation. N Engl J Med. 2011;365(10):883–891.
20. Granger CB, Alexander JH, McMurray JJV, et al. Apixaban versus Warfarin in Patients with Atrial Fibrillation. N Engl J Med. 2011;365(11):981–992.
21. Giugliano RP, Ruff CT, Braunwald E, et al. Edoxaban versus Warfarin in Patients with Atrial Fibrillation. N Engl J Med. 2013;369(22):2093–2104.
22. Cannon CP, Bhatt DL, Oldgren J, et al. Dual Antithrombotic Therapy with Dabigatran after PCI in Atrial Fibrillation. N Engl J Med. 2017;377(16):1513–1524.
23. Lopes RD, Heizer G, Aronson R, et al. Antithrombotic Therapy after Acute Coronary Syndrome or PCI in Atrial Fibrillation. N Engl J Med. 2019;380(16):1509–1524.
24. Vranckx P, Valgimigli M, Eckardt L, et al. Edoxaban-based versus vitamin K antagonist-based antithrombotic regimen after successful coronary stenting in patients with atrial fibrillation (ENTRUST-AF PCI): a randomised, open-label, phase 3b trial. Lancet. 2019;394(10206):1335–1343.
25. Lou B, Liang X, Wu Y, et al. Meta-Analysis Comparing Dual Versus Single Antiplatelet Therapy in Combination With Antithrombotic Therapy in Patients With Atrial Fibrillation Who Underwent Percutaneous Coronary Intervention With Stent Implantation. Am J Cardiol. 2018;122(4):604–611.

26. Bhatt DL. O PIONEERs! The Beginning of the End of Full-Dose Triple Therapy with Warfarin? Circulation. 2017;135(4):334–337.
27. Lopes RD, Leonardi S, Wojdyla DM, et al. Stent thrombosis in patients with atrial fibrillation undergoing coronary stenting in the AUGUSTUS trial. Circulation. 2020;141(9):781–783.
28. Ravi V, Pulipati P, Vij A, Kodumuri V. Meta-analysis comparing double versus Triple Anti-thrombotic Therapy in Patients with Atrial Fibrillation and Coronary Artery Disease. Am J Cardiol. 2020;125:19–28.
29. Lip GYH, Collet JP, Haude M, et al. 2018 Joint European consensus document on the management of antithrombotic therapy in atrial fibrillation patients presenting with acute coronary syndrome and/or undergoing percutaneous cardiovascular interventions: A joint consensus document of the Europ. Europace. 2019;21(2):192–193.
30. Calkins H, Chen LY, Cigarroa JE, et al. 2019 AHA/ACC/HRS Focused Update of the 2014 AHA/ ACC/HRS Guideline for the Management of Patients With Atrial Fibrillation. Circulation. 2019;140:e125-e151.
31. Hindricks G, Potpara T, Dagres N, et al. 2020 ESC Guidelines for the diagnosis and management of atrial fibrillation developed in collaboration with the European Association for Cardio-Thoracic Surgery (EACTS). Eur Heart J. 2021;42(5):373–498.
32. Angiolillo DJ, Goodman SG, Bhatt DL, et al. Antithrombotic Therapy in Patients With Atrial Fibrillation Treated With Oral Anticoagulation Undergoing Percutaneous Coronary Intervention. Circulation. 2018;138(5): 527–536.
33. Steffel J, Verhamme P, Potpara TS, et al. The 2018 European Heart Rhythm Association Practical Guide on the use of non-vitamin K antagonist oral anticoagulants in patients with atrial fibrillation. Eur Heart J. 2018;60:1–64.
34. Guimarães PO, Zakroysky P, Goyal A, Lopes RD, Kaltenbach LA, Wang TY. Usefulness of Antithrombotic Therapy in Patients With Atrial Fibrillation and Acute Myocardial Infarction. Am J Cardiol. 2019;123(1):12–18.
35. Wang YH, Kao HL, Wang CC, Lin SY, Lin FJ. Comparative effectiveness and safety of antithrombotic therapy in atrial fibrillation patients presenting with acute coronary syndrome or percutaneous coronary intervention. Acta Cardiol Sin. 2019;35(5):508–521.
36. Park J, Choi E-K, Han K-D, et al. Temporal trends in prevalence and antithrombotic treatment among Asians with atrial fibrillation undergoing percutaneous coronary intervention: A nationwide Korean population-based study. PLoS One. 2019;14(1):e0209593.
37. Mai L, Wu Y, Luo J, et al. A retrospective cohort study of oral anticoagulant treatment in patients with acute coronary syndrome and atrial fibrillation. BMJ Open. 2019;9(9):e031180.
38. Sabir I, Khavandi K, Brownrigg J, Camm AJ. Oral anticoagulants for Asian patients with atrial fibrillation. Nat Rev Cardiol. 2014;11(5):290–303.
39. Lamberts M, Gislason GH, Olesen JB, et al. Oral Anticoagulation and antiplatelets in atrial fibrillation patients after myocardial infarction and coronary intervention. J Am Coll Cardiol. 2013;62(11):981–989.
40. Rubboli A, Schlitt A, Kiviniemi T, et al. One-year outcome of patients with atrial fibrillation undergoing coronary artery Stenting: An analysis of the AFCAS registry. Clin Cardiol. 2014;37(6):357–364.
41. Li PK-T, Lui SL, Ng JK-C, et al. Addressing the burden of dialysis around the world: A summary of the roundtable discussion on dialysis economics at the First International Congress of Chinese Nephrologists 2015. Nephrology. 2017;22:3–8.
42. Dahal K, Kunwar S, Rijal J, Schulman P, Lee J. Stroke, major bleeding, and mortality outcomes in warfarin users with atrial fibrillation and chronic kidney disease: A meta-analysis of observational studies. Chest. 2016;149(4): 951–959.

12

Anticoagulation may contribute to antimicrobial treatment of Lemierre syndrome

Jie Ge, Peipei Zhou, Yifei Yang, Tianshu Xu and Xu Yang*

Abstract

Background: Lemierre syndrome (LS) is characterized by multisystemic infection beginning in the oropharynx, local thrombophlebitis (typically, of the internal jugular vein) and peripheral embolism. No evidence-based guidelines exist for the management of this disease, and the use of anticoagulation therapy remains particularly controversial.

Case presentation: A 61-year-old man presenting with left neck swelling, odynophagia, and dyspnea underwent emergency surgery and received intravenous antibiotics. The primary infection was controlled on hospital day 5, but on day 6 sudden leukocytosis and hypoxemia were observed. CT angiography revealed an intraluminal filling defect in the pulmonary artery on day 8. LS was diagnosed and anticoagulation therapy was initiated. The WBC count, which had maintained its peak values in the previous 2 days, decreased instantly after initiation, and follow-up controls showed thrombus resolution.

Conclusions: Our case supports the notion that anticoagulation therapy may be a valid supplement to antimicrobial therapy in LS, especially in the presence of a possibly young thrombus as suggested by clinical worsening.

Keywords: Anticoagulation, Infectious disease, Thromboembolism, Lemierre syndrome, Case report

Background

Despite its nonnegligible annual incidence of >1/100000, Lemierre syndrome (LS) often goes undiagnosed due to its non-specific symptoms [1, 2]. The most accurate definition of LS should include 1) infection that originates in the oropharynx, mastoiditis, oral cavity and sinusitis, 2) isolation of *Fusobacterium necrophorum* and 3) local thrombophlebitis, typically of the internal jugular vein, producing disseminated emboli to the periphery (often septic pulmonary emboli) [2–4]. However, as an obligate anaerobic bacterium, *Fusobacterium necrophorum* is often difficult to isolate in blood cultures. It requires a longer incubation period than other bacteria, and cultures can be false negative if antibiotics are administered before sample collection. In addition, other bacteria may cause the same clinical syndrome. Therefore, a clinical diagnosis of LS is considered to be still valid even when *Fusobacterium necrophorum* is undetected or other bacteria are detected [5–7]. Delayed treatment of LS can lead to multisystemic organ dysfunction, potential end-stage organ damage or death. Systemic emboli and septic pulmonary emboli can also be life threatening. Therefore, early diagnosis and treatment of LS are vital. The key tools of physicians are antibiotic therapy, anticoagulation therapy and drainage of abscesses [2]. The use of anticoagulation therapy remains controversial, and it is unclear whether anticoagulation treatment improves patient outcomes. Here, we report a case in which anticoagulation initiated after clinical worsening was followed by prompt clinical and

* Correspondence: Nova_gejie@163.com
Department of stomatology, Changzhou First People's Hospital, Juqian Street, Changzhou 185, Jiangsu, China

laboratory improvement, supporting a role of anticoagulation in the treatment of LS.

Case presentation

A 61-year-old man presented to the oral and maxillofacial surgery service with a 5-day history of left neck swelling, odynophagia, and dyspnea without chest pain or cough. He reported a history of 7-day odontalgia and 3-day intravenous cefotiam (1 g every 12 h) and metronidazole (500 mg every 8 h) treatment. He was otherwise healthy, with no known allergies. His weight was 65 kg. At the time of admission, the patient had an oxygen saturation (SpO) of 98% while breathing ambient air. Laboratory data revealed a white blood cell count (WBC) of 20.45×10^9 /L (Fig. 1 A), procalcitonin (PCT) of 1.142 ng/mL (Fig. 1 B), C-reactive protein (CRP) of 168.23 mg/L (Fig. 1 C), random blood glucose of 16.02 mmol/L and glycosylated hemoglobin of 8.7%. Computed tomography (CT) of the neck revealed diffusive swelling combined with pneumatosis (Fig. 2 A). The patient was then diagnosed with cervical necrotizing fasciitis.

He underwent emergency incision and drainage surgery and received empirical treatment with intravenous imipenem-cilastatin sodium (1 g every 8 h) and metronidazole (500 mg every 8 h). His blood glucose was controlled by insulin. Anaerobic cultures of pyogenic fluids and blood were obtained on admission and were sterile 5 days later, which may have been due to the antimicrobial treatment before admission. After five days of antimicrobial treatment (hospital day 5), the patient's WBC count had gradually decreased to 18.12×10^9 /L (Fig. 1 A; hospital day 5) and CRP to 8.51 mg/L (Fig. 1 C; hospital day 5). However, he had an SpO of 80% in room air and 96% with oxygen inhalation (5 L/min) on the sixth hospital day. Laboratory data showed that his WBC count increased to 21.77×10^9 /L (Fig. 1 A; hospital day 6), while his PCT level decreased to 0.211 ng/mL (Fig. 1 B; hospital day 6). A repeat CT scan revealed that the neck infection had regressed (Fig. 2 A) and that the pulmonary infection was stable (Fig. 2 B). Chest CT angiography revealed an intraluminal filling defect in the lower branch of left pulmonary artery on the eighth hospital day (Fig. 2 C). This manifestation was considered consistent with septic pulmonary embolism derived from the internal jugular vein, which was very close to the infection focus (Fig. 2 D). LS was diagnosed.

Anticoagulation therapy was performed with low molecular weight heparin (4250 U every 12 h) for the following 4 days. His WBC gradually decreased to 17.87×10^9 /L (Fig. 1 A; hospital day 13). Low molecular weight heparin was replaced with warfarin (3 mg every day) on hospital day 12. The international normalized ratio (INR) was monitored constantly and controlled between

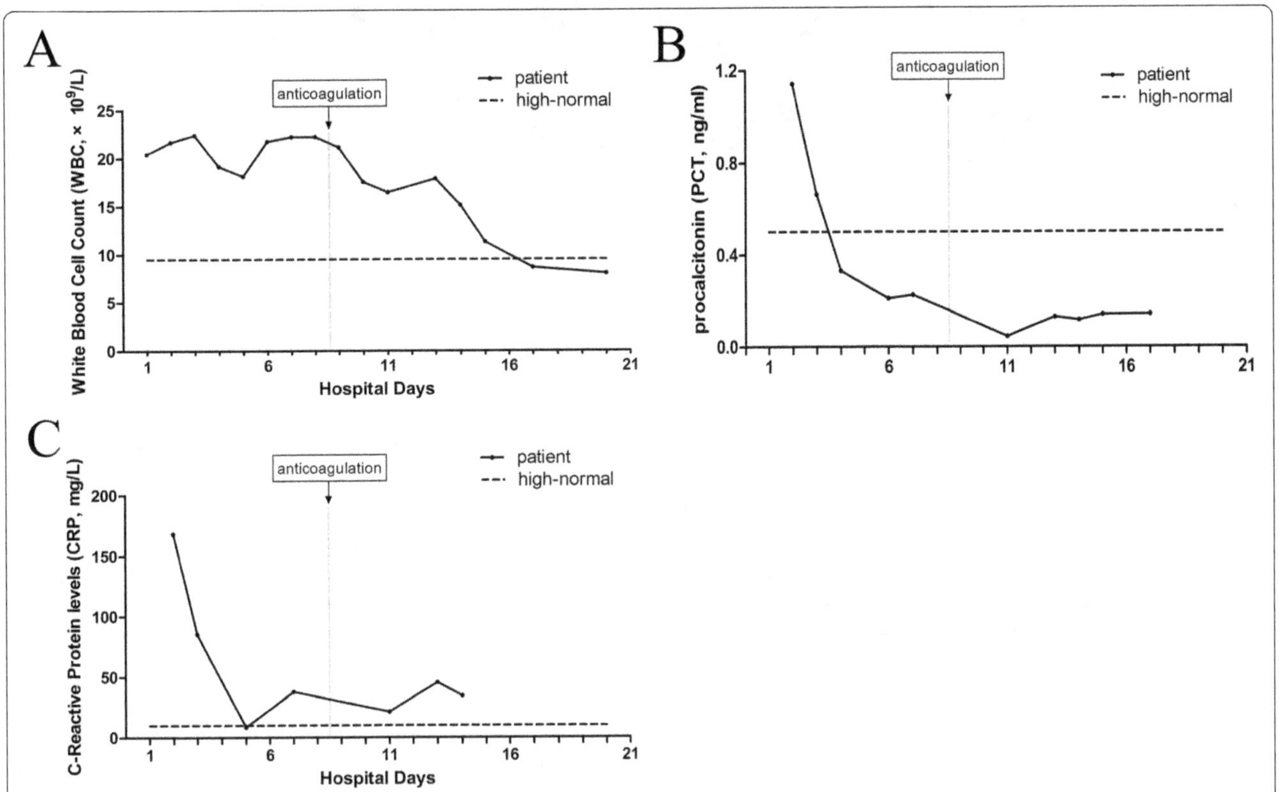

Fig. 1 Blood investigations. **A**: WBC count. **B**: PCT level. **C**: CRP level

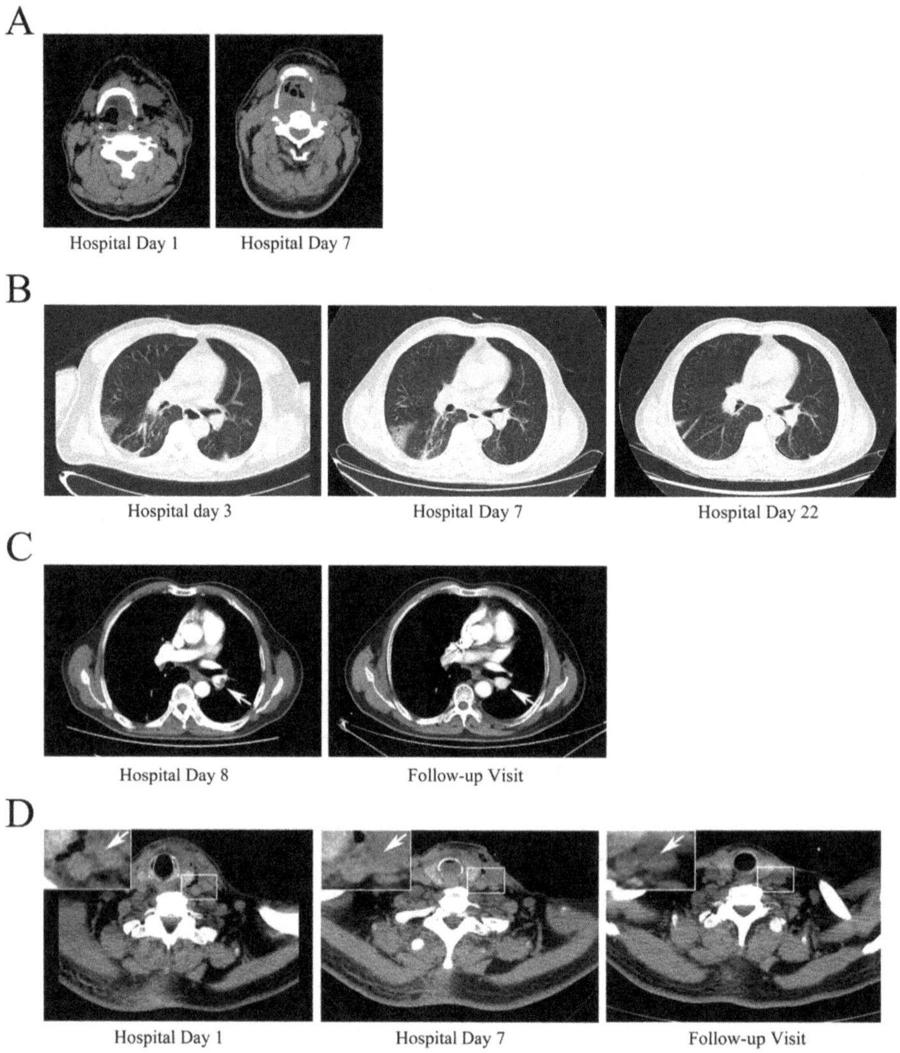

Fig. 2 Imaging. **A**: Neck CT. **B**: Chest CT. **C**: Pulmonary artery CT. White arrow: pulmonary emboli in the "Hospital Day 8" image; pulmonary emboli disappeared in the "Follow-up Visit" image. **D**: Internal jugular vein CT. White arrow: signs of inflammation next to the internal jugular vein in "Hospital Day 1" and "Hospital Day 7" images; the signs of inflammation disappeared in the "Follow-up Visit" image

2 and 2.5. The patient's WBC count decreased to 8.67 × 10^9 /L on hospital day 17 and remained normal on the following days (Fig. 1 A). Repeat chest CT showed that the pulmonary infection was cured on hospital day 22 (Fig. 2 B). He was discharged from the hospital on hospital day 24 and continued anticoagulation therapy. When he returned for a follow-up visit at the twentieth week, the embolus had dissolved (Fig. 2 C), and anticoagulation therapy was discontinued. No haemorrhage occurred during anticoagulation therapy.

Discussion and conclusions

In this case, the primary infection was controlled on hospital day 5, as proven by CT evaluation and decreased WBC and PCT levels. The sudden increase in WBC count and decrease in SpO on hospital day 6 were considered to be caused by newly formed septic pulmonary emboli. Pulmonary emboli above the subsegmental level are a possible, but rare complication of LS, and 3 days were required for diagnosis of LS. As a result, anticoagulation therapy was not initiated until hospital day 8. The WBC count maintained its peak value on hospital days 6–8 before anticoagulation therapy was initiated, but rapidly decreased after initiation. This quick response suggests that anticoagulation therapy may have contributed to the infection resolution achieved by antimicrobials.

In a review of 137 cases of LS, the authors found that 4–6 weeks of carbapenem or piperacillin/tazobactam combined with metronidazole were effective in terms of infection control, but the reason for the choice of such a duration was not explained in any of the included papers [6]. Our antimicrobial treatment was maintained until the WBC counts remained normal for 1 week and clinical symptoms improved. The duration was 24 days in total and 16 days after anticoagulation therapy proceeded, which is much shorter than the average. However, it is still unknown whether anticoagulation therapy is essential, which is an important issue especially in cases, such as the one we described, that are complicated by large intraluminal emboli.

In the past few decades, evidence remained poor regarding the management of LS, particularly regarding its potentially life-threatening thromboembolic complications. Consequently, physicians must make their decisions based on small case series or anecdotal cases when facing uncommon thromboembolic conditions, such as LS. Physicians who are opposed to anticoagulant treatment confirm that the thrombus is caused by an infection process and will be resolved at the same time when the infection is resolved. In contrast, some authors confirm that anticoagulant therapy may reduce the morbidity and mortality of serious complications, such as cavernous sinus thrombosis or pulmonary embolism. Theoretically, a septic thrombus sequesters bacteria and creates a barrier to antibiotic penetration. When the thrombus is dissolved by anticoagulants, the bacteria are exposed to a higher concentration of antibiotics, increasing accessibility [8]. Our case supports this hypothesis precisely. Unfortunately, randomized controlled trials are impractical to investigate the use of anticoagulation therapy in the treatment of LS due to the rarity of this illness. Based on small case series, the proposal has been advanced to reserve this approach to bilateral disease only; a single-center retrospective series has found no association with thrombus recanalization, although it is unclear whether recanalization is clinically relevant [9]. The improvement seen in our case despite the absence of bilateral disease and the finding of recanalization following anticoagulation could be explained by the likelihood that the thrombus had developed recently, as suggested by the sudden increase in infection parameters, and may have been more vulnerable to anticoagulation than an older, organized thrombus. This possibility is consistent with the known biology of venous thrombi [10] and should be explored by future research.

A recent European collaborative study performed an individual patient-level analysis of 712 cases published globally from 2000 to 2017 [1]. The authors could not find disease-specific elements against the safety of anticoagulation and drew the conclusion that therapeutic anticoagulation is indicated for LS if there are no contraindications. Nevertheless, the authors did not provide definitive guidelines for the duration of anticoagulation. According to the American College of Chest Physicians guidelines for provoked thrombotic events, anticoagulation therapy is recommended for a duration of at least 3 months [11], which may be available for reference to Lemierre syndrome presented pulmonary embolism. Our patient received a treatment duration of 20 weeks because his follow-up visit was delayed by the outbreak of COVID-19. A limitation of our case is the lack of microbial isolation. However, the diagnosis of LS is currently accepted even without microbial isolation in the presence of a clinical diagnosis of sepsis from an oropharyngeal focus and thrombi or emboli consistent with the primary infection location [5]. This case satisfies the broad criteria of Lemierre syndrome, that are currently accepted, but not the restrictive or classic criteria that require evidence of jugular vein thrombosis and *Fusobacterium necrophorum*, and that future management studies should report results for both subpopulations.

In conclusion, therapeutic anticoagulation may be considered in the management of LS, while further research is needed to evaluate whether the use of anticoagulant and antibiotics leads to better clinical outcomes than the use of antibiotics alone.

Patient perspective

I'm the daughter of the patient. We are grateful to the doctors' help in Changzhou First People's Hospital and happy to share the treatment experience of my father.

Abbreviations

LS: Lemierre syndrome; SpO: Oxygen saturation; WBC: White blood cell count; CRP: C-Reactive protein; PCT: Procalcitonin; CT: Computed tomography; INR: International normalized ratio

Acknowledgements

Not applicable.

Authors' contributions

JG and XY performed the literature review and drafted the manuscript. PPZ and YFY obtained the image data. TSX reviewed the report and provided important revisions. All authors read and approved the final manuscript.

References

1. Valerio L, Zane F, Sacco C, Granziera S, Nicoletti T, Russo M, et al. Patients with Lemierre syndrome have a high risk of new thromboembolic complications, clinical sequelae and death: an analysis of 712 cases. J Intern Med. 2021 Mar;289(3):325–39. https://doi.org/10.1111/joim.13114.
2. Osowicki J, Kapur S, Phuong LK, Dobson S. The long shadow of lemierre's syndrome. J Infect. 2017;74 Suppl 1:S47–53. https://doi.org/10.1016/S0163-4453(17)30191-3.
3. Schulman S. Lemierre syndrome - treat with antibiotics, anticoagulants or both? J Intern Med. 2021 Mar;289(3):437–8. https://doi.org/10.1111/joim.13100.
4. Walkty A, Embil J. Lemierre's Syndrome. N Engl J Med. 2019 Mar 21;380(12):e16. https://doi.org/10.1056/NEJMicm1808378.
5. Valerio L, Corsi G, Sebastian T, Barco S. Lemierre syndrome: current evidence and rationale of the Bacteria-associated thrombosis, thrombophlebitis and LEmierre syndrome (BATTLE) registry. Thromb Res. 2020 Dec;196:494–9. https://doi.org/10.1016/j.thromres.2020.10.002.
6. Johannesen KM, Bodtger U. Lemierre's syndrome: current perspectives on diagnosis and management. Infect Drug Resist. 2016;9:221–7. https://doi.org/10.2147/IDR.S95050.

7. Hill UG, Vallis MP, Cotter T, Hegarty MA. Has Lemierre's syndrome become a bacteriological diagnosis? Br J Hosp Med (Lond). 2010;71(3):169. https://doi.org/10.12968/hmed.2010.71.3.46983.
8. Campo F, Fusconi M, Ciotti M, Diso D, Greco A, Cattaneo CG, et al. Antibiotic and anticoagulation therapy in Lemierre's syndrome: case report and review. J Chemother. 2019 Feb;31(1):42–8. https://doi.org/10.1080/1120009X.2018.1554992.
9. Valerio L, Pleming W, Pecci A, Barco S. Management of Lemierre syndrome. Minerva Med. 2021. https://doi.org/10.23736/S0026-4806.21.07497-8.
10. Saha P, Humphries J, Modarai B, Mattock K, Waltham M, Evans CE, et al. Leukocytes and the natural history of deep vein thrombosis: current concepts and future directions. Arterioscler Thromb Vasc Biol. 2011 Mar;31(3):506–12. https://doi.org/10.1161/ATVBAHA.110.213405.
11. Kearon C, Akl EA, Ornelas J, Blaivas A, Jimenez D, Bounameaux H, et al. Antithrombotic therapy for VTE disease: CHEST guideline and expert panel report. Chest. 2016 Feb;149(2):315–52. https://doi.org/10.1016/j.chest.2015.11.026.

13

Impact of oral anticoagulation therapy on postoperative atrial fibrillation outcomes

Mariana Fragão-Marques[1,2,3*], Francisco Teixeira[3], Jennifer Mancio[1,3], Nair Seixas[4], João Rocha-Neves[2,3], Inês Falcão-Pires[1,3] and Adelino Leite-Moreira[1,2,3]

Abstract

Background: Post-operative atrial fibrillation (POAF) is the most common complication after cardiac surgery. Recent studies had shown this phenomenon is no longer considered transitory and is associated with higher risk of thromboembolic events or death. The aim of this study was to systematically review and analyze previous studies comparing oral anticoagulation therapy with no anticoagulation, regarding these long-term outcomes.

Methods: PubMed/MEDLINE, EMBASE, Web of Science and Cochrane Database were systematically searched to identify the studies comparing the risk of stroke, or thromboembolic events or mortality of POAF patients who received anticoagulation compared with those who were not anticoagulated. Incidence of stroke, thromboembolic events and all-cause mortality were evaluated up to 10 years after surgery. Time-to-event outcomes were collected through hazard ratio (HR) along with their variance and the early endpoints using frequencies or odds ratio (OR). Random effect models were used to compute statistical combined measures and 95% confidence intervals (CI). Heterogeneity was evaluated through Q statistic-related measures of variance (Tau^2, I^2, Chi-squared test).

Results: Eight observational cohort studies were selected, including 15,335 patients (3492 on Oral Anticoagulants (OAC) vs 11,429 without OAC) that met the inclusion criteria for qualitative synthesis. Patients had a wide gender distribution (38.6–82.3%), each study with a mean age above 65 years (67.5–85). Vitamin K antagonists were commonly prescribed anticoagulants (74.3–100%). OAC was associated with a protective impact on all-cause mortality at a mean of 5.0 years of follow-up (HR is 0.85 [0.72–1.01]; $p = 0.07$; $I^2 = 48\%$). Thromboembolic events did not differ between the two treatment arms (HR 0.68 [0.40–1.15], $p = 0.15$).

Conclusion: Current literature suggests a possibly protective impact of OAC therapy for all-cause mortality in patients with new-onset atrial fibrillation after cardiac surgery. However, it does not appear to impact thromboembolism rate.

Keywords: Atrial fibrillation, Cardiac surgery, Anticoagulation, Long-term outcome

* Correspondence: marianaifrm@gmail.com
[1]Cardiovascular Research and Development Center, Faculty of Medicine of the University of Porto, 4200 Porto, Portugal
[2]São João University Hospital Center, Porto, Portugal

Introduction

Postoperative atrial fibrillation (POAF) is the most common complication after cardiac surgery, with a global incidence of 20–40%. Although its pathophysiologic mechanism is still uncertain, some progress has been made. Cardiac surgery is a stressful event which generates a chain of inflammatory reactions [1], with pro-inflammatory cytokines and increased oxidative stress. Such inflammation affects atrial conduction during atrial fibrillation by changing sodium channel function through the reduction of sodium currents and consequent upstroke velocity [2–4].

Moreover, one third of patients after coronary artery bypass grafting (CABG) and almost half of patients after valve repair/replacement (VR) develop atrial fibrillation after a cardiac procedure, usually occurring early in the recovery period [5, 6]. Although this arrhythmia was previously thought as transitory and benign, patients who develop the arrhythmia have longer intensive care unit hospitalizations, higher healthcare costs, and an increased risk of postoperative complications, namely stroke, thromboembolic events and mortality, both intra-hospital and at 6 months [7–9].

While the relationship between short-term outcomes and POAF is well defined, only a few studies have demonstrated that POAF is associated with higher long-term stroke risk and mortality, contrasting to what was previously thought of POAF as a transitory and nonthreatening event [3, 10]. Indeed, surgical and anaesthetic techniques have improved over time, although patients are older and have a higher prevalence of comorbidities, possibly implying an increased structural left atrium remodelling [11–13]. Furthermore, evidence on anticoagulation therapy in this subgroup of patients is scarce, although some studies have analyzed the relationship of anticoagulation therapy in POAF management with the occurrence of adverse outcomes, namely thromboembolism and all-cause mortality [14–18]. Because of the older age of cardiac surgery patients, risks and benefits of OAC (Oral Anticoagulant) therapy should be carefully considered.

European guidelines for the management of atrial fibrillation are very clear and encourage the use of anticoagulation in AF patients for stroke prophylaxis [19]. Conversely, management of POAF is still a topic of debate in the scientific community. On one hand, 2014 AHA/ACA guidelines recommend the use of beta-blockers and nondihydropyridine calcium channel blockers, while ESC 2020 guidelines suggest amiodarone or vernakalant have been efficient in converting postoperative AF to sinus rhythm. On the other hand, the use of anticoagulation lacks good quality evidence, with no randomized clinical trials available and few observational studies. Thus, European guidelines leave the decision of anticoagulation therapy to the physician, while American guidelines (AHA/ACA) do not mention any course of action on this matter [20, 21].

The aim of this systematic review/meta-analysis was to investigate if the use of anticoagulation in patients who developed POAF undergoing cardiac surgery has an association with lower rates of long-term thromboembolic events, stroke, major bleeding and all-cause mortality; and to identify subgroups of POAF patients that can benefit more from OAC therapy.

Methods

The study protocol was registered in PROSPERO (PROSPERO ID: CRD42020208229) in accordance with standard reporting conventions. PRISMA guidelines were used in the writing of this manuscript.

Data sources and search strategy

A MEDLINE, EMBASE, Web of Science and Cochrane Database search was performed to find evidence up to the 5th August 2021 on stroke prevention with oral anticoagulants in patients who developed atrial fibrillation after cardiac surgery. The search query was constructed using the keywords *"POAF", "new onset postoperative atrial fibrillation", "new onset atrial fibrillation", "postoperative atrial fibrillation", "anticoagulants" and "stroke".* The detailed search query is reported in supplementary materials (Table 1S).

Study selection

One reviewer independently screened search records for inclusion (FT) and another checked decisions (MFM). Titles and abstracts were screened at this stage and relevant studies were selected for full-text analysis. Inclusion criteria included randomized clinical trials and cohort studies on patients submitted to cardiac surgery who developed postoperative atrial fibrillation and received oral anticoagulation therapy versus no anticoagulation. Selected studies had to include stroke, a combined outcome including stroke (example: major adverse cardiovascular events (MACE), thromboembolic events), or all-cause mortality. Exclusion criteria included manuscripts in a language other than English, no full text available, duplicate manuscripts, and absence of outcomes of interest in the published manuscript.

Data extraction and quality assessment

Two reviewers (MFM, FT) blindly and independently checked the full texts, decided on the inclusion of individual studies and extracted data about study characteristics and event rates. Disagreements between reviewers were decided by the most senior reviewer. Extracted data included event rates of long-term 1) thromboembolism, a composite outcome of ischemic stroke, transient cerebral ischemia, and thrombosis or embolism in peripheral arteries; 2) stroke; 3) all-cause mortality; and 4) major bleeding. Estimates were presented as adjusted Hazard Ratios (HR) and respective 95% Confidence Intervals (CI).

Risk of bias was assessed by two blinded reviewers (MFM, FT), independently, using the Cochrane Risk Of Bias in Non-randomized Studies - of Interventions (ROBINS-I) tool (all selected studies were observational) [22]. Evaluated bias domains included bias due to confounding, selection bias, bias in classification of interventions, bias due to deviations from intended interventions, bias due to missing data, bias in measurement of outcomes and bias in selection of the reported result.

Data analysis

Assessment of reporting bias was performed with the Egger's regression test and respective funnel plot. Heterogeneity was evaluated through Q statistic-related measures of variance (Tau^2, I^2, Chi-squared test), and a random-effects model with an inverse variance method was preferred to compute estimates for the summary effect. Forest plots were used to display results from the meta-analysis, where the measure of effect for each study is represented by a square and the respective areas are proportional to study weight.

A p value inferior to 0.05 was considered statistically significant for all analyses. Computations were conducted using Review Manager 5.3 and Stata 16.1.

Results

A total of 2890 records were identified through database searching, of which 1730 were kept after duplicates were removed. Thirty publications were assessed for eligibility through their full texts, with 8 manuscripts selected for qualitative synthesis. Two publications were excluded from quantitative analysis, since the number of patients and events was extremely low, with two additional studies excluded because their patient population was submitted to transcutaneous procedures (see below). Fig. 1 depicts the study selection process.

Included research papers were published between 2010 and 2021, with a wide range of locations (Denmark, USA, South Korea, Poland, United Kingdom, Australia, Brazil, Italy, India). All papers were observational and based on a prospective cohort (Table 1). The

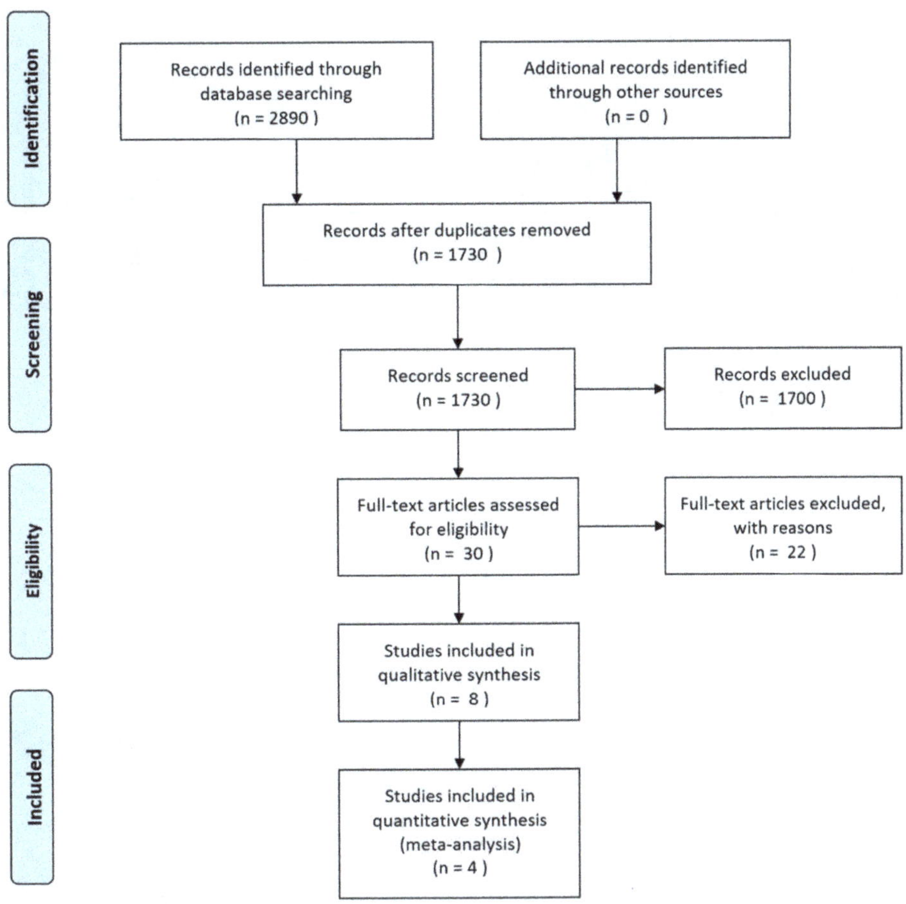

Fig. 1 Flowchart of the screening and selection process

Table 1 Included studies in qualitative synthesis

First Author	Year	Country	Patient Selection	Study Design	Anticoagulation	POAF definition	POAF (N)	OAC vs No Anticoagulants	Number	Age	Sex % (Males)	Type of Surgery		
												CABG	Valve	CABG + Valve
Butt et al. [23]	2018	Denmark	1/1/2000–30/6/2015	Prospective Cohort	83.4% Warfarin	AF rhythm requiring either medical therapy or cardioversion during hospitalization in patients without previous history of AF episodes	2108	Vitamin K or non-vitamin K antagonists	175	Median (IQR): 69.2 (63.7–74.7)	82.3	X		
								No anticoagulant	1527					
Vora et al. [24]	2018	USA	01/11/2011–30/09/2015	Prospective Cohort	83.0% Warfarin 15.2% Factor Xa inhibitor	New-onset AF following TAVR	1138	Oral Anticoagulant	329	Median (IQR): 85 (78–88)	38.6		TAVR	
					1.8% Dabigatran			No anticoagulant	809					
Butt et al. [25]	2019	Denmark	01/01/2000–30/06/2015	Prospective Cohort	97.6% Warfarin	AF rhythm requiring either medical therapy or cardioversion during hospitalization in patients without previous history of AF	675	Oral Anticoagulant	420	Median (IQR): 71 (65–77)	59.3		Aortic and/or Mitral Valve Repair/ Replacement	
								No anticoagulant	255					
El-Chami et al. [26]	2010	USA	1/1/1996–31/12/2007	Retrospective analysis of a Prospective Cohort	100% Warfarin	Occurence of new-onset POAF or atrial flutter requiring treatment	2985	Warfarin	613	Mean ± sd: 67.5 ± 9.5	73	X		
								No anticoagulant	2375					
Yoon et al. [27]	2019	South Korea	1/3/2010–1/2/2017	Prospective Cohort	Warfarin or Novel Oral Anticoagulant	Occurence of any episode of new-onset AF or flutter through hospitalization that lasted at least 30 s	31	Anticoagulant	11	Mean ± sd: 79.4 ± 5.0	52		TAVR	
								No anticoagulant	20					
Taha et al. [28]	2020	Sweden	1/1/2007–31/12/2015	Prospective Cohort	86.2% Vitamin K antagonists	POAF was defined as any new-onset atrial fibrillation during the first 30 postoperative days	7368	OAC	1770	Mean ± sd: 70 ± 8.0	81.5	X		
								No Anticoagulants	5598					
Benedetto et al. [29]	2020	Poland, UK, Austria, Australia, Brazil, Italy, India	06/2004–12/2007	Post hoc analysis of a Randomized Controlled Multicenter Trial	100% Warfarin	Occurence of any episode of AF or flutter (collectively called pAF for this analysis) after the index procedure through the time of discharge that lasted at least 30 s and was captured on a standard 12-lead ECG or cardiac telemetry	734	Warfarin	61	Mean ± sd: 66.41 ± 8.16	86,5	X		
								No Anticoagulant	662					
Madsen et al. [30]	2021	Denmark	1999–2016	Retrospective cohort	74.3% Vitamin K antagonists	AF within 30 days following STEMI	296	OAC therapy	113	Median (IQR): 71 (64–79)	69.9	PPCI		
								No Anticoagulant	183					

Table 1 Included studies in qualitative synthesis *(Continued)*

First Author	Follow-up time	Thromboembolism	Stroke	All-cause Mortality	CHA2DS2-VASc			HAS-BLED		Major bleeding	Echocardiography data
								OAC	No OAC		Left ventricle ejection fraction ≤ 30% n(%)
Butt et al. [23]	Median (IQR) 5.1 (2.2–9.2) years	HRa: 0.55 [0.32–0.95]	–	HRa: 1.09 [0.82–1.43]	**POAF:** mean ± sd: 3.2 ± 1.4			**POAF:** mean ± sd: 2.2 ± 1.1		–	-
Vora et al. [24]	1 year	–	HRa: 1.12 [0.67–1.89]	HRa: 2.08 [1.56–2.78]	**POAF:** median (IQR): 5 [5, 6]			–		HRa: 0.77 [0.61–0.98]	46 (4.0)
Butt et al. [25]	Median (IQR) 4.2 (2.0–7.1) years	HRa: 0.45 [0.22–0.90]	–	HRa: 0.64 [0.41–0.99]	**POAF:** mean ± sd: 2.9 ± 1.7			Mean ± sd: 2.1 ± 1.2	Mean ± sd: 2.2 ± 1.2	–	–
El-Chami et al. [26]	Mean 6 years (range 0–12)	–	–	HRa: 0.78 [0.66–0.92]	–			–		–	–
Yoon et al. [27]	12 months	OR: 0.67	–	–	**POAF:** mean ± sd: 4.1 ± 1.4			–		–	1 (3.2)
First Author	**Follow-up time**	**Thromboembolism**	**Stroke**	**All-cause Mortality**	**CHA2DS2-VASc**			**HAS-BLED**		**Major bleeding**	**Echocardiography data**
						OAC	**No OAC**	**OAC**	**No OAC**		**Left ventricle ejection fraction ≤ 30% n(%)**
Taha et al. [28]	4.5 years (range 0–9)	HRa: 1.01 [0.77–1.33]	HRa: 1.08 [0.80–1.45]	HRa: [0.73–1.09]	**≥2**	n(%) 1637 (95.5)	n(%) 5201 (94.2)	–	–	HRa: 1.40 [1.08–1.82]	–
					≥4	n(%) 925 (54.0)	n(%) 2738 (50.3)				
Benedetto et al. [29]	10 years	–	Cumulative incidence (OAC): 3.6% [95% CI 0.0–8.4%]	-	**POAF:** mean ± sd: 3.46 ± 1.31			–	–	Cumulative Incidence (OAC): 3.4 [95% CI 0.0–8.1]	21 (2.9)
			Cumulative incidence (No OAC): 5.3% [95% CI 3.5–7.0%]							Cumulative Incidence (No OAC): 4.1 [95% CI 2.6–5.7]	
Madsen et al. [30]	Median (IQR) 4.7 (2.8–7.4) years	–	HRa: 0.70 [0.33–1.49]	HRa: 0.69 [0.47–1.00]	**≥2**	n(%) 105 (92.9%)	n(%) 169 (92.4%)	**≥3:** n(%) 77 (68.1)	**≥3:** n(%) 92 (50.3)	HRa: 1.31 [0.75–2.27]	–

HRa adjusted Hazard Ratio with 95% Confidence Intervals

total number of included patients with POAF for quantitative synthesis was 12,733 (2978 with Oral Anticoagulants (OAC) vs 9755 without OAC). Vitamin K antagonists represented the majority of prescribed oral anticoagulants across all studies (74.3–100%), although Yoon et al. 2019 lacked information concerning this issue [27].

While POAF definitions included only new-onset episodes, Vora et al. 2018 and Yoon et al. 2019 considered all cases of POAF, in contrast with the remaining studies, which exclusively selected episodes requiring treatment. All studies had a mean age above 65 years (67.5–85), even though gender distribution varied significantly across studies (38.6–82.3% of males), with male gender being more common in CABG surgery. Selected research papers included both CABG [23, 26] and valve repair/replacement [24, 25, 27].

Risk of bias is represented in Fig. 1S and Fig. 2S (supplementary content). Yoon et al. 2019 presented their results as a percentage of events between therapeutic groups, without an adjusted measure of effect or an adequate time-dependent analysis. In the OAC group, there was no description of which specific anticoagulants were used and only 2 thromboembolic events were reported. Thus, this study was considered as having a serious risk of bias and was excluded from quantitative analysis. Benedetto et al. 2020 is a post-hoc analysis of a well-designed randomized clinical trial, although it did not present time-dependent adjusted estimates; thus, this study was not included in the quantitative synthesis and had a serious risk of bias in domain 1, thus presenting an overall serious risk of bias. The remaining studies had a moderate risk of bias due to confounding, as all measures of effect were adjusted (see below), despite not being randomized controlled trials. The selected papers for quantitative synthesis all had time-dependent adjusted estimates and were exclusively from cohorts submitted to conventional cardiac surgery (Vora et al. and Madsen et al. were excluded). Moreover, considering papers with more than one reported outcome, Butt et al. 2018 and Butt et al. 2019 had into account competing risks in their outcome analysis. Taha et al. 2020, on the other hand, does not clarify this potential source of confounding.

Furthermore, there was little information concerning deviations from intended interventions or missing data. However, Butt et al. 2019 reported a decrease to 55.0% at 3 months of patients who were initially in the OAC treatment arm, to 31.7% at 6 months and 22.1% at 1 year of follow-up, being attributed a serious risk of bias concerning deviations from intended treatment. Benedetto et al. 2020 and El Chami et al. 2010 used multiple imputation to eliminate missing values, the latter considering absent data as missing at random; thus, a low risk of bias was considered in these cases. Apart from Yoon et al. 2019, all selected studies were classified as having an overall moderate risk of bias.

All-cause mortality

All-cause mortality was reported in all selected studies for quantitative analysis. The median or mean follow-up varied between 4.2–6 years and the pooled HR is 0.85 [0.72–1.01] ($p = 0.07$; $I^2 = 48\%$), with 2978 vs 9755 (OAC vs control) analyzed patients (Fig. 2). Covariates used in the adjusted model are presented in Table 2S.

Publication bias

Publication bias for this outcome was evaluated by a funnel plot and Egger's regression test ($p = 0.85$), which suggests absence of bias – Fig. 3.

Thromboembolism

Thromboembolism was reported in 3 of the selected studies [23, 25, 28] and was defined as a composite of ischemic stroke, transient cerebral ischemia, and thrombosis or embolism in peripheral arteries in all the research papers (Table 3S). A total of 2365 vs 7380 (OAC vs control) patients were included in the analysis and median follow-up time varied between 4.2–5.1 years. HR and 95% CI were adjusted for comorbidities and other concomitant medical therapy (Table 2S). The pooled estimate was HR 0.68 [0.40–1.15] ($p = 0.15$; $I^2 = 72\%$) and the respective forest plot is represented in Fig. 4.

Study or Subgroup	log[Hazard Ratio]	SE	OAC Total	Control Total	Weight	Hazard Ratio IV, Random, 95% CI
Butt et al 2018	0.0862	0.1452	175	1527	21.5%	1.09 [0.82, 1.45]
Butt et al 2019	-0.4463	0.2272	420	255	11.4%	0.64 [0.41, 1.00]
El Chami 2010	-0.2485	0.0852	613	2375	35.7%	0.78 [0.66, 0.92]
Taha et al 2020	-0.1165	0.1011	1770	5598	31.3%	0.89 [0.73, 1.09]
Total (95% CI)			**2978**	**9755**	**100.0%**	**0.85 [0.72, 1.01]**

Heterogeneity: Tau² = 0.01; Chi² = 5.72, df = 3 (P = 0.13); I² = 48%
Test for overall effect: Z = 1.83 (P = 0.07)

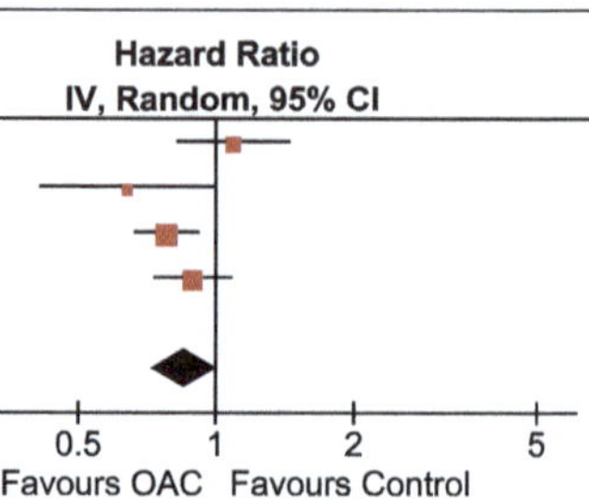

Fig. 2 Pooled estimate of all-cause mortality with OAC therapy

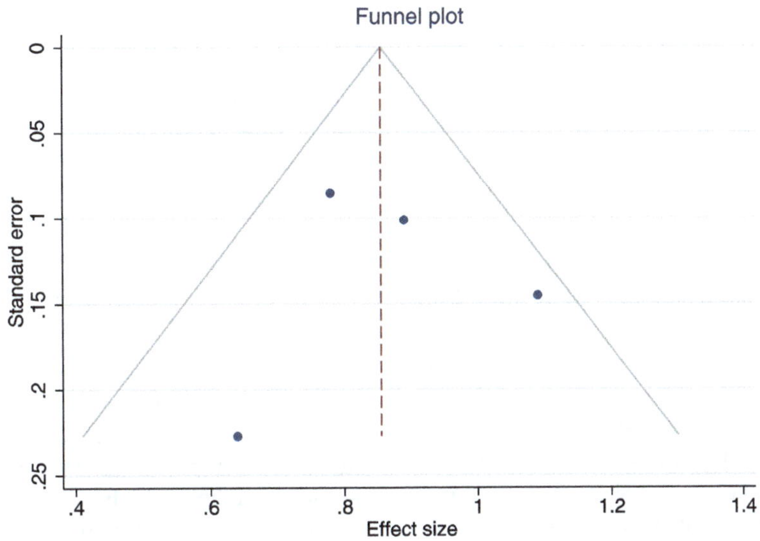

Fig. 3 Funnel plot and Egger's regression test

Stroke

Stroke was reported as a separate outcome in 3 studies – Madsen et al. (Primary Percutaneous Coronary Intervention - PPCI), Taha et al. (CABG) and Vora et al. (Transcatheter Aortic Valve Replacement - TAVR). The results were similar between studies, with no reported impact of OAC on stroke rates (Madsen et al. HR 0.70 [0.33–1.48]; Taha et al. HR 1.08 [0.80–1.46]; and Vora et al. HR 1.12 [0.67–1.87]). Table 2S presents the covariates included in each study's multivariate cox regression.

Major bleeding

This outcome was reported in 3 of the included studies (Madsen et al., Taha et al. and Vora et al.), with conflicting results between publications. Taha et al. found an association between OAC therapy and major bleeding (HR 1.40 [1.08–1.81]), with Madsen et al. reporting no significant impact of OACs in bleeding events (HR 1.31 [0.75–2.29]). However, Vora et al. reported a protective effect of this therapy – HR 0.77 [0.61–0.97]. The covariates used in each of the 3 studies are present in Table 2S and the respective definitions for major bleeding are in Table 3S.

Discussion

In this meta-analysis, POAF patients treated with OACs appear to have a reduction in long-term all-cause mortality ($p = 0.07$, non-significant). Furthermore, these patients had a tendency towards a reduction in risk of long-term thromboembolic events ($p = 0.15$).

This work combined the available research papers on OAC therapy, resulting in estimates with a high number of patients (12,733 in total) corresponding to high-quality observational studies. AF has long been implicated in the incidence of stroke, with a fivefold increase in risk of ischemic stroke, namely, cardioembolic, which has particularly high mortality and residual disability [31]. Cryptogenic strokes may have AF as an underdiagnosed underlying cause, as demonstrated by monitoring with an insertable cardiac monitor in a randomized controlled trial [32]. In addition to stroke, prevention of systemic thromboembolic events is part of the fundamental management of AF [33]; AF represents a significant cause of mortality, with increasing incidence due to aging demographics [4, 34]. As far as AF management is concerned, anticoagulation therapy with vitamin K antagonists (VKA) reduces stroke and mortality by 64 and 26%, respectively [35]. On the other hand, the novel oral

Study or Subgroup	log[Hazard Ratio]	SE	OAC Total	Control Total	Weight	Hazard Ratio IV, Random, 95% CI
Butt et al 2018	-0.5978	0.2763	175	1527	32.0%	0.55 [0.32, 0.95]
Butt et al 2019	-0.7985	0.3651	420	255	25.7%	0.45 [0.22, 0.92]
Taha et al 2020	0.01	0.1384	1770	5598	42.4%	1.01 [0.77, 1.32]
Total (95% CI)			**2365**	**7380**	**100.0%**	**0.68 [0.40, 1.15]**

Heterogeneity: Tau² = 0.16; Chi² = 7.04, df = 2 (P = 0.03); I² = 72%
Test for overall effect: Z = 1.44 (P = 0.15)

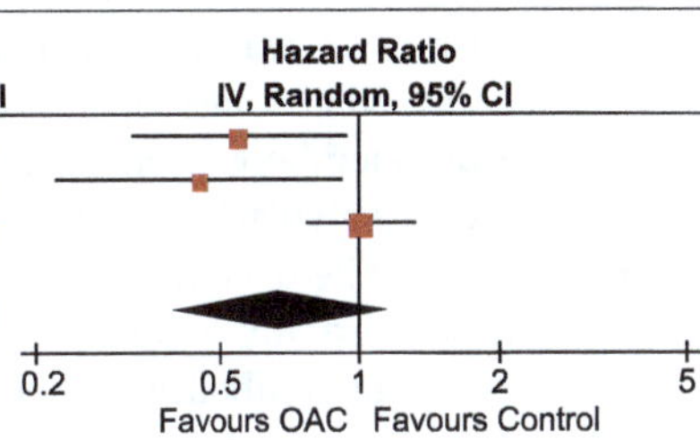

Fig. 4 Pooled estimate of thromboembolism event with OAC therapy

anticoagulants (NOAC) are a reasonable alternative for thromboembolic event prevention in non-valvular AF, with a 19% reduction in risk of stroke/systemic embolism, and 51% reduction in haemorrhagic stroke when compared with VKAs [36].

Nevertheless, paroxysmal AF classification remains elusive, with diverse patterns possibly requiring and presenting different treatments and outcomes [7, 37]. POAF is a subtype of paroxysmal AF linked to increased early stroke and 30-day mortality risk [38]. Concerning long-term results, POAF is associated with an increased risk of stroke and mortality, as demonstrated in a meta-analysis of patients submitted to both cardiac and non-cardiac surgery, where the latter presented a higher risk of stroke when compared to cardiac surgery. These patients presented a 37% increase in risk of both long-term stroke and mortality [39]. In this work, OAC therapy appears to prevent long-term mortality ($p = 0.07$, non-significant), with a tendency to reduce long-term thromboembolic events ($p = 0.15$).

It is necessary to further understand if short and long POAF episodes present the same stroke risk, and if they benefit in a similar way from OAC therapy. Similarly, there is no evidence in which type of anticoagulation therapy should be used, as all research papers considered OAC therapy without discriminating NOAC vs VKA. Currently, guidelines recommend considering the overall presence of stroke and bleeding risk factors, although the definition of AF burden at which to initiate OAC therapy is poorly defined, and consequently, this knowledge gap results in significant variation in clinical practice [34, 40]. In this meta-analysis, bleeding risk varied between heterogeneous studies, which could be related both to the underlying disease (coronary artery disease or valvular disease) and to the type of procedure (CABG, PPCI or TAVR).

Thromboembolic events are one of the most serious complications of AF, and without anticoagulation therapy, stroke occurrence varies between 1.9 and 18.2%, depending on comorbidities [41]. The potential decrease in mortality in OAC-treated POAF patients could be related to cardiovascular events. Additionally, POAF is a risk factor for AF occurrence at follow-up, which could also help to explain these findings [41]. However, thromboembolism risk was not decreased significantly with OAC-therapy. Main causes of mortality in AF could be not only thromboembolic events but also heart failure (either ischemic or valvular) and bleeding due to anticoagulation therapy. The overall measure of effect (hazard ratio) in all-cause mortality was 0.85 [0.72–1.01] vs 0.68 [0.40–1.15] in thromboembolism. There were less studies reporting thromboembolism, with the ones reporting it, presenting estimates with greater standard errors, resulting in a larger confidence interval for thromboembolism when compared with all-cause mortality - [0.40–1.15] vs [0.72–1.01]. In addition, there could be a degree of under reporting of thromboembolic events when compared to mortality. Acute myocardial infarction is also a possible cause of death in these patients which was not included in the thromboembolism outcome (composite of ischemic stroke, transient cerebral ischemia, and thrombosis or embolism in peripheral arteries) [42]. These factors could have contributed to the discrepancy in results concerning all-cause mortality and thromboembolic events.

This systematic review and meta-analysis focused on different types of cardiac surgery with a relatively low number of studies, therefore increasing heterogeneity, despite including a high number of patients. Two of the manuscripts were from the same database, even though included patients were submitted to different types of surgery, limiting generalizability, counterbalanced by the wide range of locations (Denmark, USA, South Korea, Sweden, Poland, UK, India, Austria, Australia, Brazil, Italy). As all selected papers were observational, there is a risk of indication bias. Still, pooled estimates were adjusted for a vast number of covariates. Deviation from intended interventions was reported in three studies, with only one reporting a significant deviation in the treatment arm over time, which was accounted for in the statistical analysis [25]. Furthermore, Taha et al. did not have competing risks into account in their analysis, which could be a source of bias. Finally, although the estimates were adjusted, each study had a different pool of covariates in their regression models, increasing heterogeneity.

Conclusions

Current literature suggests a possibly protective impact of OAC therapy for all-cause mortality in patients with new-onset atrial fibrillation after cardiac surgery. However, it does not appear to impact stroke, thromboembolism and major bleeding.

Abbreviations

AF: Atrial Fibrillation; AHA/ACA: American Heart Association/American College of Cardiology; POAF: Post-Operative Atrial Fibrillation; CABG: Coronary artery bypass grafting; CI: Confidence Intervals; ESC: European Society of Cardiology; FT: Francisco Teixeira; MACE: Major Adverse Cardiovascular Events; MFM: Mariana Fragão-Marques; NOAC: Novel Oral Anticoagulants; OAC: Oral Anticoagulants; OR: Odds Ratio; PPCI: Percutaneous Coronary Intervention; TAVR: Transcatheter Aortic Valve Replacement; VKA: Vitamin K Antagonists; VR: Valve repair/replacement

Supplementary Information

Additional file 1. Supplementary Methods and Results.

Acknowledgements
Not applicable.

Authors' contributions
Conceptualization and design, MFM; *Methodology*, MFM, FT and JM; *Analysis*, MFM and FT; *Data acquisition*, MFM and FT; *Original draft preparation*, MFM and FT; *Review and editing*, JM, JRN, NS, ALM, IFP; *Project administration*, MFM. All authors have read and agreed to the published version of the manuscript.

Author details
[1]Cardiovascular Research and Development Center, Faculty of Medicine of the University of Porto, 4200 Porto, Portugal. [2]São João University Hospital Center, Porto, Portugal. [3]Faculty of Medicine of the University of Porto, Porto, Portugal. [4]Vila Nova de Gaia Hospital Center, Vila Nova de Gaia, Portugal.

References

1. Racca V, Torri A, Grati P, Panzarino C, Marventano I, Saresella M, et al. Inflammatory Cytokines During Cardiac Rehabilitation After Heart Surgery and Their Association to Postoperative Atrial Fibrillation. Sci Rep 2020;10(1) 8618.
2. Ishii Y, Schuessler RB, Gaynor SL, Yamada K, Fu AS, Boineau JP, et al. Inflammation of Atrium After Cardiac Surgery Is Associated With Inhomogeneity of Atrial Conduction and Atrial Fibrillation. Circulation. 2005; 111(22):2881.
3. Wang GK, Wang SY. Modifications of Human Cardiac Sodium Channel Gating by UVA Light. J Membr Biol. 2002;189(2):153.
4. Proebstle T, Mitrovics M, Schneider M, Hombach V, Rüdel R. Recombinant interleukin-2 acts like a class I antiarrhythmic drug on human cardiac sodium channels. Pflügers Archiv Eur J Physiol. 1995;429(4):462.
5. Seo C, Michie C, Hibbert B, Davis DR. Systematic review of pre-clinical therapies for post-operative atrial fibrillation. PLoS One. 2020;15(11): e0241643.
6. Fragão-Marques M, Mancio J, Oliveira J, Falcão-Pires I, Leite-Moreira A. Gender differences in predictors and long-term mortality of new-onset postoperative atrial fibrillation following isolated aortic valve replacement surgery. Ann Thoracic Cardiovasc Surgery. 2020;26(6):342–51 Available from: https://pubmed.ncbi.nlm.nih.gov/32350163/.
7. Creswell LL, Schuessler RB, Rosenbloom M, Cox JL. Hazards of postoperative atrial arrhythmias. Ann Thorac Surg. 1993;56(3):539.
8. Eikelboom R, Sanjanwala R, Le M-L, Yamashita MH, Arora RC. Postoperative Atrial Fibrillation After Cardiac Surgery: A Systematic Review and Meta-analysis. Ann Thorac Surg. 2020.
9. Shen J, Lall S, Zheng V, Buckley P, Damiano RJ, Schuessler RB. The persistent problem of new-onset postoperative atrial fibrillation: A single-institution experience over two decades. J Thorac Cardiovasc Surg. 2011;141(2):559.
10. Lin MH, Kamel H, Singer DE, Wu YL, Lee M, Ovbiagele B. Perioperative/ Postoperative Atrial Fibrillation and Risk of Subsequent Stroke and/or Mortality: A Meta-Analysis. Stroke. 2019;50(6):1364–71 Available from: https:// pubmed.ncbi.nlm.nih.gov/31043148/.
11. Fragão-Marques M, Miranda I, Martins D, Barroso I, Mendes C, Pereira-Neves A, et al. Atrial matrix remodeling in atrial fibrillation patients with aortic stenosis. BMC Cardiovasc Disord. 2020;20(1):468 Available from: https:// pubmed.ncbi.nlm.nih.gov/33129260/.
12. Pessoa-Amorim G, Mancio J, Vouga L, Ribeiro J, Gama V, Bettencourt N, et al. Impaired Left Atrial Strain as a Predictor of New-onset Atrial Fibrillation After Aortic Valve Replacement Independently of Left Atrial Size. Revista Española de Cardiología (English Edition). 2018;71(6):466–76 Available from: https://pubmed.ncbi.nlm.nih.gov/29146482/.
13. Fragão-Marques M, Saraiva F, Oliveira J, Lourenço AP, Leite-Moreira A, Falcão-Pires I. De novo atrial fibrillation following aortic valve replacement surgery is associated with decreased creatinine clearance and increased C-reactive protein levels. Porto Biomed J. 2017;2(5):189 Available from: https:// pubmed.ncbi.nlm.nih.gov/32258646/.
14. Butt JH, Olesen JB, Gundlund A, Kümler T, Olsen PS, Havers-Borgersen E, et al. Long-term Thromboembolic Risk in Patients with Postoperative Atrial Fibrillation after Left-Sided Heart Valve Surgery. JAMA Cardiol. 2019;4(11): 1139–47.
15. Butt JH, Xian Y, Peterson ED, Olsen PS, Rørth R, Gundlund A, et al. Long-Term thromboembolic risk in patients with postoperative atrial fibrillation after coronary artery bypass graft surgery and patients with nonvalvular atrial fibrillation. JAMA Cardiol. 2018;3:417–24.
16. Mariscalco G, Klersy C, Zanobini M, Banach M, Ferrarese S, Borsani P, et al. Atrial Fibrillation After Isolated Coronary Surgery Affects Late Survival. Circulation. 2008;118(16):1612.
17. Horwich P, Buth KJ, Légaré J-F. New Onset Postoperative Atrial Fibrillation is Associated with a Long-Term Risk for Stroke and Death Following Cardiac Surgery. J Card Surg. 2013;28(1):8.
18. Gialdini G, Nearing K, Bhave PD, Bonuccelli U, Iadecola C, Healey JS, et al. Perioperative Atrial Fibrillation and the Long-term Risk of Ischemic Stroke. JAMA. 2014;312(6):616.
19. Hindricks G, Potpara T, Dagres N, Arbelo E, Bax JJ, Blomström-Lundqvist C, et al. 2020 ESC Guidelines for the diagnosis and management of atrial fibrillation developed in collaboration with the European Association of Cardio-Thoracic Surgery (EACTS). Eur Heart J. 2020;29.
20. Fuster V, Rydén LE, Asinger RW, Cannom DS, Crijns HJ, Frye RL, et al. ACC/ AHA/ESC Guidelines for the Management of Patients With Atrial Fibrillation: Executive Summary A Report of the American College of Cardiology/ American Heart Association Task Force on Practice Guidelines and the European Society of Cardiology Committee for Practice Guidelines and Policy Conferences (Committee to Develop Guidelines for the Management of Patients With Atrial Fibrillation) Developed in Collaboration With the North American Society of Pacing and Electrophysiology. Circulation. 2001; 104(17):2118.
21. Kirchhof P, Benussi S, Kotecha D, Ahlsson A, Atar D, Casadei B, et al. 2016 ESC Guidelines for the management of atrial fibrillation developed in collaboration with EACTS. Eur Heart J. 2016;37(38):2893.
22. Sterne JA, Hernán MA, Reeves BC, Savović J, Berkman ND, Viswanathan M, et al. ROBINS-I: A tool for assessing risk of bias in non-randomised studies of interventions. BMJ. 2016;355:i4919 Available from: 10.1136/bmj.i4919.
23. Butt JH, Xian Y, Peterson ED, Olsen PS, Rørth R, et al. Long-Term thromboembolic risk in patients with postoperative atrial fibrillation after coronary artery bypass graft surgery and patients with nonvalvular atrial fibrillation. JAMA Cardiol. 2018;3(5):417–24.
24. Vora AN, Dai D, Matsuoka R, Harrison JK, Hughes GC, Sherwood MW, et al. Incidence, Management, and Associated Clinical Outcomes of New-Onset Atrial Fibrillation Following Transcatheter Aortic Valve Replacement. J Am Coll Cardiol Intv. 2018;11(17):1746.
25. Butt JH, Olesen JB, Gundlund A, Kümler T, Olsen PS, et al. Long-term Thromboembolic Risk in Patients with Postoperative Atrial Fibrillation after Left-Sided Heart Valve Surgery. JAMA Cardiol. 2019;4(11):1139–47.
26. El-Chami MF, Kilgo P, Thourani V, Lattouf OM, Delurgio DB, Guyton RA, et al. New-Onset Atrial Fibrillation Predicts Long-Term Mortality After Coronary Artery Bypass Graft. J Am Coll Cardiol. 2010;55(13):1370.
27. Yoon Y-H, Ahn J-M, Kang D-Y, Ko E, Lee PH, Lee S-W, et al. Incidence, Predictors, Management, and Clinical Significance of New-Onset Atrial Fibrillation After Transcatheter Aortic Valve Implantation. Am J Cardiol. 2019; 123(7):1127.
28. Taha A, Nielsen SJ, Bergfeldt L, Ahlsson A, Friberg L, Björck S, et al. New-onset atrial fibrillation after coronary artery bypass grafting and long-term outcome: A population-based nationwide study from the SWEDEHEART registry. J Am Heart Assoc. 2021;10(1):1–9.
29. Benedetto U, Gaudino MF, Dimagli A, Gerry S, Gray A, Lees B, et al. Postoperative atrial fibrillation and long-term risk of stroke after isolated coronary artery bypass graft surgery. Circulation. 2020;142(14):1320–9.
30. Madsen JM, Jacobsen MR, Sabbah M, Topal DG, Jabbari R, Glinge C, et al. Long-term prognostic outcomes and implication of oral anticoagulants in patients with new-onset atrial fibrillation following st-segment elevation myocardial infarction. Am Heart J. 2021;238:89–99.
31. Pistoia F, Sacco S, Tiseo C, Degan D, Ornello R, Carolei A. The Epidemiology of Atrial Fibrillation and Stroke. Cardiol Clin. 2016;34(2):255.
32. Sanna T, Diener H-C, Passman RS, di Lazzaro V, Bernstein RA, Morillo CA, et al. Cryptogenic Stroke and Underlying Atrial Fibrillation. N Engl J Med. 2014;370(26):2478.
33. Jame S, Barnes G. Stroke and thromboembolism prevention in atrial fibrillation. Heart. 2020;106(1):10.
34. Hindricks G, Potpara T, Dagres N, Arbelo E, Bax JJ, Blomström-Lundqvist C, et al. 2020 ESC Guidelines for the diagnosis and management of atrial

fibrillation developed in collaboration with the European Association for Cardio-Thoracic Surgery (EACTS). Eur Heart J. 2021;42(5):546.
35. Hart RG, Pearce LA, Aguilar MI. Meta-analysis: Antithrombotic Therapy to Prevent Stroke in Patients Who Have Nonvalvular Atrial Fibrillation. Ann Intern Med. 2007;146(12):857.
36. Ruff CT, Giugliano RP, Braunwald E, Hoffman EB, Deenadayalu N, Ezekowitz MD, et al. Comparison of the efficacy and safety of new oral anticoagulants with warfarin in patients with atrial fibrillation: a meta-analysis of randomised trials. Lancet. 2014;383(9921):955.
37. de With RR, Marcos EG, Dudink EAMP, Spronk HM, Crijns HJGM, Rienstra M, et al. Atrial fibrillation progression risk factors and associated cardiovascular outcome in well-phenotyped patients: data from the AF-RISK study. EP Europace. 2020;22(3):352.
38. Dobrev D, Aguilar M, Heijman J, Guichard J-B, Nattel S. Postoperative atrial fibrillation: mechanisms, manifestations and management. Nat Rev Cardiol. 2019;16(7):417.
39. Lin M-H, Kamel H, Singer DE, Wu Y-L, Lee M, Ovbiagele B. Perioperative/Postoperative Atrial Fibrillation and Risk of Subsequent Stroke and/or Mortality. Stroke. 2019;50(6):1364.
40. Perino AC, Fan J, Askari M, Heidenreich PA, Keung E, Raitt MH, et al. Practice Variation in Anticoagulation Prescription and Outcomes After Device-Detected Atrial Fibrillation. Circulation. 2019;139(22):2502.
41. Yadava M, Hughey AB, Crawford TC. Postoperative atrial fibrillation: incidence, mechanisms, and clinical correlates. Cardiol Clin. 2014;32(4):627.
42. John RM, Michaud GF, Stevenson WG. Atrial fibrillation hospitalization, mortality, and therapy. Eur Heart J. 2018;39(44):3958–60.

14

Intermediate-to-therapeutic versus prophylactic anticoagulation for coagulopathy in hospitalized COVID-19 patients

Sirui Zhang[1†], Yupei Li[2,3†], Guina Liu[1] and Baihai Su[1,2,3,4,5*]

Abstract

Background: Anticoagulation in hospitalized COVID-19 patients has been associated with survival benefit; however, the optimal anticoagulant strategy has not yet been defined. The objective of this meta-analysis was to investigate the effect of intermediate-to-therapeutic versus prophylactic anticoagulation for thromboprophylaxis on the primary outcome of in-hospital mortality and other patient-centered secondary outcomes in COVID-19 patients.

Methods: MEDLINE, EMBASE, and Cochrane databases were searched from inception to August 10th 2021. Cohort studies and randomized clinical trials that assessed the efficacy and safety of intermediate-to-therapeutic versus prophylactic anticoagulation in hospitalized COVID-19 patients were included. Baseline characteristics and relevant data of each study were extracted in a pre-designed standardized data-collection form. The primary outcome was all-cause in-hospital mortality and the secondary outcomes were incidence of thrombotic events and incidence of any bleeding and major bleeding. Pooled analysis with random effects models yielded relative risk with 95 % CIs.

* Correspondence: subaihai@scu.edu.cn
[†]Sirui Zhang and Yupei Li contributed equally to this work.
[1]West China School of Medicine, Sichuan University, 610041 Chengdu, China
[2]Department of Nephrology, Med+ Biomaterial Institute, West China Hospital, Sichuan University, 610041 Chengdu, China

Results: This meta-analysis included 42 studies with 28,055 in-hospital COVID-19 patients totally. Our pooled analysis demonstrated that intermediate-to-therapeutic anticoagulation was not associated with lower in-hospital mortality (RR=1.12, 95 %CI 0.99-1.25, p=0.06, I^2=77 %) and lower incidence of thrombotic events (RR=1.30, 95 %CI 0.79-2.15, p=0.30, I^2=88 %), but increased the risk of any bleeding events (RR=2.16, 95 %CI 1.79-2.60, p<0.01, I^2=31 %) and major bleeding events significantly (RR=2.10, 95 %CI 1.77-2.51, p<0.01, I^2=11 %) versus prophylactic anticoagulation. Moreover, intermediate-to-therapeutic anticoagulation decreased the incidence of thrombotic events (RR=0.71, 95 %CI 0.56-0.89, p=0.003, I^2=0 %) among critically ill COVID-19 patients admitted to intensive care units (ICU), with increased bleeding risk (RR=1.66, 95 %CI 1.37-2.00, p<0.01, I^2=0 %) and unchanged in-hospital mortality (RR=0.94, 95 %CI 0.79-1.10, p=0.42, I^2=30 %) in such patients. The Grading of Recommendation, Assessment, Development, and Evaluation certainty of evidence ranged from very low to moderate.

Conclusions: We recommend the use of prophylactic anticoagulation against intermediate-to-therapeutic anticoagulation among unselected hospitalized COVID-19 patients considering insignificant survival benefits but higher risk of bleeding in the escalated thromboprophylaxis strategy. For critically ill COVID-19 patients, the benefits of intermediate-to-therapeutic anticoagulation in reducing thrombotic events should be weighed cautiously because of its association with higher risk of bleeding.

Trial registration: The protocol was registered at PROSPERO on August 17th 2021 (CRD42021273780).

Keywords: COVID-19, Anticoagulation, Mortality, Bleeding, Thromboprophylaxis, Meta-analysis

Background

Coronavirus disease 2019 (COVID-19), provoked by severe acute respiratory syndrome coronavirus-2 infection, is currently the most serious public health crisis worldwide [1]. Patients who are hospitalized with COVID-19 frequently have macrovascular and microvascular thrombosis and inflammation, which may contribute to high morbidity and mortality [2–7]. In a recent meta-analysis of 49 studies enrolling 18,093 hospitalized patients with COVID-19, the overall estimated pooled incidence of venous thromboembolism was 17.0 %, with a higher incidence (27.9 %) among those admitted to intensive care unit (ICU) [8]. Mechanisms of hypercoagulable state in these patients have not been fully elucidated yet, and may potentially attribute to immunothrombosis that is mediated by abnormal endothelial dysfunction and platelet activation [9–11]. Accordingly, several national and international clinical guidance reports have recommended the use of prophylactic anticoagulation in hospitalized COVID-19 patients who do not have a contraindication to anticoagulant administration for thromboprophylaxis [12–15].

However, increasing evidence demonstrated that some COVID-19 patients, especially those with critical illness, still developed severe thrombotic complications despite the use of prophylactic anticoagulant [16–18]. Enhanced-dose anticoagulation strategies have thus been recommended by some guidance statements in critically ill COVID-19 patients [19–21], though patients may also develop bleeding complications on elevated anticoagulation treatment. The effectiveness and safety of intermediate-to-therapeutic anticoagulation are still uncertain [22].

Previous meta-analyses that investigated the optimal anticoagulation strategy only included limited studies and reported inconsistent conclusions [23–25]. As more evidence from high-quality randomized controlled trials (RCTs) and observational cohort studies have become available recently, we conducted an updated meta-analysis to investigate the efficacy and safety of intermediate-to-therapeutic versus prophylactic anticoagulation in COVID-19 patients with subsequent subgroup analyzes being performed in critically ill COVID-19 patients further.

Methods

This review was conducted following the Preferred Reporting Items for Systemic Reviews and Meta-Analyses (PRISMA) Statement [26] and registered on the Open PROSPERO Framework (registration number: CRD42021273780).

Search strategy

Literature search was conducted strictly and comprehensively in MEDLINE, EMBASE, and Cochrane databases. Two independent investigators (ZSR and LYP) searched studies available from database inception to August 10th 2021 without language limitation. The following key words and/or medical subject heading terms were used: 'COVID', 'COVID-19', '2019 novel coronavirus infection', 'SARS-CoV-2', '2019-nCoV disease', 'anticoagulation', 'anticoagulants', 'anticoagulant', 'unfractionated heparin', 'UFH', 'fondaparinux', 'enoxaparin', 'low-molecular-weight heparin', 'LMWH', 'heparin, low molecular weight', 'heparin', 'antithrombotic', and 'anti-thrombosis', 'thromboprophylaxis' [see Additional file 1 for the detailed search strategy].

Study selection

Two independent investigators (ZSR and LYP) performed the initial screening of titles and abstracts. Full-length articles of identified studies were retrieved to assess eligibility. Any discrepancies were adjudicated by a third reviewer (SBH). The inclusion criteria of our meta-analysis were as follows: (1) cohort studies and RCTs, (2) studies that enrolled COVID-19 patients admitted to general wards or ICUs, and (3) studies that compared the efficacy or safety of intermediate-to-therapeutic versus prophylactic anticoagulation. The exclusion criteria were as follows: (1) studies enrolling out-hospital COVID-19 patients, or (2) animal experiments, case reports, reviews, comments, editorial comments, or (3) no relevant and sufficient data on preferred outcomes. In case a same patient population was enrolled in a few articles, we only selected the most comprehensive study.

Data extraction

After study selection, the following data were extracted: author, publication year, study type, study location, patient characteristics, numbers of patients in different groups, in-hospital mortality, incidence of any bleeding events, incidence of major bleeding events, and incidence of thrombotic events using a predesigned standardized data-collection form by two researchers (ZSR and LYP) independently.

Quality assessment

Quality assessment of studies were conducted by two independent reviewers (ZSR and LYP). The Cochrane Collaboration tool was used to assess the risk of bias in randomized controlled trials [27]. The quality of cohort studies was assessed using the Newcastle–Ottawa Scale (NOS) [28], evaluating three aspects: (1) selection of study groups, (2) comparability of study groups, and (3) outcome ascertainment. Meanwhile, we rated the quality of evidence for each outcome in the pooled analysis as high, moderate, low, and very low quality by the Grading of Recommendations Assessment, Development and Evaluation (GRADE) framework [29].

Study outcomes

Our primary outcome was all-cause mortality during hospitalization for COVID-19. Secondary patient-centered outcomes included the incidence of bleeding events and thrombotic complications during hospitalization for COVID-19. We also investigated these outcomes in critically ill COVID-19 patients who were admitted to ICU exclusively. Definitions of bleeding events depended on the variable definitions of each study, mostly in accordance with Myocardial Infarction (TIMI) bleeding [30] or the World health organization bleeding scale [31, 32]. Major bleeding was mostly defined by the criteria of the International Society on Thrombosis and Haemostasis (ISTH) [33]. Thrombotic complications mainly included deep venous thrombosis and pulmonary embolism, or jointly venous thromboembolism.

Statistical analysis

Risk ratios (RR) with 95 % confidence interval (CI) were calculated for dichotomous outcomes such as mortality, bleeding events and thrombotic complications. A random effects model was applied for meta-analyses due to the heterogeneity of study populations and design. Heterogeneity among studies was assessed by the chi-square test and shown as an I^2 index (25–50 %: low heterogeneity; 50–75 %: moderate heterogeneity; greater than 75 %: high heterogeneity). Sensitivity analysis was conducted by omitting each study at a time to determine whether each study affected the overall estimate and to identify studies that potentially drove the results. Publication bias was assessed with funnel plots and Egger test. A two-side P-value <0.05 was considered to be of statistical significance. All statistical analyses were carried out using the meta package in R 3.6.2 and Review Manager software (version 5.4).

Results

Study Selection

From 6,002 yielded studies, we retained 74 studies after removing duplications and screening titles and abstracts. Forty-two studies involving 28,055 subjects met the inclusion criteria and were finally included in this meta-analysis after full-text review. The PRISMA flow diagram demonstrates the process of study screening and selection in detail, as shown in Fig. 1.

Study Characteristics

Of the forty-two included studies, 6 studies [34–39] were RCTs and 36 studies [40–75] were cohort studies. Thirteen studies [34, 38, 39, 41, 43, 52, 55, 58, 61, 64, 67, 69, 70] were performed exclusively in patients admitted to ICU. Eighteen studies [34, 40, 42, 48, 51, 53–55, 57, 62–66, 68–70, 73] reported results from the United States and two [37, 38] were international studies. Other studies originated from eleven countries (Italy [47, 49, 56, 58, 60, 72, 75], France [41, 61, 67], Brazil [35, 36], England [59], Greek [46], China [45], Japan [43], Mexico [44], United Arab Emirates [52, 71], Turkey [74], Iran [39] and Spain [50]).

We included a pooled population of 23,579 hospitalized COVID-19 patients [34–49, 51–61, 63–68, 70–75] with reported information related to in-hospital mortality,

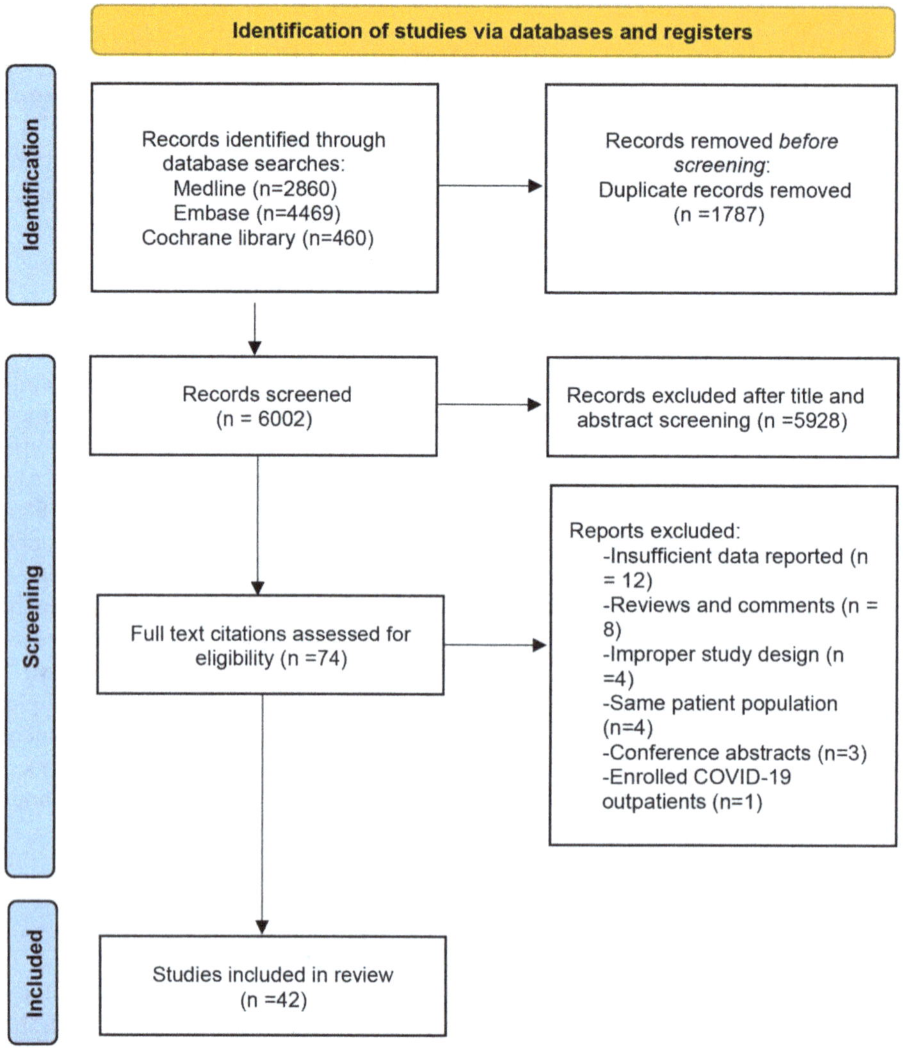

Fig. 1 Flowchart of selection of studies

19,275 patients [34–41, 44, 46–48, 50, 51, 53, 55, 58, 59, 61, 62, 64–67, 70, 71, 73] with reported information related to bleeding events and 8492 patients [34–39, 41–43, 47, 56, 58, 60–62, 64, 66] with reported information related to thrombotic events. The mean age in most studies was over 60 years. The proportion of male subjects ranged from 38.1 to 82.2 %. The types of administered anticoagulants, exact anticoagulation dosages and anticoagulation treatment duration varied widely across studies. Enoxaparin and unfractionated heparin were the most used anticoagulants in the included studies. Additional file 2 further summarized the detailed baseline characteristics of each study and the details of anticoagulation administration in each study were listed in Additional file 3.

Assessment of study quality

The score by NOS for the included cohort studies ranged from 6 to 9, while 10 studies were of high quality scoring 9. A full assessment is shown in Additional file 4. Cochrane Collaboration Risk of Bias assessing bias of RCTs indicated low bias in the majority of included RCTs (Additional file 5).

In-hospital mortality

Data regarding in-hospital mortality of COVID-19 patients receiving prophylactic anticoagulation or intermediate-to-therapeutic anticoagulation were available from 39 studies [34–49, 51–61, 63–68, 70–75] (23,579 patients) which included both ICU and non-ICU patients. In-hospital mortality ranged widely across studies with an average of 22.1 % for prophylactic anticoagulation group and 22.6 % for intermediate-to-therapeutic anticoagulation group in non-ICU patients, while the average incidence of in-hospital death was 31.7 % in prophylactic anticoagulation group and 31.1 % in intermediate-to-therapeutic anticoagulation group in ICU patients. Figure 2a a

Study or Subgroup	I-TAC Events	I-TAC Total	PAC Events	PAC Total	Weight	Risk Ratio M-H, Random, 95% CI
Bikedeli 2021	127	276	123	286	4.2%	1.07 [0.89, 1.29]
Bolzetta 2021	12	24	29	57	2.7%	0.98 [0.61, 1.58]
Canoglu 2020	10	56	44	98	2.1%	0.40 [0.22, 0.73]
Daughety 2020	10	27	24	99	2.1%	1.53 [0.84, 2.79]
Di Castelnuovo 2021	62	418	114	983	3.7%	1.28 [0.96, 1.70]
Elmelhat 2020	3	39	0	20	0.2%	3.67 [0.20, 67.85]
Ferguson 2020	12	46	28	95	2.2%	0.89 [0.50, 1.58]
Goligher 2021	199	534	200	564	4.3%	1.05 [0.90, 1.23]
Hanif 2020	86	191	218	672	4.2%	1.39 [1.15, 1.68]
Helms 2021	11	71	20	108	1.8%	0.84 [0.43, 1.64]
Hsu 2020	20	64	56	377	2.8%	2.10 [1.36, 3.25]
Ionescu 2021	307	998	702	2121	4.5%	0.93 [0.83, 1.04]
Jean-François 2020	2	18	1	8	0.3%	0.89 [0.09, 8.44]
Jonmarker 2020	17	85	26	67	2.4%	0.52 [0.31, 0.87]
Kaur 2020	109	381	132	652	4.0%	1.41 [1.13, 1.76]
Lemos 2020	2	10	5	10	0.6%	0.40 [0.10, 1.60]
Longhitano 2020	10	47	2	27	0.6%	2.87 [0.68, 12.15]
Lopes 2021	35	310	23	304	2.5%	1.49 [0.90, 2.46]
Lynn 2021	53	152	38	250	3.2%	2.29 [1.59, 3.30]
Marco 2021	40	149	73	287	3.4%	1.06 [0.76, 1.47]
Martinelli 2021	12	127	21	151	1.9%	0.68 [0.35, 1.33]
Meizlish 2021	19	191	37	191	2.5%	0.51 [0.31, 0.86]
Moll 2021	12	47	13	47	1.8%	0.92 [0.47, 1.81]
Motta 2020	29	75	43	299	3.1%	2.69 [1.81, 4.00]
Musoke 2020	42	101	33	216	3.1%	2.72 [1.84, 4.02]
Nadeem 2021	23	42	23	34	3.3%	0.81 [0.56, 1.16]
Nadkarni 2020	257	900	424	1959	4.4%	1.32 [1.15, 1.51]
Paolisso 2020	4	89	75	361	1.1%	0.22 [0.08, 0.58]
Paranjpe 2020	179	786	445	1987	4.4%	1.02 [0.87, 1.18]
Patrick 2021	86	1180	86	1046	3.7%	0.89 [0.67, 1.18]
Perepu 2021	13	87	18	86	1.9%	0.71 [0.37, 1.37]
Pesavento 2020	14	84	27	240	2.1%	1.48 [0.82, 2.69]
Poulakou 2021	2	54	1	26	0.2%	0.96 [0.09, 10.14]
Qin 2021	25	77	19	109	2.4%	1.86 [1.11, 3.13]
Rodolfo 2021	12	212	9	109	1.4%	0.69 [0.30, 1.58]
Takayama 2021	0	33	5	29	0.2%	0.08 [0.00, 1.39]
Vaughn 2021	58	216	211	966	3.9%	1.23 [0.96, 1.58]
Voicu 2021	20	43	18	50	2.6%	1.29 [0.79, 2.11]
Yu 2021	80	133	131	215	4.3%	0.99 [0.83, 1.18]
Total (95% CI)		**8373**		**15206**	**100.0%**	**1.12 [0.99, 1.25]**
Total events	2014		3497			

Heterogeneity: $Tau^2 = 0.08$; $Chi^2 = 160.71$, df = 38 ($P < 0.00001$); $I^2 = 76\%$
Test for overall effect: Z = 1.85 (P = 0.06)

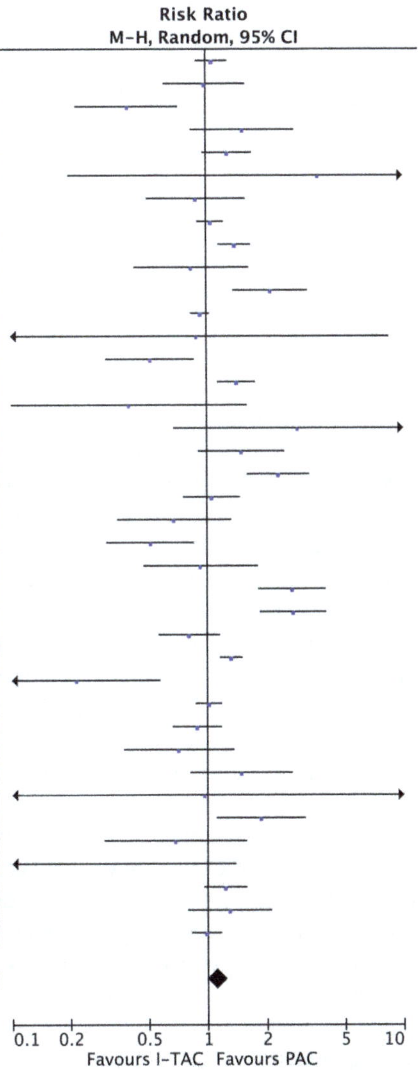

b

Study or Subgroup	I-TAC Events	I-TAC Total	PAC Events	PAC Total	Weight	Risk Ratio M-H, Random, 95% CI
Bikedeli 2021	127	276	123	286	26.1%	1.07 [0.89, 1.29]
Ferguson 2020	12	46	28	95	6.7%	0.89 [0.50, 1.58]
Goligher 2021	199	534	200	564	28.8%	1.05 [0.90, 1.23]
Helms 2021	11	71	20	108	5.2%	0.84 [0.43, 1.64]
Jean-François 2020	2	18	1	8	0.5%	0.89 [0.09, 8.44]
Jonmarker 2020	17	85	26	67	7.9%	0.52 [0.31, 0.87]
Martinelli 2021	12	127	21	151	5.2%	0.68 [0.35, 1.33]
Moll 2021	12	47	13	47	5.2%	0.92 [0.47, 1.81]
Perepu 2021	13	87	18	86	5.5%	0.71 [0.37, 1.37]
Takayama 2021	0	33	5	29	0.3%	0.08 [0.00, 1.39]
Voicu 2021	20	43	18	50	8.7%	1.29 [0.79, 2.11]
Total (95% CI)		**1367**		**1491**	**100.0%**	**0.94 [0.79, 1.10]**
Total events	425		473			

Heterogeneity: $Tau^2 = 0.02$; $Chi^2 = 14.25$, df = 10 (P = 0.16); $I^2 = 30\%$
Test for overall effect: Z = 0.80 (P = 0.42)

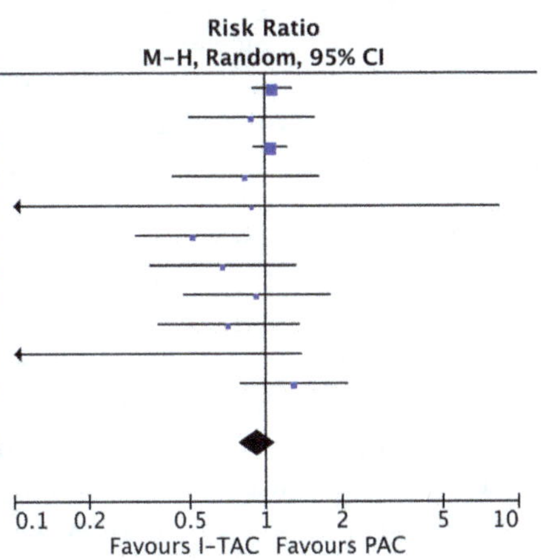

Fig. 2 a Forest plot of the effect of intermediate-to-therapeutic versus prophylactic anticoagulation on in-hospital mortality in general COVID -19 patients; **b** Forest plot of the effect of intermediate-to-therapeutic versus prophylactic anticoagulation on in-hospital mortality in COVID -19 patients admitted to ICU demonstrated that intermediate-to-therapeutic anticoagulation was not significantly associated with reduced in-hospital mortality compared to prophylactic anticoagulation in unselected hospitalized COVID-19 patients (RR= 1.12, 95 %CI 0.99-1.25, p=0.06, I^2=77 %). The sensitivity analysis by leave-one-out approach indicated that the result was relatively stable because the risk ratio remained unchangeable though p value fluctuated around 0.05, as shown in Additional file 6. The funnel plot and Egger test (p=0.79) showed no evidence of significant publication bias, as shown in Additional file 7. The quality of evidence for in-hospital mortality for general COVID patients was rated as very low using GRADE framework in view of high heterogeneity and potential selection bias (Additional file 8).

Eleven studies [34, 38, 39, 41, 43, 55, 58, 61, 64, 67, 70] exclusively investigated in-hospital mortality of critically ill COVID-19 patients admitted to ICU. The subgroup analysis of ICU patients also indicated that intermediate-to-therapeutic anticoagulation was not significantly associated with reduced in-hospital mortality when compared with prophylactic anticoagulation and heterogeneity across the studies decreased significantly (RR=0.94, 95 %CI 0.79-1.10, p=0.42, I^2=30 %, see Fig. 2b). The quality of evidence for subgroup analysis of ICU settings regarding in-hospital mortality were rated as moderate-quality, as shown in Additional file 8. In the subgroup analysis stratified by study regions, we also did not observe a significant survival benefit in patients receiving intermediate-to-therapeutic anticoagulation as compared with those receiving prophylactic anticoagulation although the heterogeneity across different subgroups was high (see Additional file 9).

Bleeding events

A total of 27 studies [34–41, 44, 46–48, 50, 51, 53, 55, 58, 59, 61, 62, 64–67, 70, 71, 73] including 19,275 patients assessed the incidence of any bleeding events in intermediate-to-therapeutic anticoagulation group and prophylactic anticoagulation group. COVID-19 patients admitted to general wards, the average incidence of any bleeding events was 2.27 % in prophylactic anticoagulation and 5.50 % in intermediate-to-therapeutic anticoagulation group. In ICU settings, the average bleeding incidence was 7.14 % in prophylactic anticoagulation group and 10.2 % in intermediate-to-therapeutic anticoagulation group. As shown in Fig. 3a, intermediate-to-therapeutic anticoagulation was significantly associated an increased incidence of any bleeding events when compared to prophylactic anticoagulation (RR=2.16, 95 %CI 1.79-2.60, p<0.01, I^2=31 %). The predefined sensitivity analyses did not change the overall effect and the results remained stable (Additional file 10). Besides, evidence of publication bias was not found according to the funnel plot and following Egger test (p=0.757) (Additional file 11). The quality of evidence for bleeding events was rated as moderate using GRADE framework, as shown in Additional file 12. Figure 3b further showed that intermediate-to-therapeutic anticoagulation was also associated with higher incidence of major bleeding events significantly (RR=2.11, 95 %CI 1.77-2.51, p<0.01, I^2=11 %).

Subgroup analysis of bleeding risk related to thromboprophylaxis in ICU settings included 10 studies [34, 38, 39, 41, 50, 55, 58, 61, 64, 70] and 4596 patients totally, showing that intermediate-to-therapeutic anticoagulation was significantly associated with increased incidence of any bleeding events with low heterogeneity (RR=1.66, 95 %CI 1.37-2.00, p<0.01, I^2=0 %, Fig. 3c). The quality of evidence for subgroup analyses of ICU settings regarding bleeding incidence were rated as moderate-quality evidence respectively, as shown in Additional file 12.

Thrombotic complication events

Incidence of thrombotic events was reported in 17 studies [34–39, 41–43, 47, 56, 58, 60–62, 64, 66] which included a total of 8,492 admitted patients with COVID-19. The results ranged widely across studies with an average incidence of 3.75 % for prophylactic anticoagulation group and 6.45 % for intermediate-to-therapeutic anticoagulation group in non-critically ill patients, while 13.0 % for prophylactic group and 8.58 % for intermediate-to-therapeutic anticoagulation group in ICU patients. As shown in Fig. 4a, the current meta-analysis found that the pooled risk ratio of thrombotic events risk did not favor either of two groups with high heterogeneity (RR=1.30, 95 %CI 0.79-2.15, p=0.30, I^2=88 %). The predefined sensitivity analysis conformed the stability of the results in this meta-analysis, as shown in Additional file 13. The funnel plot and following Egger test (p=0.45) further indicated no evidence of significant publication bias (Additional file 14). The quality of evidence for thrombotic events was rated as very low using GRADE framework, as shown in Additional file 15.

Subgroup analysis of studies exclusively enrolling critically ill COVID-19 patients admitted to ICU indicated that patients receiving intermediate-to-therapeutic anticoagulation were associated with reduced risk of thrombotic events compared with prophylactic anticoagulation (RR=0.71, 95 %CI 0.56-0.89, p =0.03, I^2=0 %), as shown in Fig. 4b. The quality of evidence for these subgroup analyses were rated as moderate-quality for ICU settings, as shown in Additional file 15.

Discussion

In this systemic review and meta-analysis, we included 42 studies with 28,055 COVID-19 patients admitted to hospital in total. By analyzing data of 23,579 hospitalized

a

Study or Subgroup	I-TAC Events	I-TAC Total	PAC Events	PAC Total	Weight	Risk Ratio M-H, Random, 95% CI
Bikedeli 2021	17	276	10	286	4.2%	1.76 [0.82, 3.78]
Daughety 2020	1	27	3	99	0.7%	1.22 [0.13, 11.29]
Elmelhat 2020	3	39	0	20	0.4%	3.67 [0.20, 67.85]
Ferguson 2020	12	46	8	95	3.8%	3.10 [1.36, 7.05]
Goligher 2021	20	539	13	562	4.9%	1.60 [0.81, 3.19]
Helms 2021	1	71	2	108	0.6%	0.76 [0.07, 8.23]
Hsu 2020	7	64	10	377	3.1%	4.12 [1.63, 10.44]
Ionescu 2021	81	998	46	2121	9.6%	3.74 [2.63, 5.33]
Jonmarker 2020	8	85	8	67	3.2%	0.79 [0.31, 1.99]
Kodama 2021	8	82	18	498	4.0%	2.70 [1.21, 6.00]
Lemos 2020	6	10	2	10	1.7%	3.00 [0.79, 11.44]
Lopes 2021	26	310	7	304	3.8%	3.64 [1.61, 8.27]
Lynn 2021	13	152	8	250	3.6%	2.67 [1.13, 6.30]
Marco 2021	2	21	3	65	1.1%	2.06 [0.37, 11.53]
Martinelli 2021	4	127	0	151	0.4%	10.69 [0.58, 196.63]
Moll 2021	5	47	2	47	1.2%	2.50 [0.51, 12.25]
Musoke 2020	12	122	7	178	3.3%	2.50 [1.01, 6.17]
Nadkarni 2020	27	900	33	1959	7.1%	1.78 [1.08, 2.94]
Pablo 2021	112	618	132	1215	12.0%	1.67 [1.32, 2.10]
Paranjpe 2020	24	786	38	1987	7.1%	1.60 [0.96, 2.64]
Patrick 2021	22	1180	9	1047	4.2%	2.17 [1.00, 4.69]
Perepu 2021	8	87	8	86	3.1%	0.99 [0.39, 2.51]
Pesavento 2020	18	84	15	240	5.4%	3.43 [1.81, 6.49]
Poulakou 2021	2	54	1	26	0.6%	0.96 [0.09, 10.14]
Rodolfo 2021	15	212	7	109	3.5%	1.10 [0.46, 2.62]
Voicu 2021	11	43	7	50	3.6%	1.83 [0.78, 4.30]
Yu 2021	18	133	8	215	3.9%	3.64 [1.63, 8.13]
Total (95% CI)		**7113**		**12172**	**100.0%**	**2.16 [1.79, 2.60]**
Total events	483		405			

Heterogeneity: Tau² = 0.06; Chi² = 37.91, df = 26 (P = 0.06); I² = 31%
Test for overall effect: Z = 8.12 (P < 0.00001)

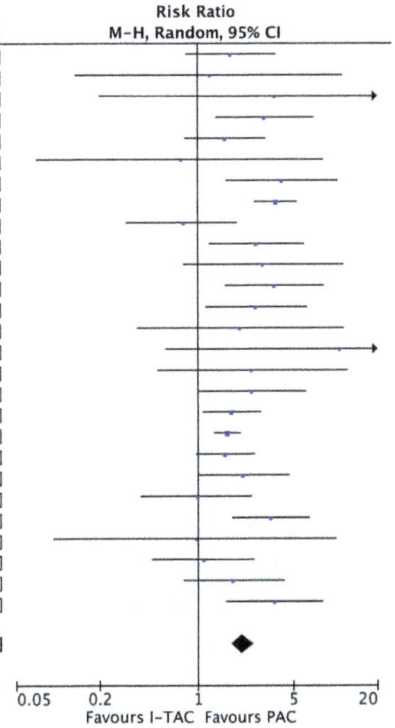

b

Study or Subgroup	I-TAC Events	I-TAC Total	PAC Events	PAC Total	Weight	Risk Ratio M-H, Random, 95% CI
Perepu 2021	2	87	2	86	0.8%	0.99 [0.14, 6.86]
Jonmarker 2020	3	85	2	67	1.0%	1.18 [0.20, 6.87]
Halaby 2021	31	211	26	216	10.2%	1.22 [0.75, 1.98]
Daughety 2020	1	27	3	99	0.6%	1.22 [0.13, 11.29]
Paranjpe 2020	24	786	38	1987	9.6%	1.60 [0.96, 2.64]
Goligher 2021	20	539	13	562	5.7%	1.60 [0.81, 3.19]
Nadkarni 2020	27	900	33	1959	9.6%	1.78 [1.08, 2.94]
Bikedeli 2021	7	276	4	286	2.0%	1.81 [0.54, 6.13]
Voicu 2021	11	43	7	50	3.8%	1.83 [0.78, 4.30]
Marco 2021	1	149	1	287	0.4%	1.93 [0.12, 30.58]
Pablo 2021	53	618	59	1347	15.8%	1.96 [1.37, 2.80]
Rodolfo 2021	4	212	1	109	0.6%	2.06 [0.23, 18.18]
Patrick 2021	22	1180	9	1047	4.6%	2.17 [1.00, 4.69]
Hsu 2020	3	64	8	377	1.7%	2.21 [0.60, 8.11]
Lopes 2021	10	310	4	304	2.2%	2.45 [0.78, 7.73]
Musoke 2020	12	122	7	178	3.5%	2.50 [1.01, 6.17]
Kodama 2021	8	82	18	498	4.4%	2.70 [1.21, 6.00]
Pesavento 2020	8	84	8	240	3.2%	2.86 [1.11, 7.37]
Yu 2021	18	133	8	215	4.3%	3.64 [1.63, 8.13]
Ionescu 2021	81	998	46	2121	16.0%	3.74 [2.63, 5.33]
Total (95% CI)		**6906**		**12035**	**100.0%**	**2.10 [1.77, 2.51]**
Total events	346		297			

Heterogeneity: Tau² = 0.02; Chi² = 21.46, df = 19 (P = 0.31); I² = 11%
Test for overall effect: Z = 8.32 (P < 0.00001)

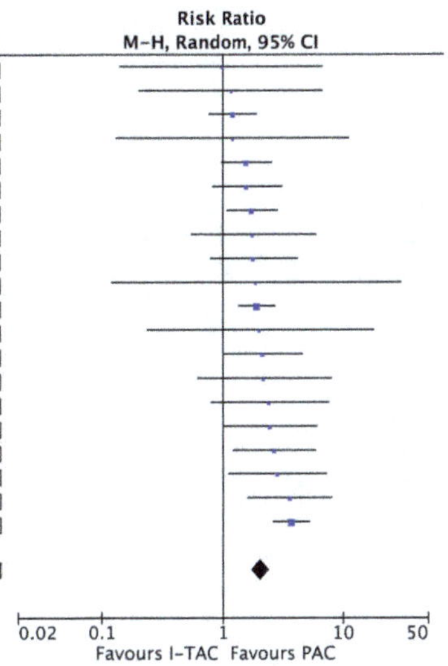

c

Study or Subgroup	I-TAC Events	I-TAC Total	PAC Events	PAC Total	Weight	Risk Ratio M-H, Random, 95% CI
Bikedeli 2021	17	276	10	286	6.1%	1.76 [0.82, 3.78]
Ferguson 2020	12	46	8	95	5.2%	3.10 [1.36, 7.05]
Goligher 2021	20	539	13	562	7.5%	1.60 [0.81, 3.19]
Helms 2021	1	71	2	108	0.6%	0.76 [0.07, 8.23]
Jonmarker 2020	8	85	8	67	4.1%	0.79 [0.31, 1.99]
Martinelli 2021	4	127	0	151	0.4%	10.69 [0.58, 196.63]
Moll 2021	5	47	2	47	1.4%	2.50 [0.51, 12.25]
Pablo 2021	112	618	132	1215	65.7%	1.67 [1.32, 2.10]
Perepu 2021	8	87	8	86	4.1%	0.99 [0.39, 2.51]
Voicu 2021	11	43	7	50	4.8%	1.83 [0.78, 4.30]
Total (95% CI)		**1939**		**2667**	**100.0%**	**1.66 [1.37, 2.00]**
Total events	198		190			

Heterogeneity: Tau² = 0.00; Chi² = 8.20, df = 9 (P = 0.51); I² = 0%
Test for overall effect: Z = 5.26 (P < 0.00001)

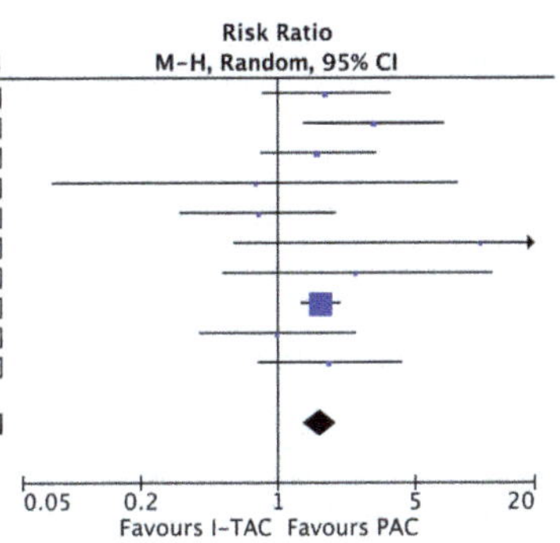

Fig. 3 (See legend on next page.)

(See figure on previous page.)

Fig. 3 a Forest plot of the effect of intermediate-to-therapeutic versus prophylactic anticoagulation on any bleeding events in general COVID -19 patients; **b** Forest plot of the effect of intermediate-to-therapeutic versus prophylactic anticoagulation on major bleeding events in general COVID-19 patients; **c** Forest plot of the effect of intermediate-to-therapeutic versus prophylactic anticoagulation on any bleeding events in COVID-19 patients admitted to ICU

COVID -19 patients from 33 cohort studies and 6 RCTs reporting in-hospital mortality, intermediate-to-therapeutic anticoagulation did not improve the primary outcome of in-hospital mortality in unselected hospitalized COVID-19 patients when compared with prophylactic anticoagulation. Additionally, a subgroup analysis of critically ill COVID-19 patients admitted to ICU also showed no significant survival benefit of intermediate-to-therapeutic anticoagulation against standard thromboprophylaxis. These results were inconsistent with earlier studies which reported a significant association between enhanced-dose anticoagulation and improved outcomes [51, 65]. It is noteworthy that the average in-hospital mortality for non-critically ill COVID-19 patients was 22.1 % for prophylactic anticoagulation group and 22.6 % for intermediate-to-therapeutic anticoagulation group in our meta-analysis, suggesting a relatively moderate-to-severe illness in such patients where the underlying thrombotic states and inflammatory damage may have been too advanced to be influenced and improved by higher doses of anticoagulants. In contrast, the latest adaptive, multiplatform, controlled trial (ATTACC, ACTIV-4a and REMAP-CAP) found that therapeutic-dose anticoagulation was associated with

a

Study or Subgroup	I-TAC Events	I-TAC Total	PAC Events	PAC Total	Weight	Risk Ratio M-H, Random, 95% CI
Bikedeli 2021	9	276	10	286	5.9%	0.93 [0.38, 2.26]
Goligher 2021	38	530	62	559	6.9%	0.65 [0.44, 0.95]
Helms 2021	15	71	42	108	6.7%	0.54 [0.33, 0.90]
Hsu 2020	13	64	38	377	6.6%	2.02 [1.14, 3.57]
Jonmarker 2020	10	85	12	67	6.2%	0.66 [0.30, 1.43]
Kodama 2021	17	82	9	498	6.2%	11.47 [5.29, 24.86]
Lemos 2020	2	10	2	10	3.8%	1.00 [0.17, 5.77]
Longhitano 2020	11	47	10	27	6.3%	0.63 [0.31, 1.29]
Lopes 2021	23	310	30	304	6.7%	0.75 [0.45, 1.26]
Marco 2021	19	149	3	287	5.1%	12.20 [3.67, 40.56]
Martinelli 2021	16	127	20	151	6.5%	0.95 [0.51, 1.76]
Patrick 2021	13	1180	22	1046	6.4%	0.52 [0.27, 1.03]
Perepu 2021	11	87	8	86	6.0%	1.36 [0.57, 3.21]
Pesavento 2020	3	84	6	240	4.7%	1.43 [0.37, 5.59]
Takayama 2021	1	33	4	29	3.1%	0.22 [0.03, 1.86]
Vaughn 2021	32	219	16	970	6.6%	8.86 [4.95, 15.85]
Voicu 2021	11	43	12	50	6.3%	1.07 [0.52, 2.17]
Total (95% CI)		**3397**		**5095**	**100.0%**	**1.30 [0.79, 2.15]**
Total events	244		306			

Heterogeneity: $Tau^2 = 0.90$; $Chi^2 = 132.38$, df = 16 ($P < 0.00001$); $I^2 = 88\%$
Test for overall effect: Z = 1.04 (P = 0.30)

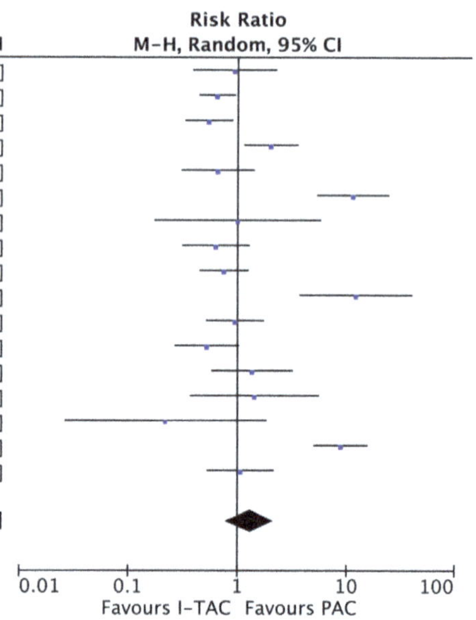

b

Study or Subgroup	I-TAC Events	I-TAC Total	PAC Events	PAC Total	Weight	Risk Ratio M-H, Random, 95% CI
Bikedeli 2021	9	276	10	286	6.9%	0.93 [0.38, 2.26]
Goligher 2021	38	530	62	559	36.5%	0.65 [0.44, 0.95]
Helms 2021	15	71	42	108	21.1%	0.54 [0.33, 0.90]
Jonmarker 2020	10	85	12	67	9.0%	0.66 [0.30, 1.43]
Martinelli 2021	16	127	20	151	14.4%	0.95 [0.51, 1.76]
Takayama 2021	1	33	4	29	1.2%	0.22 [0.03, 1.86]
Voicu 2021	11	43	12	50	10.8%	1.07 [0.52, 2.17]
Total (95% CI)		**1165**		**1250**	**100.0%**	**0.71 [0.56, 0.89]**
Total events	100		162			

Heterogeneity: $Tau^2 = 0.00$; $Chi^2 = 4.99$, df = 6 ($P = 0.54$); $I^2 = 0\%$
Test for overall effect: Z = 2.93 (P = 0.003)

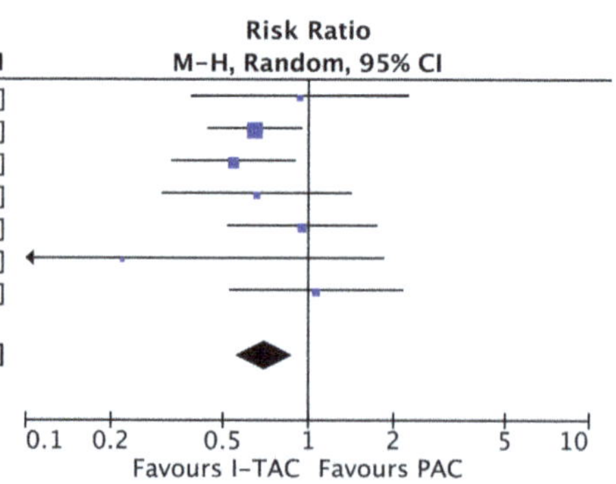

Fig. 4 a Forest plot of the effect of intermediate-to-therapeutic versus prophylactic anticoagulation on thrombotic events in general COVID-19 patients; **b** Forest plot of the effect of intermediate-to-therapeutic versus prophylactic anticoagulation on thrombotic events in COVID-19 patients admitted to ICU lower mortality until hospital discharge with a reduced need for organ support in the moderately ill COVID-19 patients with a crude 28-day in-hospital mortality of only 8.2 % for prophylactic anticoagulation group and 7.3 % for intermediate-to-therapeutic anticoagulation group [37]. Beyond clinical settings, different study countries might also have different discernible outcomes. As shown in Additional file 9, our subgroup analysis classified by study regions found that intermediate-to-therapeutic anticoagulation was not associated with lower in-hospital mortality in the pooled analysis of studies from South America, Europe, East Asia and West Asia. Data from North America even showed a significant survival benefit of prophylactic anticoagulation in unselected hospitalized COVID-19 patients as compared with intermediate-to-therapeutic anticoagulation. In general, the available evidence showed that therapeutic anticoagulation did not reduce in-hospital mortality in both critically ill and non-selected patients with COVID-19, and the evidence was of moderate quality for severe COVID-19 patients admitted to ICU and of very low quality for general COVID-19 patients admitted to hospital. Heterogeneity across the included studies was high, which might derive from different study design, imbalances in baseline characteristics, varied anticoagulation therapy (e.g., drug type, exact dosage, and route), diverse disease severity or different study countries.

Additionally, meta-analysis of data from 11 cohort studies and 6 RCTs reporting thrombotic events indicated that intermediate-to-therapeutic anticoagulation did not reduce relative risk of thrombotic events either versus prophylactic anticoagulation in general COVID-19 patients. However, a subgroup analysis of critically ill patients admitted to ICU found intermediate-to-therapeutic anticoagulation significantly reduced the incidence of thrombotic events by 30 %. These results should be interpreted with caution considering that possible insufficient thrombosis screening in patients admitted to general wards might inevitably influence the reliability of this evidence [76].

Recent studies have also reported high incidences of hemorrhage among inpatients with COVID-19. In this meta-analysis, we observed a significant increase of incidence of any bleeding events and major bleeding events in both general and critically ill patients receiving intermediate-to-therapeutic anticoagulation when compared with prophylactic anticoagulation. Especially, in critically ill COVID-19 patients, use of intermediate-to-therapeutic dose anticoagulants significantly reduced incidence of thrombotic events by 30 % but increased incidence of bleeding events by nearly 70 %, without a beneficial effect on patient survival. Therefore, the potential profit of elevated dose anticoagulation of thromboprophylaxis on thrombosis prevention are associated with an increase in bleeding events and should thus be weighed against the risk of bleeding.

Growing evidences have arisen to determine the optimal anticoagulation strategy that weighs thrombotic events and consequent bleeding risk in hospitalized patients with COVID-19. In the updated guidelines on the use of anticoagulants for thromboprophylaxis in COVID-19 patients, the American Society of Hematology recommended prophylactic anticoagulation over intermediate anticoagulation in COVID-19 patients with no confirmed or suspected thromboembolism based on low certainty of the evidence [77]. The latest NICE guideline also recommended a standard prophylactic dose of a low molecular weight heparin to young people and adults with COVID-19 who need low-flow or high-flow oxygen, continuous positive airway pressure, non-invasive ventilation or invasive mechanical ventilation within 14 h of admission [78]. Consistently, our meta-analysis further confirmed the insufficient beneficial effects of high-dose anticoagulation in general COVID-19 patients admitted to hospital. It is also noteworthy that the main outcomes in the included RCTs were typically composite endpoints [35, 37, 38, 79], which were not necessarily all related to the same end goal and limited the potential impact of these results in our daily clinical practice [76]. We instead focused on single endpoints like in-hospital mortality, thrombotic events and bleeding events. Therefore, the fact that therapeutic anticoagulation improved the composite outcome involving survival and receipt of organ support among non-critically ill patients in the multiplatform trials [37] is not as such recognized in the present review.

COVID-19 patients may exhibit complex coagulopathy states. Thrombotic and bleeding events are staggered in time and hypercoagulable states are not always consistent in the course of disease. A recent literature review by Tacquard, et al. demonstrated that thrombotic events occurred primarily in the first ten days after admission while bleeding events occurred most often late [76]. Hardy et al. also found an increase in thrombin generation with a decrease in overall fibrinolytic capacity during the first week of hospitalization, resulting in a strong procoagulant state. After this early stage of the disease, inflammatory markers and D-dimer levels gradually decreased in survivors, probably in relation to a decrease in the intensity of processes leading to microthrombosis [80]. Thromboprophylaxis strategy in hospitalized COVID-19 patients should thus be related to the disease progression and vary according to the severity of illness. D-dimers and fibrin monomers, another fibrin-related biomarker, have been extensively studied in COVID-19, and elevated levels of such biomarkers are associated with increased disease severity and mortality [81–83]. Recently, Godon, et al. showed that D-dimers and fibrin monomers were both useful to predict thrombotic events in COVID-19 patients [82]. The optimal cutoff value was determined at 5700 μg/L for fibrin monomers to predict thrombotic events with a sensitivity of 67 % and a specificity of 77 %, while the optimal cutoff value for D-dimers was 3300 μg/L with a sensitivity of 75 % and a specificity of 71 % [82]. Besides, these biomarkers are also of great value to adapt thromboprophylaxis protocol for coagulopathy in COVID-19 patients. Tassiopoulos et al. found D-dimer-driven anticoagulation protocol significantly reduced the overall mortality (31 % vs. 57 %) in intubated COVID-19 patients using a propensity-matched analysis [84]. Julie et al. further established an individualized, targeted-intensity pharmacologic thromboprophylaxis protocol evaluating degree of illness severity, total body weight, and biomarkers (involving D-dimers and thromboelastography max amplitude) in 803 COVID-19 patients admitted to hospital, and found that patients in the targeted-intensity thromboprophylaxis protocol group experienced significantly fewer thrombotic events, fewer major bleeding events, and lower mortality versus patients treated by standard thromboprophylaxis protocol [85]. These results encouraged the clinicians to adopt an individualized and targeted approach to escalated anticoagulation regimens for coagulopathy in COVID-19 patients admitted to both ICU and ward settings in future studies.

Importantly, the choices of different anticoagulation doses mainly follow local institutional protocols and were decided by the physicians in most studies, which resulted in the inconsistent anticoagulation dosage within the same group leading to potential bias [86]. For instance,in the ATTACC, ACTIV-4a and REMAP-CAP trial including critically ill COVID-19 patients, 22.4 % patients among therapeutic-dose group did not receive therapeutic-dose anticoagulation, whereas 51.7 % patients among control group received an intermediate dose, which may blunt the potential benefit of therapeutic-dose anticoagulation [38, 86]. Another challenge of precise anticoagulation in some COVID-19 patients is heparin resistance that occurs with unfractionated heparin only and entails the need of huge unfractionated heparin dosages to reach the therapeutic target [87, 88]. Therefore, monitoring of anticoagulation with anti-Xa activity is warranted to prevent a possible increased bleeding risk when high dosages of heparin are administered [87, 89].

This study has several limitations. Firstly, we included 36 cohort studies and only 6 RCTs. In those cohort studies, selection bias exists. Patients with higher disease severity and risk of thrombotic events were more likely to be treated by intermediate-to-therapeutic anticoagulation, which might lead to undervaluation of potential benefit. Secondly, most patients enrolled in the included studies were over 60 years old and it will be more reasonable to include patients with a wider age scope considering mortality is significantly higher in the elderly inpatients with COVID-19. Thirdly, the criteria for admission to hospital, definition of in-hospital mortality, bleeding and thrombotic events, follow-up periods and exact dosage of two groups might vary from region to region during different stages of the pandemic, affecting risk of both thrombotic and fatal outcomes. Results of the current meta-analysis should therefore be interpreted with caution considering these limitations.

Conclusions

Among unselected in-hospital patients with COVID-19, the current meta-analysis showed that intermediate-to-therapeutic anticoagulation was not associated with lower in-hospital mortality and incidence of thrombotic events, but increased the risk of bleeding events versus prophylactic anticoagulation. In contrast, intermediate-to-therapeutic anticoagulation reduced the risk of thrombotic events with increased incidence of bleeding events in critically COVID-19 patients admitted to ICU. We recommended the use of prophylactic anticoagulation against empirical intermediate-to-therapeutic anticoagulation among unselected hospitalized COVID-19 patients based on low certainty in the evidence. For those with severer illness, the benefits to reduce thrombotic events of intermediate-to-therapeutic anticoagulation should also be weighed cautiously by clinicians because of the significantly increased risk of bleeding associated with higher dose of anticoagulant use. Furthermore, the optimal timing of anticoagulation initiation and treatment duration remains unexplored in this field. More well-designed RCTs that effectively stratify included patients by disease severity, timing of anticoagulation initiation, and treatment duration are highly encouraged to provide high-quality evidence regarding the safety and efficacy of higher dose anticoagulation in different clinical settings.

Abbreviations

ICU: Intensive care unit; COVID-19: Coronavirus disease; RR: Risk ratio; RCT: Randomized clinical trail; CI: Confidence interval; UFH: Unfractionated heparin; LMWH: Low-molecular-weight heparin; I-TAC: Intermediate-to-therapeutic anticoagulation; PAC: Prophylactic anticoagulation

Supplementary Information

Additional file 1. Detailed search strategy.

Additional file 2. Baseline characteristics of each study.

Additional file 3. Details of anticoagulation administration in each study.

Additional file 4. Quality assessment of cohort studies by NOS score.

Additional file 5. Quality assessment of RCTs by Cochrane Collaboration tool.

Additional file 6. Sensitivity analysis of in-hospital mortality outcome.

Additional file 7. Funnel plot for the assessment risk of publication bias of in-hospital mortality outcome.

Additional file 8. The quality of evidence for in-hospital mortality assessed by GRADE framework.

Additional file 9. Subgroup analysis of in-hospital mortality stratified by study regions.

Additional file 10. Sensitivity analysis of bleeding events outcome.

Additional file 11. Funnel plot for the assessment risk of publication bias of bleeding events outcome.

Additional file 12. The quality of evidence for bleeding events assessed by GRADE framework.

Additional file 13. Sensitivity analysis of thrombotic complication events outcome.

Additional file 14. Funnel plot for the assessment risk of publication bias of thrombotic complication events outcome.

Additional file 15. The quality of evidence for thrombotic complication events assessed by GRADE framework.

Acknowledgements

Not applicable.

Authors' contributions

ZSR and LYP searched the relevant literature, collected the data and performed data analyses. LYP and SBH contributed to the design of study and data interpretation. ZSR and LGN wrote the first draft. LYP and SBH critically revised the manuscript. All authors read and approved the manuscript.

Author details

[1]West China School of Medicine, Sichuan University, 610041 Chengdu, China. [2]Department of Nephrology, Med+ Biomaterial Institute, West China Hospital, Sichuan University, 610041 Chengdu, China. [3]Institute for Disaster Management and Reconstruction, Sichuan University, 610207 Chengdu, China. [4]The first People's Hospital of Shuangliu District, 610200 Chengdu, China. [5]Med-X Center for Materials, Sichuan University, 610041 Chengdu, China.

References

1. Zhu N, Zhang D, Wang W, Li X, Yang B, Song J, Zhao X, Huang B, Shi W, Lu R, et al. A Novel Coronavirus from Patients with Pneumonia in China, 2019. N Engl J Med. 2020;382(8):727–33.
2. Middeldorp S, Coppens M, van Haaps TF, Foppen M, Vlaar AP, Müller MCA, Bouman CCS, Beenen LFM, Kootte RS, Heijmans J, et al. Incidence of venous thromboembolism in hospitalized patients with COVID-19. J Thromb Haemost. 2020;18(8):1995–2002.
3. Zhang L, Feng X, Zhang D, Jiang C, Mei H, Wang J, Zhang C, Li H, Xia X, Kong S, et al. Deep Vein Thrombosis in Hospitalized Patients With COVID-19 in Wuhan, China: Prevalence, Risk Factors, and Outcome. Circulation. 2020; 142(2):114–28.
4. Klok FA, Kruip M, van der Meer NJM, Arbous MS, Gommers D, Kant KM, Kaptein FHJ, van Paassen J, Stals MAM, Huisman MV, et al. Confirmation of the high cumulative incidence of thrombotic complications in critically ill ICU patients with COVID-19: An updated analysis. Thromb Res. 2020;191: 148–50.
5. Mirsadraee S, Gorog DA, Mahon CF, Rawal B, Semple TR, Nicol ED, Arachchillage DRJ, Devaraj A, Price S, Desai SR, et al. Prevalence of Thrombotic Complications in ICU-Treated Patients With Coronavirus Disease 2019 Detected With Systematic CT Scanning. Crit Care Med. 2021;49(5):804–15.
6. Xiong X, Chi J, Gao Q: Prevalence and risk factors of thrombotic events on patients with COVID-19: a systematic review and meta-analysis. Thromb J. 2021, 19(1):32.
7. Fontelo P, Bastola MM, Zheng Z, Baik SH: A review of thromboembolic events in hospitalized COVID-19 patients. Thromb J. 2021, 19(1):47.
8. Jiménez D, García-Sanchez A, Rali P, Muriel A, Bikdeli B, Ruiz-Artacho P, Le Mao R, Rodríguez C, Hunt BJ, Monreal M: Incidence of VTE and Bleeding Among Hospitalized Patients With Coronavirus Disease 2019: A Systematic Review and Meta-analysis. Chest 2021, 159(3):1182–1196.
9. Varga Z, Flammer AJ, Steiger P, Haberecker M, Andermatt R, Zinkernagel AS, Mehra MR, Schuepbach RA, Ruschitzka F, Moch H: Endothelial cell infection and endotheliitis in COVID-19. Lancet 2020, 395(10234):1417–1418.
10. Nicolai L, Leunig A, Brambs S, Kaiser R, Weinberger T, Weigand M, Muenchhoff M, Hellmuth JC, Ledderose S, Schulz H et al: Immunothrombotic Dysregulation in COVID-19 Pneumonia Is Associated With Respiratory Failure and Coagulopathy. Circulation 2020, 142(12):1176–1189.
11. Iba T, Levy JH, Levi M, Thachil J: Coagulopathy in COVID-19. J Thromb Haemost 2020, 18(9):2103–2109.
12. Rochwerg B, Agarwal A, Siemieniuk RA, Agoritsas T, Lamontagne F, Askie L, Lytvyn L, Leo YS, Macdonald H, Zeng L et al: A living WHO guideline on drugs for covid-19. BMJ (Clinical research ed) 2020,370:m3379.
13. Cuker A, Tseng EK, Nieuwlaat R, Angchaisuksiri P, Blair C, Dane K, Davila J, DeSancho MT, Diuguid D, Griffin DO et al: American Society of Hematology 2021 guidelines on the use of anticoagulation for thromboprophylaxis in patients with COVID-19. Blood adv 2021, 5(3):872–888.
14. Gerotziafas GT, Catalano M, Colgan MP, Pecsvarady Z, Wautrecht JC, Fazeli B, Olinic DM, Farkas K, Elalamy I, Falanga A et al: Guidance for the Management of Patients with Vascular Disease or Cardiovascular Risk Factors and COVID-19: Position Paper from VAS-European Independent Foundation in Angiology/Vascular Medicine. Thromb Haemost 2020, 120(12):1597–1628.
15. Kyriakoulis KG, Kollias A, Kyriakoulis IG, Kyprianou IA, Papachrysostomou C, Makaronis P, Kotronias RA, Terentes-Printzios D, Toskas I, Mikhailidis DP: Thromboprophylaxis in Patients with COVID-19: Systematic Review of National and International Clinical Guidance Reports. Curr Vasc Pharmacol 2021.
16. Klok FA, Kruip M, van der Meer NJM, Arbous MS, Gommers D, Kant KM, Kaptein FHJ, van Paassen J, Stals MAM, Huisman MV et al: Incidence of thrombotic complications in critically ill ICU patients with COVID-19. Thromb Res 2020, 191:145–147.
17. Helms J, Tacquard C, Severac F, Leonard-Lorant I, Ohana M, Delabranche X, Merdji H, Clere-Jehl R, Schenck M, Fagot Gandet F et al: High risk of thrombosis in patients with severe SARS-CoV-2 infection: a multicenter prospective cohort study. Intensive Care Med 2020, 46(6):1089–1098.
18. Santoro F, Núñez-Gil IJ, Viana-Llamas MC, Maroun Eid C, Romero R, Fernández Rozas I, Aparisi A, Becerra-Muñoz VM, García Aguado M, Huang J et al: Anticoagulation Therapy in Patients With Coronavirus Disease 2019: Results From a Multicenter International Prospective Registry (Health Outcome Predictive Evaluation for Corona Virus Disease 2019 [HOPE-COVID19]). Crit Care Med 2021, 49(6):e624-e633.
19. Rosovsky RP, Sanfilippo KM, Wang TF, Rajan SK, Shah S, Martin KA, F NÁ, Huisman M, Hunt BJ, Kahn SR et al: Anticoagulation Practice Patterns in COVID-19: A Global Survey. Res Pract Thromb Haemost 2020, 4(6):969–983.
20. Susen S, Tacquard CA, Godon A, Mansour A, Garrigue D, Nguyen P, Godier A, Testa S, Levy JH, Albaladejo P et al: Prevention of thrombotic risk in hospitalized patients with COVID-19 and hemostasis monitoring. Crit care (Lond, Engl) 2020, 24(1):364.
21. Lavinio A, Ercole A, Battaglini D, Magnoni S, Badenes R, Taccone FS, Helbok R, Thomas W, Pelosi P, Robba C: Safety profile of enhanced thromboprophylaxis strategies for critically ill COVID-19 patients during the first wave of the pandemic: observational report from 28 European intensive care units. Crit care (Lond, Engl) 2021, 25(1):155.
22. Flaczyk A, Rosovsky RP, Reed CT, Bankhead-Kendall BK, Bittner EA, Chang MG: Comparison of published guidelines for management of coagulopathy and thrombosis in critically ill patients with COVID 19: implications for clinical practice and future investigations. Crit care (Lond, Engl) 2020, 24(1):559.
23. Patell R, Chiasakul T, Bauer E, Zwicker JI: Pharmacologic Thromboprophylaxis and Thrombosis in Hospitalized Patients with COVID-19: A Pooled Analysis. Thromb Haemost 2021, 121(1):76–85.
24. Abdel-Maboud M, Menshawy A, Elgebaly A, Bahbah EI, El Ashal G, Negida A: Should we consider heparin prophylaxis in COVID-19 patients? a systematic review and meta-analysis. J Thromb Thrombolysis 2020.
25. Wijaya I, Andhika R, Huang I: The Use of Therapeutic-Dose Anticoagulation

and Its Effect on Mortality in Patients With COVID-19: A Systematic Review. Clin Appl Thromb Hemost 2020, 26.

26. Liberati A, Altman DG, Tetzlaff J, Mulrow C, Gøtzsche PC, Ioannidis JP, Clarke M, Devereaux PJ, Kleijnen J, Moher D: The PRISMA statement for reporting systematic reviews and meta-analyses of studies that evaluate healthcare interventions: explanation and elaboration. BMJ (Clinical research ed) 2009, 339:b2700.
27. Higgins JP, Altman DG, Gøtzsche PC, Jüni P, Moher D, Oxman AD, Savovic J, Schulz KF, Weeks L, Sterne JA: The Cochrane Collaboration's tool for assessing risk of bias in randomised trials. BMJ (Clinical research ed) 2011, 343:d5928.
28. Stang A: Critical evaluation of the Newcastle-Ottawa scale for the assessment of the quality of nonrandomized studies in meta-analyses. Eur J Epidemiol 2010, 25(9):603–605.
29. Guyatt GH, Oxman AD, Vist GE, Kunz R, Falck-Ytter Y, Alonso-Coello P, Schünemann HJ: GRADE: an emerging consensus on rating quality of evidence and strength of recommendations. BMJ (Clinical research ed) 2008, 336(7650):924–926.
30. Mehran R, Rao SV, Bhatt DL, Gibson CM, Caixeta A, Eikelboom J, Kaul S, Wiviott SD, Menon V, Nikolsky E et al: Standardized bleeding definitions for cardiovascular clinical trials: a consensus report from the Bleeding Academic Research Consortium. Circulation 2011, 123(23):2736–2747.
31. Fogarty PF, Tarantino MD, Brainsky A, Signorovitch J, Grotzinger KM: Selective validation of the WHO Bleeding Scale in patients with chronic immune thrombocytopenia. Curr Med Res Opin 2012, 28(1):79–87.
32. Slichter SJ, Kaufman RM, Assmann SF, McCullough J, Triulzi DJ, Strauss RG, Gernsheimer TB, Ness PM, Brecher ME, Josephson CD et al: Dose of prophylactic platelet transfusions and prevention of hemorrhage. N Engl J Med 2010, 362(7):600–613.
33. Schulman S, Angerås U, Bergqvist D, Eriksson B, Lassen MR, Fisher W: Definition of major bleeding in clinical investigations of antihemostatic medicinal products in surgical patients. J Thromb Haemost 2010, 8(1):202–204.
34. Perepu US, Chambers I, Wahab A, Ten Eyck P, Wu C, Dayal S, Sutamtewagul G, Bailey SR, Rosenstein LJ, Lentz SR: Standard prophylactic versus intermediate dose enoxaparin in adults with severe COVID-19: A multi-center, open-label, randomized controlled trial. J Thromb Haemost 2021.
35. Lopes RD, de Barros ESPGM, Furtado RHM, Macedo AVS, Bronhara B, Damiani LP, Barbosa LM, de Aveiro Morata J, Ramacciotti E, de Aquino Martins P et al: Therapeutic versus prophylactic anticoagulation for patients admitted to hospital with COVID-19 and elevated D-dimer concentration (ACTION): an open-label, multicentre, randomised, controlled trial. Lancet 2021, 397(10291):2253–2263.
36. Lemos ACB, do Espírito Santo DA, Salvetti MC, Gilio RN, Agra LB, Pazin-Filho A, Miranda CH: Therapeutic versus prophylactic anticoagulation for severe COVID-19: A randomized phase II clinical trial (HESACOVID). Thromb Res 2020, 196:359–366.
37. Lawler PR, Goligher EC, Berger JS, Neal MD, McVerry BJ, Nicolau JC, Gong MN, Carrier M, Rosenson RS, Reynolds HR et al: Therapeutic Anticoagulation with Heparin in Noncritically Ill Patients with Covid-19. N Engl J Med 2021.
38. Goligher EC, Bradbury CA, McVerry BJ, Lawler PR, Berger JS, Gong MN, Carrier M, Reynolds HR, Kumar A, Turgeon AF et al: Therapeutic Anticoagulation with Heparin in Critically Ill Patients with Covid-19. N Engl J Med 2021.
39. Bikdeli B, Talasaz AH, Rashidi F, Bakhshandeh H, Rafiee F, Rezaeifar P, Baghizadeh E, Matin S, Jamalkhani S, Tahamtan O et al: Intermediate-Dose versus Standard-Dose Prophylactic Anticoagulation in Patients with COVID-19 Admitted to the Intensive Care Unit: 90-Day Results from the INSPIRATION Randomized Trial. Thromb Haemost 2021.
40. Yu B, Gutierrez VP, Carlos A, Hoge G, Pillai A, Kelly JD, Menon V: Empiric use of anticoagulation in hospitalized patients with COVID-19: a propensity score-matched study of risks and benefits. Biomark Res 2021, 9(1):29.
41. Voicu S, Chousterman BG, Bonnin P, Deye N, Malissin I, Gall AL, Barthélémy R, Sutterlin L, Naim G, Mrad A et al: Increased anticoagulation reduces proximal deep vein thrombosis in mechanically ventilated COVID-19 patients: Venous thrombosis prevention & COVID-19. J Infect 2021, 82(5):186–230.
42. Vaughn VM, Yost M, Abshire C, Flanders SA, Paje D, Grant P, Kaatz S, Kim T, Barnes GD: Trends in Venous Thromboembolism Anticoagulation in Patients Hospitalized With COVID-19. JAMA netw open 2021, 4(6):e2111788.
43. Takayama W, Endo A, Otomo Y: Anticoagulation therapy using unfractionated heparin at a therapeutic dose for coronavirus disease 2019 patients with severe pneumonia: a retrospective historical control study. Acute Med Surg 2021, 8(1):e679.
44. Rodolfo., Aguilar-Soto M, Rodríguez-Toledo CA, Camiro-Zúñiga A, Demichelis R: The impact of different prophylactic anticoagulation doses on the outcomes of patients with COVID-19. Thromb Res 2021, 202:14–16.
45. Qin W, Dong F, Zhang Z, Hu B, Chen S, Zhu Z, Li F, Wang X, Zhang Y, Wang Y et al: Low molecular weight heparin and 28-day mortality among patients with coronavirus disease 2019: A cohort study in the early epidemic era. Thromb Res 2021, 198:19–22.
46. Poulakou G, Dimakakos E, Kollias A, Kyriakoulis KG, Rapti V, Trontzas I, Thanos C, Abdelrasoul M, Vantana T, Leontis K et al: Beneficial Effects of Intermediate Dosage of Anticoagulation Treatment on the Prognosis of Hospitalized COVID-19 Patients: The ETHRA Study. In vivo (Athens, Greece) 2021, 35(1):653–661.
47. Pesavento R, Ceccato D, Pasquetto G, Monticelli J, Leone L, Frigo A, Gorgi D, Postal A, Marchese GM, Cipriani A et al: The hazard of (sub)therapeutic doses of anticoagulants in non-critically ill patients with Covid-19: The Padua province experience. J Thromb Haemost 2020, 18(10):2629–2635.
48. Paranjpe I, Fuster V, Lala A, Russak AJ, Glicksberg BS, Levin MA, Charney AW, Narula J, Fayad ZA, Bagiella E et al: Association of Treatment Dose Anticoagulation With In-Hospital Survival Among Hospitalized Patients With COVID-19. J Am Coll Cardiol 2020, 76(1):122–124.
49. Paolisso P, Bergamaschi L, D'Angelo EC, Donati F, Giannella M, Tedeschi S, Pascale R, Bartoletti M, Tesini G, Biffi M et al: Preliminary Experience With Low Molecular Weight Heparin Strategy in COVID-19 Patients. Front Pharmacol 2020, 11:1124.
50. Pablo P, Farfán-Sedano AI, Pedrajas JM, Llamas P, Sigüenza P, Jaras MJ, Quintana-Diaz M, Fernández-Capitán C, Bikdeli B, Jiménez D et al: Bleeding risk in hospitalized patients with COVID-19 receiving intermediate- or therapeutic doses of thromboprophylaxis. J Thromb Haemost 2021.
51. Nadkarni GN, Lala A, Bagiella E, Chang HL, Moreno PR, Pujadas E, Arvind V, Bose S, Charney AW, Chen MD et al: Anticoagulation, Bleeding, Mortality, and Pathology in Hospitalized Patients With COVID-19. J Am Coll Cardiol 2020, 76(16):1815–1826.
52. Nadeem R, Thomas SJ, Fathima Z, Palathinkal AS, Alkilani YE, Dejan EA, Darwish IMI, Alsubousi AA, Backour AM, Kandeel H et al: Pattern of anticoagulation prescription for patients with Covid-19 acute respiratory distress syndrome admitted to ICU. Does it impact outcome? Heart Lung 2021, 50(1):1–5.
53. Musoke N, Lo KB, Albano J, Peterson E, Bhargav R, Gul F, DeJoy R, 3rd, Salacup G, Pelayo J, Tipparaju P et al: Anticoagulation and bleeding risk in patients with COVID-19. Thromb Res 2020, 196:227–230.
54. Motta JK, Ogunnaike RO, Shah R, Stroever S, Cedeño HV, Thapa SK, Chronakos JJ, Jimenez EJ, Petrini J, Hegde A: Clinical Outcomes With the Use of Prophylactic Versus Therapeutic Anticoagulation in Coronavirus Disease 2019. Crit Care Explor 2020, 2(12):e0309.
55. Moll M, Zon RL, Sylvester KW, Rimsans J, Chen EC, Ghosh AJ, Abston E, Kim A, Rutherford H, Mitre X et al: Intermediate versus standard dose heparin prophylaxis in COVID-19 ICU patients: A propensity score-matched analysis. Thromb Res 2021, 203:57–60.
56. Mennuni MG, Renda G, Grisafi L, Rognoni A, Colombo C, Lio V, Foglietta M, Petrilli I, Pirisi M, Spinoni E et al: Clinical outcome with different doses of low-molecular-weight heparin in patients hospitalized for COVID-19. J Thromb Thrombolysis 2021:1–9.
57. Meizlish ML, Goshua G, Liu Y, Fine R, Amin K, Chang E, DeFilippo N, Keating C, Liu Y, Mankbadi M et al: Intermediate-dose anticoagulation, aspirin, and in-hospital mortality in COVID-19: A propensity score-matched analysis. Am J Hematol 2021, 96(4):471–479.
58. Martinelli I, Ciavarella A, Abbattista M, Aliberti S, De Zan V, Folli C, Panigada M, Gori A, Artoni A, Ierardi AM et al: Increasing dosages of low-molecular-weight heparin in hospitalized patients with Covid-19. Intern Emerg Med 2021, 16(5):1223–1229.
59. Lynn L, Reyes JA, Hawkins K, Panda A, Linville L, Aldhahri W, Kango G, Shah S, Ayanian S, Teufel K: The effect of anticoagulation on clinical outcomes in novel Coronavirus (COVID-19) pneumonia in a U.S. cohort. Thromb Res 2021, 197:65–68.
60. Longhitano Y, Racca F, Zanza C, Muncinelli M, Guagliano A, Peretti E, Minerba AC, Mari M, Boverio R, Salio M et al: Venous Thrombo-Embolism in Hospitalized SARS-CoV-2 Patients Treated with Three Different Anticoagulation Protocols: Prospective Observational Study. Biology 2020, 9(10).
61. Llitjos JF, Leclerc M, Chochois C, Monsallier JM, Ramakers M, Auvray M, Merouani K: High incidence of venous thromboembolic events in anticoagulated severe COVID-19 patients. J Thromb Haemost 2020, 18(7):1743–1746.
62. Kodama R, Kalsi A, Singh A, Vishnuvardhan N, Nimkar N, Paul S, Usta S, Ashraf F, Mazloom A, Ashfaq A et al: Outcomes in COVID-19 patients on

treatment dose anti- coagulation compared to prophylactic dose anti-coagulation. Blood 2020, 136(SUPPL 1):40–41.

63. Kaur J, Sule AA, Koehler T, Krishnamoorthy G, DeLongpre J: Anticoagulation management and outcomes in COVID-19 patients: A multi-center retrospective cohort study. Blood 2020, 136(SUPPL 1):34.
64. Jonmarker S, Hollenberg J, Dahlberg M, Stackelberg O, Litorell J, Everhov Å H, Järnbert-Pettersson H, Söderberg M, Grip J, Schandl A et al: Dosing of thromboprophylaxis and mortality in critically ill COVID-19 patients. Crit care (Lond, Engl) 2020, 24(1):653.
65. Ionescu F, Jaiyesimi I, Petrescu I, Lawler PR, Castillo E, Munoz-Maldonado Y, Imam Z, Narasimhan M, Abbas AE, Konde A et al: Association of anticoagulation dose and survival in hospitalized COVID-19 patients: A retrospective propensity score-weighted analysis. Eur J Haematol 2021, 106(2):165–174.
66. Hsu A, Liu Y, Zayac AS, Olszewski AJ, Reagan JL: Intensity of anticoagulation and survival in patients hospitalized with COVID-19 pneumonia. Thromb Res 2020, 196:375–378.
67. Helms J, Severac F, Merdji H, Schenck M, Clere-Jehl R, Baldacini M, Ohana M, Grunebaum L, Castelain V, Anglés-Cano E et al: Higher anticoagulation targets and risk of thrombotic events in severe COVID-19 patients: bi-center cohort study. Ann Intensive Care 2021, 11(1):14.
68. Hanif A, Khan S, Mantri N, Hanif S, Saleh M, Alla Y, Chinta S, Shrestha N, Ji W, Attwood K et al: Thrombotic complications and anticoagulation in COVID-19 pneumonia: a New York City hospital experience. Ann Hematol 2020, 99(10):2323–2328.
69. Halaby R, Cuker A, Yui J, Matthews A, Ishaaya E, Traxler E, Domenico C, Cooper T, Tierney A, Niami P et al: Bleeding risk by intensity of anticoagulation in critically ill patients with COVID-19: A retrospective cohort study. J Thromb Haemost 2021, 19(6):1533–1545.
70. Ferguson J, Volk S, Vondracek T, Flanigan J, Chernaik A: Empiric Therapeutic Anticoagulation and Mortality in Critically Ill Patients With Respiratory Failure From SARS-CoV-2: A Retrospective Cohort Study. J Clin Pharmacol 2020, 60(11): 1411–1415.
71. Elmelhat A, Elbourai E, Dewedar H, Elgergawi T, Alkhanbouli M, Ahmed S, Malik Z, Nugud A, Mohammed S, Mohammad H et al: Comparison between Prophylactic versus Therapeutic Doses of Low-Molecular-Weight Heparin in Severely Ill Coronavirus Disease 2019 Patients in Relation to Disease Progression and Outcome. Dubai Med J 2020, 3(4):162–169.
72. Di Castelnuovo A, Costanzo S, Antinori A, Berselli N, Blandi L, Bonaccio M, Cauda R, Guaraldi G, Menicanti L, Mennuni M et al: Heparin in COVID-19 Patients Is Associated with Reduced In-Hospital Mortality: the Multicenter Italian CORIST Study. Thromb Haemost 2021.
73. Daughety MM, Morgan A, Frost E, Kao C, Hwang J, Tobin R, Patel B, Fuller M, Welsby I, Ortel TL: COVID-19 associated coagulopathy: Thrombosis, hemorrhage and mortality rates with an escalated-dose thromboprophylaxis strategy. Thromb Res 2020, 196:483–485.
74. Canoglu K, Saylan B: Therapeutic dosing of low-molecular-weight heparin may decrease mortality in patients with severe COVID-19 infection. Ann Saudi Med 2020, 40(6):462–468.
75. Bolzetta F, Maselli M, Formilan M, Busonera F, Albanese P, Chiaromanni F, Romano A, Veronese N: Prophylactic or therapeutic doses of heparins for COVID-19 infection? A retrospective study. Aging Clin Exp Res 2021, 33(1): 213–217.
76. Tacquard C, Mansour A, Godon A, Gruel Y, Susen S, Godier A, Albaladejo P: Anticoagulation in COVID-19: not strong for too long? Anaest Crit Care Pain Med 2021, 40(2):100857.
77. Cuker A, Tseng EK, Nieuwlaat R, Angchaisuksiri P, Blair C, Dane K, Davila J, DeSancho MT, Diuguid DL, Griffin DO et al: American Society of Hematology living guidelines on the use of anticoagulation for thromboprophylaxis in patients with COVID-19: May 2021 update on the use of intermediate intensity anticoagulation in critically ill patients. Blood adv 2021, 5 (20): 3951–3959.
78. National Institute for Health and Care Excellence. COVID-19 rapid guideline: Managing COVID-19. https://www.nice.org.uk/guidance/NG191. Accessed 02 November 2021.
79. Sadeghipour P, Talasaz AH, Rashidi F, Sharif-Kashani B, Beigmohammadi MT, Farrokhpour M, Sezavar SH, Payandemehr P, Dabbagh A, Moghadam KG et al: Effect of Intermediate-Dose vs Standard-Dose Prophylactic Anticoagulation on Thrombotic Events, Extracorporeal Membrane Oxygenation Treatment, or Mortality Among Patients With COVID-19 Admitted to the Intensive Care Unit: The INSPIRATION Randomized Clinical Trial. JAMA 2021, 325(16):1620–1630.
80. Hardy M, Michaux I, Lessire S, Douxfils J, Dogné JM, Bareille M, Horlait G, Bulpa P, Chapelle C, Laporte S et al: Prothrombotic disturbances of hemostasis of patients with severe COVID-19: A prospective longitudinal observational study. Thromb Res 2021, 197:20–23.
81. Liao DY, Zhou F, Luo LL, Xu M, Wang HB, Xia JH, Gao Y, Cai LQ, Wang ZH, Yin P et al: Haematological characteristics and risk factors in the classification and prognosis evaluation of COVID-19: a retrospective cohort study. Lancet Haematol 2020, 7(9):E671-E678.
82. Godon A, Durand Z, Agier L, Lecompte T, Mullier F, Marlu R, de Maistre E, Tacquard C, Levy JH, Godier A et al: Comparison of Fibrin Monomers and D-dimers to predict thrombotic events in critically ill patients with COVID-19 pneumonia: A retrospective study. Thromb Res 2021, 205:8–10.
83. Moosavi M, Wooten M, Goodman A, Nahab FB, Duncan A, Maier C, Guarner J: Retrospective Analyses Associate Hemostasis Activation Biomarkers With Poor Outcomes in Patients With COVID-19. Am J Clin Pathol 2021, 155(4): 498–505.
84. Tassiopoulos AK, Mofakham S, Rubano JA, Labropoulos N, Bannazadeh M, Drakos P, Volteas P, Cleri NA, Alkadaa LN, Asencio AA et al: D-Dimer-Driven Anticoagulation Reduces Mortality in Intubated COVID-19 Patients: A Cohort Study With a Propensity-Matched Analysis. Front Med 2021, 8:10.
85. Farrar JE, Trujillo TC, Mueller SW, Beltran L, Nguyen C, Hassell K, Kiser TH: Evaluation of a patient specific, targeted-intensity pharmacologic thromboprophylaxis protocol in hospitalized patients with COVID-19. J Thromb Thrombolysis 2021.
86. Ten Cate H: Surviving Covid-19 with Heparin? N Engl J Med 2021, 385(9): 845–846.
87. Novelli C, Borotto E, Beverina I, Punzi V, Radrizzani D, Brando B: Heparin dosage, level, and resistance in SARS-CoV2 infected patients in intensive care unit. Int J Lab Hematol 2021.
88. White D, MacDonald S, Bull T, Hayman M, de Monteverde-Robb R, Sapsford D, Lavinio A, Varley J, Johnston A, Besser M et al: Heparin resistance in COVID-19 patients in the intensive care unit. J Thromb Thrombolysis 2020, 50(2):287–291.
89. Beun R, Kusadasi N, Sikma M, Westerink J, Huisman A: Thromboembolic events and apparent heparin resistance in patients infected with SARS-CoV-2. Int J Lab Hematol 2020, 42:19–20.

15

The impact on renal function after long-term use of anticoagulants in atrial fibrillation patients

Wei-Chieh Lee[1,2], Pai-Wei Lee[3], Po-Jui Wu[2], Yen-Nan Fang[2], Huang-Chung Chen[2], Yu-Sheng Lin[4], Hsiu-Yu Fang[2], Shang-Hung Chang[3], Ping-Yen Liu[1*] and Mien-Cheng Chen[2*]

Abstract

Objective: Long-term oral anticoagulant should be considered or recommended in patients with atrial fibrillation (AF) and CHA2DS2VASc score ≥ 1 for stroke prevention. Warfarin and different direct oral anticoagulants (DOACs) are metabolized differently by the kidney. The impact on renal function after long-term use of anticoagulants in the patients with AF remains unclear. This study aimed to compare DOACs and warfarin's impact on the decline in renal function from a large cohort with AF.

Methods: This study included patients with nonvalvular AF from 2000 to 2018, mainly through the medical history (ICD code) of the Chang Gung Research Database. Baseline estimated glomerular filtration rate (eGFR), follow-up eGFR and the change in eGFR between 2-year eGFR and baseline eGFR were compared between different DOACs and warfarin after propensity score matching. The primary study endpoint was acute kidney injury (AKI).

Results: 3657 patients were enrolled in this study and the mean observation time was 3.3 ± 0.9 years. During the observation period, there was a significantly higher incidence of AKI during follow-up in the warfarin group than in the different DOAC groups before and after propensity score matching (before: warfarin vs. DOAC: 9.2% vs. 5.2%, $p < 0.001$; after: warfarin vs. DOAC: 8.9% vs. 4.4%, $p < 0.001$). There was no difference in the incidence of AKI between dabigatran group and anti-factor Xa inhibitor group after propensity score matching. The incidence of AKI was similar among rivaroxaban, apixaban and edoxaban groups after propensity score matching. The change in eGFR between 2-year eGFR and baseline eGFR did not differ between the warfarin and DOAC groups after propensity score matching (warfarin vs. DOAC: − 1.27 ± 20.32 vs. -1.94 ± 17.24 mL/min/1.73 m^2, $p = 0.461$).

Conclusions: During the mean observation time of 3.3 ± 0.9 years, warfarin was associated with a higher incidence of AKI compared with DOACs. The decline in renal function did not differ among warfarin and different DOAC groups.

Keywords: Atrial fibrillation, Acute kidney injury, Estimated glomerular filtration rate, Warfarin, Non-vitamin K oral anticoagulant

* Correspondence: larry@mail.ncku.edu.tw; chenmien@ms76.hinet.net
[1]Institute of Clinical Medicine, College of Medicine, National Cheng Kung University, Tainan, Taiwan
[2]Division of Cardiology, Department of Internal Medicine, Kaohsiung Chang Gung Memorial Hospital, Chang Gung University College of Medicine, 123 Ta Pei Road, Niao Sung District, Kaohsiung City 83301, Taiwan

Background

Due to the aging population, increasing number of patients experiences atrial fibrillation (AF). Long-term oral anticoagulant should be considered in AF patients with CHA2DS2VASc score = 1 and is strongly recommended in patients with CHA2DS2-VASc score ≥ 2 for stroke prevention. Warfarin has been reported to cause arterial calcification and microthrombus, which contribute to worsening renal function in warfarin users [1, 2]. Direct oral anticoagulants (DOACs) have predictable anticoagulant effects, infrequent monitoring requirements and less drug-food interactions compared to warfarin [3]. Moreover, warfarin and different DOACs are metabolized differently by the kidney [3]. The optimal regimen for patients with chronic kidney disease (CKD) needing anticoagulants is currently debated [4]. In the Randomized Evaluation of Long-Term Anticoagulation Therapy (RE-LY) study, after an average of 30 months, AF patients taking warfarin exhibited a greater decline in renal function compared with those taking dabigatran (warfarin vs. dabigatran 150 mg vs. dabigatran 110 mg; -3.68 ± 0.24 vs. -2.46 ± 0.23 vs. -2.57 ± 0.24 ml/min; $p = 0.0002$ and $p = 0.0009$, respectively) [5]. However, there was a small, statistically significant decline in creatinine clearance (CrCl) among patients receiving rivaroxaban compared with patients receiving warfarin in the subgroup analysis of ROCKET-AF trial (Rivaroxaban Once Daily Oral Direct Factor Xa Inhibition Compared with Vitamin K Antagonism for Prevention of Stroke and Embolism Trial in Atrial Fibrillation) (warfarin vs. rivaroxaban; -3.5 ± 15.1 vs. -4.3 ± 14.6 mL/min; $P < 0.001$) [6, 7]. On the contrary, in the US medical care database, rivaroxaban was associated with a 19% reduction in the hazard of acute kidney injury (AKI) and an 18% reduction in progression to stage 5 CKD or hemodialysis compared with warfarin in patients with AF [8]. Moreover, in a recent multicenter prospective cohort study, patients taking direct oral anticoagulants (DOACs) showed a slower decline in renal function compared with those taking warfarin, but the favorable association between DOAC use and decline of renal function was partially lost in patients with diabetes [9]. Thus, there are different impacts of DOACs and warfarin on renal decline in different population with AF. Moreover, there are limited data in terms of different impacts on renal decline of long-term use of the four different DOACs and warfarin in AF patients in the Asian population [10].

According, we conducted this study to compare DOACs and warfarin's impact on the decline in renal function from a large Chang Gung Research Database (CGRD), which had detailed laboratory data for comparison.

Methods

Patient population

This study included patients with AF from January 2000 to December 2018, mainly through the medical history obtained from the CGRD. The CGRD is based on the largest healthcare system in Taiwan, which comprises four tertiary care medical centers and three major teaching hospitals with a total of 10,050 beds [11]. The CGRD contains data of detailed laboratory values and drug use.

The inclusion criteria were as follows: patients aged ≥18 years and diagnosed with AF (International Classification of Diseases, Ninth Revision, Clinical Modification (ICD-9-CM) code 427.31 or Tenth Revision (ICD-10) codes I480, I481, I482, and I4891), and patients who were prescribed the same oral anticoagulant (warfarin or DOACs) for more than 2 years. All patients in the DOAC groups had their dosage adjustment according to dosing criteria of each DOAC, especially while renal function declined.

Exclusion criteria were as follows: patients who had taken oral anticoagulants for mechanical valves, rheumatic mitral stenosis, pulmonary embolism, venous thromboembolism, or preventive use after orthopedic surgery and patients with baseline estimated glomerular filtration rate (eGFR) < 30 mL/min. The flowchart of the study population is illustrated in Fig. 1.

Data on general demographics, comorbidities, baseline, and follow-up eGFR, medication use, presence of AKI, the need for hemodialysis, and renal death were obtained and compared between the warfarin and DOAC groups, among warfarin, dabigatran, and anti-factor Xa inhibitors, and between different anti-factor Xa inhibitors.

The patients and the public did not involve in the design of this study but involved in the process of review of institutional review committee.

Ethical statement

This retrospective study conformed to the ethical guidelines of the 1975 Declaration of Helsinki and was approved for human research by the institutional review committee of Kaohsiung Chang Gung Memorial Hospital (number: 202000917B0).

Definition

Renal function was estimated using as modification of diet in renal disease *equation*. AKI was defined as increase in serum Cr by ≥0.3 mg/dL within 48 h or increase in serum Cr to ≥1.5 times the baseline, which was known or presumed to have occurred within the past 7 days [12]. The need for hemodialysis was defined as patients presenting with oliguria or anuria and receiving hemodialysis. Renal death was defined as death due to renal disease.

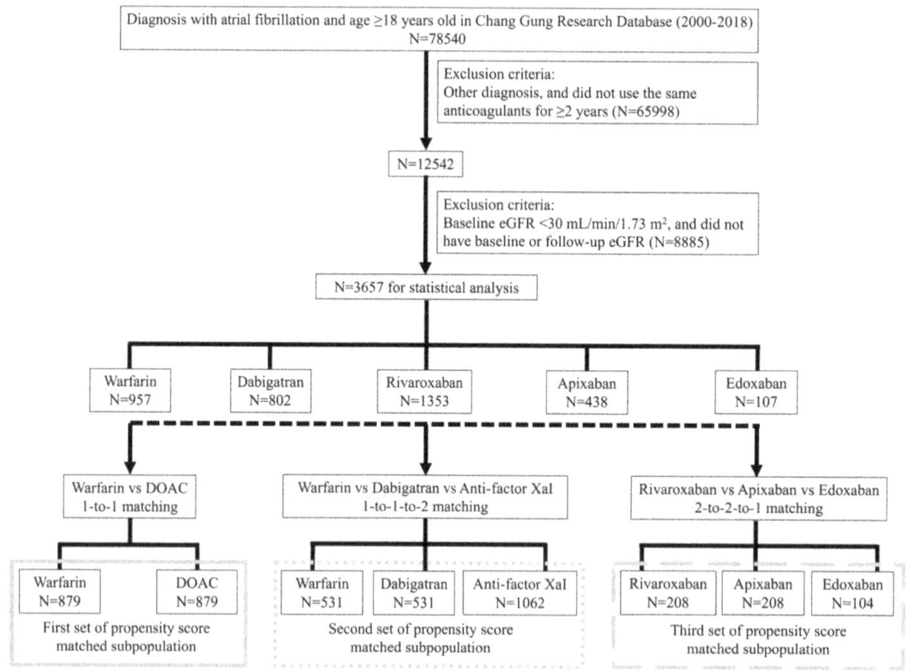

Fig. 1 Flow chart of the study population
eGFR: estimated glomerular filtration rate; DOAC: direct oral anticoagulants.

Study endpoint

The primary study endpoint was AKI, and the secondary endpoints were the need for hemodialysis and renal death.

Statistical analysis

Data are presented as mean ± standard deviation or numbers (percentages). The clinical characteristics of the two groups were compared using the independent samples t-test or analysis of variance test for continuous variables and the chi-squared test or Fisher's exact test for categorical variables. Propensity score matching was performed using a multivariate logistic regression model to adjust for differences in baseline characteristics (sex, age, diabetes mellitus, hypertension, hyperlipidemia, heart failure, serum Cr, eGFR, and angiotensin-converting enzyme inhibitors [ACEIs]/angiotensin-receptor blockers [ARBs]) for 1-to-1 or 1-to-1-to 2 or 2-to-2-to-1 matched analysis. Using the estimated logits, the different groups had the closest estimated logit values for comparison between different groups. Matching quality was analyzed using the absolute value of the standardized mean difference (ASMD) between the groups after matching, where a value lower than 0.1 represented negligible difference between the groups. Statistical significance was set at p-value < 0.05. All analyses were performed using SAS version 9.4 (SAS Institute Inc., Cary, NC, USA).

Results

Baseline characteristics and renal outcomes between warfarin and DOAC groups (before propensity score matching)

3657 patients were enrolled in this study and the mean observation time was 3.3 ± 0.9 years. The baseline characteristics and renal outcomes of the study population before propensity score matching are shown in Table 1. There were more male patients in the DOACs group (62.5%) compared with warfarin group (54.2%) ($p < 0.001$). Patients in the warfarin group were younger than those in the DOAC groups (warfarin vs. DOACs; 66 ± 11.3 vs. 70 ± 9.6; $p < 0.001$). Patients in the warfarin group had a lower prevalence of hypertension and hyperlipidemia, and a higher prevalence of heart failure than those in the DOAC groups. Patients in the warfarin group had a higher prevalence of CKD stage ≥3 (warfarin vs. DOACs; 37.1% vs. 24.6%; $p = 0.009$) than those in the DOAC groups. CHA2DS2-VASc scores significantly differ among warfarin and different DOAC groups ($p < 0.001$). Patients in the warfarin group had a lower prevalence of ACEI/ARB use than those in the DOAC groups. The average level of international normalized ratio (INR) in the warfarin group was 1.69 ± 0.93 at the 1-year follow-up and 1.56 ± 0.99 at the 2-year follow-up.

Although baseline serum Cr level significantly differ among warfarin and different DOAC groups (warfarin vs. DOACs; 1.09 ± 0.36 mg/dL vs. 1.06 ± 0.31 mg/dL; $p < 0.001$), baseline eGFR did not significantly differ

Table 1 Baseline characteristics and renal outcomes (before propensity score matching)

Variables	Warfarin group	DOAC group				*p* value (NOACs vs. Warfarin)
	Warfarin	Dabigatran	Rivaroxaban	Apixaban	Edoxaban	
N	957	802	1353	438	107	
Gender (male)	519 (54.2)	526 (65.6)	807 (59.6)	282 (64.4)	73 (68.2)	< 0.001
Mean age	66 ± 11.3	69 ± 9.6	70 ± 9.5	71 ± 9 .8	69 ± 10.0	< 0.001
Medical history						
Type 2 DM	179 (18.7)	166 (20.7)	289 (21.4)	104 (23.7)	24 (22.4)	0.065
Hypertension	346 (36.2)	336 (41.9)	625 (46.2)	230 (52.5)	50 (46.7)	< 0.001
Hyperlipidemia	184 (19.2)	171 (21.3)	303 (22.4)	126 (28.8)	35 (32.7)	0.007
Heart failure	136 (14.2)	62 (7.7)	135 (10.0)	28 (13.2)	9 (8.4)	< 0.001
Prior stroke	40 (4.2)	50 (6.2)	79 (5.8)	20 (4.6)	5 (4.7)	0.085
Vascular disease	20 (2.1)	11 (1.4)	24 (1.8)	20 (4.6)	0 (0)	1.000
Chronic kidney disease						
Stage < 3	602 (62.9)	597 (74.4)	897 (66.3)	272 (62.1)	60 (56.1)	0.009
Stage ≥3	355 (37.1)	205 (25.6)	246 (18.2)	166 (37.9)	47 (43.9)	
CHA2DS2-VASc	2.17 ± 1.33	2.42 ± 1.39	2.62 ± 1.33	2.6 2 ± 1.30	2.45 ± 1.40	< 0.001
Medication						
ACEI/ARB	528 (55.2)	472 (58.9)	803 (59.3)	254 (58.0)	72 (67.3)	0.029
Spironolactone	0 (0)	0 (0)	0 (0)	2 (0.5)	1 (0.9)	0.572
Renal function						
The average serum Cr (mg/dL)	1.09 ± 0.36	1.02 ± 0.27	1.06 ± 0.31	1.11 ± 0.34	1.14 ± 0.36	0.017
Baseline eGFR (mL/min/1.73 m^2)	70.51 ± 24.95	74.98 ± 22.17	71.38 ± 23.38	68.51 ± 21.34	68.06 ± 21.89	0.128
1-year eGFR (mL/min/1.73 m^2)	69.26 ± 23.86	73.33 ± 22.59	68.74 ± 22.55	66.71 ± 21.72	69.03 ± 23.49	0.553
2-year eGFR (mL/min/1.73 m^2)	69.52 ± 26.89	72.73 ± 25.14	68.14 ± 23.01	65.80 ± 22.80	67.05 ± 22.78	0.657
Renal outcomes						
Acute kidney injury (%)	88 (9.2)	40 (5.0)	69 (5.1)	27 (6.2)	4 (3.7)	< 0.001
Renal failure requiring HD (%)	3 (0.3)	0 (0)	2 (0.1)	1 (0.2)	0 (0)	0.188
Renal death (%)	5 (0.5)	3 (0.4)	4 (0.3)	1 (0.2)	1 (0.9)	0.378
Observation time (years)	3.9 ± 1.5	3.8 ± 1.1	3.5 ± 0.8	2.9 ± 0.3	2.6 ± 0.4	< 0.001

Data were presented as mean ± standard deviation or numbers (percentages)
Abbreviation: *N* number, *DOAC* direct oral anticoagulants, *DM* diabetes mellitus, *Cr* creatinine, *eGFR* estimated glomerular filtration rate, *ACEI* Angiotensin-converting enzyme inhibitor, *ARB* angiotensin receptor blocker, *HD* hemodialysis

among warfarin and different DOAC groups (warfarin vs. DOACs; 70.51 ± 24.95 mL/min vs. 71.85 ± 22.75 mL/min; $p = 0.128$). Moreover, follow-up 1-year and 2-year eGFR did not significantly differ among warfarin and different DOAC groups (Table 1). However, during the observation period, there was a significantly higher incidence of AKI in the warfarin group than in the different DOAC groups (warfarin vs. DOACs; 9.2% vs. 5.2%; $p < 0.001$). During the observation period, there were no significant differences in the need for hemodialysis and renal death among warfarin and different DOAC groups.

Baseline characteristics and renal outcomes between warfarin and DOAC groups (after propensity score matching)

The baseline characteristics and renal outcomes of the warfarin and DOAC groups after propensity score matching are shown in Table 2. Age, gender, and the prevalence of all comorbidities were similar between warfarin and DOAC groups. The prevalence of CKD stage ≥3 and the mean CHA2DS2-VASc score did not differ between warfarin and DOAC groups. The prevalence of ACEI/ARB use was similar between warfarin and DOAC groups.

There was no significant difference in serum Cr level, baseline eGFR, 1-year and 2-year follow-up eGFR between the warfarin and DOAC groups after propensity score matching (Table 2) (Fig. 2A). Moreover, the change in eGFR between 2-year eGFR and baseline eGFR did not differ between warfarin and DOAC groups (warfarin vs. DOAC: − 1.27 ± 20.32 vs. -1.94 ± 17.24 mL/min/1.73 m^2, $p = 0.461$) (Fig. 2B). In the subgroups analysis, including age ≥ 70 or < 70 years, with or without diabetes mellitus, with or without heart failure, with or

Table 2 Baseline characteristics and renal outcomes (after warfarin and DOACs 1:1 propensity score matching)

Variables	Warfarin group	DOAC group	*p* value	ASMD
N	879	879		
Gender (male)	490 (55.7)	502 (57.1)	0.597	0.002
Mean age	67 ± 10.6	67 ± 10.3	0.967	0.002
Medical history 1				
Type 2 DM	160 (18.2)	166 (18.9)	0.759	0.002
Hypertension	335 (38.1)	334 (38.0)	1.000	0.0002
Hyperlipidemia	172 (19.6)	181 (20.6)	0.634	0.002
Heart failure	109 (12.4)	115 (13.1)	0.721	0.002
Previous stroke	38 (4.3)	49 (5.6)	0.272	0.006
Vascular disease	19 (2.2)	16 (1.8)	0.733	0.002
Chronic kidney disease				
Stage < 3	556 (63.3)	550 (62.6)	0.805	0.001
Stage ≥3	323 (36.7)	329 (37.4)		0.001
CHA2DS2-VASc	2.23 ± 1.34	2.29 ± 1.37	0.351	0.044
Medication				
ACEI/ARB	494 (56.2)	476 (54.2)	0.415	0.003
Spironolactone	0 (0)	0 (0)	–	–
Renal function				
The average serum Cr (mg/dL)	1.08 ± 0.35	1.09 ± 0.35	0.912	0.029
Baseline eGFR (mL/min/1.73 m^2)	70.33 ± 24.21	70.54 ± 24.67	0.861	0.009
1-year eGFR (mL/min/1.73 m^2)	68.98 ± 23.57	69.56 ± 24.09	0.613	0.024
2-year eGFR (mL/min/1.73 m^2)	69.06 ± 26.46	68.60 ± 24.84	0.708	0.018
Renal outcomes				
Acute kidney injury (%)	78 (8.9)	39 (4.4)	< 0.001	0.017
Renal failure requiring HD (%)	2 (0.2)	2 (0.2)	1.000	0
Renal death (%)	4 (0.5)	3 (0.3)	1.000	0.002

Data were presented as mean ± standard deviation or numbers (percentages)
Abbreviation: *DOAC* direct oral anticoagulants, *ASMD* absolute standardized mean difference, *N* number, *DM* diabetes mellitus, *Cr* creatinine, *eGFR* estimated glomerular filtration rate, *ACEI* Angiotensin-converting enzyme inhibitor, *ARB* angiotensin receptor blocker, *HD* hemodialysis

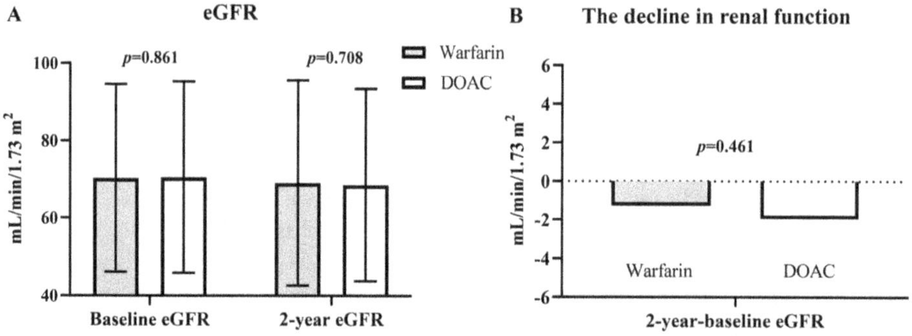

Fig. 2 (**A**) Comparison of baseline and 2-year follow-up estimated glomerular filtration rate (eGFR) between warfarin and DOAC groups after propensity score matching. (**B**) Comparison of the change in eGFR between 2-year eGFR and baseline eGFR between warfarin and DOAC groups after propensity score matching

without hypertension, with or without ACEI/ARB use, or CKD stage ≥3 or < 3, the change in eGFR between 2-year eGFR and baseline eGFR did not differ between warfarin and DOAC groups (Supplemental Fig. 1). However, during the observation period, there was a higher incidence of AKI during follow-up in the warfarin group than in the DOAC group (8.9% vs. 4.4%; $p < 0.001$). During the observation period, the incidence of hemodialysis and renal death did not differ between warfarin and DOAC groups.

Baseline characteristics and renal outcomes among warfarin, dabigatran, and anti-factor Xa inhibitor groups (after propensity score matching)

The baseline characteristics and renal outcomes of warfarin, dabigatran, and anti-factor Xa inhibitor groups after propensity score matching are listed in Table 3. Patients in the dabigatran group were younger and had a lower prevalence of hypertension and CKD stage ≥3 compared with warfarin and anti-factor Xa inhibitor groups.

Patients in the dabigatran group had a lower serum Cr level and higher baseline and follow-up eGFR compared with warfarin and anti-factor Xa inhibitor groups (Fig. 3A). There was no difference in serum Cr level, and baseline and follow-up eGFR between warfarin and anti-factor Xa inhibitor groups. Of note, the change in eGFR between 2-year eGFR and baseline eGFR did not differ among dabigatran, warfarin, and anti-factor Xa inhibitor groups (Fig. 3B). In the subgroups analysis, including age ≥ 70 or < 70 years, with or without diabetes mellitus, with or without heart failure, with or without hypertension, with or without ACEI/ARB use, or CKD stage ≥3 or < 3, the change in eGFR between 2-year eGFR and baseline eGFR did not differ among dabigatran, warfarin, and anti-factor Xa inhibitor groups (Supplemental Fig. 2). However, during the observation period, the incidence of AKI was significantly higher in the warfarin group compared with dabigatran and anti-factor Xa inhibitor groups (10.2% vs. 4.3% vs. 5.4%; $p < 0.001$) (Table 3). There was no difference in the incidence of AKI between dabigatran and anti-factor Xa inhibitor groups. The incidences of hemodialysis and renal death were similar among warfarin, dabigatran, and anti-factor Xa inhibitor groups (Table 3).

Baseline characteristics and renal outcomes among three different anti-factor Xa inhibitor groups (after propensity score matching)

The baseline characteristics and renal outcomes of rivaroxaban, apixaban and edoxaban groups after propensity score matching are listed in Table 4. Vascular disease was the only comorbidity to be significantly different among the three groups.

There was no significant difference in baseline eGFR, 1-year and 2-year follow-up eGFR among rivaroxaban, apixaban and edoxaban groups after propensity score matching (Table 4) (Fig. 4A). Moreover, the change in eGFR between 2-year eGFR and baseline eGFR did not differ among rivaroxaban, apixaban and edoxaban groups (Fig. 4B). In the subgroups analysis, including age ≥ 70 or < 70 years, with or without diabetes mellitus, with or without heart failure, with or without hypertension, with or without ACEI/ARB use, or CKD stage ≥3 or < 3, the change in eGFR between 2-year eGFR and baseline eGFR did not differ among rivaroxaban, apixaban and edoxaban groups (Supplemental Fig. 3). During the observation period, the incidence of AKI, hemodialysis, and renal death were similar among rivaroxaban, apixaban and edoxaban groups (Table 4).

Discussion

The significance of this study

As the frequency of anticoagulation use is increasing due to increasing number of patients experiencing AF and the dosages of DOACs during the follow-up period might need to be adjusted according to renal function, the issue of renal function decline or acute kidney injury associated with anticoagulant use in AF patients is very important and clinically relevant. In this study, during the observation period, warfarin group had a higher incidence of AKI compared with different DOAC groups before and after propensity score matching. However, the incidence of the need for hemodialysis and renal death did not differ among warfarin group and different DOACs groups. The incidences of AKI, hemodialysis and renal death were similar between dabigatran, and anti-factor Xa inhibitor groups. The incidence of AKI, hemodialysis, and renal death were similar among rivaroxaban, apixaban and edoxaban groups. The change in eGFR between 2-year eGFR and baseline eGFR did not differ between the warfarin and DOAC groups during the observation period.

Anticoagulant-related nephropathy

For a long time, warfarin has been widely used as an anticoagulant therapy to prevent primary and secondary thromboembolic events in patients with AF. However, labile INR has been frequently observed in clinical practice. Adverse effects of warfarin therapy on the kidney have been reported and warfarin-related nephropathy is defined as unexplained AKI and hematuria (visible or nonvisible) while receiving warfarin therapy [13, 14]. Warfarin-related nephropathy is a significant risk factor for the progression of CKD and mortality [15]. Many case reports have mentioned that DOACs (dabigatran, apixaban, or rivaroxaban) could also cause AKI due to the induction of tubular red blood cell (RBC) casts and

Table 3 Baseline characteristics and renal outcomes (after warfarin, dabigatran, and anti-factor Xa inhibitors 1:1:2 propensity score matching)

Variable	Warfarin	Dabigatran	Anti-factor Xa inhibitors	*p* value	ASMD		
					W vs D	W vs Xal	D vs Xal
N	531	531	1062				
Gender (male)	344 (64.8)	358 (67.4)	660 (62.1)	0.110	0.003	0.003	0.007
Mean age	71 ± 8.8[a, b]	70 ± 8.7[a]	71 ± 8.6[b]	0.004	0.108	0.068	0.177
Medical history							
Type 2 DM	111 (20.9)	104 (19.6)	238 (22.4)	0.415	0.003	0.003	0.006
Hypertension	258 (48.6)[a]	214 (40.3)[b]	524 (49.3)[a]	0.002	0.012	0.001	0.014
Hyperlipidemia	127 (23.9)	118 (22.2)	267 (25.1)	0.436	0.004	0.002	0.006
Heart failure	34 (6.4)	34 (6.4)	87 (8.2)	0.285	0	0.007	0.002
Previous stroke	30 (5.6)	31 (5.8)	58 (5.5)	0.952	0.001	0.001	0.002
Vascular disease	14 (2.6)	6 (1.1)	24 (2.3)	0.188	0.011	0.002	0.009
Chronic kidney disease							
Stage < 3	355 (66.9)[a]	407 (76.6)[b]	678 (63.8)[a]	< 0.001	0.012	0.004	0.015
Stage ≥3	176 (33.1)[a]	124 (23.4)[b]	384 (36.2)[a]		0.018	0.005	0.024
CHA2DS2-VASc	2.55 ± 1.30[a]	2.40 ± 1.33[a]	3.26 ± 1.33[b]	< 0.001	0.114	0.106	0.218
Medication							
ACEI/ARB	329 (62.0)	310 (58.4)	669 (63.0)	0.199	0.005	0.001	0.006
Spironolactone	0 (0)	0 (0)	2 (0.4)	0.500	–	0.006	0.006
Renal function							
The average serum Cr (mg/dL)	1.06 ± 0.30[a]	1.00 ± 0.26[b]	1.07 ± 0.30[a]	< 0.001	0.214	0.033	0.249
Baseline eGFR (mL/min/1.73 m^2)	71.47 ± 22.42[a]	76.00 ± 21.91[b]	69.65 ± 21.24[a]	< 0.001	0.204	0.083	0.294
1-year eGFR (mL/min/1.73 m^2)	68.90 ± 21.78[a]	73.85 ± 22.02[b]	67.82 ± 21.21[a]	< 0.001	0.226	0.050	0.279
2-year eGFR (mL/min/1.73 m^2)	68.87 ± 24.74[a]	73.68 ± 25.72[b]	66.91 ± 21.82[a]	< 0.001	0.191	0.084	0.284
Renal outcomes							
Acute kidney injury (%)	54 (10.2)[a]	23 (4.3)[b]	57 (5.4)[b]	< 0.001	0.022	0.017	0.005
Renal failure requiring HD (%)	0 (0)	0 (0)	1 (0.1)	1.000	–	0.004	0.004
Renal death (%)	3 (0.6)	0 (0)	4 (0.4)	0.288	0.011	0.003	0.009

Data were presented as mean ± standard deviation or numbers (percentages)
Different letters (a, b) associated with different groups indicate significant difference (at 0.05 level) by Bonferroni multiple comparison procedure
Abbreviation: *ASMD* absolute standardized mean difference, *W* warfarin, *D* dabigatran, *Xal* anti-factor Xa inhibitor, *N* number, *DM* diabetes mellitus, *Cr* creatinine, *eGFR* estimated glomerular filtration rate, *ACEI* Angiotensin-converting enzyme inhibitor, *ARB* angiotensin receptor blocker, *HD* hemodialysis

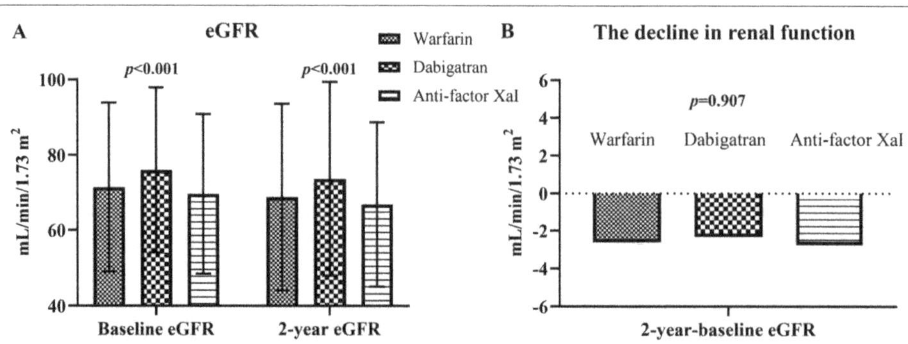

Fig. 3 (**A**) Comparison of baseline and 2-year follow-up estimated glomerular filtration rate (eGFR) among warfarin, dabigatran, and anti-factor Xa inhibitor groups after propensity score matching. (**B**) Comparison of the change in eGFR between 2-year eGFR and baseline eGFR among warfarin, dabigatran, and anti-factor Xa inhibitor groups after propensity score matching

Table 4 Baseline characteristics and renal outcomes (after rivaroxaban, apixaban, and edoxaban 2:2:1 propensity score matching)

Variable	Rivaroxaban	Apixaban	Edoxaban	p value	ASMD		
					R vs A	R vs E	A vs E
N	208	208	104				
Gender (male)	128 (61.5)	137 (65.9)	71 (68.3)	0.447	0.005	0.008	0.003
Mean age	70 ± 10.3	70 ± 10.0	69 ± 10.0	0.967	0.004	0.026	0.030
Medical history							
Type 2 DM	49 (23.6)	49 (23.6)	23 (22.1)	0.953	0	0.003	0.003
Hypertension	101 (48.6)	101 (48.6)	47 (45.2)	0.828	0	0.005	0.005
Hyperlipidemia	57 (27.4)	57 (27.4)	34 (32.7)	0.565	0	0.010	0.010
Heart failure	19 (9.1)	13 (6.3)	9 (8.7)	0.523	0.010	0.002	0.009
Previous stroke	11 (5.3)	9 (4.3)	5 (4.8)	0.900	0.004	0.002	0.002
Vascular disease	6 (2.9)	2 (1.0)	0 (0)	0.018	0.014	0.024	0.014
Chronic kidney disease							
Stage < 3	130 (62.5)	131 (63.0)	59 (56.7)	0.527	0.001	0.007	0.008
Stage ≥3	78 (37.5)	77 (37.0)	45 (43.3)		0.001	0.009	0.010
CHA2DS2-VASc	2.59 ± 1.34	2.52 ± 1.35	2.44 ± 1.40	0.652	0.052	0.109	0.058
Medication							
ACEI/ARB	131 (63.0)	112 (53.8)	69 (66.3)	0.055	0.012	0.004	0.016
Spironolactone	0 (0)	1 (0.5)	1 (1.0)	0.160	0.010	0.014	0.006
Renal function							
The average serum Cr (mg/dL)	1.08 ± 0.32	1.10 ± 0.35	1.13 ± 0.35	0.504	0.060	0.149	0.086
Baseline eGFR (mL/min/1.73 m^2)	70.04 ± 22.25	69.57 ± 22.49	68.55 ± 21.88	0.856	0.021	0.068	0.046
1-year eGFR (mL/min/1.73 m^2)	67.53 ± 22.23	67.02 ± 20.75	69.60 ± 23.43	0.608	0.024	0.091	0.117
2-year eGFR (mL/min/1.73 m^2)	67.13 ± 22.39	66.87 ± 23.40	67.37 ± 22.69	0.983	0.011	0.011	0.022
Renal outcomes							
Acute kidney injury (%)	5 (2.4)	10 (4.8)	4 (3.8)	0.423	0.013	0.008	0.005
Renal failure requiring HD (%)	1 (0.5)	0 (0)	0 (0)	0.400	0.010	0.010	–
Renal death (%)	1 (0.5)	0 (0)	1 (1.0)	0.160	0.010	0.006	0.014

Data were presented as mean ± standard deviation or numbers (percentages)
Abbreviation: *ASMD* absolute standardized mean difference, *R* rivaroxaban, *A* apixaban, *E* edoxaban, *N* number, *DM* diabetes mellitus, *Cr* creatinine, *eGFR* estimated glomerular filtration rate, *ACEI* Angiotensin-converting enzyme inhibitor, *ARB* angiotensin receptor blocker, *HD* hemodialysis

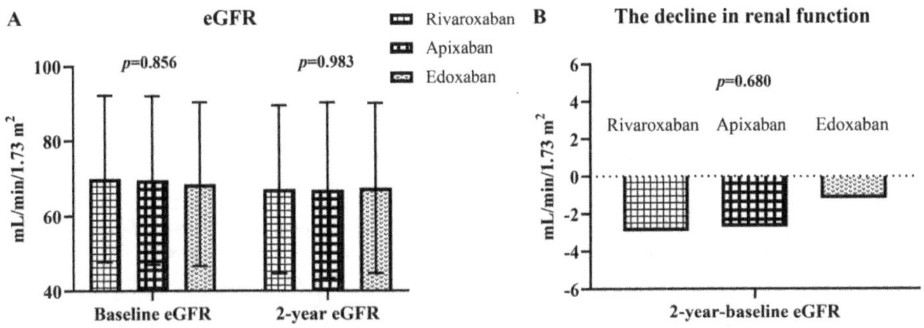

Fig. 4 (**A**) Comparison of baseline and 2-year follow-up estimated glomerular filtration rate (eGFR) among rivaroxaban, apixaban, and edoxaban groups after propensity score matching. (**B**) Comparison of the change in eGFR between 2-year eGFR and baseline eGFR among rivaroxaban, apixaban, and edoxaban groups after propensity score matching

tubular necrosis or interstitial nephritis [16–18]. Therefore, all anticoagulants can cause anticoagulant-related nephropathy (ARN). Pathological findings of ARN revealed the presence of RBCs in Bowman's space and in tubules and occlusive RBC casts predominantly in distal nephron segments with dysmorphic RBCs in the glomerulus on electron microscopy, implying injury to the glomerular filtration barrier [19]. Accordingly, the main pathological mechanism of ARN was attributed to hemorrhage in the glomerulus and tubular obstruction by RBC. Chan et al. reported that apixaban, dabigatran, and rivaroxaban were associated with a lower risk of AKI than warfarin in a large cohort of Taiwanese patients who did or did not have CKD [10]. However, they did not provide detailed serial follow-up eGFR values under different anticoagulants treatment due to the lack of laboratory data in that registry database, and the diagnoses of AKI and CKD were made according to the ICD code. Moreover, they did not provide information in terms of impact of edoxaban on the decline in renal function in AF patients. In our study, edoxaban group had a significantly lower incidence of AKI compared with warfarin group and had a similar incidence of AKI compared with rivaroxaban and, apixaban groups.

The AKI period represents the time window wherein critical interventions might be initiated to alter the natural history of kidney disease [20]. Therefore, it is possible to observe recovery of renal function with critical intervention after AKI. Moreover, the association between AKI and subsequent renal function decline is amplified by pre-existing severity of CKD [21]. In our study, patients with advanced stage of CKD (eGFR < 30 ml/min) was excluded and more than 60% of patients with CKD were in stage < 3 before and after propensity score matching. In this study, we observed that during the observation period, the change in eGFR between 2-year eGFR and baseline eGFR did not differ among warfarin, dabigatran, and anti-factor Xa inhibitor groups.

Anticoagulants use and the decline in renal function

The decline of renal function is common in patients with AF, regardless of treatment with warfarin or DOACs. In the analysis from the RE-LY study, dabigatran may provide slower progression of renal function when compared with warfarin use [5]. There was a small, statistically significant decline in renal function among patients receiving rivaroxaban compared with patients receiving warfarin in the subgroup analysis of ROCKET-AF trial [6, 7]. In a recent multicenter prospective cohort study, Pastori et al. reported that DOACs provided a slower decline in renal function compared to those using warfarin [9]. Therefore, the results about the decline in renal function after long-term anticoagulants use is still controversial and the underlying mechanism is not clear.

In our study, we still noted a higher incidence of AKI in patients with AF using warfarin when compared those using DOACs. However, the decline in renal function did not differ between warfarin and DOAC use during the observation period. Randomized studies are warranted to clarify the issues of the association of long-term anticoagulants use and renal function decline in AF patients treated with different anticoagulants. Despite the observed trends in AKI incidence and eGFR decline, anticoagulation for stroke prevention in AF patients remains indicated because the benefits outweigh the risks.

Study limitations

The first limitation of this study was its retrospective nature. Second, this is not a randomized study, and this study still has selective bias even though propensity score matching was performed. Third, the ICD-9 M and ICD-10 M codes were relied on each physician's choice in clinical practice. However, we used laboratory data in the database to confirm the diagnosis of AKI and the decline in renal function. Fourth, we could not totally exclude or explore all renal toxic materials during the follow-up period. Some confounders including more hospitalization, progression of diabetes, hypertension management beyond ACEI/ARB, or progression of HF could influence the results, but were not available in our study. Finally, we only enrolled patients using the same anticoagulants for 2 years, who also had regular follow-ups of renal function during the observation period. Therefore, only a limited number of patients were finally enrolled in this study. However, this study provided the incidence of AKI and the changes in eGFR under the same anticoagulant during the long observation period. Further large prospective studies are warranted to validate our findings.

Conclusions

During the mean observation time of 3.3 ± 0.9 years, warfarin was associated with a higher incidence of AKI compared with DOACs. The decline in renal function did not differ among warfarin and different DOAC groups.

Abbreviations

AF: atrial fibrillation; DOAC: direct oral anticoagulant; CrCl: creatinine clearance; RE-LY: Randomized Evaluation of Long-Term Anticoagulation Therapy; ROCKET-AF: Rivaroxaban Once Daily Oral Direct Factor Xa Inhibition Compared with Vitamin K Antagonism for Prevention of Stroke and Embolism Trial in Atrial Fibrillation; AKI: acute kidney injury; CGRD: Chang Gung Research Database; ICD: International Classification of Diseases; CM: Clinical Modification; eGFR: estimated glomerular filtration rate; ACEI: angiotensin-converting enzyme inhibitor; ARB: angiotensin-receptor blocker; ASMD: absolute value of the standardized mean difference; CKD: chronic kidney disease; INR: international normalized ratio; RBC: red blood cell; ARN: anticoagulant-related nephropathy

Supplementary Information

Additional file 1. Supplemental Fig. 1 Comparison of the change in estimated glomerular filtration rate (eGFR) between 2-year eGFR and baseline eGFR between warfarin and DOAC groups after propensity score matching. In the subgroups analyses, including age ≥ 70 (A) or < 70 years old (B), with (C) or without (D) diabetes mellitus (DM), with (E) or without (F) heart failure (HF), with (G) or without (H) hypertension (HTN), with (I) or without (J) angiotensin-converting enzyme inhibitor (ACEI)/angiotensin-receptor blocker (ARB) and chronic kidney disease (CKD) stage ≥3 (K) or < 3 (L). ACE: angiotensin-converting enzyme inhibitor. ARB: angiotensin-receptor blocker. Supplemental Fig. 2 Comparison of the change in estimated glomerular filtration rate (eGFR) between 2-year eGFR and baseline eGFR among warfarin, dabigatran, and anti-factor Xa inhibitor groups after propensity score matching. In the subgroups analyses, including age ≥ 70 (A) or < 70 years old (B), with (C) or without (D) diabetes mellitus (DM), with (E) or without (F) heart failure (HF), with (G) or without (H) hypertension (HTN), with (I) or without (J) angiotensin-converting enzyme inhibitor (ACEI)/angiotensin-receptor blocker (ARB) and chronic kidney disease (CKD) stage ≥3 (K) or < 3 (L). Supplemental Fig. 3 Comparison of the change in estimated glomerular filtration rate (eGFR) between 2-year eGFR and baseline eGFR among rivaroxaban, apixaban and edoxaban groups. In the subgroups analyses, including age ≥ 70 (A) or < 70 years old (B), with (C) or without (D) diabetes mellitus (DM), with (E) or without (F) heart failure (HF), with (G) or without (H) hypertension (HTN), with (I) or without (J) angiotensin-converting enzyme inhibitor (ACEI)/angiotensin-receptor blocker (ARB) and chronic kidney disease (CKD) stage ≥3 (K) or < 3 (L).

Acknowledgments
The authors thank the statistical assistance and wish to acknowledge the support of the Maintenance Project of the Center for Big Data Analytics and Statistics (Grant CMRPG8K0821) at Chang Gung Memorial Hospital for the study design and monitoring, data analysis, and interpretation.

Authors' contributions
WC Lee designed the study and wrote the manuscript. WC Lee, HC Chen, and YS Lin set the study rationale. WC Lee and PW Lee performed the comprehensive analysis. PJ wu, YN Fang, and HY Fang prepared Figs. SH Chang, PY Liu, and MC Chen did the final revision. All authors reviewed the manuscript. All authors read and approved the final manuscript.

Author details
[1]Institute of Clinical Medicine, College of Medicine, National Cheng Kung University, Tainan, Taiwan. [2]Division of Cardiology, Department of Internal Medicine, Kaohsiung Chang Gung Memorial Hospital, Chang Gung University College of Medicine, 123 Ta Pei Road, Niao Sung District, Kaohsiung City 83301, Taiwan. [3]Center for Big Data Analytics and Statistics, Chang-Gung University and Hospital, Taipei, Taiwan. [4]Division of Cardiology, Chang Gung Memorial Hospital, Chiayi, Taiwan.

References

1. van Gorp RH, Schurgers LJ. New insights into the pros and cons of the clinical use of vitamin K antagonists (VKAs) versus direct Oral anticoagulants (DOACs). Nutrients. 2015;7(11):9538–57. https://doi.org/10.3390/nu7115479.
2. Willems BA, Vermeer C, Reutelingsperger CP, Schurgers LJ. The realm of vitamin K dependent proteins: shifting from coagulation toward calcification. Mol Nutr Food Res. 2014;58(8):1620–35. https://doi.org/10.1002/mnfr.201300743.
3. Heidbuchel H, Verhamme P, Alings M, Antz M, Diener HC, Hacke W, et al. Updated European heart rhythm association practical guide on the use of non-vitamin K antagonist anticoagulants in patients with non-valvular atrial fibrillation. Europace. 2015;17(10):1467–507. https://doi.org/10.1093/europace/euv309.
4. Königsbrügge O, Ay C. Atrial fibrillation in patients with end-stage renal disease on hemodialysis: magnitude of the problem and new approach to oral anticoagulation. Res Pract Thromb Haemost. 2019;3(4):578–88. https://doi.org/10.1002/rth2.12250.
5. Böhm M, Ezekowitz MD, Connolly SJ, Eikelboom JW, Hohnloser SH, Reilly PA, et al. Changes in renal function in patients with atrial fibrillation: an analysis from the RE-LY trial. J Am Coll Cardiol. 2015;65(23):2481–93. https://doi.org/10.1016/j.jacc.2015.03.577.
6. Fordyce CB, Hellkamp AS, Lokhnygina Y, Lindner SM, Piccini JP, Becker RC, et al. On-treatment outcomes in patients with worsening renal function with rivaroxaban compared with warfarin: insights from ROCKET AF. Circulation. 2016;134(1):37–47. https://doi.org/10.1161/CIRCULATIONAHA.116.021890.
7. On-Treatment Outcomes in Patients With Worsening Renal Function With Rivaroxaban Compared With Warfarin: Insights From ROCKET AF. Circulation. 2020;141(8):e98. https://doi.org/10.1161/CIR.0000000000000763. Epub 2020 Feb 24. Erratum for: Circulation. 2016 Jul 5;134(1):37-47. PMID: 32091925.
8. Coleman CI, Kreutz R, Sood N, Bunz TJ, Meinecke AK, Eriksson D, et al. Rivaroxaban's impact on renal decline in patients with Nonvalvular atrial fibrillation: a US MarketScan claims database analysis. Clin Appl Thromb Hemost. 2019;25:1076029619868535. https://doi.org/10.1177/1076029619868535.
9. Pastori D, Ettorre E, Lip GYH, Sciacqua A, Perticone F, Melillo F, et al. Association of different oral anticoagulants use with renal function worsening in patients with atrial fibrillation: a multicentre cohort study. Br J Clin Pharmacol. 2020;86(12):2455–63. https://doi.org/10.1111/bcp.14350.
10. Chan YH, Yeh YH, Hsieh MY, Chang CY, Tu HT, Chang SH, et al. The risk of acute kidney injury in Asians treated with apixaban, rivaroxaban, dabigatran, or warfarin for non-valvular atrial fibrillation: a nationwide cohort study in Taiwan. Int J Cardiol. 2018;265:83–9. https://doi.org/10.1016/j.ijcard.2018.02.075.
11. Tsai MS, Lin MH, Lee CP, Yang YH, Chen WC, Chang GH, et al. Chang gung research database: a multi-institutional database consisting of original medical records. Biom J. 2017;40(5):263–9. https://doi.org/10.1016/j.bj.2017.08.002.
12. KDIGO Clinical Practice Guideline for Acute Kidney Injury. Summary of Recommendation Statements. Kidney Int Suppl. 2012;2(1):8–12. https://doi.org/10.1038/kisup.2012.7.
13. Ryan M, Ware K, Qamri Z, Satoskar A, Wu H, Nadasdy G, et al. Warfarin-related nephropathy is the tip of the iceberg: direct thrombin inhibitor dabigatran induces glomerular hemorrhage with acute kidney injury in rats. Nephrol Dial Transplant. 2014;29(12):2228–34. https://doi.org/10.1093/ndt/gft380.
14. Glassock RJ. Anticoagulant-related nephropathy: It's the real McCoy. Clin J Am Soc Nephrol. 2019;14(6):935–7. https://doi.org/10.2215/CJN.02470319.
15. Brodsky SV. Anticoagulants and acute kidney injury: clinical and pathology considerations. Kidney Res Clin Pract. 2014;33(4):174–80. https://doi.org/10.1016/j.krcp.2014.11.001.
16. Marcelino G, Hemett OM, Descombes E. Acute renal failure in a patient with rivaroxaban-induced hypersensitivity syndrome: a case report with a review of the literature and of pharmacovigilance registries. Case Rep Nephrol. 2020;2020:6940183–6. https://doi.org/10.1155/2020/6940183.
17. Brodsky SV, Mhaskar NS, Thiruveedi S, Dhingra R, Reuben SC, Calomeni E, et al. Acute kidney injury aggravated by treatment initiation with apixaban: another twist of anticoagulant-related nephropathy. Kidney Res Clin Pract. 2017;36(4):387–92. https://doi.org/10.23876/j.krcp.2017.36.4.387.
18. DiMaria C, Hanna W, Murone J, Reichart J. Direct oral anticoagulant and AKI: apixaban-induced acute interstitial nephritis. BMJ Case Rep. 2019;12(6): e230371. https://doi.org/10.1136/bcr-2019-230371.
19. L'Imperio V, Guarnieri A, Pieruzzi F, Sinico RA, Pagni F. Anticoagulant-related nephropathy: a pathological note. J Thromb Thrombolysis. 2018;46(2):260–3. https://doi.org/10.1007/s11239-018-1669-3.
20. Chawla LS, Bellomo R, Bihorac A, Goldstein SL, Siew ED, Bagshaw SM, et al. Acute kidney disease and renal recovery: consensus report of the acute disease quality initiative (ADQI) 16 workgroup. Nat Rev Nephrol. 2017;13(4): 241–57. https://doi.org/10.1038/nrneph.2017.2.
21. Hsu RK, Hsu CY. The role of acute kidney injury in chronic kidney disease. Semin Nephrol. 2016;36(4):283–92. https://doi.org/10.1016/j.semnephrol.2016.05.005.

An optimal window of platelet reactivity by LTA assay for patients undergoing percutaneous coronary intervention

Jing Wang[1,2†], Jing Wang[1†], Zhou Dong[1†], Jiazheng Ma[1†], Jianzhen Teng[1], Tong Wang[1,3], Xiaofeng Zhang[1,4], Qian Gu[1], Zekang Ye[1], Inam Ullah[1], Chuchu Tan[1], Samee Abdus[1], Lu Shi[1], Xiaoxuan Gong[1] and Chunjian Li[1*]

Abstract

Objective: This study was aimed to determine how platelet reactivity (PR) on dual antiplatelet therapy predicts ischemic and bleeding events in patients underwent percutaneous coronary intervention (PCI).

Design: A total of 2768 patients who had received coronary stent implantation and had taken aspirin 100 mg in combination with clopidogrel 75 mg daily for > 5 days were consecutively screened and 1885 were enrolled. The recruited patients were followed-up for 12 months. The primary end-point was the net adverse clinical events (NACE) of cardiovascular death, nonfatal myocardial infarction (MI), target vessel revascularization (TVR), stent thrombosis (ST) and any bleeding.

Result: 1709 patients completed the clinical follow-up. By using the receiver operating characteristic (ROC) curve analysis, the optimal cut-off values were found to be 37.5 and 25.5% respectively in predicting ischemic and bleeding events. Patients were classified into 2 groups according to PR: inside the window group (IW) [adenosine diphosphate (ADP) induced platelet aggregation (PL_{ADP}) 25.5–37.4%)] and outside the window group (OW) (PL_{ADP} < 25.5% or ≥ 37.5%). The incidence of NACE was 16.8 and 23.1% respectively in the IW and OW group. The hazard ratio of NACE in IW group was significantly lower [0.69 (95% CI, 0.54–0.89, $P = 0.004$)] than that in the OW group during 12-month follow-up.

Conclusion: An optimal therapeutic window of 25.5–37.4% for PL_{ADP} predicts the lowest risk of NACE, which could be referred for tailored antiplatelet treatment while using LTA assay.

Keywords: Light transmittance aggregometry, Platelet reactivity, Percutaneous coronary intervention, Therapeutic window

* Correspondence: lijay@njmu.edu.cn
†Jing Wang, Jing Wang, Zhou Dong and Jiazheng Ma contributed equally to this work.
[1]Departments of Cardiology, the First Affiliated Hospital of Nanjing Medical University, 300 Guangzhou Road, Nanjing 210029, Jiangsu, China

Introduction

Dual antiplatelet therapy with aspirin and an adenosine diphosphate (ADP)-receptor ($P2Y_{12}$) inhibitor is a cornerstone of the pharmacological treatment for patients with coronary artery disease undergoing percutaneous coronary intervention (PCI) [1].

Clopidogrel is one of the most widely used $P2Y_{12}$ inhibitors, which undergoes a two-step metabolic transformation before binding to the platelet $P2Y_{12}$ receptor [2]. Studies have shown wide variability of platelet clopidogrel response [3], indicating that a substantial proportion of patients have inappropriate platelet inhibition at a regular dose of clopidogrel 75 mg once daily. It has been reported that high on-treatment platelet reactivity (HOPR) detected by platelet aggregometry leads to increased risk of thrombotic events [4–8], while low on-treatment platelet reactivity (LOPR) leads to increased risk of bleeding after PCI [9, 10]. Thus, it is important to identify an optimal platelet inhibition or on-treatment platelet reactivity (PR) by platelet aggregometry [11, 12].

This study was to investigate an optimal therapeutic window for PR determined by light transmission aggregometry (LTA) to predict the lowest ischemic and bleeding risks in patients underwent PCI and treated with dual antiplatelet agents.

Methods

This is a prospective, single-center, registration study conducted at the First Affiliated Hospital of Nanjing Medical University, Nanjing, China. The study was registered at URL: https://www.clinicaltrials.gov (Unique identifier: NCT01968499) and was approved by the ethics committee of the First Affiliated Hospital of Nanjing Medical University. Written informed consent was obtained from each patient.

Study population

A total of 2768 patients were consecutively screened from April 2011 to October 2016 in the First Affiliated Hospital of Nanjing Medical University, among which 883 declined to participate, and the remaining 1885 patients were enrolled in the study (Fig. 1).

The inclusion criteria were patients who had undergone coronary stent implantation and taken aspirin 100 mg in combination with clopidogrel 75 mg daily for > 5 days [7]. Exclusion criteria were patients: 1) intolerant to aspirin or clopidogrel (e.g. history of allergic reactions or gastrointestinal bleeding); 2) taking any other antiplatelet agents in addition to aspirin and clopidogrel (e.g. cilostazol); 3) taking any anticoagulant agents (e.g. vitamin K antagonists, new oral anticoagulants); 4) with myelodysplastic syndrome or abnormal baseline platelet counts of $< 80 \times 10^9$/L or $> 450 \times 10^9$/L; 5) with hemoglobin < 90 g/L; 6) with cancer or any other complications that may not suitable to be recruited at the discretion of the investigators.

PR measurements

Six milliliter venous blood was collected into 3.2% citrate vacutainer tubes in the morning 2 h after the patients'

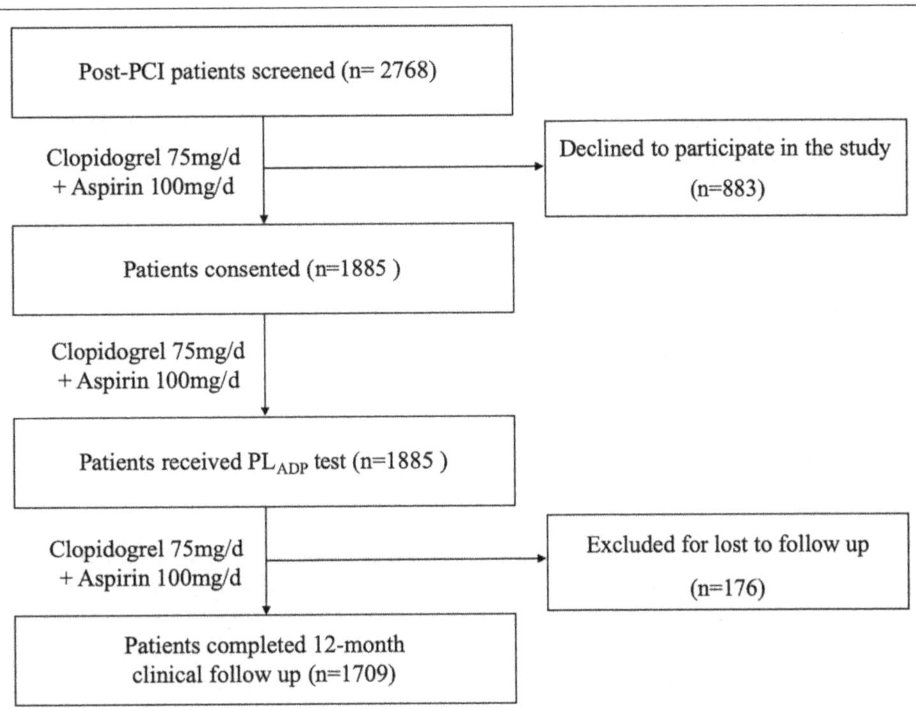

Fig. 1 Study Flow Chart

taking clopidogrel (if glycoprotein (GP) IIb/IIIa inhibitors were used, testing would be performed 24 h after drug discontinuation). Blood samples were subjected to platelet function test by LTA within 2 h as previously described [13]. In brief, samples were centrifuged at 200 g for 8 min to obtain platelet-rich plasma (PRP). Platelet-poor plasma (PPP) was prepared by centrifuging the remaining blood at 2465 g for 10 min. Platelet counts were adjusted by the addition of PPP to the PRP to achieve a count of 250×10^9/L. The ADP-induced platelet aggregation (PL_{ADP}) was recorded using the maximum platelet aggregation within 8 min after addition of ADP (final concentration 5 μmol/L) by a Chronolog Model 700 aggregometer (Chrono-log Corporation, Havertown, PA, USA) [13].

Study end-points

The primary end-point was set as the net adverse clinical events (NACE), a composite of ischemic events including cardiovascular death, nonfatal myocardial infarction (MI), target vessel revascularization (TVR), stent thrombosis (ST) and any bleeding defined by the Thrombolysis in Myocardial Infarction (TIMI) criteria [14]. MI was defined in accordance with the Third Universal Definition proposed in 2007 [15]. ST was defined as definite or probable according to the Academic Research Consortium definitions [16]. All the clinical events were independently adjudicated by two investigators blinded to the results of PR tests. Disagreements were resolved by discussion or consultation with a third investigator (Li).

The outcome data were collected by 2 investigators who were blinded to the results of platelet reactivity testing. The patients were followed up in the clinic and less preferably by telephone call if they were unable to attend the clinic. A standard case report form was used to record the outcome.

Statistical analysis

Statistical analysis was performed using SPSS 22.0 software (SPSS, Chicago, IL, USA). Continuous variables are expressed as means ± standard deviations (SD) or medians (range [or Inter Quartile Range]). Categorical variables are expressed as frequencies and percentages. Two-sided Mann–Whitney tests were used to compare PL_{ADP} between groups. The time to primary endpoint between groups was compared using the Kaplan–Meier method. Survival curves were compared using the log-rank test and hazard ratios were calculated using Cox's regression models. Sensitivity and specificity of PL_{ADP} in predicting thrombotic events were calculated at different thresholds by receiver operating characteristic (ROC) curve analysis. A two-sided $P < 0.05$ was statistically significant.

Results

Among the enrolled patients, 1709 completed the 12-month clinical follow-up (Fig. 1). There were 45 (2.6%) ischemic events and 328 (19.2%) bleeding events. Ischemic events included 20 deaths, 20 MI, 21 ST and 11 TVR. Bleeding events included 5 major bleeding, 27 minor bleeding and 296 minimal bleeding.

Relationship between PR and 1-year outcome

The average time from PCI to PR test reached 2.50 days. Patients with ischemic events during follow-up had a higher PL_{ADP} level compared to those without (36% [IQR: 25–45] vs.29% [IQR: 20–40]; $P = 0.054$). ROC analysis was performed to evaluate the value of PL_{ADP} in predicting ischemic events. As a result, a PL_{ADP} cut-off value of 37.5% provided a sensitivity of 48.9%, specificity of 70%, and the largest area under the curve value of 0.58 (Fig. 2a). By comparison, the recommended cut-off value of 46% by LTA provides a sensitivity of 20% and a specificity of 84.3% [12]. While adopting 37.5% as a new cut-off value, 521 patients (30.5%) were defined with HOPR, who experienced a higher rate of ischemic events compared with those without (4.2% vs. 1.9%; $P = 0.007$, Fig. 3a).

On the other hand, patients who experienced bleeding events had significantly lower PL_{ADP} compared with those without bleeding (25% [IQR 18–38] vs.30% [IQR 21–41]; $P < 0.001$). By ROC analysis, a cut-off value of 25.5% provided a sensitivity of 50.3%, a specificity of 62.6%, and the largest area under the curve of 0.57 in predicting bleeding (Fig. 2b). Using this new cut-off value, 682 (39.9%) patients were defined with LOPR, who experienced a higher rate of bleeding events compared to those without (24.2% vs. 15.9%; $P < 0.001$, Fig. 3b).

The risk of ischemic events and NACE was non-significantly higher in patients with HOPR compared with those in normal responders (4.2% vs. 2.2%; HR 1.99; $P = 0.063$ and 19.8% vs. 16.8%; HR 1.19; $P = 0.247$, for ischemic events and NACE, respectively) (Table 1, Fig. 4), while the risk of total bleeding and NACE was significantly higher in patients with LOPR compared with those in normal responders (24.2% vs. 15.8%; HR 1.61; $P = 0.001$ and 25.7% vs. 16.8%; HR 1.64; $P < 0.001$, for bleeding and NACE, respectively) (Table 1, Fig. 4).

Optimal PR or therapeutic window of PR to prevent ischemic and bleeding events

According to the ROC curve analysis, we defined an optimal window of PL_{ADP} between 25.5 and 37.5% after dual antiplatelet treatment. As a result, 29.6% of the study population was comprised within this therapeutic window in this study.

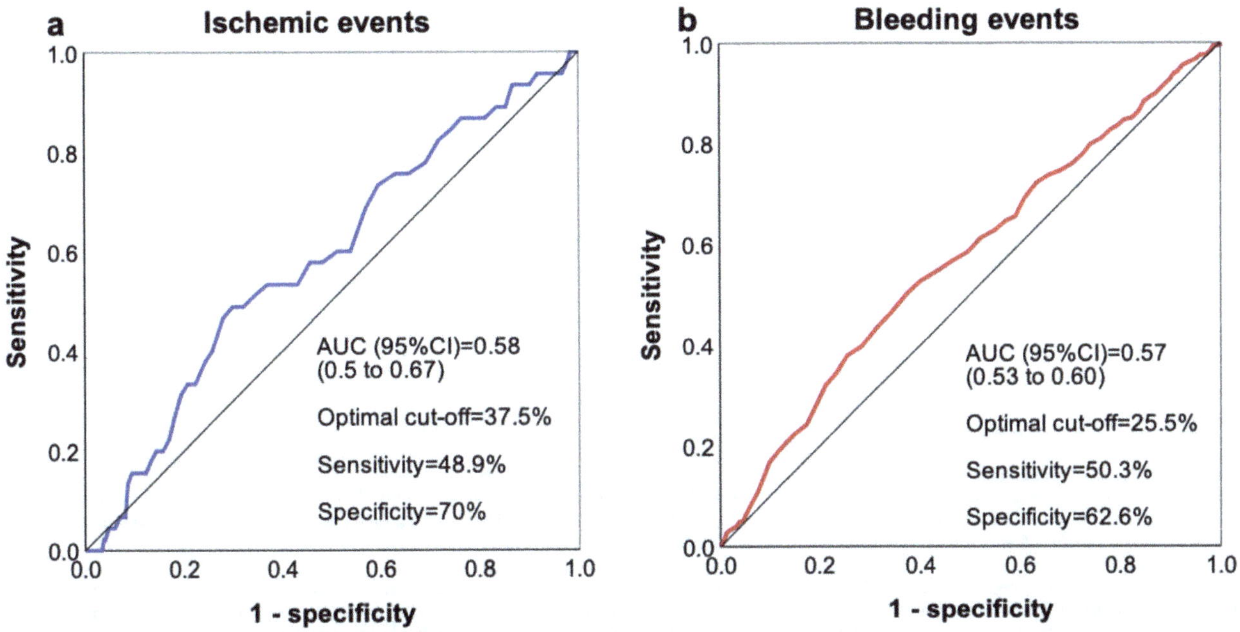

Fig. 2 ROC Curves for Ischemic and Bleeding Events. (a) Receiver operating characteristic (ROC) analysis for ischemic events. (b) ROC analysis for bleeding events. AUC, area under the curve; CI, confidence interval; PL_{ADP}, ADP induced platelet aggregation

We classified the patients into 2 groups according to PR: inside the window group (IW) [PL_{ADP}(25.5–37.4%)] and outside the window group (OW) ($PL_{ADP} < 25.5\%$ or $\geq 37.5\%$). The baseline demographic characteristics, clinical, angiographic and biological characteristics and medication history were described in Table 2. There were no significant differences in all the baseline characteristics between the 2 groups.

We further analyzed the prognosis according to the newly defined therapeutic window. The NACE rate of the IW group patients was lower than that of the OW group patients (16.8% vs. 23.1%; $P = 0.004$) (Fig. 3c). Kaplan-Meier analysis showed a significant difference in NACE and bleeding between patients within and outside the window, although no significant difference was found in ischemic events ($P = 0.438$, 0.024 and 0.004, for ischemic events, bleeding and NACE, respectively)(Fig. 5). The hazard ratio of NACE for OW group was significantly higher during the 12-month follow-up compared with IW group [1.44 (95% CI: 1.12–1.85; $P = 0.004$)] after adjusting for age, gender, body mass index (BMI), history of

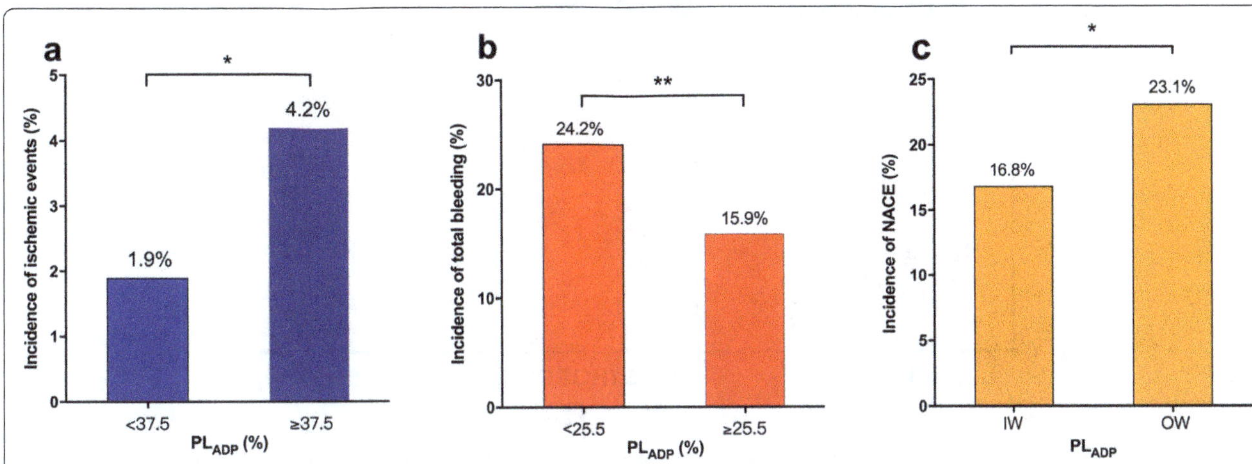

Fig. 3 Incidence of Ischemic, Bleeding Events and NACE Stratified by Platelet Reactivity. (a) Incidence of Ischemic events; (b) Incidence of Bleeding events; (c) Incidence of NACE. *$P < 0.05$; **$P < 0.001$. PL_{ADP}, ADP induced platelet aggregation; NACE, net adverse clinical events; IW, inside the window; OW, outside the window

Table 1 Multivariate analysis based on PL_{ADP} tri-classification

One-year outcome	PL_{ADP}						
	Normal responder* *n* = 506	HOPR† *n* = 521			LOPR‡ *n* = 682		
	n(%)	n(%)	HR(95%CI)	P	n(%)	HR(95%CI)	*P*
Net adverse clinical events	85 (16.8)	103 (19.8)	1.19 (0.89,1.61)	0.247	175 (25.7)	1.64 (1.25,2.14)	0.000
Ischemic events	11 (2.2)	22 (4.2)	1.99 (0.96,4.10)	0.063	12 (1.8)	0.83 (0.37,1.89)	0.660
Death	5 (1.0)	12 (2.3)	2.34 (0.82,6.66)	0.111	3 (0.4)	0.45 (0.11,1.88)	0.273
MI	5 (1.0)	9 (1.7)	1.78 (0.60,5.31)	0.303	6 (0.9)	0.93 (0.28,3.05)	0.903
ST	5 (1.0)	11 (2.1)	2.23 (0.77,6.43)	0.138	5 (0.7)	0.78 (0.23,2.70)	0.693
TVR	1 (0.2)	6 (1.2)	5.86 (0.70,48.86)	0.102	4 (0.6)	3.33 (0.37,29.89)	0.282
Bleeding events	80 (15.8)	83 (16.1)	0.99 (0.73,1.36)	0.967	165 (24.2)	1.61 (1.23,2.12)	0.001
Major + Minor	10 (2.0)	5 (1.0)	0.47 (0.16,1.39)	0.172	17 (2.5)	1.17 (0.53,2.60)	0.701
Minimal	70 (13.8)	78 (15.1)	1.09 (0.78,1.52)	0.603	148 (21.7)	1.59 (1.19,2.13)	0.002

Risk factors included in the analysis of net clinical outcome: Sex, age, BMI, Smoking, Hypertension, Diabetes, CABG history, PCI history, Hemoglobin, Platelet count, eGFR, APTT, INR; Risk factors included in the analysis of MACE: Sex, Age, BMI, Smoking, Hypertension, Diabetes, CABG history, PCI history; Risk factors included in the analysis of bleeding: Sex, Age, Hypertension, Diabetes, Hemoglobin, Platelet count, eGFR, INR, APTT

*Normal responder: $25.5\% \leq PL_{ADP} < 37.5\%$ (control group); † HOPR: $PL_{ADP} \geq 37.5\%$; ‡ LOPR: $PL_{ADP} < 25.5\%$

PL_{ADP} ADP induced platelet aggregation, *HOPR* high on-treatment platelet reactivity, *LOPR* low on-treatment platelet reactivity, *HR* hazard ratio, *CI* confidence interval, *MI* myocardial infarction, *ST* stent thrombosis, *TVR* target vessel revascularization, *BMI* body mass index, *CABG* coronary artery bypass grafting, *PCI* percutaneous coronary intervention, *eGFR* estimated glomerular filtration rate, *APTT* activated partial thromboplastin time, *INR* international normalized ratio

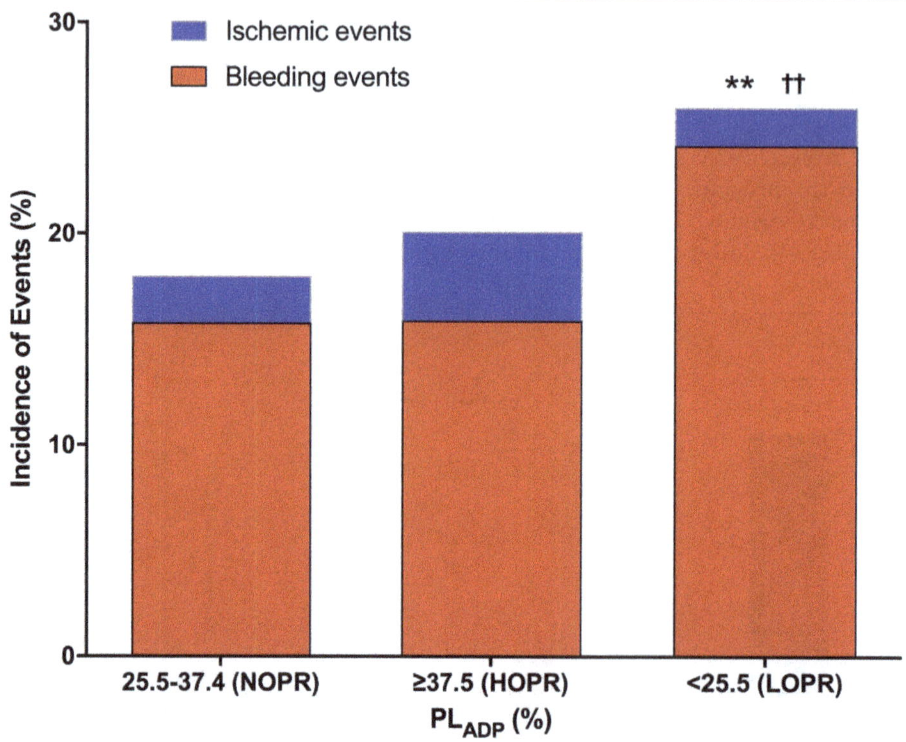

Fig. 4 1-year Adverse Events in Groups of Different Level of PL_{ADP}. Patients were stratified into groups of NOPR (25.5–37.4%), HOPR (≥37.5%) and LOPR (< 25.5%). ** represents $P < 0.001$ for bleeding events compared with the NOPR group. †† represents $P < 0.001$ for net adverse clinical events compared with the NOPR group. PL_{ADP}, ADP induced platelet aggregation; NOPR, normal on-treatment platelet reactivity; HOPR, high on-treatment platelet reactivity; LOPR, low on-treatment platelet reactivity

Table 2 Baseline characteristics and medications

	IW*	OW†	P
	n = 506	n = 1203	
Age	65 (58,72)	64 (56,71)	0.104
Gender (%)	74.70	75.40	0.763
BMI (kg/cm^2)	24.73 (22.84,26.60)	24.51 (22.76,26.54)	0.702
History of CABG (%)	1.20	0.70	0.376
History of PCI (%)	10.50	8.10	0.122
Cardiovascular risk factor			
Smoking (%)	46.20	46.30	0.983
Hypertension (%)	68.00	64.70	0.188
Diabetes (%)	26.50	25.10	0.551
Angiography and intervention			
SYNTAX score	15 (9,21.50)	15 (9,21.50)	0.44
Length of stent	39 (24,66)	39 (24,62)	0.856
Number of stent	2 (1,3)	2 (1,3)	0.737
Biology			
HB(g/L)	136 (125,146)	136 (125,146)	0.988
PLT (×10^9)	186 (157,227)	186 (155,222)	0.996
LDL (mmol/L)	2.57 (2.06,3.24)	2.49 (2.04,3.12)	0.382
eGFR (ml/min.1.732)	89.51 (77.34,103.95)	89.59 (76.43,104.85)	0.93
APTT (s)	25.90 (23.50,28.40)	25.70 (23.60,28.20)	0.787
INR	1.02 (0.98,1.07)	1.02 (0.98,1.06)	0.609
Medications			
ACEI/ARB (%)	57.70	56.20	0.564
β blocker (%)	66.80	65.10	0.497
Statin (%)	96.40	96.20	0.815
IIb/IIIa inhibitor (%)	2.20	1.20	0.108

Data are presented as median (interquartile range) or percentage as appropriate. * IW: 25.5% ≤ PL_{ADP} < 37.5%; † OW: PL_{ADP} < 25.5% or ≥ 37.5%
IW inside the window, *OW* outside the window, *BMI* body mass index, *CABG* coronary artery bypass grafting, *PCI* percutaneous coronary intervention, *MACE* major adverse clinical events, *HB* Hemoglobin, *PLT* platelet count, *LDL* low density lipoprotein, *eGFR* estimated glomerular filtration rate, *APTT* activated partial thromboplastin time, *INR* international normalized ratio, *ACEI/ARB* angiotension converting enzyme inhibitors/ angiotension receptor blocker, *IIb/IIIa* glycoprotein IIb/IIIa inhibitors

smoking, hypertension, diabetes, coronary artery bypass grafting (CABG), PCI, hemoglobin, platelet count, estimated glomerular filtration rate (eGFR), activated partial thromboplastin time (APTT), and international normalized ratio (INR) (Table 3). The total bleeding rate was also significantly higher in OW than IW after adjusting for the confounders [1.33 (95% CI: 1.03–1.72; P = 0.028)], which turned out to be the main contributor to NACE (Table 3).

Discussion

In this study, we identified an optimal range of platelet reactivity as 25.5–37.4% for PL_{ADP} while determined by LTA for patients underwent PCI and on the treatment of regular-dose aspirin and clopidogrel, and approximately one third (29.6%) of the patients meet this therapeutic window. Patients inside the window presented significantly lower risk of NACE than those outside the window during 12-month follow-up.

Several studies have tried to identify a threshold of PR that could stratify patients at risk of ischemic events. Bliden et al. [17] found that HOPR (defined as PL_{ADP} ≥ 50% measured by LTA with ADP concentration of 5 μmol/L) was the only variable being significantly related to ischemic events after adjusting for hypertension, diabetes and use of calcium channel inhibitors. Gurbel et al. [6] demonstrated that HOPR (defined as PL_{ADP} ≥ 46% measured by LTA [12] with ADP concentration of 5 μmol/L) was an independent risk factor for ischemic events within 2 years of non-emergent PCI (OR = 3.9, P< 0.001).

The cut-off value of PL_{ADP} in our study is 37.5%, which is lower than the previous study. However, as demonstrated by the GRAVITAS trial, when HOPR was defined as ≥230 $P2Y_{12}$ reaction units (PRU) by VerifyNow $P2Y_{12}$ test, high-dose clopidogrel compared with standard-dose clopidogrel did not reduce the incidence of major adverse cardiovascular events [18], while the post-hoc analysis found that the achievement of a PRU < 208 was associated with significantly improved clinical

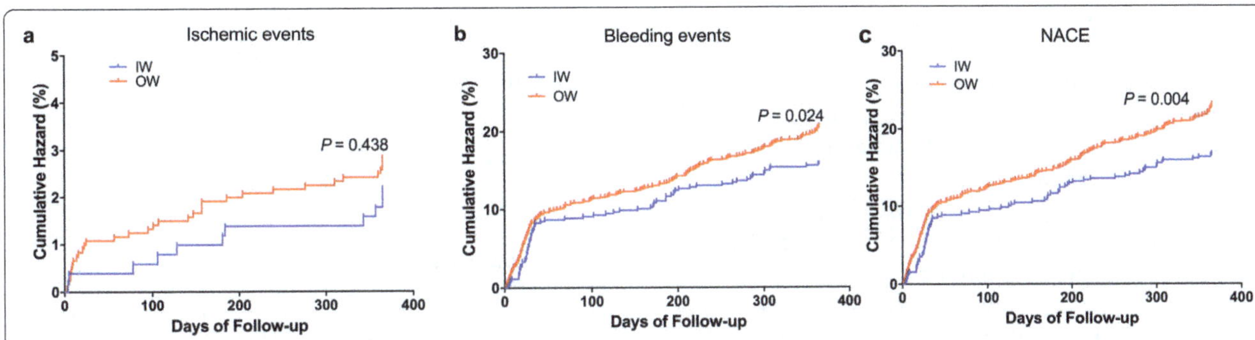

Fig. 5 Kaplan-Meier Analysis of Clinical Events. (a) Kaplan-Meier Analysis of Ischemic events; (b) Kaplan-Meier Analysis of Bleeding events; (c) Kaplan-Meier Analysis of NACE. NACE, net adverse clinical events; IW, inside the window; OW, outside the window

Table 3 Multivariate analysis based on the therapeutic window

One-year outcome	IW* 506 n(%)	OW† 1203 n(%)	HR	95%CI	P
Net adverse clinical events	85 (16.8)	278 (23.1)	1.44	1.12–1.85	0.004
Ischemic events	11 (2.2)	34 (2.8)	1.34	0.68–2.64	0.403
Death	5 (1.0)	15 (1.2)	1.27	0.46–3.51	0.640
MI	5 (1.0)	15 (1.2)	1.30	0.47–3.59	0.608
ST	5 (1.0)	16 (1.3)	1.41	0.52–3.87	0.500
TVR	1 (0.2)	10 (0.8)	4.49	0.57–35.17	0.150
Bleeding events	80 (15.8)	248 (20.6)	1.33	1.03–1.72	0.028
Major + Minor	10 (2.0)	221 (1.8)	0.86	0.40–1.84	0.700
Minimal	70 (13.8)	226 (18.8)	1.38	1.05–1.81	0.022

Risk factors included in the analysis of net clinical outcome: Sex, age, BMI, Smoking, Hypertension, Diabetes, CABG history, PCI history, Hemoglobin, Platelet count, eGFR, APTT, INR; Risk factors included in the analysis of MACE: Sex, Age, BMI, Smoking, Hypertension, Diabetes, CABG history, PCI history; Risk factors included in the analysis of bleeding: Sex, Age, Hypertension, Diabetes, Hemoglobin, Platelet count, eGFR, INR, APTT

* IW: 25.5% $\leq PL_{ADP} < 37.5\%$; † OW: $PL_{ADP} < 25.5\%$ or $\geq 37.5\%$

outcomes. Consistent with the GRAVITAS trial, our result suggests that a lower cut-off value of PL_{ADP} might bring more low responders to the intensified antiplatelet treatment and consequently reduce ischemic events.

In addition to recurrent ischemic events, the prognostic importance of bleeding complications following PCI has also been established. ADAPT-DES trial showed that HOPR (defined by > 208 PRU, by VerifyNow $P2Y_{12}$ test) was inversely related to TIMI major bleeding (adjusted HR: 0.73, 95% CI: 0.61 to 0.89, $P = 0.002$) [3]. Studies suggested a possible link between LOPR and bleeding [7–9, 18–23]. With the LTA method, Tsukahara et al. [24] found that high-responsiveness was the independent predictor of major bleeding in patients receiving drug-eluting stents and treated with thienopyridine. Parodi et al. [25] reported that LOPR ($PL_{ADP} < 40\%$, 10 μmol/L ADP, LTA assay) were the independent predictor of bleeding events. Consistent with previous studies, we confirmed the predictive value of PR on the occurrence of bleeding events after PCI as measured with the LTA assay, and we suggested a cut-off value of $PL_{ADP} < 25.5\%$ to predict the bleeding events.

The optimal therapeutic window of PL_{ADP} is uncertain, Campo [26] and Mangiacapra et al. [1] have reported two therapeutic windows for PR measured with the VerifyNow $P2Y_{12}$ assay. However, in Campo's study, they reported all clinical events (ischemic and bleeding) after 1 month and up to 1 year of follow-up. Patients with adverse events during the first month were excluded. In Mangiacapra's study, only short-term outcome of 1-month clinical events were analyzed. By contrast, using the two thresholds for ischemic and bleeding events, we found an optimal therapeutic window for PL_{ADP} by LTA assay, ranging from 25.5 to 37.4%, which was associated with the lowest 1-year incidence of NACE. To the best of our knowledge, our study was the first that use LTA method to demonstrate an optimal therapeutic window for PL_{ADP} regarding the 1-year clinical outcome.

Our study has important clinical implications. According to the results, post-PCI evaluation of PR carries important prognostic information, and the antiplatelet treatment should be guided referring to optimal therapeutic window of PR instead of single cut-off value. In particular, for patients with HOPR and higher ischemic risk, more aggressive antiplatelet strategies might be useful. On the other hand, for patients with LOPR and higher bleeding risk, conservative antiplatelet therapies should also be indicated until PR falls within the desired range.

The present study has potential limitations. First, the limited funding support prevented us to perform another cohort to validate the study results. Thus, a prospective study would be needed before using such an assay to try to predict outcomes. Second, the sample size was modest, so we could not analyze the optimal ranges of platelet reactivity for different age groups. Third, platelet reactivity could vary while patients taking clopidogrel treatment for longer term. However, we could not further extend the time of platelet reactivity test due to the limited hospitalization period. Besides, patients would be on high risk of thrombotic events early after PCI, so clopidogrel response in early stage of stent implantation would be more important to overcome or predict the thrombotic events.

Conclusion

An optimal therapeutic window of 25.5–37.4% for PL_{ADP} predicts the lowest risk of net adverse cardiovascular events, which could be referred for tailored antiplatelet treatment while using platelet aggregation assay by light transmittance aggregometry.

Code availability
Not applicable.

Authors' contributions
Jing Wang, Jing Wang, Tong Wang, Jiazheng Ma and Jianzhen Teng analyzed data and wrote the manuscript; Xiaofeng Zhang, Jing Wang, Qian Gu, Zekang Ye, Inam Ullah, Chuchu Tan, Samee Abdus, Lu Shi and Xiaoxuan Gong provided patients, collected data, and critically reviewed the manuscript; Chunjian Li designed the study and critically reviewed the manuscript. All authors approved the manuscript for submission.

Author details
[1]Departments of Cardiology, the First Affiliated Hospital of Nanjing Medical University, 300 Guangzhou Road, Nanjing 210029, Jiangsu, China. [2]Department of Cardiology, the Affiliated Huaian No.1 People's Hospital of Nanjing Medical University, Huai'an, Jiangsu, China. [3]Department of Cardiology, the First People's Hospital of Yancheng, Yancheng, Jiangsu, China. [4]Department of Cardiology, the Second Hospital of Nanjing, Nanjing University of Chinese Medicine, Nanjing, Jiangsu, China.

References

1. Mangiacapra F, Patti G, Barbato E, Peace AJ, Ricottini E, Vizzi V, et al. A therapeutic window for platelet reactivity for patients undergoing elective percutaneous coronary intervention: results of the ARMYDA-PROVE (antiplatelet therapy for reduction of MYocardial damage during angioplasty-platelet reactivity for outcome validation effort) study. JACC Cardiovasc Interv. 2012;5(3):281–9. https://doi.org/10.1016/j.jcin.2012.01.009.
2. Herbert JM, Savi P. P2Y12, a new platelet ADP receptor, target of clopidogrel. Semin Vasc Med. 2003;3(2):113–22. https://doi.org/10.1055/s-2003-40669.
3. Stone GW, Witzenbichler B, Weisz G, Rinaldi MJ, Neumann FJ, Metzger DC, et al. Platelet reactivity and clinical outcomes after coronary artery implantation of drug-eluting stents (ADAPT-DES): a prospective multicentre registry study. Lancet. 2013;382(9892):614–23. https://doi.org/10.1016/s0140-6736(13)61170-8.
4. Gurbel PA, Bliden KP, Saucedo JF, Suarez TA, DiChiara J, Antonino MJ, et al. Bivalirudin and clopidogrel with and without eptifibatide for elective stenting: effects on platelet function, thrombelastographic indexes, and their relation to periprocedural infarction results of the CLEAR PLATELETS-2 (Clopidogrel with Eptifibatide to arrest the reactivity of Platelets) study. J Am Coll Cardiol. 2009;53(8):648–57. https://doi.org/10.1016/j.jacc.2008.10.045.
5. Gurbel PA, Bliden KP, Samara W, Yoho JA, Hayes K, Fissha MZ, et al. Clopidogrel effect on platelet reactivity in patients with stent thrombosis: results of the CREST study. J Am Coll Cardiol. 2005;46(10):1827–32. https://doi.org/10.1016/j.jacc.2005.07.056.
6. Gurbel PA, Antonino MJ, Bliden KP, Dichiara J, Suarez TA, Singla A, et al. Platelet reactivity to adenosine diphosphate and long-term ischemic event occurrence following percutaneous coronary intervention: a potential antiplatelet therapeutic target. Platelets. 2008;19(8):595–604. https://doi.org/10.1080/09537100802351065.
7. Breet NJ, van Werkum JW, Bouman HJ, Kelder JC, Ruven HJ, Bal ET, et al. Comparison of platelet function tests in predicting clinical outcome in patients undergoing coronary stent implantation. JAMA. 2010;303(8):754–62. https://doi.org/10.1001/jama.2010.181.
8. Cuisset T, Frere C, Quilici J, Gaborit B, Castelli C, Poyet R, et al. Predictive values of post-treatment adenosine diphosphate-induced aggregation and vasodilator-stimulated phosphoprotein index for stent thrombosis after acute coronary syndrome in clopidogrel-treated patients. Am J Cardiol. 2009;104(8):1078–82. https://doi.org/10.1016/j.amjcard.2009.06.007.
9. Patti G, Pasceri V, Vizzi V, Ricottini E, Di Sciascio G. Usefulness of platelet response to clopidogrel by point-of-care testing to predict bleeding outcomes in patients undergoing percutaneous coronary intervention (from the antiplatelet therapy for reduction of myocardial damage during angioplasty-bleeding study). Am J Cardiol. 2011;107(7):995–1000. https://doi.org/10.1016/j.amjcard.2010.11.025.
10. Sibbing D, Steinhubl SR, Schulz S, Schömig A, Kastrati A. Platelet aggregation and its association with stent thrombosis and bleeding in clopidogrel-treated patients: initial evidence of a therapeutic window. J Am Coll Cardiol. 2010;56(4):317–8. https://doi.org/10.1016/j.jacc.2010.03.048.
11. Price MJ. Bedside evaluation of thienopyridine antiplatelet therapy. Circulation. 2009;119(19):2625–32. https://doi.org/10.1161/circulationaha.107.696732.
12. Bonello L, Tantry US, Marcucci R, Blindt R, Angiolillo DJ, Becker R, et al. Consensus and future directions on the definition of high on-treatment platelet reactivity to adenosine diphosphate. J Am Coll Cardiol. 2010;56(12):919–33. https://doi.org/10.1016/j.jacc.2010.04.047.
13. Li C, Hirsh J, Xie C, Johnston MA, Eikelboom JW. Reversal of the anti-platelet effects of aspirin and clopidogrel. J Thromb Haemost. 2012;10(4):521–8. https://doi.org/10.1111/j.1538-7836.2012.04641.x.
14. Rao AK, Pratt C, Berke A, Jaffe A, Ockene I, Schreiber TL, et al. Thrombolysis in myocardial infarction (TIMI) trial--phase I: hemorrhagic manifestations and changes in plasma fibrinogen and the fibrinolytic system in patients treated with recombinant tissue plasminogen activator and streptokinase. J Am Coll Cardiol. 1988;11(1):1–11. https://doi.org/10.1016/0735-1097(88)90158-1.
15. Thygesen K, Alpert JS, White HD. Universal definition of myocardial infarction. J Am Coll Cardiol. 2007;50(22):2173–95. https://doi.org/10.1016/j.jacc.2007.09.011.
16. Cannon CP, Battler A, Brindis RG, Cox JL, Ellis SG, Every NR, et al. American College of Cardiology key data elements and definitions for measuring the clinical management and outcomes of patients with acute coronary syndromes. A report of the American College of Cardiology Task Force on clinical data standards (acute coronary syndromes writing committee). J Am Coll Cardiol. 2001;38(7):2114–30. https://doi.org/10.1016/s0735-1097(01)01702-8.
17. Bliden KP, DiChiara J, Tantry US, Bassi AK, Chaganti SK, Gurbel PA. Increased risk in patients with high platelet aggregation receiving chronic clopidogrel therapy undergoing percutaneous coronary intervention: is the current antiplatelet therapy adequate? J Am Coll Cardiol. 2007;49(6):657–66. https://doi.org/10.1016/j.jacc.2006.10.050.
18. Price MJ, Berger PB, Teirstein PS, Tanguay JF, Angiolillo DJ, Spriggs D, et al. Standard- vs high-dose clopidogrel based on platelet function testing after percutaneous coronary intervention: the GRAVITAS randomized trial. JAMA. 2011;305(11):1097–105. https://doi.org/10.1001/jama.2011.290.
19. SIBBING D, SCHULZ S, BRAUN S, MORATH T, STEGHERR J, Mehilli J, et al. Antiplatelet effects of clopidogrel and bleeding in patients undergoing coronary stent placement. 2010;8(2):250–6. https://doi.org/10.1111/j.1538-7836.2009.03709.x.
20. BONELLO L, MANCINI J, PANSIERI M, MAILLARD L, ROSSI P, COLLET F, et al. Relationship between post-treatment platelet reactivity and ischemic and bleeding events at 1-year follow-up in patients receiving prasugrel. 2012;10(10):1999–2005. https://doi.org/10.1111/j.1538-7836.2012.04875.x.
21. Collet J-P, Cuisset T, Rangé G, Cayla G, Elhadad S, Pouillot C, et al. Bedside Monitoring to Adjust Antiplatelet Therapy for Coronary Stenting. 2012;367(22):2100–9. https://doi.org/10.1056/NEJMoa1209979.
22. Gurbel PA, Bliden KP, Navickas IA, Mahla E, Dichiara J, Suarez TA, et al. Adenosine diphosphate–induced platelet-fibrin clot strength: A new thrombelastographic indicator of long-term poststenting ischemic events. Am Heart J. 2010;160(2):346–54. https://doi.org/10.1016/j.ahj.2010.05.034.
23. Mokhtar OA, Lemesle G, Armero S, Mancini J, Bonello C, Tahirou I, et al. Relationship between platelet reactivity inhibition and non-CABG related major bleeding in patients undergoing percutaneous coronary intervention. Thromb Res. 2010;126(2):e147–e9. https://doi.org/10.1016/j.thromres.2010.01.013.
24. Tsukahara K, Kimura K, Morita S, Ebina T, Kosuge M, Hibi K, et al. Impact of high-responsiveness to dual antiplatelet therapy on bleeding complications in patients receiving drug-eluting stents. Circ J. 2010;74(4):679–85. https://doi.org/10.1253/circj.cj-09-0601.
25. Parodi G, Bellandi B, Venditti F, Carrabba N, Valenti R, Migliorini A, et al. Residual platelet reactivity, bleedings, and adherence to treatment in patients having coronary stent implantation treated with prasugrel. Am J Cardiol. 2012;109(2):214–8. https://doi.org/10.1016/j.amjcard.2011.08.034.
26. Campo G, Parrinello G, Ferraresi P, Lunghi B, Tebaldi M, Miccoli M, et al. Prospective evaluation of on-clopidogrel platelet reactivity over time in patients treated with percutaneous coronary intervention relationship with gene polymorphisms and clinical outcome. J Am Coll Cardiol. 2011;57(25):2474–83. https://doi.org/10.1016/j.jacc.2010.12.047.

17

Clopidogrel versus ticagrelor in the treatment of Chinese patients undergoing percutaneous coronary intervention: Effects on platelet function assessed by platelet function tests and mean platelet volume

Yang Zhang[1†], Rui Peng[1†], Xiaojuan Li[2], Gaowa Cheng[1], Ximing Wang[1], Jinxing Yu[1], Muxing Hua[2], Xi Chen[1*] and Zhou Zhou[1*]

Abstract

Background: Knowledge on the pharmacodynamic effects of antiplatelet drugs including clopidogrel and ticagrelor on Asian patients is scarce. We aim to evaluate the effects of the two drugs on platelet reactivity in the treatment of Chinese patients who underwent percutaneous coronary intervention (PCI), using two platelet function tests (PFT). Meanwhile, the relationship between mean platelet volume (MPV), a routine index of platelet size, and high on-treatment platelet reactivity (HPR) is also investigated.

Methods: Patients receiving dual antiplatelet therapy (DAPT) were scheduled for the assessment of platelet reactivity at 2–3 days after PCI. Two PFTs, light transmission aggregometry (LTA) and vasodilator-stimulated phosphoprotein (VASP)-FCM assay, were applied in the evaluation of platelet reactivity. The MPV was measured simultaneously with EDTA plasma using a Sysmex XN 2000 automated hematology analyzer.

Results: The final study population included the aspirin + clopidogrel group ($n = 46$) and the aspirin + ticagrelor group ($n = 66$). In the aspirin + ticagrelor group, the maximal light transmittance (LT) changes in response to 5 μM ADP assessed by LTA was obviously lower than that in the aspirin + clopidogrel group ($P < 0.001$). The platelet reactivity index (PRI) level in the VASP test was also markedly lower in the group given aspirin and ticagrelor ($P < 0.001$). There was a significant difference in HPR between the two groups. MPV showed a potent ability to predict the presence of HPR at VASP assay (AUC = 0.788, 95% CI: 0.701–0.875, $P < 0.001$) in receiver-operating characteristic curve analysis.

* Correspondence: chenxifw@pumc.edu.cn; zhouzhou@fuwaihospital.org
†Yang Zhang and Rui Peng contributed equally to this work.
[1]Diagnostic Laboratory Service, State Key Laboratory of Cardiovascular Disease, Fuwai Hospital, National Center for Cardiovascular Diseases, Chinese Academy of Medical Sciences, Peking Union Medical College, No.167, Beilishi Road, Xicheng District, Beijing 100037, China

Conclusions: Compared with clopidogrel, ticagrelor has dramatically greater antiplatelet effect, with a superiority in suppressing platelet function and a lower HPR rate. In addition, there existed a significant independent association between MPV and high prevalence of HPR in the VASP assay.

Keywords: Dual antiplatelet therapy, Platelet function tests, High on-treatment platelet reactivity, Mean platelet volume

Introduction

It is known that dual antiplatelet therapy (DAPT) which consists of aspirin and one of the P2Y12 receptor antagonists has been used for secondary prevention of thrombotic events, particularly in acute coronary syndromes (ACS) and percutaneous coronary intervention (PCI) with stenting [1, 2]. Clopidogrel, a popular P2Y12 receptor inhibitor, is most widely used. However, the wide inter- and intra-individual variability in clopidogrel response represents a significant clinical limitation [3, 4], and high on-treatment platelet reactivity (HPR) to adenosine diphosphate (ADP) is now regarded as a well-established marker reflecting the thrombotic recurrence risk [5, 6]. In comparison with clopidogrel (a thienopyridine P2Y12R antagonist), which can bind irreversibly to the ADP receptor, ticagrelor, a novel non-thienopyridine ADP antagonist, reversibly inhibits the ADP P2Y12 receptor located on platelets, preventing platelet activation and aggregation [7]. To date, most clinical studies have demonstrated that ticagrelor can provide a more rapid effect on platelet inhibition and a more favorable pharmacodynamic profile when compared with clopidogrel [8, 9]. In addition, it has been recommended in the current guideline that new DAPT with aspirin and ticagrelor can be administered to patients with ACS after stenting (IIA) [10].

It has been suggested that ethnic differences in the response to P2Y12 inhibitors could influence the pharmacodynamic effects in different races. East Asian patients are at a higher bleeding risk under DAPT, compared with non-East Asians [11]. In Korean and Japanese patients with ACS, ticagrelor presented a higher incidence of significant bleeding, compared with clopidogrel [12, 13]. Unfortunately, few Chinese patients were included in the studies that investigated the responses to clopidogrel and ticagrelor. Therefore, exploring the effects of the two popular antiplatelet drugs on platelet function in Asian/Chinese patients is increasingly urgent and will provide more potent clinical and experimental evidence to guide the use of these antiplatelet drugs among East Asian populations.

Platelet activation by ADP is central to the development of atherothrombosis. Platelet function tests (PFT) play an important role in evaluating individual antiplatelet drug responses and the therapeutic effects of different treatments. Therefore, PFT are recommended to guide the clinical treatment of patients with high risk factors for ischemia and those undergoing PCI or who have poor drug compliance [14]. In recent years, platelet reactivity has been measured by various systems in PFT [15]. Modern laboratory techniques, including the platelet function analyzer (PFA), the VerifyNow P2Y12 assay, light-transmission aggregometry (LTA), multiple electrode platelet aggregometry (MEA), thromboelastography (TEG) and vasodilator-stimulated phosphoprotein (VASP) assay, are all applied to measure different properties associated with platelet reactivity, with different detection principles. LTA, invented by Born [16, 17] and O'Brien [18], is the oldest available method for assessment of platelet activation and was regarded as the "gold standard" [19]. The VASP assay was based on flow cytometric measurement of the VASP phosphorylation level [20]. Furthermore, mean platelet volume (MPV), which is a common index indicating platelet size, has been recommended as a marker of platelet activity [21]. However, the role of MPV in evaluating HPR rates in patients with stents is still debated, because contrasting results have been reported so far on the relationship between platelet size and aggregation [22–24].

Therefore, our present study aimed to evaluate the pharmacodynamic effects of clopidogrel and ticagrelor on Chinese patients undergoing PCI, with LTA and VASP assay used to assess platelet function. We also investigated the relationship between MPV and HPR among patients receiving DAPT.

Methods

Study design

For this prospective study, we consecutively enrolled 112 patients presenting to Fuwai Hospital (Beijing, China) who were scheduled to undergo PCI for the assessment of platelet function from March 2017 to June 2017. The procedure followed in this study was in accordance with standard ethical principles according to the Declaration of Helsinki. Consecutive participants were enrolled in line with the following inclusion criteria: age > 18 years; had undergone PCI with drug-eluting stenting. The exclusion criteria were as follows: a history of coronary artery bypass graft or heart transplantation; use of glycoprotein IIb/IIIa receptor inhibitors or other ADP receptor antagonists;

infection; renal failure undergoing dialysis; history of drug allergy; bleeding; family history and platelet count < 100 × 10^9 cells/L. Diagnosis and performance of PCI were based on standard practices. The participants were divided into two groups: the aspirin + clopidogrel group ($n = 46$) and the aspirin + ticagrelor group ($n = 66$) according to different clinical therapy methods. The choice of DAPT depended on patients' clinical characteristics and evaluations of clinicians, in accordance with 2017 ESC guideline [25]. For those who had received maintenance antiplatelet therapy comprising aspirin 100 mg (BAYASPIRIN®, Bayer Healthcare Manufacturing S.r.l., Garbagnate Milanese, Italy) and clopidogrel 75 mg (PLAVIX®, Sanofi Winthrop Industrie, Carbon Blanc Cedex, France) for longer than five days, clopidogrel 300-mg loading dose (LD) was administered at least 12 h before PCI. An LD of clopidogrel 300 mg and 200 mg aspirin was administered at least 12 h before PCI for those who had not received aspirin and clopidogrel antiplatelet maintenance therapy. Then daily thereafter PCI, all patients were given a maintenance dose of clopidogrel and aspirin (75 mg and 100 mg once daily) at least 1 year. An LD of ticagrelor 180 mg and a maintenance dose (90 mg twice daily) were also administered. Additional file 1 (Fig. S1) shows the flow chart of our study design.

Clinical data collection

Patients' basic information including age and sex was recorded on admission. The clinical characteristic information including body mass index (BMI), left ventricular ejection fraction (LVEF), history of diseases and medication were also recorded simultaneously. Patients were scheduled for biochemistry and platelet function testing at 2–3 days after drug intake, on the day of PCI. Patients took clopidogrel and aspirin after breakfast daily and were collected blood before breakfast. The timing of last ticagrelor intake was after dinner and blood collection was at next day before breakfast. The hemoglobin (Hb), platelet count (PLT) and MPV were measured using a Sysmex XN 2000 automated hematology analyzer (Sysmex, Kobe, Japan) and appropriate reagents with EDTA plasma, within 2 h after blood draw; serum low-density lipoprotein-cholesterol (LDL-C), high-sensitivity C-reactive protein (hsCRP), alanine transaminase (ALT) and aspartate transaminase (AST) were assayed using an Olympus AU-5400 biochemistry autoanalyzer (Olympus Corporation, Mishama, Japan); the value of LVEF was determined via chest X-radiography and echocardiography.

Platelet function measurement

Light transmittance aggregometry

Blood samples were collected in 3.2% sodium citrate tubes (Becton-Dickinson, San Jose, CA, USA) and tests conducted within 2 h [26]. The blood was centrifuged at 120×*g* for 10 min to acquire the supernatant as platelet-rich plasma (PRP). The platelet count of PRP was unadjusted according to recommendation of ISTH consensus [27]. Subsequently, platelet-poor plasma was obtained after another centrifugation at 1500×*g* for 15 min for the remaining blood. An AG800 automatic platelet aggregation analyzer (Techlink, Biomedical Technology Co., Ltd., Beijing, China) was applied to detect platelet aggregation at 37 °C, and 5 μM ADP was used to stimulate platelets. The maximal light transmittance (LT) changes in response to 5 μM ADP from baseline, based on the reference of platelet-poor plasma, was regarded as the result of aggregation.

Vasodilator-stimulated phosphoprotein assay

The VASP assay was carried out by an experienced technician within 24 h. Platelet VASP kits were used to determine VASP phosphorylation according to the manufacturer's instructions (Diagnostica Stago, Asnières, France). Briefly, blood samples were collected in 3.2% sodium citrate tubes. Fixation was performed after incubation with ADP and/or prostaglandin E_1 (PGE_1) in vitro. In the process of indirect immunolabeling, each sample was incubated with 16C2 monoclonal antibody and then stained with a goat anti-mouse fluorescein isothiocyanate polyclonal antibody. Flow cytometric measurement was performed via a cytometer (Mindray Bio-Medical Electronics Co., Ltd., Shenzhen, China). EPICSXL software was used to gate and analyze the mean fluorescence intensity (MFI) of platelet events. A ratio directly associated with VASP phosphorylation state was established by determining an MFI corresponding to experimental conditions. A platelet reactivity index (PRI) was calculated according to the formula: $PRI = [(MFI(PGE_1) - MFI(PGE_1) + ADP)/MFI(PGE_1)] \times 100$. The intra- and inter-assay coefficients of variation (CV) were < 5 and < 8%, respectively.

The HPR rates in the two DAPT groups were also compared. HPR was defined as those situations in which 5 μM ADP maximum platelet aggregation was ≥46% [5], or the VASP result was > 50% PRI [28].

Statistical analysis

SPSS version 21.0 (SPSS Inc., Chicago, Illinois) was used to analyze the data statistically. For continuous variables, the results were shown as mean ± standard deviation (SD) if in a normal distribution or as median and interquartile range (IQR, percentiles 25–75) if the distribution was skewed. Statistical significance was assessed by independent-samples *t*-test, one-way analysis of variance (ANOVA), or the Mann–Whitney U test. Chi-square or Fisher exact tests were used for categorical variables and expressed as number, n (proportions, %). Bivariate correlation analysis was assessed with Pearson's or

Spearman's correlation analysis. To identify the independent associations between MPV and HPR adjusted for hypertension, dyslipidemia, diabetes, previous PCI, angiotensin converting enzyme inhibitor (ACEI), β-blocker, LDL-C, hsCRP, and AST, multivariate logistic regression analysis was performed. Receiver-operating characteristic (ROC) curves were assessed to evaluate the predictive value of MPV for HPR. The optimal cut-off value was determined by Youden's index (YI) calculated as (sensitivity + specificity − 1). A 2-tailed P-value < 0.05 indicated statistical significance.

Results

Study population and baseline characteristics

In total, 112 consecutive participants were enrolled in this study. Table 1 shows the baseline characteristics of the two DAPT groups. There were no significant differences in mean age, BMI and proportion of males between the two groups. The patients receiving aspirin and clopidogrel had higher LVEF, more history of hypertension and less history of diabetes. The patients treated with aspirin and ticagrelor had more previous PCI and myocardial infarction (MI) and more frequent use of ACEI. In the laboratory data acquired after PCI, the levels of hsCRP, ALT and AST were markedly higher in the group given aspirin and ticagrelor. Interestingly, patients in the aspirin + clopidogrel group had a significantly higher value of MPV (11.4 ± 1.4 vs 10.2 ± 0.9 fL, $P <$ 0.001). Nevertheless, no significant difference was found in PLT count between the two groups.

Platelet function testing in patients of the two DAPT groups

As measured by LTA, the maximal light transmittance (LT) changes in response to 5 μM ADP in the aspirin + clopidogrel group was dramatically higher than that in the

Table 1 Demographics of the study population

Variables	Aspirin + clopidogrel group (n = 46)	Aspirin + ticagrelor group (n = 66)	P
Age, yrs.	58.1 ± 9.1	56.3 ± 11.6	0.401
Male, n (%)	36(78.3)	55(83.3)	0.499
BMI, kg/m^2	25.9 ± 3.3	25.9 ± 3.2	0.963
LVEF, %	63.0(60.0, 66.0)	60.0(52.8, 65.0)	< 0.001
Risk factors			
Hypertension, n (%)	33(71.7)	31(47.0)	0.009
Diabetes, n (%)	9(19.6)	26(39.4)	0.026
Hyperlipidemia, n (%)	43(93.5)	58(89.2)	0.441
Past history			
Previous PCI, n (%)	9(19.6)	28(42.4)	0.011
Previous MI, n (%)	17(37.0)	56(84.8)	< 0.001
Previous stroke, n (%)	10(22.2)	4(6.1)	0.012
Medications			
Statins, n (%)	46(100.0)	66(100.0)	1.000
ACEI, n (%)	11(24.4)	29(46.0)	0.022
ARB, n (%)	8(18.2)	7(11.1)	0.300
β-blocker, n (%)	38(84.4)	60(93.8)	0.112
Laboratory			
Hemoglobin, g/L	147.7 ± 14.0	143.5 ± 12.4	0.095
LDL-C, mmol/L	2.0(1.7, 2.8)	2.2(1.5, 2.7)	0.708
HsCRP, mg/L	1.1(0.5, 3.0)	2.6(1.2, 7.2)	0.006
AST, U/L	22.0(19.0, 27.5)	27.0(20.0, 85.0)	0.007
ALT, U/L	27.0(17.0, 39.2)	32.5(22.8, 52.5)	0.022
Platelet, 10^9 cells/L	223.1 ± 60.2	244.7 ± 69.7	0.091
MPV, fL	11.4 ± 1.4	10.2 ± 0.9	< 0.001

Values are mean ± SD if the distribution is normal; median (interquartile range) if skewed; number, n (proportions, %) for categorical variables
ACEI Angiotensin converting enzyme inhibitor, *ALT* Alanine transaminase, *AST* Aspartate transaminase, *ARB* Angiotensin receptor blocker, *BMI* Body mass index, *CABG* Coronary artery bypass graft, *hsCRP* highly sensitive C-reactive protein, *LDL-C* Low-density lipoprotein cholesterol, *LVEF* Left ventricular ejection fraction, *MI* Myocardial infarction, *MPV* Mean platelet volume, *PCI* Percutaneous coronary intervention

aspirin + ticagrelor group (38.8 ± 16.2% vs 18.5 ± 9.5%, $P < 0.001$; Fig. 1A). According to the results of the VASP test, the aspirin + ticagrelor group presented a significantly lower PRI level than the aspirin + clopidogrel group (23.9 ± 15.9% vs 63.5 ± 21.5%, $P < 0.001$; Fig. 1B).

Using the criteria which have been reported in the literature [14, 29], the HPR rates were compared between the different DAPT groups and platelet function results (Fig. 2). In the LTA assay, the HPR rate differed significantly between the two groups (aspirin + clopidogrel: aspirin + ticagrelor = 21.7:1.5, $P < 0.001$; Fig. 2A). Similar results could also be observed in the VASP assay, with a higher HPR rate in those given aspirin and clopidogrel (aspirin + clopidogrel: aspirin + ticagrelor = 73.9:7.6, P < 0.001; Fig. 2B).

In addition, as shown in Additional file 2 (Fig. S2), a significant positive correlation was observed between the results for LTA and VASP assay (r = 0.660, $P < 0.001$). Multivariate regression analysis for prediction of HPR by the LTA and VASP assay is presented in Additional file 3 (Table S1). After multivariate adjustment for previous percutaneous coronary intervention, previous stroke, MPV, hsCRP, left ventricular ejection fraction, and aspartate transaminase, dual antiplatelet therapy remained independently significant in predicting HPR in the LTA and VASP assay.

Association between mean platelet volume and high on-treatment platelet reactivity

To investigate whether MPV could indicate the level of HPR in patients receiving DAPT, the participants were divided into three groups, according to MPV tertiles (< 10.0 fL; 10.0–11.0 fL; ≥ 11.0 fL). Table 2 shows the main clinical characteristics and biochemistry results according to the MPV values. Larger platelets were associated with higher LVEF ($P = 0.026$), higher Hb ($P = 0.011$), lower AST levels ($P = 0.010$) and lower PLT count ($P = 0.001$), and with less history of previous MI ($P = 0.031$). Notably, more patients in the highest MPV tertile received aspirin and clopidogrel ($P < 0.001$). With regard to the platelet function results, ADP-mediated platelet aggregation ($P = 0.006$) and PRI ($P < 0.001$) was much higher in patients of the highest MPV tertile. A higher percentage of HPR was observed at VASP assay in patients with higher MPV ($P < 0.001$), and this was also true for ADP-induced aggregation at LTA test ($P = 0.048$). Furthermore, analysis showed that there existed a positive correlation between MPV levels and PRI (r = 0.488, $P < 0.001$), as well as maximal LT changes in response to 5 μM ADP (r = 0.343, $P < 0.001$) (Fig. 3). There was also an inverse relationship between MPV and platelet count (r = − 0.413, $P < 0.001$).

As can be seen in Table 3, the independence of MPV and MPV tertiles in predicting HPR at VASP assay was subsequently determined using univariate and multivariable logistic regression analysis. Results indicated that there was an independent association between MPV level and the increased prevalence of HPR in the VASP assay, as well as MPV tertiles. As the increasing trend of MPV tertiles, it also presented higher OR values which indicating a higher prevalence of HPR. After adjustment for percutaneous coronary intervention, previous stroke, dual antiplatelet therapy, left ventricular ejection fraction and aspartate transaminase, MPV was significantly and

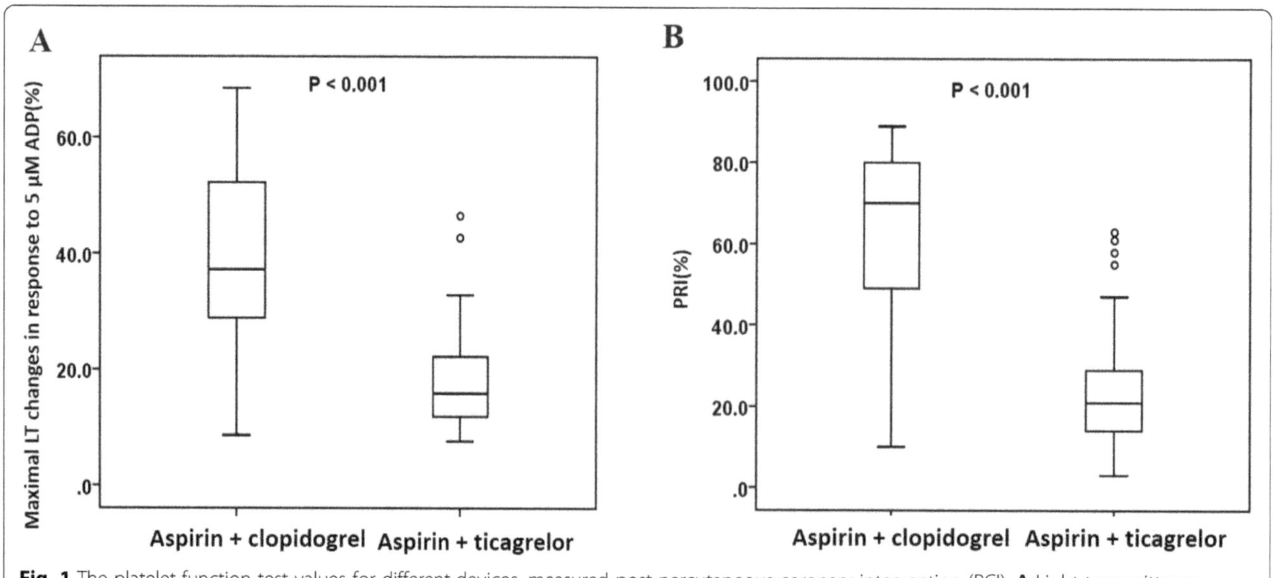

Fig. 1 The platelet function test values for different devices, measured post-percutaneous coronary intervention (PCI). **A** Light transmittance aggregometry (maximal LT changes in response to 5 μM ADP, %); **B** Vasodilator - stimulated phosphoprotein test (PRI, %). Error bars indicate SD. Abbreviations: ADP, adenosine diphosphate; PRI, platelet response index

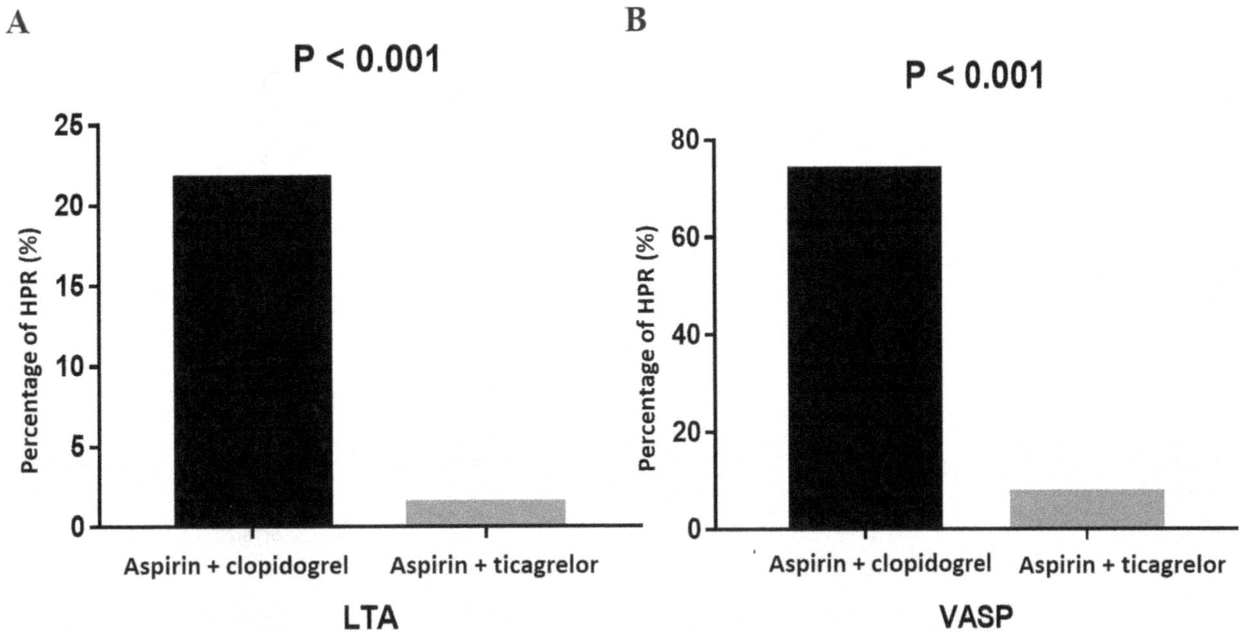

Fig. 2 The percentage of high platelet reactivity (HPR) measured post-percutaneous coronary intervention (PCI) in different groups. **A** ADP-Light transmittance aggregometry (LTA); **B** Vasodilator-stimulated phosphoprotein (VASP) test

independently associated with HPR (OR = 2.105, 95% CI: 1.175–3.771, $P = 0.012$), and the results of MPV tertile 3 were marginally significant (OR = 5.446, 95% CI:0.936–31.690, $P = 0.059$). Nevertheless, MPV and MPV tertiles did not present significant independence in predicting HPR at LTA testing. In addition, analysis of ROC curves showed a potent ability of MPV in predicting the presence of HPR at VASP assay in patients undergoing PCI and receiving DAPT (area under curve [AUC] = 0.788, 95% CI: 0.701–0.875, $P < 0.001$) (Fig. 4A). The cut-off value of MPV in predicting HPR was 10.55 fL. Furthermore, analysis of ROC curves was also conducted in patients given aspirin and clopidogrel (Fig. 4B). MPV could predict HPR at VASP assay for those patients (area under curve [AUC] = 0.729, 95% CI: 0.552–0.906, $P = 0.019$) with a cut-off value of 11.65 fL.

Finally, Fig. 5 displays the MPV levels of the two groups given aspirin and clopidogrel or ticagrelor. It was found that the levels of MPV were significantly higher in those patients given aspirin and clopidogrel than those given aspirin and ticagrelor ($P < 0.001$), which was also shown in Table 1.

Discussion

Our study, for the first time, characterized the effects of clopidogrel and ticagrelor on platelet function, using LTA and VASP assay, in a Chinese population undergoing PCI. This study provides evidence that MPV is independently associated with HPR at VASP assay and could also be used to evaluate the platelet reactivity of patients receiving clopidogrel or ticagrelor. The three major findings in this study are as follows. (1) The effect of ticagrelor on platelet reactivity was significantly greater than that of clopidogrel, with a more potent inhibition of platelet activity measured by LTA and VASP assay. (2) Patients with ACS undergoing PCI who were received standard-of-care treatment with ticagrelor, on a basis of aspirin, had a lower prevalence of HPR when compared with those given clopidogrel. (3) MPV can independently indicate HPR in patients, measured by VASP assay, and was much higher in patients using clopidogrel, which potentially reflects a higher prevalence of HPR.

Many studies have previously assessed the pharmacodynamic effects of clopidogrel and ticagrelor in patients with ST-segment elevation myocardial infarction (STEMI) undergoing early PCI using different PFTs, and have reported that ticagrelor provided more potent and prompt platelet inhibition than clopidogrel [30]. In particular, several clinical trials demonstrated that the primary efficacy end point and clinical benefits favored ticagrelor compared with clopidogrel in patients with ACS; the former markedly reduced the mortality due to stroke, vascular causes, and myocardial infarction [31, 32]. In this study, the effect on platelet function of ticagrelor and clopidogrel in Chinese patients agreed with the findings reported in Western populations. Although there have been several studies investigating the pharmacology and bleeding risk associated with two antiplatelet drugs among Asian populations [33–36], few studies have concentrated on their different effects on

Table 2 Clinical characteristics and chemistry results according to mean platelet volume

Variables	I tert < 10.0 fL (*n* = 37)	II tert 10.0–11.0 fL (*n* = 42)	III tert ≥11.0 fL (*n* = 33)	*P*
Age, yrs.	58.2 ± 10.3	55.7 ± 12.1	57.4 ± 9.2	0.566
Male, n (%)	33(89.2)	31(73.8)	27(81.8)	0.216
BMI, kg/m^2	26.1 ± 3.5	25.9 ± 3.4	25.5 ± 2.6	0.758
LVEF, %	60.0(53.0, 65.0)	63.0(60.0, 65.0)	65.0(58.0, 68.0)	0.026
Risk factors				
Hypertension, n (%)	20(54.1)	20(47.6)	24(72.7)	0.083
Diabetes, n (%)	14(37.8)	14(33.3)	7(21.2)	0.304
Hyperlipidemia, n (%)	34(91.9)	38 (90.5)	29(87.9)	0.850
Past history				
Previous PCI, n (%)	15(40.5)	12(28.6)	10(30.3)	0.489
Previous MI, n (%)	29(78.4)	28(66.7)	16(48.5)	0.031
Previous stroke, n (%)	4(10.8)	4(9.5)	6(18.2)	0.494
Medications				
Statins, n (%)	37(100.0)	42(100.0)	33(100.0)	1.000
ACEI, n (%)	17(45.9)	14(33.3)	9(27.3)	0.245
ARB, n (%)	6(16.2)	3(7.1)	6(18.2)	0.313
β-blocker, n (%)	36(97.3)	34(81.0)	28(84.8)	0.078
Laboratory				
Hemoglobin, g/L	140.0 ± 13.0	147.0 ± 13.2	148.8 ± 11.9	0.011
LDL-C, mmol/L	2.4(1.7, 2.8)	2.2(1.6, 2.8)	2.0(1.7, 2.2)	0.457
HsCRP, mg/L	3.1(1.2, 8.4)	1.8(0.9, 4.7)	1.5(0.5, 6.7)	0.232
AST, U/L	25.0(20.5, 85.0)	25.5(20.8, 38.2)	21.0(16.5, 28.0)	0.010
ALT, U/L	26.0(22.0, 42.5)	32.0(21.5, 52.0)	29.0(17.0, 40.0)	0.474
Platelet, 10^9 cells/L	257.3 ± 73.4	243.9 ± 63.2	201.4 ± 48.3	0.001
Maximal LT changes in response to 5 μM ADP, %	17.0(12.4, 25.7)	20.6(12.1, 36.5)	32.0(16.4, 51.5)	0.006
PRI, %	21(11.5, 28.0)	31.0(23.0, 66.5)	61.0(30.5, 79.0)	< 0.001
Percentage of HPR-LTA, %	0(0)	6(14.3)	5(15.2)	0.049
Percentage of HPR-VASP, %	4(10.8)	15(35.7)	20(60.6)	< 0.001
Dual antiplatelet therapy				
Traditional therapy, n (%)	6(16.2)	18(42.9)	22(66.7)	< 0.001
New therapy, n (%)	31(83.8)	24(57.1)	11(33.3)	< 0.001

Values are mean ± SD if the distribution is normal; median (interquartile range) if skewed; number, n (proportions, %) for categorical variables
ADP Adenosine diphosphate, *HPR* High on-treatment platelet reactivity, *LT* Light transmittance, *PRI* Platelet response index. Others were as Table 1

platelet function in such populations, using different PFTs including LTA and VASP test, even though only Verify Now was applied to evaluate the platelet inhibition with ticagrelor versus clopidogrel in diabetic patients after PCI in the study of Zhenyu Liu et al. [37].

Various kinds of PFT have been applied to monitor platelet activity in the setting of DAPT (aspirin and clopidogrel or ticagrelor) in large clinical trials. Verify Now, LTA, MEA and flow cytometry are most intensively used among those techniques. LTA, as a traditional technique, has always been acknowledged as the most classical method. VASP phosphorylation measures activation-dependent platelet signaling. This assay requires small sample volumes and whole blood, maintaining high stability, and is dependent on the P2Y12 receptor, the site of action for clopidogrel and ticagrelor [38]. Therefore, the VASP assay has been used in many clinical trials on the background of the above characteristics. Meanwhile, it has shown a relatively good correlation with LTA results, which was also seen in our results in Fig. S2. In our study, we used LTA and VASP assay and found evidence for a significant effect of

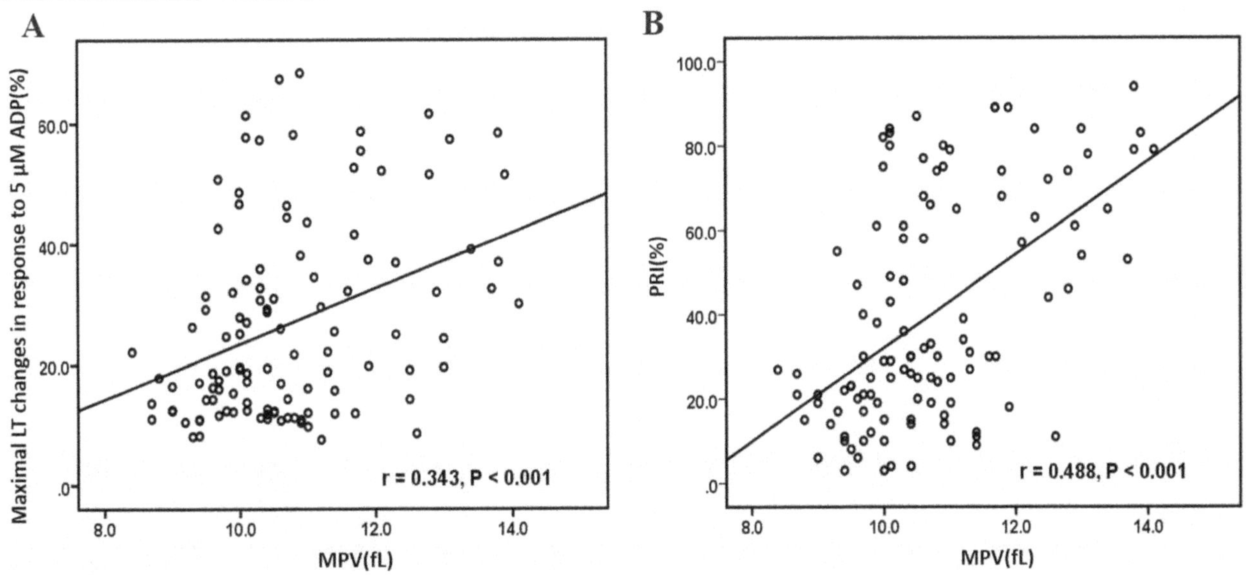

Fig. 3 Relationships between mean platelet volume (MPV) and platelet aggregation results. **A** LTA after ADP stimulation; **B** VASP test. Correlation coefficient (r) was calculated using Pearson's method

ticagrelor on platelet inhibition. In addition, use of LTA and VASP testing may identify patients who are at high risk of thrombotic events such as cardiac death and stent thrombosis during follow up [39]. However, the difference in HPR prevalence with the two tests was relatively large. According to studies reported, the results of platelet aggregation and HPR remained difference with various PFTs. It was considered that the definition standard of HPR influenced our results, especially HPR in the VASP assay which was referenced with the definition of France but not Asian population. Therefore, the definition of HPR at VASP assay might be adjusted with the data of Asians in further investigations. The association between the HPR with the two tests and the ending of patients should be followed up and the study population need to be enlarged as recommended in consensus [40, 41].

Furthermore, a higher HPR rate in patients receiving clopidogrel was observed in our study. This finding indicated that clopidogrel was more prone to induce drug resistance in Chinese individuals. This could guide a more efficient tailored therapy for those patients who were identified as at very high risk. On the genetic level, CYP2C19 polymorphism have been identified as the most prominent effector on platelet activity after clopidogrel treatment [42]. According to literature reported [43, 44], as compared with Africans and whites, East Asian population has a high prevalence of the CYP2C19 loss-of-function (LOF) genotype with CYP2C19*3 variant which was in accordance with previous results found in our laboratory center with Chinese population [45]. Additionally, the prevalence of the LOF mutations among different Asian populations also presented difference, and ticagrelor could become a substitute for

Table 3 Regression analysis to assess HPR according to MPV and MPV tertiles[a]

Variables	Univariate		Multivariate	
	OR (95% CI)	P	OR (95% CI)	P
MPV	**2.797(1.813, 4.313)**	**< 0.001**	**2.105(1.175, 3.771)**	**0.012**
MPV tertiles tertiles				
Tertile 1	**1**		**1**	
Tertile 2	**4.583(1.361, 15.440)**	**0.014**	**3.537(0.644, 19.442)**	**0.146**
Tertile 3	**12.692(3.634, 44.333)**	**< 0.001**	**5.446(0.936, 31.690)**	**0.059**

[a] Adjusted for previous of percutaneous coronary intervention, previous of stroke, dual antiplatelet therapy, left ventricular ejection fraction, and aspartate transaminase

HPR High on-treatment platelet reactivity, *MPV* Mean platelet volume

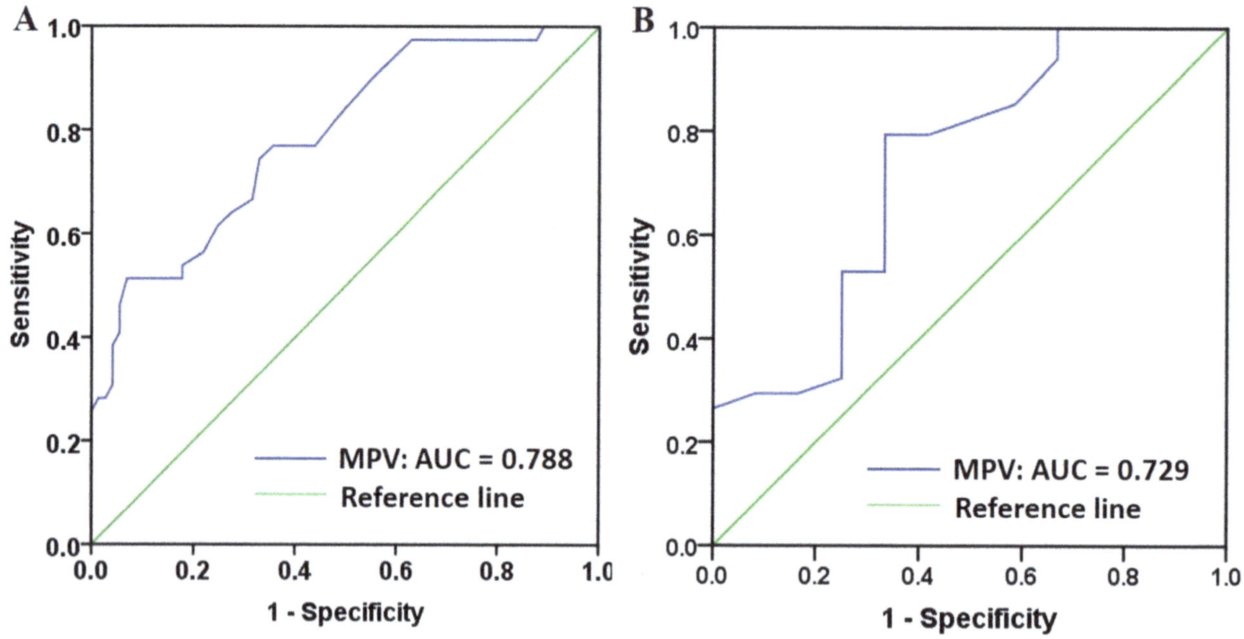

Fig. 4 Receiver operating characteristic (ROC) curve of MPV for predicting HPR at VASP assay in different groups. **A** The whole study population. **B** Patients given aspirin and clopidogrel

clopidogrel in those with LOF mutations [46].Therefore, it could be implied that our results in Chinese population may provide additional information to Asian population. Of note, patients in this study were not assigned by randomization to clopidogrel or ticagrelor because the choice of anti-platelet drugs should obey the clinical guidelines and should be evaluated by clinicians according to patients' symptoms. The data in Table S1 demonstrate that the results of HPR might not be influenced by differences in hsCRP, transaminases, MPV and other variables between the two groups.

Further, we provided evidence that MPV, which has been proposed as a cheap and easy-to-obtain marker of platelet size, could indicate platelet reactivity and the level of HPR in patients receiving DAPT. The inverse relationship between MPV and platelet count in our

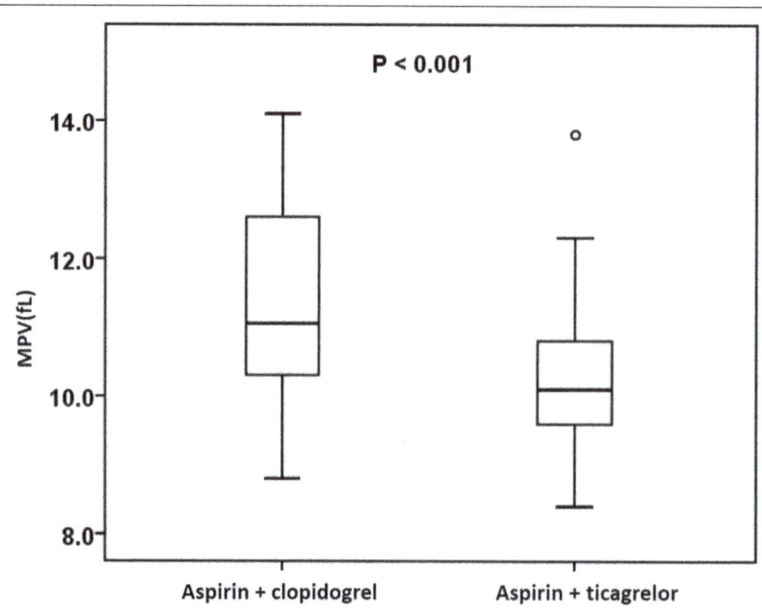

Fig. 5 The comparison of MPV levels in the groups given aspirin and clopidogrel or ticagrelor

results proved the reliability of this study, which was in accordance with reported findings. A close relationship has been demonstrated between MPV and cardiovascular risk factors including obesity, diabetes mellitus, hypertension, hypercholesterolemia and other factors [47, 48]. However, data relating MPV with acute coronary and cerebrovascular events are still contrasting. Lippi et al. [49] demonstrated that there was a significant increase of MPV levels in ACS patients when compared with non-ACS patients. In addition, platelet size could predict impaired angiographic reperfusion and the death rate in patients with STEMI undergoing PCI [50]. In contrast, Tavil et al. demonstrated that MPV was related to central obesity, hypertension and hypercholesterolemia, but not to coronary artery disease (CAD), in patients referred for coronary angiography [51]. The role of MPV in indicating the response to antiplatelet drugs has also raised great debate. Asher et al. [52] documented a higher rate of HPR with larger platelets after clopidogrel loading dose received by patients with acute myocardial infarction. Kubica et al. [53] reported similar findings in patients undergoing PCI. In addition, larger-sized platelets could independently predict the risk of high residual platelet reactivity for treatment with aspirin + clopidogrel, also in patients treated with PCI [54]. However, Monica et al. [24] found no impact of larger platelet volume on the majority of platelet function tests, and in particular on ADP-mediated aggregation or the response to clopidogrel or ticagrelor. Our present study evaluated the association between MPV and platelet function in patients with DAPT and confirmed the well-established strict association of MPV with other platelet function parameters, including ADP-induced aggregation conducted by LTA and PRI in the VASP assay. Regarding the variation in the role of MPV in indicating platelet function, it has been considered that this may be related to the various PFTs used in different studies. We found that MPV was related to HPR only at the VASP test but not at the LTA assay. Similar results for the association between MPV and HPR could be found at MEA test, according to Kim et al. [54]. Of note, there was a very low correlation between the results of the MEA test and platelet volume indices, although there was a strong correlation between VASP test parameters and MPV. It could be noted that there was a significant difference in the baseline value of MPV in the two treatment arms. To avoid drawing questionable conclusions on MPV, the dual antiplatelet therapy was included in the multivariate regression analysis to assess the independence of MPV and MPV tertiles in predicting HPR. Therefore, the results obtained are rational and the conclusion we drew is also reasonable. In this study, the present results of multivariable logistic regression analysis showed that MPV as a continuous variable could independently indicate HPR at VASP assay and the results of MPV tertile 3 were marginally significant. This might because the sample size of the study is not large enough to ensure enough number of samples in MPV tertiles. It could be inferred that MPV tertiles would be significantly and independently associated with HPR if the sample size were enlarged. Therefore, the sample size should be enlarged to verify the results and investigate the role of MPV tertiles in indicating HPR in the further study. Based on the results of ROC analysis, a threshold could be found (MPV = 11.65 fL) for which a switch from clopidogrel to ticagrelor should be considered. This provided additional information and evidence regarding to the role of MPV in guiding clinical practice and anti-platelet drugs using. Of note, the swelling effect of EDTA on blood cells especially on platelet volume over the first two hours should be addressed. A significant increase in MPV could be observed in blood samples anticoagulated with EDTA over time [55]. In our study, it was recommended that MPV test should be conducted within 2 h after blood draw. Therefore, time elapsed between blood collection and testing is quite important for the accuracy of testing results which should be paid more attention [55].

It has been demonstrated that ticagrelor had superiority over clopidogrel in suppressing platelet function in patients with ACS, with a more pronounced antiplatelet effect during the initial treatment phase and during maintenance therapy [56]. Our present study is consistent with previous research. Recently, the EROSION study [57] reported that DAPT with aspirin and ticagrelor without stenting may be an option for patients with ACS caused by plaque erosion. Therefore, the potential clinical application of ticagrelor in anti-thrombotic therapy for ACS patients should not be ignored.

In this study, several limitations of the design should be stated. First, the absence of long-term follow-up of our patients should be considered, and, therefore, we cannot evaluate the impact of the two different types of DAPT on clinical outcome. Furthermore, we need to enlarge the dataset in order to improve the representativeness and reliability of the results. In addition, the impact of genetic factors, such as CYP2C19 polymorphism, on anti-platelet drug responsiveness was not evaluated in this study; the response to clopidogrel is closely associated with the polymorphism of CYP2C19. The results of this study may therefore have been confounded by the prevalence of CYP2C19 polymorphism.

Conclusions

Our study investigated the antiplatelet effect of clopidogrel and ticagrelor in Chinese patients undergoing PCI, using two platelet function tests, LTA and VASP assay. Ticagrelor has markedly greater antiplatelet effect than clopidogrel, with a superiority in inhibiting platelet activity and a lower HPR rate. In addition, an independent association between MPV and high HPR prevalence in the VASP assay was found. Clinicians should be aware that MPV could be another potential marker to reflect the platelet reactivity in response to anti-platelet drugs and take it into consideration during antiplatelet therapy.

Abbreviations

ACEI: Angiotensin converting enzyme inhibitor; ACS: Acute coronary syndromes; ADP: Adenosine diphosphate; ALT: Alanine transaminase; ANOVA: One-way analysis of variance; AST: Aspartate transaminase; BMI: Body mass index; CAD: Coronary artery disease; CV: Coefficient of variation; DAPT: Dual antiplatelet therapy; Hb: Hemoglobin; HPR: High on-treatment platelet reactivity; hsCRP: High-sensitivity C-reactive protein; IQR: Interquartile range; LDL-C: Low-density lipoprotein-cholesterol; LTA: Light-transmission aggregometry; LVEF: Left ventricular ejection fraction; MEA: Multiple electrode platelet aggregometry; MFI: Mean fluorescence intensity; MI: Myocardial infarction; MPV: Mean platelet volume; PCI: Percutaneous coronary intervention; PFA: Platelet function analyzer; PFT: Platelet function test; PGE_1: Prostaglandin E_1; PLT: Platelet count; PRI: Platelet reactivity index; ROC: Receiver-operating characteristic; SD: Standard deviation; STEMI: ST-segment elevation myocardial infarction; TEG: Thromboelastography; VASP: Vasodilator-stimulated phosphoprotein; YI: Youden's index

Supplementary Information

Additional file 1: Fig. S1. Study flow diagram.

Additional file 2: Fig. S2. Relationships between the results obtained by light transmittance aggregometry (LTA, %) and vasodilator-stimulated phosphoprotein (VASP) (PRI, %) assay systems post-percutaneous coronary intervention (PCI). Correlation coefficient (r) was calculated using Pearson's method.

Additional file 3: Table S1. Multivariate regression analysis for prediction of HPR at LTA and VASP assay.

Authors' contributions

YZ was key in the design of the work and had major input in writing the manuscript. RP was a major contributor to the clinical work and drafted the manuscript. XJL and GWC provided technical contributions in platelet function tests. XMW and JXY helped in screening patients and recording of laboratory data. MXH provided technical suggestions and supervised the study. XC and ZZ supervised the study and revised the manuscript. All authors read and approved the final manuscript.

Author details

[1]Diagnostic Laboratory Service, State Key Laboratory of Cardiovascular Disease, Fuwai Hospital, National Center for Cardiovascular Diseases, Chinese Academy of Medical Sciences, Peking Union Medical College, No.167, Beilishi Road, Xicheng District, Beijing 100037, China. [2]Department of Laboratory Medicine, Yunnan Fuwai Cardiovascular Hospital, Kunming 650000, China.

References

1. Steinhubl SR, Berger PB, Mann JT 3rd, Fry ET, DeLago A, Wilmer C, et al. Early and sustained dual oral antiplatelet therapy following percutaneous coronary intervention: a randomized controlled trial. Jama. 2002;288:2411–20.
2. Yusuf S, Zhao F, Mehta SR, Chrolavicius S, Tognoni G, Fox KK. Effects of clopidogrel in addition to aspirin in patients with acute coronary syndromes without ST-segment elevation. N Engl J Med. 2001;345:494–502.
3. Gurbel PA, Bliden KP, Hiatt BL, O'Connor CM. Clopidogrel for coronary stenting: response variability, drug resistance, and the effect of pretreatment platelet reactivity. Circulation. 2003;107:2908–13.
4. van der Heijden DJ, Westendorp IC, Riezebos RK, Kiemeneij F, Slagboom T, van der Wieken LR, et al. Lack of efficacy of clopidogrel pre-treatment in the prevention of myocardial damage after elective stent implantation. J Am Coll Cardiol. 2004;44:20–4.
5. Bonello L, Tantry US, Marcucci R, Blindt R, Angiolillo DJ, Becker R, et al. Consensus and future directions on the definition of high on-treatment platelet reactivity to adenosine diphosphate. J Am Coll Cardiol. 2010;56: 919–33.
6. Marcucci R, Gori AM, Paniccia R, Giusti B, Valente S, Giglioli C, et al. Cardiovascular death and nonfatal myocardial infarction in acute coronary syndrome patients receiving coronary stenting are predicted by residual platelet reactivity to ADP detected by a point-of-care assay: a 12-month follow-up. Circulation. 2009;119:237–42.
7. Vang JJ, Nilsson L, Berntsson P, Wissing BM, Giordanetto F, Tomlinson W, et al. Ticagrelor binds to human P2Y(12) independently from ADP but antagonizes ADP-induced receptor signaling and platelet aggregation. J Thromb Haemost. 2009;7:1556–65.
8. May CH, Lincoff AM. Safety profile and bleeding risk of ticagrelor compared with clopidogrel. Expert Opin Drug Saf. 2012;11:959–67.
9. Franchi F, Faz GT, Rollini F, Park Y, Cho JR, Thano E, et al. Pharmacodynamic effects of switching from Prasugrel to Ticagrelor: results of the prospective, randomized SWAP-3 study. JACC Cardiovasc Interv. 2016;9:1089–98.
10. Levine GN, Bates ER, Bittl JA, Brindis RG, Fihn SD, Fleisher LA, et al. 2016 ACC/AHA guideline focused update on duration of dual antiplatelet therapy in patients with coronary artery disease: a report of the American College of Cardiology/American Heart Association task force on clinical practice guidelines: an update of the 2011 ACCF/AHA/SCAI guideline for percutaneous coronary intervention, 2011 ACCF/AHA guideline for coronary artery bypass graft surgery, 2012 ACC/AHA/ACP/AATS/PCNA/SCAI/STS guideline for the diagnosis and Management of Patients with Stable Ischemic Heart Disease, 2013 ACCF/AHA guideline for the management of ST-elevation myocardial infarction, 2014 AHA/ACC guideline for the Management of Patients with non-ST-elevation acute coronary syndromes, and 2014 ACC/AHA guideline on perioperative cardiovascular evaluation and Management of Patients Undergoing Noncardiac Surgery. Circulation. 2016;134:e123–55.
11. Kang J, Park KW, Palmerini T, Stone GW, Lee MS, Colombo A, et al. Racial differences in Ischaemia/bleeding risk trade-off during anti-platelet therapy: individual patient level landmark Meta-analysis from seven RCTs. Thromb Haemost. 2019;119:149–62.
12. Park DW, Kwon O, Jang JS, Yun SC, Park H, Kang DY, et al. Clinically significant bleeding with Ticagrelor versus Clopidogrel in Korean patients with acute coronary syndromes intended for invasive management: a randomized clinical trial. Circulation. 2019;140:1865–77.
13. Goto S, Huang CH, Park SJ, Emanuelsson H, Kimura T. Ticagrelor vs. clopidogrel in Japanese, Korean and Taiwanese patients with acute coronary syndrome -- randomized, double-blind, phase III PHILO study. Circ J. 2015;79:2452–60.
14. Gorog DA, Fuster V. Platelet function tests in clinical cardiology: unfulfilled expectations. J Am Coll Cardiol. 2013;61:2115–29.
15. Kong R, Trimmings A, Hutchinson N, Gill R, Agarwal S, Davidson S, et al. Consensus recommendations for using the multiplate((R)) for platelet function monitoring before cardiac surgery. Int J Lab Hematol. 2015;37:143–7.
16. Born GV, Cross MJ. The aggregation of blood platelets. J Physiol. 1963;168: 178–95.
17. Born GV. Aggregation of blood platelets by adenosine diphosphate and its reversal. Nature. 1962;194:927–9.
18. O'Brien JR. Platelet aggregation: part II some results from a new method of study. J Clin Pathol. 1962;15:452–5.
19. Breddin HK. Can platelet aggregometry be standardized? Platelets. 2005;16: 151–8.
20. Schwarz UR, Geiger J, Walter U, Eigenthaler M. Flow cytometry analysis of intracellular VASP phosphorylation for the assessment of activating and inhibitory signal transduction pathways in human platelets--definition and detection of ticlopidine/clopidogrel effects. Thromb Haemost. 1999;82: 1145–52.
21. Chu SG, Becker RC, Berger PB, Bhatt DL, Eikelboom JW, Konkle B, et al. Mean platelet volume as a predictor of cardiovascular risk: a systematic review and meta-analysis. J Thromb Haemost. 2010;8:148–56.
22. Jakl M, Sevcik R, Ceral J, Fatorova I, Horacek JM, Vojacek J. Mean platelet volume and platelet count: overlooked markers of high on-treatment

platelet reactivity and worse outcome in patients with acute coronary syndrome. Anadolu Kardiyol Derg. 2014;14:85–6.

23. Beyan C, Kaptan K, Ifran A. Platelet count, mean platelet volume, platelet distribution width, and plateletcrit do not correlate with optical platelet aggregation responses in healthy volunteers. J Thromb Thrombolysis. 2006; 22:161–4.
24. Verdoia M, Pergolini P, Rolla R, Nardin M, Barbieri L, Schaffer A, et al. Mean platelet volume and high-residual platelet reactivity in patients receiving dual antiplatelet therapy with clopidogrel or ticagrelor. Expert Opin Pharmacother. 2015;16:1739–47.
25. Valgimigli M, Bueno H, Byrne RA, Collet JP, Costa F, Jeppsson A, et al. 2017 ESC focused update on dual antiplatelet therapy in coronary artery disease developed in collaboration with EACTS: the task force for dual antiplatelet therapy in coronary artery disease of the European Society of Cardiology (ESC) and of the European Association for Cardio-Thoracic Surgery (EACTS). Eur Heart J. 2018;39:213–60.
26. Kim IS, Jeong YH, Kang MK, Koh JS, Park Y, Hwang SJ, et al. Correlation of high post-treatment platelet reactivity assessed by light transmittance aggregometry and the VerifyNow P2Y12 assay. J Thromb Thrombolysis. 2010;30:486–95.
27. Cattaneo M, Cerletti C, Harrison P, Hayward CP, Kenny D, Nugent D, et al. Recommendations for the standardization of light transmission Aggregometry: a consensus of the working party from the platelet physiology subcommittee of SSC/ISTH. J Thromb Haemost. 2013;11:1183–9.
28. Barragan P, Bouvier JL, Roquebert PO, Macaluso G, Commeau P, Comet B, et al. Resistance to thienopyridines: clinical detection of coronary stent thrombosis by monitoring of vasodilator-stimulated phosphoprotein phosphorylation. Catheter Cardiovasc Interv. 2003;59:295–302.
29. Marcucci R, Gori AM, Paniccia R, Giusti B, Valente S, Giglioli C, et al. High on-treatment platelet reactivity by more than one agonist predicts 12-month follow-up cardiovascular death and non-fatal myocardial infarction in acute coronary syndrome patients receiving coronary stenting. Thromb Haemost. 2010;104:279–86.
30. Dehghani P, Lavoie A, Lavi S, Crawford JJ, Harenberg S, Zimmermann RH, et al. Effects of ticagrelor versus clopidogrel on platelet function in fibrinolytic-treated STEMI patients undergoing early PCI. Am Heart J. 2017; 192:105–12.
31. Wallentin L, Becker RC, Budaj A, Cannon CP, Emanuelsson H, Held C, et al. Ticagrelor versus clopidogrel in patients with acute coronary syndromes. N Engl J Med. 2009;361:1045–57.
32. Held C, Asenblad N, Bassand JP, Becker RC, Cannon CP, Claeys MJ, et al. Ticagrelor versus clopidogrel in patients with acute coronary syndromes undergoing coronary artery bypass surgery: results from the PLATO (platelet inhibition and patient outcomes) trial. J Am Coll Cardiol. 2011;57:672–84.
33. Kang HJ, Clare RM, Gao R, Held C, Himmelmann A, James SK, et al. Ticagrelor versus clopidogrel in Asian patients with acute coronary syndrome: a retrospective analysis from the platelet inhibition and patient outcomes (PLATO) trial. Am Heart J. 2015;169:899–905.e891.
34. Li H, Butler K, Yang L, Yang Z, Teng R. Pharmacokinetics and tolerability of single and multiple doses of ticagrelor in healthy Chinese subjects: an open-label, sequential, two-cohort, single-Centre study. Clin Drug Investig. 2012;32:87–97.
35. Wang Y, Wu H, Chen Y, Wang Q, Qian J, Ge J. Ticagrelor pharmacokinetics and pharmacodynamics in Chinese patients with STEMI and NSTEMI without opioid administration. Adv Ther. 2020;37:4220–32.
36. Tang XF, Han YL, Zhang JH, Wang J, Zhang Y, Xu B, et al. Comparing of light transmittance aggregometry and modified thrombelastograph in predicting clinical outcomes in Chinese patients undergoing coronary stenting with clopidogrel. Chin Med J. 2015;128:774–9.
37. Liu Z, Tian R, Wang Y, Chen Q, Li J, Xu L, et al. Platelet inhibition with Ticagrelor versus Clopidogrel in diabetic patients after percutaneous coronary intervention for chronic coronary syndromes. Thromb Haemost. 2020;120:1221–9.
38. Spurgeon BE, Aburima A, Oberprieler NG, Tasken K, Naseem KM. Multiplexed phosphospecific flow cytometry enables large-scale signaling profiling and drug screening in blood platelets. J Thromb Haemost. 2014;12: 1733–43.
39. Valenti R, Marcucci R, Capodanno D, De Luca G, Migliorini A, Gori AM, et al. Residual platelet reactivity to predict long-term clinical outcomes after clopidogrel loading in patients with acute coronary syndromes: comparison of different cutoff values by light transmission aggregometry from the responsiveness to clopidogrel and stent thrombosis 2-acute coronary syndrome (RECLOSE 2-ACS) study. J Thromb Thrombolysis. 2015;40:76–82.
40. Tantry US, Bonello L, Aradi D, Price MJ, Jeong YH, Angiolillo DJ, et al. Consensus and update on the definition of on-treatment platelet reactivity to adenosine diphosphate associated with ischemia and bleeding. J Am Coll Cardiol. 2013;62:2261–73.
41. Aradi D, Kirtane A, Bonello L, Gurbel PA, Tantry US, Huber K, et al. Bleeding and stent thrombosis on P2Y12-inhibitors: collaborative analysis on the role of platelet reactivity for risk stratification after percutaneous coronary intervention. Eur Heart J. 2015;36:1762–71.
42. Jeong YH, Tantry US, Kim IS, Koh JS, Kwon TJ, Park Y, et al. Effect of CYP2C19*2 and *3 loss-of-function alleles on platelet reactivity and adverse clinical events in east Asian acute myocardial infarction survivors treated with clopidogrel and aspirin. Circ Cardiovasc Interv. 2011;4:585–94.
43. Li S, Choi JL, Guo LZ, Goh RY, Kim BR, Woo KS, et al. Correlation between the CYP2C19 phenotype status and the results of three different platelet function tests in cardiovascular disease patients receiving antiplatelet therapy: an emphasis on newly introduced platelet function analyzer-200 P2Y test. Ann Lab Med. 2016;36:42–8.
44. Man M, Farmen M, Dumaual C, Teng CH, Moser B, Irie S, et al. Genetic variation in metabolizing enzyme and transporter genes: comprehensive assessment in 3 major east Asian subpopulations with comparison to Caucasians and Africans. J Clin Pharmacol. 2010;50:929–40.
45. Wang Z, Liu Z, Wang W, Fu Y, Chen W, Li W, et al. Two common mutations within CYP2C19 affected platelet aggregation in Chinese patients undergoing PCI: a one-year follow-up study. Pharmacogenomics J. 2019;19: 157–63.
46. Narasimhalu K, Ang YK, Tan DSY, De Silva DA, Tan KB. Cost effectiveness of genotype-guided antiplatelet therapy in Asian ischemic stroke patients: Ticagrelor as an alternative to Clopidogrel in patients with CYP2C19 loss of function mutations. Clin Drug Investig. 2020;40:1063–70.
47. Nadar SK, Blann AD, Kamath S, Beevers DG, Lip GY. Platelet indexes in relation to target organ damage in high-risk hypertensive patients: a substudy of the Anglo-Scandinavian cardiac outcomes trial (ASCOT). J Am Coll Cardiol. 2004;44:415–22.
48. Ozder A, Eker HH. Investigation of mean platelet volume in patients with type 2 diabetes mellitus and in subjects with impaired fasting glucose: a cost-effective tool in primary health care? Int J Clin Exp Med. 2014;7:2292–7.
49. Lippi G, Meschi T, Borghi L. Mean platelet volume increases with aging in a large population study. Thromb Res. 2012;129:e159–60.
50. Huczek Z, Kochman J, Filipiak KJ, Horszczaruk GJ, Grabowski M, Piatkowski R, et al. Mean platelet volume on admission predicts impaired reperfusion and long-term mortality in acute myocardial infarction treated with primary percutaneous coronary intervention. J Am Coll Cardiol. 2005;46:284–90.
51. Tavil Y, Sen N, Yazici HU, Hizal F, Abaci A, Cengel A. Mean platelet volume in patients with metabolic syndrome and its relationship with coronary artery disease. Thromb Res. 2007;120:245–50.
52. Asher E, Fefer P, Shechter M, Beigel R, Varon D, Shenkman B, et al. Increased mean platelet volume is associated with non-responsiveness to clopidogrel. Thromb Haemost. 2014;112:137–41.
53. Kubica A, Kasprzak M, Siller-Matula J, Kozinski M, Pio Navarese E, Obonska K, et al. Time-related changes in determinants of antiplatelet effect of clopidogrel in patients after myocardial infarction. Eur J Pharmacol. 2014; 742:47–54.
54. Kim YG, Suh JW, Yoon CH, Oh IY, Cho YS, Youn TJ, et al. Platelet volume indices are associated with high residual platelet reactivity after antiplatelet therapy in patients undergoing percutaneous coronary intervention. J Atheroscler Thromb. 2014;21:445–53.
55. Hardy M, Lessire S, Kasikci S, Baudar J, Guldenpfennig M, Collard A, et al. Effects of time-interval since blood draw and of anticoagulation on platelet testing (count, indices and impedance aggregometry): a systematic study with blood from healthy volunteers. J Clin Med. 2020;9:994–7.
56. Storey RF, Angiolillo DJ, Patil SB, Desai B, Ecob R, Husted S, et al. Inhibitory effects of ticagrelor compared with clopidogrel on platelet function in patients with acute coronary syndromes: the PLATO (PLATelet inhibition and patient outcomes) PLATELET substudy. J Am Coll Cardiol. 2010;56:1456–62.
57. Jia H, Dai J, Hou J, Xing L, Ma L, Liu H, et al. Effective anti-thrombotic therapy without stenting: intravascular optical coherence tomography-based management in plaque erosion (the EROSION study). Eur Heart J. 2017;38:792–800.

18

Fibrinolytic markers could be useful predictors of severity in patients with pulmonary arterial hypertension

Makoto Shoji*, Taiju Matsui, Hideaki Tanaka, Kosuke Nomura, Hiroaki Tsujita, Yusuke Kodama, Shinji Koba, Youichi Kobayashi and Toshiro Shinke

Abstract

Background: The severity of pulmonary arterial hypertension (PAH) is classified based on mean pulmonary artery pressure (mPAP) levels. However, other markers have not been elucidated. Fibrinolytic markers, such as total plasminogen activator inhibitor-1 (tPAI-1) and thrombomodulin (TM), are known to reflect arterial endothelial function. However, the relationship between serum tPAI-1, TM and pulmonary circulation has not been completely determined.

Methods: This study included 100 consecutive patients (38 men), with a mean age of 68.9 ± 12.0 years, with cardiac diseases who underwent right heart catheterization. Serum coagulation and fibrinolytic marker levels were measured.

Results: The average mPA*P* value was 25.1 ± 13.1 mmHg for all patients. The mPAP levels revealed a significant positive correlation with serum tPAI-1 ($\rho = 0.24$, $p = 0.042$) and uric acid ($\rho = 0.29$, $p = 0.0031$) levels. In the group with mPAP levels less than 25 mmHg ($n = 58$, ave. 17.3 ± 4.3 mmHg), mPAP levels showed a significant positive correlation with serum tPA-1 ($\rho = 0.34$, $p = 0.034$) and TM ($\rho = 0.34$, $p = 0.043$) values. The mean tPAI-1 (29.8 ± 23.3 ng/ml, $p = 0.047$) and uric acid (5.7 ± 1.8 mg/dl, $p = 0.026$) levels were significantly less in those with lower mPAP levels. A multivariate analysis revealed that tPAI-1 alone was a significant independent characteristic marker of PAH (odds ratio 1.02, 95%CI 1.000–1.036, $p = 0.034$).

Conclusions: These results indicate that serum tPAI-1 and TM may be useful predictors of severity, similar to mPAP in patients with PAH. They could be beneficial in predicting PAH among patients in the early stage of the disease.

Keywords: tPAI-1, Thrombomodulin, Pulmonary artery hypertension

* Correspondence: mashoji@hotmail.com
Department of Medicine, Division of Cardiology, Showa University School of Medicine, 1-5-8 Hatanodai, Shinagawa-ku, Tokyo 142-8666, Japan

Background

The severity of pulmonary artery hypertension (PAH) is classified based on the mean pulmonary artery pressure (mPAP) levels that are evaluated by right heart catheterization (RHC). It is a fetal disease that is reported to have a poor prognosis despite the development in medication [1, 2]. The mPAP has been established as an accurate prognostic marker for PAH in previous reports [3, 4]. However, the patients require RHC to evaluate mPAP, which is an invasive procedure. Thus, non-invasive and alternative predictors for prognosis are needed.

The fibrinolytic marker, total plasminogen activator inhibitor-1 (tPAI-1) is a major inhibitor of plasminogen activator in plasma. It is stored in platelets and has several sources, including the vascular endothelium [5]. tPAI-1 is known to be associated with a proinflammatory atherosclerotic risk. Moreover, there are reports that tPAI-1 is independently associated with the degree of intima media thickness (IMT) [6, 7]. Thrombomodulin (TM) has an anticoagulant effect that is activating protein C, and this is corroborated by reports about elevated blood levels of TM in patients with acute pulmonary embolism [8, 9]. It is also known that TM is metabolized by the liver and excreted through the kidneys, and its level is elevated in a variety of diseases [10].

These fibrinolytic markers, tPAI-1 and TM, are known to reflect arterial endothelial function. However, the relationship between serum tPAI-1, TM and pulmonary circulation has not been completely elucidated. In the present study, we aimed to evaluate if tPAI-1 and TM could be used as predictors of severity in patients with PAH.

Methods

We retrospectively reviewed the medical records of all consecutive patients who underwent RHC to assess cardiac function in Showa University Hospital between January 1, 2012, and March 31, 2018. This study was approved by the ethics committee of Showa University School of Medicine.

The details about patient history, physical examination, blood investigations, and echocardiography were evaluated. Patients with the following diseases that could affect serum tPAI-1 and TM levels were excluded from the study: (1) those on hemodialysis [11]; (2) those currently under treatment for malignant neoplasms; (3) those with hepatic failure [12, 13]; (4) those with congestive heart failure (CHF) NYHA grade III or more.

Blood samples were collected from patients at admission before RHC was performed. Fibrinolytic and coagulation marker levels, including tPAI-1, TM, D-dimer, thrombin-antithrombin complex (TAT), plasmin-α2 plasmin inhibitor complex (PIC), and prothrombin fragment 1 + 2 (PTF 1 + 2) were also measured. The tPAI-1 level was measured using the latex agglutination test (JCA-BM9130, JEOL Ltd., Tokyo, Japan). The TM level was measured using an enzyme-linked immunoassay (ELISA) kit, AP-X (Kyowa Medex Co Ltd., Tokyo, Japan) [14].

Statistical analysis

Data are reported as mean ± standard deviation. Continuous and categorical variables were compared using the Mann-Whitney *U* test or chi-squared test, as appropriate. We performed Cox's stepwise logistic regression analysis to identify significant independent characteristic markers that were related to mPAP. We then calculated the odds ratios (ORs) and 95% confidence intervals (CIs). Correlation analysis was performed using Spearman's rank correlation. We considered p values less than 0.05 to be statistically significant. JMP software version

Table 1 Patient characteristics

	Total Patients
N	100
Baseline characteristics	
Age (years)	68.9 ± 12.0
Male	38 (38%)
BMI	21.8 ± 4.2
Hypertension	42 (42%)
Diabetes mellitus	11 (11%)
Heart failure	30 (30%)
Collagen diseases	21 (21%)
Valvular diseases	11 (11%)
Pulmonary embolism	11 (11%)
Congenital heart diseases	9 (9%)
Respiratory diseases	7 (7%)
Ischemic heart diseases	6 (6%)
Idiopathic pulmonary hypertension	5 (5%)
Taking anticoagulants	41 (41%)
Hemodynamics	
Mean pulmonary artery pressure (mmHg)	25.1 ± 13.2
Pulmonary capillary wedge pressure (mmHg)	13.4 ± 9.0
Right ventricular pressure (mmHg)	40.7 ± 20.4
Echocardiography	
Ejection Fraction (%)	56.3 ± 12.8
Right Ventricular systolic pressure (mmHg)	51.2 ± 21.5
BNP (pg/ml)	464.8 ± 1367
Uric Acid (mg/dl)	6.1 ± 1.9
Estimated GFR (ml/min)	61.4 ± 21.8

Data are presented as mean ± SD or n (%)
BMI Body mass index

Table 2 Coagulation and Fibrinolytic markers

Makers	
D-dimer (μg/ml)	**3.24 ± 11.5**
Thrombomodulin (FU/ml)	3.0 ± 1.3
tPAI-1 (ng/ml)	38.0 ± 39.8
TAT (μg/l)	6.33 ± 11.1
PIC (μg/ml)	1.5 ± 2.8
PT F1 + 2 (pmol/l)	258 ± 217

Data are presented as mean ± SD or n (%)
tPAI-1 Total plasminogen activator inhibitor-1; *TAT* Thrombin antithrombin complex, *PIC* plasmin-α plasmin inhibitor complex, *PT F1 + 2* Prothrombin-fragment 1 + 2

14.0 (SAS, Cary, NC, USA) was used for the statistical analysis.

Results

We reviewed the medical records of 111 consecutive patients who underwent RHC. Of these, 4 were excluded because of ongoing hemodialysis, 3 for currently undergoing treatment of a malignant neoplasm, 2 for hepatic failure, and 2 for worsening CHF (NYHA grade III or more). The remaining 100 patients were included in the study, and their clinical characteristics are shown in Tables 1, 2.

The mean age of the participants was 68.9 ± 12.0 years, and thirty-eight patients (38%) were men. The underlying conditions comprised heart failure in 30 patients (30%), collagen diseases in 21 (21%), valvular diseases in 11 (11%), pulmonary embolism in 11 (11%), congenital heart diseases in 9 (9%), respiratory diseases in 7 (7%), ischemic heart diseases in 6 (6%), and idiopathic pulmonary hypertension in 5 (5%) (Table 1).

The average mPAP value was 25.1 ± 13.1 mmHg. The mPAP values had significant positive correlation with serum tPAI-1 ($\rho = 0.24$, $p = 0.042$) and uric acid ($\rho = 0.29$, $p = 0.0031$) levels (Table 1, Fig. 1). After categorizing the patients based on their mPAP values, those in the group with average mPAP values less than 25 mmHg (17.3 ± 4.3 mmHg) were observed to have a significant positive correlation between serum tPA-1 ($\rho = 0.34$, $p = 0.034$) and TM ($\rho = 0.34$, $p = 0.043$) levels and mPAP values (Fig. 2).

Both mean tPAI-1 (29.8 ± 23.3 ng/ml, $p = 0.047$) and uric acid (5.7 ± 1.8 mg/dl, $p = 0.026$) levels were significantly less in the group with lower mPAP values. A multivariate analysis, adjusted for age, gender, and BMI, revealed that tPAI-1 level alone was an independent characteristic marker (odds ratio 1.02, 95%CI 1.000–1.036, $p = 0.034$) of the severity of PAH (Tables 3, 4).

Discussion

The study results indicate that mPAP values have a significant positive correlation with serum tPAI-1 and uric acid levels in all enrolled patients. Among patients with mPAP values less than 25 mmHg PAP, a significant positive correlation is observed with serum tPAI-1 and TM levels. The uric acid levels revealed a lower degree of association than the tPAI-1 levels, which was found to be

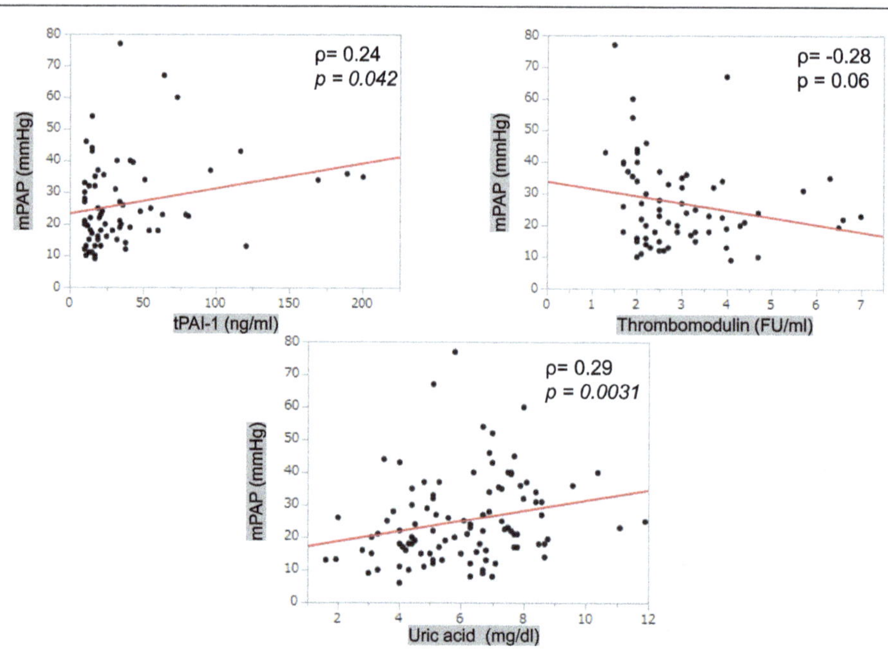

Fig. 1 Relationship between the mPAP levels and serum markers. A significant positive correlation is noted between the mPAP levels with serum tPAI-1 and uric acid values

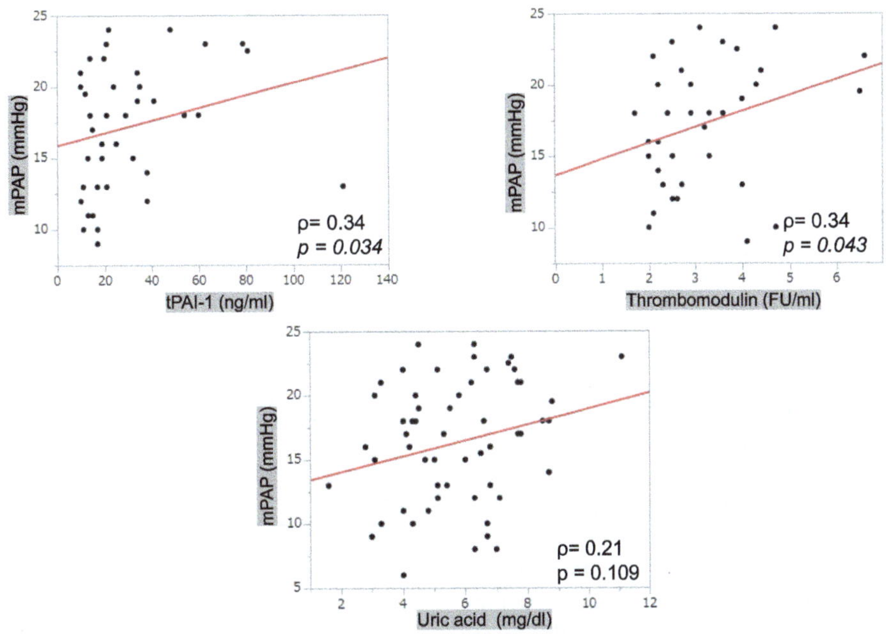

Fig. 2 Relationship between the mPAP and serum markers in those with levels less than 25 mmHg. The mPAP levels had significant positive correlation with serum tPAI-1 and TM values

an independent marker in the group with lower mPAP values.

The severity of PAH in patients is indicated by the mPAP levels evaluated by RHC, which is an invasive examination. Therefore, less-invasive and reliable biomarkers that reflect the disease status accurately are desired. Serum uric acid is a traditional biomarker that reflects endothelial function and is a potential risk factor for arteriosclerotic change [15, 16]. In the present study, uric acid levels revealed a significant positive correlation with mPAP values in all enrolled patients. This result is supported by the findings in some previous studies on atherosclerosis. However, in the group with mPAP values less than 25 mmHg, uric acid levels did not show a significant association with mPAP.

Table 3 Comparison of biomarkers, mPAP< 25 or not

	mPAP< 25	mPAP≥25	*P* value
N	58	42	
D-dimer	2.0 ± 2.4	4.9 ± 18	N.S.
Thrombomodulin	3.3 ± 1.3	2.6 ± 1.1	N.S.
tPAI-1	29.8 ± 23.3	49.0 ± 52.5	0.047
TAT	5.0 ± 9.2	8.1 ± 12.9	N.S.
PIC	1.2 ± 0.7	1.9 ± 4.1	N.S.
PT F1 + 2	262.7 ± 171.1	252.7 ± 260.7	N.S.
BNP	249.2 ± 294.9	752.2 ± 2024	N.S.
Uric Acid	5.7 ± 1.8	6.6 ± 2.0	0.026
Estimated GFR	63.9 ± 22.5	58.1 ± 20.4	N.S.

According to the diagnostic criteria for PAH, an mPAP level of 25 mmHg is the cut-off value. Many clinicians focus on the preclinical stage of PAH predominantly, and the patients with mPAP levels less than 25 mmHg should be on intensive, careful follow-up because the response to treatment changes dramatically according to the state of the disease [1–4]. Hence, we focused our investigations in this group. The results indicate that unlike serum uric acid levels, tPAI-1 levels alone are an independent characteristic marker in the group with lower mPAP levels. Additionally, the mPAP levels reveal a significant positive association with serum tPAI-1 and TM but not uric acid levels, which means that these markers could be potential predictors of severity in patients with PAH in their early stages.

tPAI-1 is an inhibitor of plasminogen, which regulates the systemic fibrinolytic system, and the levels indicate microvascular injury due to various conditions, including diabetes mellitus [17]. It complements the activities of protein anticoagulants and endothelial-derived platelet

Table 4 Multivariate logistic regression adjusted to age, gender, BMI

	Multivariate logistic regression	
	OR (95% CI)	*P* value
tPAI-1	1.02 (1.000–1.036)	0.034
UA	1.07 (0.793–1.434)	N.S.

Multivariate logistic regression adjusted to age, gender, BMI
OR Odds ratio, *CI* Confidence interval

inhibitors, such as proteins C, S, anti-thrombin III, and nitric oxide [5]. It is an endogenous defense mechanism for the prevention of atherosclerotic change, and there are some reports that the tPAI-1 levels are positively and independently associated with the degree of IMT [6, 7].

In contrast, TM is a factor that regulates the anticoagulation system by capturing thrombin and activating protein C. Once damage to endothelial cells occurs, TM expressed on endothelial cells is cleaved from the membrane, and the product is detectable in a soluble form in circulating peripheral blood. This indicates that TM can be a marker of endothelial cell damage [18–20]. The mechanism in advanced PAH is speculated to involve an increased release of tPAI-1 and TM from smooth muscle and endothelial cells caused by pulmonary vascular damage. This could result in elevated serum tPAI-1 and TM levels, as indicated in the present study. Ogawa et al. suggested that thrombin modulates pulmonary circulation through activation of the Akt pathway in smooth muscle cells among patients with PAH and chronic thromboembolic pulmonary hypertension (CTEPH) [21]. It also meant that TM levels could be altered due to endothelial dysfunction in the pulmonary artery. However, the concentration of circulating serum TM in peripheral blood would be saturated and the rest would be recruited by the kidney. In fact, there were no significant differences in the concentration of TM between the groups with mPAP levels less than or more than 25 mmHg.

We have demonstrated that mPAP levels have a significant positive correlation with serum tPAI-1 and TM but not uric acid values, which means that these markers could be potential predictors of severity in patients with PAH, especially in their early stages with mPAP levels less than 25 mmHg.

This study has few limitations. First, this study was retrospective in nature with its inherent defects; therefore, a prospective study is needed in the future to confirm the results. Second, the population size is small, and the patients were from heterogeneous backgrounds. A larger sample size that includes a larger cohort of severe cases would allow a more reliable statistical evaluation. Third, not plasma but serum was used to evaluate tPAI-1 and other markers in this study based on previous study [14]. Serum is the supernatant of clotted blood where platelets have released their contents. Hence there is a possibility that the value of tPAI-1 is overestimated since it is a component of the platelet releasate.

Conclusion

These results reveal that serum tPAI-1 and TM may be useful predictors that are similar to mPAP in patients with PAH. They could be beneficial in predicting severity in patients with PAH, especially in their early stages.

Abbreviations

BMI: Body mass index; CHF: Congestive heart failure; CI: Confidence intervals; CTEPH: Chronic thromboembolic pulmonary hypertension; ELISA: Enzyme-linked immune sorbent assay; IMT: Intima media thickness; OR: Odds ratio; PIC: Plasmin-α2 plasmin inhibitor complex; PT F1 + 2: Prothrombin-fragment 1 + 2; RHC: Right heart catheterization; SD: Standard deviation; TAT: Thrombin antithrombin; tPAI-1: Total plasminogen activator inhibitor-1; TM: Thrombomodulin

Authors' information (optional)

Showa University School of Medicine, Department of Medicine, Division of Cardiology.

Authors' contributions

M.S.: Design of the work, Drafting the manuscript. T.M.: Interpretation of data. H.T.: Interpretation of data. K.N.: Interpretation of data. H.T.: Interpretation of data. S.K.: Manuscript Drafting. Y.K.: Interpretation of data. T.S.: Manuscript Editing. The author(s) read and approved the final manuscript.

References

1. Galiè N, Humbert M, Vachiery JL, Gibbs S, Lang I, Torbicki A, et al. 2015 ESC/ERS Guidelines for the diagnosis and treatment of pulmonary hypertension: The Joint Task Force for the Diagnosis and Treatment of Pulmonary Hypertension of the European Society of Cardiology (ESC) and the European Respiratory Society (ERS): Endorsed by: Association for European Paediatric and Congenital Cardiology (AEPC), International Society for Heart and Lung Transplantation (ISHLT). Eur Heart J. 2016;37(1):67–119. https://doi.org/10.1093/eurheartj/ehv317.
2. Tamura Y, Kumamaru H, Satoh T, Miyata H, Ogawa A, Tanabe N, et al. Effectiveness and outcome of pulmonary arterial hypertension-specific therapy in Japanese patients with pulmonary arterial hypertension. Circ J. 2017;82(1):275–82. https://doi.org/10.1253/circj.CJ-17-0139.
3. Galiè N, Channick RN, Frantz RP, Grünig E, Jing ZC, Moiseeva O, et al. Risk stratification and medical therapy of pulmonary arterial hypertension. Eur Respir J. 2019;53(1):1801889. https://doi.org/10.1183/13993003.01889-2018.
4. Ogawa A, Ejiri K, Matsubara H. Long-term patient survival with idiopathic/heritable pulmonary arterial hypertension treated at a single center in Japan. Life Sci. 2014;118(2):414–9. https://doi.org/10.1016/j.lfs.2014.01.077.
5. Vaughan DE. PAI-1 and atherothrombosis. J Thromb Haemost. 2005;3(8):1879–83. https://doi.org/10.1111/j.1538-7836.2005.01420.x.
6. Carratala A, Martinez-Hervas S, Rodriguez-Borja E, Benito E, Real JT, Saez GT, et al. PAI-1 levels are related to insulin resistance and carotid atherosclerosis in subjects with familial combined hyperlipidemia. J Investig Med. 2018;66(1):17–21. https://doi.org/10.1136/jim-2017-000468.
7. Sakata T, Mannami T, Baba S, Kokubo Y, Kario K, Okamoto A, et al. Potential of free-form TFPI and PAI-1 to be useful markers of early atherosclerosis in a Japanese general population (the Suita study): association with the intimal-medial thickness of carotid arteries. Atherosclerosis. 2004;176(2):355–60. https://doi.org/10.1016/j.atherosclerosis.2004.05.017.
8. Li YH, Shi GY, Wu HL. The role of thrombomodulin in atherosclerosis: from bench to bedside. Cardiovasc Hematol Agents Med Chem. 2006;4(2):183–7. https://doi.org/10.2174/187152506776369953.
9. Chen PS, Wang KC, Chao TH, Chung HC, Tseng SY, Luo CY, et al. Recombinant Thrombomodulin exerts anti-autophagic action in endothelial cells and provides anti-atherosclerosis effect in apolipoprotein E deficient mice. Sci Rep. 2017 Jun 12;7(1):3284. https://doi.org/10.1038/s41598-017-03443-z.
10. Takano S, Kimura S, Ohdama S, Aoki N. Plasma thrombomodulin in health and diseases. Blood. 1990;76(10):2024–9. https://doi.org/10.1182/blood.V76.10.2024.2024.
11. Mizutani M, Yuzawa Y, Maruyama I, Sakamoto N, Matsuo S. Glomerular localization of thrombomodulin in human glomerulonephritis. Lab Investig. 1993;69(2):193–202.
12. Takatori M, Iwabuchi S, Ro S, Murayama M, Maeyama S, Uchikoshi T, et al. Increased serum levels and sinusoidal expression of thrombomodulin in acute liver damage. Thromb Res. 1999;93(3):113–20. https://doi.org/10.1016/S0049-3848(98)00167-4.
13. Biguzzi E, Franchi F, Bucciarelli P, Colombo M, Romeo R. Endothelial protein C receptor plasma levels increase in chronic liver disease, while

thrombomodulin plasma levels increase only in hepatocellular carcinoma. Thromb Res. 2007;120(2):289–93. https://doi.org/10.1016/j.thromres.2006.09.009.

14. Ochi A, Adachi T, Inokuchi K, Ogawa K, Nakamura Y, Chiba Y, et al. Effects of aging on the coagulation fibrinolytic system in outpatients of the cardiovascular department. Circ J. 2016;80(10):2133–40. https://doi.org/10.1253/circj.CJ-16-0530.
15. Iribarren C, Folsom AR, Eckfeldt JH, McGovern PG, Nieto FJ. Correlates of uric acid and its association with asymptomatic carotid atherosclerosis: the ARIC study. Atherosclerosis Risk in Communities. Ann Epidemiol. 1996;6(4):331–40. https://doi.org/10.1016/S1047-2797(96)00052-X.
16. Song M, Li N, Yao Y, Wang K, Yang J, Cui Q, et al. Longitudinal association between serum uric acid levels and multiterritorial atherosclerosis. J Cell Mol Med. 2019;23(8):4970–9. https://doi.org/10.1111/jcmm.14337.
17. Adly AA, Elbarbary NS, Ismail EA, Hassan SR. Plasminogen activator inhibitor-1 (PAI-1) in children and adolescents with type 1 diabetes mellitus: relation to diabetic micro-vascular complications and carotid intima media thickness. J Diabetes Complicat. 2014;28(3):340–7. https://doi.org/10.1016/j.jdiacomp.2014.01.011.
18. Abe H, Okajima K, Okabe H, Takatsuki K, Binder BR. Granulocyte proteases and hydrogen peroxide synergistically inactivate thrombomodulin of endothelial cells in vitro. J Lab Clin Med. 1994;123(6):874–81.
19. Ishii H, Uchiyama H, Kazama M. Soluble thrombomodulin antigen in conditioned medium is increased by damage of endothelial cells. Thromb Haemost. 1991;65(05):618–23. https://doi.org/10.1055/s-0038-1648199.
20. Boffa MC, Karochkine M, Bérard M. Plasma thrombomodulin as a marker of endothelium damage. Nouv Rev Fr Hematol. 1991;33(6):529–30.
21. Ogawa A, Firth AL, Ariyasu S, Yamadori I, Matsubara H, Song S, et al. Thrombin-mediated activation of Akt signaling contributes to pulmonary vascular remodeling in pulmonary hypertension. Physiol Rep. 2013;1(7):e00190.

19

Monitoring coagulation-fibrinolysis activation prompted timely diagnosis of hemophagocytic lymphohistiocytosis-related disseminated intravascular coagulation

Liqin Ling, Xunbei Huang, Chaonan Liu, Juan Liao and Jing Zhou*

Abstract

Background: Timely diagnosis of disseminated intravascular coagulation (DIC) in hemophagocytic lymphohistiocytosis (HLH) patients is crucial but challenging, as HLH interferes with the results of the laboratory tests included in the DIC score system.

Case presentation: Here, we reported a case of lymphoma-associated HLH, in which coagulation-fibrinolysis activation /inhibition markers (TAT, tPAIC, and PIC), prompted timely diagnosis of early stage DIC (initial phase of microvascular thrombosis, yet non-overt), prior to the development of organ failures and/or bleedings.

Conclusions: This report highlights the importance of the implementation of new biomarkers (such as TAT, tPAIC, and PIC), into the diagnostic work-up for coagulation disorders. These biomarkers are directly suggestive of microthrombus formation, therefore they can be of paramount importance in diagnosing DIC with complicated etiologies, such as hematological diseases-related DIC.

Keywords: Coagulation, Fibrinolysis, Hemophagocytic lymphohistiocytosis, Disseminated intravascular coagulation

Background

Disseminated intravascular coagulation (DIC) has been observed in hemophagocytic lymphohistiocytosis (HLH) patients in nearly 50 % of cases [1, 2]. DIC is approved to be associated with higher mortality in HLH patients [2]. Therefore, it is vital to diagnose DIC early in HLH patients to take timely treatments options. However, it is challenging to diagnose DIC in HLH patients, as HLH has been shown to interfere with the major indices used in the DIC score system, including platelet count and fibrinogen concentration [1, 2]. Therefore, much effort has been given to the development of more specific biomarkers to support DIC diagnosis. Here, we have discussed the value of coagulation-fibrinolysis activation /inhibition markers in the early diagnosis of DIC before the manifestation of obvious clinical symptoms.

Case presentation

A 47-year-old man was diagnosed with $CD30^+$ lymphoma with HLH complications one year ago. He had already been through four courses of chemotherapy, including one course of CHOP (cyclophosphamide, doxorubicin, vincristine, and prednisone) and three courses of BV-CHP (brentuximab vedotin in combination with cyclophosphamide, doxorubicin, and prednisone). He

* Correspondence: zhoujinghuaxi@163.com
Department of Laboratory Medicine, West China Hospital, Sichuan University, No. 37 Guo Xue Alley, Sichuan 610041 Chengdu, China

was scheduled for his fifth chemotherapy on Nov 19, 2020. However, on the day of the hospitalization, his HLH was still significantly active (interleukin-2 receptor 32,560 U /mL, ferritin 12,573 ng /mL). Moreover, he was febrile and thus suspected with infection. Therefore, his clinicians decided to suspend his chemotherapy until his HLH and infection got controlled with corresponding treatments. The patient was therefore given etoposide and dexamethasone (treatment of HLH in accordance to the HLH-2004 protocol [3]), antibiotics (treatment of infection), and further symptomatic treatments.

However, his condition was not improving during this hospitalization. He had started to demonstrate refractory fibrinogenemia since Nov 22, 2020, and he was given fibrinogen infusion accordingly. The cause of his fibrinogenemia was thought to be primary fibrinolysis at that time, considering that primary fibrinolysis frequently occurs in HLH patients due to a massive endogenous release of tissue plasminogen activator from activated monocytes [1]. Therefore, antifibrinolytic therapy was commenced since Nov 27, 2020 (tranexamic acid 1 g per day) to prevent bleeding complications (the patient had suffered gastrointestinal hemorrhage during his last chemotherapy). Unfortunately, his fibrinogenemia was still rapidly progressing, his plasma fibrinogen concentration decreased to an undetectable level (<0.5 g/L) on Dec 13, 2020, even though the antifibrinolytic therapy was effective (his plasma levels of fibrinogen/fibrin degradation products, including FDP and D-dimer, had been decreasing since the antifibrinolytic therapy was commenced) (shown in supplementary Table 1).

During this period, his platelet count was decreasing over time (from 23×10^9 /L on Nov 22, to 2×10^9 /L on Dec 13), his red blood cell (RBC) count was slightly decreasing (from 2.42×10^{12} /L on Nov 22, to 2.07×10^{12} /L on Dec 13), and his white blood cell (WBC) count was fluctuating due to multiple infusions of recombinant human granulocyte colony-stimulating factor (G-CSF) (shown in supplementary Table 1). And there had been no clinical signs of thrombosis or bleeding, or liver dysfunction yet.

It seems incomprehensible that his fibrinogenemia was not accompanied by either thrombosis /hyperfibrinolysis (excessive consumption) or hepatic impairment (decreased synthesis). His fibrinogenemia could not be improved until we found the answer to this puzzling question.

Discussion and Conclusions

Acquired fibrinogenemia is most frequently caused by decreased synthesis, hemodilution, or excessive consumption [4]. In our patient, decreased synthesis was excluded, because on Dec 13, 2020, his coagulation factor VII (103 %), a marker of hepatocellular synthetic function [5], was still within the normal range (70-150 %). Besides, his albumin level had been stable since hospitalization (around 30 g/L), although it was lower than the normal range (40-55 g/L), it could be explained by his overall unhealthy status. Hemodilution was also ruled out as there wasn't any presence of a massive fluid infusion. Therefore, excessive consumption was suspected. Both thrombin and plasmin can use fibrinogen as a substrate, consequently both coagulation activation and fibrinolysis activation can result in excessive consumption of fibrinogen [6, 7]. Since fibrinolysis was inhibited by tranexamic acid in this patient, systemic coagulation activation, which can result in microvascular thrombosis (the early or compensatory stage of DIC) [8], seemed to be a reasonable cause of his fibrinogenemia.

However, diagnosing DIC in this patient was very challenging, especially during the early stage (initial phase of microvascular thrombosis). Clinically, microvascular thrombosis is not readily apparent as clot formation primarily involves the microvasculature. It usually gets noticed during the presentation of organ failures [9], when it is already too late. Therefore, timely diagnosis of DIC, especially at an early stage, should not be relied on clinical manifestations. The diagnosis of DIC was further exacerbated in this case due to the issues that occurred in the standard laboratory diagnostic work-up. Primarily, his fibrinogenemia had already impaired global coagulation parameters (prothrombin time, PT; international normalized ratio, INR; activated partial thromboplastin time, aPTT; and thrombin time, TT), which are the most prevalent tests implemented in a coagulation lab. Secondly, his antifibrinolytic therapy had influenced FDP /D-dimer testing, which could also be indicative of ongoing coagulation activation otherwise [10]. Lastly and most importantly, platelet phagocytosis in his HLH background could confound thrombocytopenia caused by coagulation activation [11], diminishing the value of thrombocytopenia.

Theoretically, regardless of the underlying conditions, unbalanced coagulation-fibrinolysis activation (more thrombin, less plasmin) is inherent to the early stage of DIC [9], which is a prerequisite for microthrombus formation. Thus coagulation-fibrinolysis activation /inhibition markers could be specific measures of DIC. Consistent with this theory, thrombin activation marker (thrombin-antithrombin complex, TAT, normal range: < 4.0 ng /mL) and plasmin inhibition marker (tissue plasminogen activator-plasminogen activator inhibitor complex, t-PAIC, normal range: < 10.5 ng /mL) were elevated in this patient on Dec 13, 2020 (TAT, 52 ng /mL; t-PAIC, 95.6 ng /mL), while plasmin activation marker (plasmin-α2-plasmin inhibitor complex, PIC, normal range: < 0.8 μg /mL) was within the normal range (PIC, 0.27 μg /mL). These results highly suggested a prothrombotic state (early stage of DIC) in this patient, even though there was no specific clinical signs yet.

However, the diagnostic value of these markers in DIC has not been well-defined, DIC diagnosis in this case could not be confirmed yet, besides, the patient refused to take a biopsy. Anyway, these results reminded us to focus on the course of the disease in this patient, which resulted in finding additional evidence to support a diagnosis of early DIC stage in this case. First, we performed tests for his coagulation factors on Dec 16, 2020. We found that several coagulation factors were diminished (FV 55 %, FIX 69 %, FX 46 %, FXI 46 %, FXII 43 %) and TAT was more elevated (75.2 ng /mL), suggesting that thrombin was chronically consuming coagulation factors in the patient, indicating a chronic systemic coagulation activation. Secondly, after carefully reviewing his routine blood test results, we found an increasing percentage of schistocytes since his hospitalization (from 0.1 % on Nov 22, to 1.5 % on Dec 16, shown in Fig. 1), which was an important marker of microthrombus formation [12]. Lastly, even though there was no prevalent clinical manifestations of renal/liver dysfunction, we found that renal/liver function markers were changing over time which indicated organ impairments (not classified as organ failures as most of the markers were still within the normal ranges) (shown in Fig. 2). Eventually, the diagnosis of DIC in this patient was confirmed on Dec 16, 2020. However, there was still no prevalent clinical signs of renal/liver dysfunction. Our report here demonstrates that coagulation-fibrinolysis activation /inhibition markers could help to prompt timely diagnosis of the early stage of DIC before it could progress to organ failures and/or bleedings.

After his DIC was diagnosed, his antifibrinolytic therapy was stopped immediately, so that his fibrinolysis could get ameliorated, and therefore avoid more microvascular thrombosis. Besides, his DIC could signify that his HLH was not under control with treatments aimed at HLH itself. His clinicians decided to start his fifth chemotherapy course immediately, because his lymphoma was the root cause of his HLH. It should be noted that the fifth chemotherapy was ABVD course (adriamycin, bleomycin, vinblastin, dacarbazine), then changed to AVD because the patient was allergic to bleomycin. This course was different from his previous chemotherapies, because his clinicians thought that prior chemotherapies might not be practical due to his worsening condition. The patients' condition improved after these treatments, several days after he finished his fifth chemotherapy, on Dec 24, 2020, his TAT decreased to 19.6 ng /mL, PIC increased to 2.49 μg /mL and and t-PAIC decreased to 15.6 ng /mL. And his fibrinogenemia had been ameliorated ever since the above-mentioned managements were instituted (shown in supplementary Table 1). Other laboratory test results were also improving, including platelet counts, renal/liver function markers, et al. (shown in supplementary Table 1).

It is challenging to diagnose DIC early in patients with HLH, as HLH interferes with the major indices used in the DIC score system. HLH itself shares two coagulation abnormalities (thrombocytopenia, hypofibrinogenemia) with DIC [1, 2]. Besides, as mentioned above, HLH related antifibrinolytic therapy can diminish the diagnostic value of FDP/D-dimer. In addition to HLH, several other clinical conditions may also interfere with the current diagnostic work-up for DIC. Examples include hepatic cirrhosis (instead of coagulation activation, thrombocytopenia might be caused by hypersplenism, coagulation factor deficiency (including

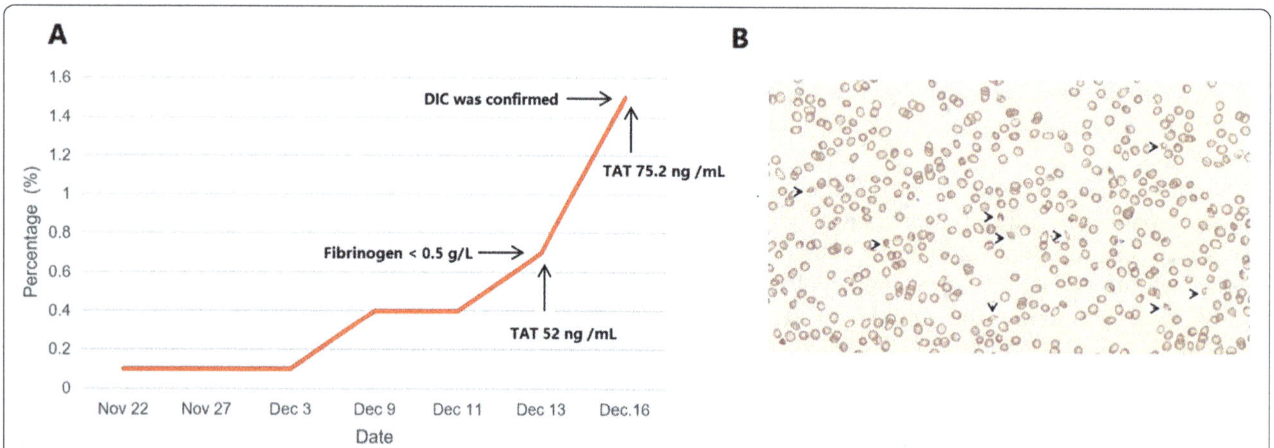

Fig. 1 Schistocytes in the peripheral smear as a supplementary evidence of microthrombus formation during early stage DIC. **A** the percentage of schistocyte was increasing over time; **B** a representative image of schistocytes in the peripheral smear on Dec 16, 2020, black arrows (schistocytes)

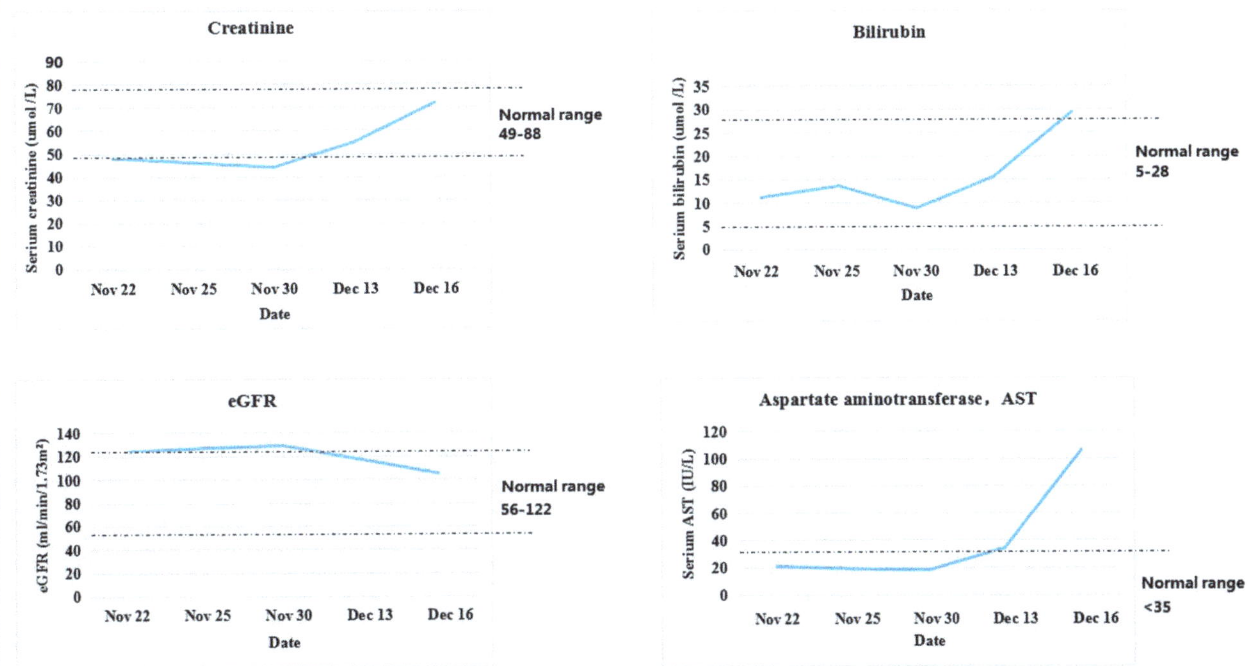

Fig. 2 Change of some serum biochemical indicators as another supplementary evidence of microthrombus formation during early stage DIC. All parameters seemed stable until Dec 13, 2020, but got worse on Dec 16, 2020, indicating organ impairments

hypofibrinogenemia) might caused by decreased synthesis) [13], or bone marrow suppression (thrombocytopenia due to less thrombopoiesis) [14], or heparin-induced thrombocytopenia (thrombocytopenia due to excess platelet consumption) [15].

To compensate for the aforementioned issues, parameters directly suggestive of coagulation activation might be more relevant [9, 16], such as prothrombin fragment 1 + 2 (F1 + 2), *ex vivo* thrombin generation assay, and TAT testing. Besides, disturbed fibrinolysis is also an essential contributor to the progress of DIC. In the early phase of DIC, fibrinolysis might be impaired so that microthrombus forms, but fibrinolysis might be over-activated at the late stage of DIC, which leads to bleeding tendency [9, 17]. Therefore, markers of fibrinolysis should also be considered, such as t-PAIC and PIC. Tests for TAT, PIC, t-PAIC have already been standardized, automated, and implemented in some routine coagulation laboratories in Asian countries such as China and Japan [18]. We measured these markers via qualitative chemiluminescence enzyme immunoassay performed on HISCL automated analyzers (HISCL-5000, Sysmex, Japan) [18]. TAT is considered a sensitive marker of thrombin generation, while PIC is an indicator of plasmin generation. There are already studies demonstrating that TAT could predict DIC development in sepsis patients at inclusion [18, 19], TAT was higher in patients who subsequently developed DIC than in patients who did not develop DIC. Moreover, TAT in combination with PIC was more potent than TAT alone [20], compared to patients with elevated TAT plus elevated PIC, which indicated a new balance of thrombin/plasmin generation, patients with elevated TAT alone (PIC was not elevated) had a poorer prognosis (higher risk to develop multiple organ failures). This is consistent with the theory that unbalanced coagulation-fibrinolysis activation is inherent to DIC development [9].

It has been proved that the prognosis of DIC becomes very poor if not treated timely before clinical symptoms manifest (organ failures and/or bleedings) [21, 22]. Currently, there are several well-known scoring systems for DIC diagnosis, all these systems include laboratory indices like platelet count, PT, fibrinogen, FDP/D-dimer [9]. However, as discussed above, these markers can be easily influenced, making it challenging to diagnose DIC at an early stage. Our report here demonstrated that coagulation-fibrinolysis activation /inhibition markers (TAT, t-PAIC, PIC) helped diagnose DIC at an early stage despite some indices (platelet count, PT, FDP/D-dimer) in the DIC score system being influenced. Combined with literature reviewing, it would be prudent to pioneer the implementation of coagulation-fibrinolysis activation /inhibition markers into the diagnostic work-up for DIC so that timely diagnosis and personalized management of DIC can be achieved. In addition, the Japanese Society on thrombosis and hemostasis is proposing a new DIC diagnostic criteria, in which TAT is included as a major index [22].

Abbreviations

DIC: Disseminated intravascular coagulation; HLH: Hemophagocytic lymphohistiocytosis; TAT: Thrombin-antithrombin complex; tPAIC: Tissue plasminogen activator-plasminogen activator inhibitor complex; PIC: Plasmin-α2-plasmin inhibitor complex; FDP: Fibrinogen/fibrin degradation products; PT: Prothrombin time; aPTT: Activated partial thromboplastin time; TT: Thrombin time; INR: International normalized ratio; CHOP: Cyclophosphamide, doxorubicin, vincristine, and prednisone; BV-CHP: Brentuximab vedotin in combination with cyclophosphamide, doxorubicin, and prednisone; ABVD: Adriamycin, bleomycin, vinblastin, dacarbazine

Supplementary Information

Additional file 1: Supplementary Table 1. Laboratory tests results.

Acknowledgements

We thank Swati Dass and Vivin Karthik for helping to improve the English language within this manuscript.

Authors' contributions

Liqin Ling and Jing Zhou wrote the manuscript. Xunbei and Chaonan Liu performed the laboratory tests mentioned in this report. Juan Liao collected all related clinical information of this patient. The author(s) read and approved the final manuscript.

References

1. Valade S, Mariotte E, Azoulay E. Coagulation disorders in hemophagocytic lymphohistiocytosis/macrophage activation syndrome. Crit Care Clin. 2020; 36(2):415–26.
2. Valade S, Azoulay E, Galicier L, Boutboul D, Zafrani L, Stepanian A, et al. Coagulation disorders and bleedings in critically ill patients with hemophagocytic lymphohistiocytosis. Medicine (Baltimore). 2015;94(40): e1692.
3. Henter JI, Horne A, Aricó M, Egeler RM, Filipovich AH, Imashuku S, et al. HLH-2004: diagnostic and therapeutic guidelines for hemophagocytic lymphohistiocytosis. Pediatr Blood Cancer. 2007;48(2):124–31.
4. Besser MW, MacDonald SG. Acquired hypofibrinogenemia: current perspectives. J Blood Med. 2016;7:217–225.
5. Rodríguez-Iñigo E, Bartolomé J, Quiroga JA, Hedner U, Suárez A, Tomás JF, et al. Expression of factor VII in the liver of patients with liver disease: correlations with the disease severity and impairment in the hemostasis. Blood Coagul Fibrinolysis. 2001;12(3):193–9.
6. Mosesson MW. Fibrinogen and fibrin structure and functions. J Thromb Haemost. 2005;3(8):1894–1904.
7. Jian JW, Chiu WC, Chang HT, Hsu PH, Huang CC. Fibrinolysis and thrombosis of fibrinogen-modified gold nanoparticles for detection of fibrinolytic-related proteins. Anal Chim Acta. 2013;24:67–72.
8. Taylor FB Jr, Toh CH, Hoots WK, Wada H, Levi M. Towards definition, clinical and laboratory criteria, and a scoring system for disseminated intravascular coagulation. Thromb Haemost. 2001;86(5):1327–30.
9. Adelborg K, Larsen JB, Hvas AM. Disseminated intravascular coagulation: epidemiology, biomarkers, and management. Br J Haematol. 2021;192(5): 803–18.
10. Pabinger I, van Es N, Heinze G, Posch F, Riedl J, Reitter EM, et al. A clinical prediction model for cancer-associated venous thromboembolism: a development and validation study in two independent prospective cohorts. Lancet Haematol. 2018;5(7):e289-98.
11. Aricò M, Danesino C, Pende D, Moretta L. Pathogenesis of haemophagocytic lymphohistiocytosis. Br J Haematol. 2001;114(4):761–9.
12. Lesesve JF, Martin M, Banasiak C, André-Kerneïs E, Bardet V, Lusina D, et al. Schistocytes in disseminated intravascular coagulation. Int J Lab Hematol. 2014;36(4):439–43.
13. Drolz A, Horvatits T, Roedl K, Rutter K, Staufer K, Kneidinger N, et al. Coagulation parameters and major bleeding in critically ill patients with cirrhosis. Hepatology. 2016;64(2):556–68.
14. Shin SY, Cho OH, Bae IG. Bone marrow suppression and hemophagocytic histiocytes are common findings in Korean severe fever with thrombocytopenia syndrome patients. Yonsei Med J. 2016;57(5):1286–9.
15. Lovecchio F. Heparin-induced thrombocytopenia. Clin Toxicol (Phila). 2014; 52(6):579–83.
16. Berry LR, Chan AK. Thrombin generation. Methods Mol Biol. 2013;992:139–54.
17. Levi M. Pathogenesis and diagnosis of disseminated intravascular coagulation. Int J Lab Hematol. 2018;40(Suppl 1):15–20.
18. Mei H, Jiang Y, Luo L, Huang R, Su L, Hou M, et al. Evaluation the combined diagnostic value of TAT, PIC, tPAIC, and sTM in disseminated intravascular coagulation: a multi-center prospective observational study. Thromb Res. 2019;173:20–6.
19. Koyama K, Madoiwa S, Nunomiya S, Koinuma T, Wada M, Sakata A, et al. Combination of thrombin-antithrombin complex, plasminogen activator inhibitor-1, and protein C activity for early identification of severe coagulopathy in initial phase of sepsis: a prospective observational study. Crit Care. 2014;13(1):R13.
20. Asakura H, Ontachi Y, Mizutani T, Kato M, Saito M, Kumabashiri I, et al. An enhanced fibrinolysis prevents the development of multiple organ failure in disseminated intravascular coagulation in spite of much activation of blood coagulation. Crit Care Med. 2001;29(6):1164–8.
21. Wada H, Hasegawa K, Watanabe M, Rinsho Ketsueki. DIC: an update on diagnosis and treatment. Rinsho Ketsueki. 2017;58(5):523–9.
22. Asakura H, Takahashi H, Uchiyama T, Eguchi Y, Okamoto K, Kawasugi K, et al. Proposal for new diagnostic criteria for DIC from the Japanese Society on Thrombosis and Hemostasis. Thromb J. 2016;14:42.

20

Association of circulating proprotein convertase subtilisin/kexin type 9 concentration, prothrombin time and cardiovascular outcomes

Jia Peng, Ming-Ming Liu, Hui-Hui Liu, Yuan-Lin Guo, Na-Qiong Wu, Qian Dong, Jie Qian, Ke-Fei Dou, Cheng-Gang Zhu* and Jian-Jun Li*

Abstract

Background: Proprotein convertase subtilisin/kexin type 9 (PCSK9) is considered to have multiple roles in the development of atherosclerosis, which is recently reported to participate in the thrombotic process. We aimed to examine the relationship between PCSK9 concentration, coagulation indexes and cardiovascular events.

Methods: A total of 2293 consecutive patients with angina-like chest pain and without lipid-lowering drugs treatment were enrolled and followed up for major adverse cardiovascular events (MACEs). Circulating PCSK9 concentration was determined by ELISA. The routine coagulation tests including activated partial thromboplastin time (APTT), prothrombin time (PT) and thrombin time were performed. The associations between PCSK9 concentration, routine coagulation indicators and MACEs were analyzed.

Results: Patients with high PCSK9 levels had lower PT and APTT levels (all $p < 0.05$). However, PCSK9 concentration was only independently and negatively correlated with PT ($\beta = -0.115$, $p < 0.001$). During a mean of 38.3 months, 186 (8.1%) MACEs were occurred. Multiple Cox regression analysis indicated high PCSK9 or low PT levels as risk factors related to MACEs. When the prognosis was analyzed by the combination of PCSK9 and PT levels, patients with high PCSK9 and low PT had higher incidence of MACEs compared to those with low PCSK9 and high PT.

Conclusions: Our study firstly suggested that PCSK9 concentration was negatively correlated with plasma levels of PT. Furthermore, high PCSK9 and low PT were associated with MACEs and the combination of PCSK9 with PT had an addictive effect on predicting cardiovascular outcomes in patients with chest pain, which was useful for further subdivision of cardiovascular risks.

Keywords: PCSK9, Coagulation, PT, Atherosclerosis, Cardiovascular risks

* Correspondence: fuwaizcg@126.com; lijianjun938@126.com
Cardiometabolic Medicine Center, State Key Laboratory of Cardiovascular Disease, Fu Wai Hospital, National Center for Cardiovascular Diseases, Chinese Academy of Medical Sciences and Peking Union Medical College, No 167 BeiLiShi Road, XiCheng District, Beijing 100037, China

Introduction

Atherosclerotic cardiovascular disease (ASCVD) has become the one of major cause of mortality through the world. Currently, there is more convincing evidence that clotting activation resulting in hypercoagulability participates the formation of thrombi after rupture of atherosclerotic lesion, therefore, promoting development of coronary artery disease (CAD) [1–3]. Activated partial thromboplastin time (APTT), prothrombin time (PT) and thrombin time (TT) are contained in routine coagulation screening tests, reflecting activation of coagulation system and thrombotic state by quantified numbers, which is related to the formation of thrombosis and acute ischemic events [4]. APTT and PT are involved in intrinsic and extrinsic coagulation pathway respectively, which is associated not only with venous thromboembolism but also with arterial thrombosis. Moreover, a large-scale genome-wide association study (GWAS) has suggested that APTT and PT are relevant to the elevated risks of CAD in gene level [5]. However, the role of coagulation in predicting cardiovascular risks need to further evaluate.

Recently, proprotein convertase subtilisin/kexin type 9 (PCSK9) is considered as a major risk factor for CAD, which plays an important role in cholesterol metabolism by increasing the degradation of hepatic low density lipoprotein cholesterol receptors (LDLR), thereby resulting in increasing circulating low density lipoprotein cholesterol (LDL-C) levels [6, 7]. Thereafter, PCSK9 inhibitors have been recommended to apply in patients with severe hypercholesterolemia or with statin intolerance to reduce lipid-related cardiovascular risk according to guideline for the management of dyslipidemia [8]. More importantly, PCSK9 has been prompted to be associated with pro-coagulation to aggravate atherosclerosis, apart from regulating plasma LDL-C levels [9]. Furthermore, our previous study, found that circulating PCSK9 concentration was independently correlated with fibrinogen, a major coagulation-related protein in circulation, in stable CAD patients [10]. Nevertheless, there are no studies concerning the correlation between circulating PCSK9 concentration and routine coagulation tests and their relationship with major adverse cardiovascular events (MACEs) until now .

The aim of this present study was to explore the potential association between PCSK9 and routine coagulation indexes including APTT, PT and TT, and to evaluate the predictive ability of PCSK9 and routine coagulation indexes in MACEs among untreated patients with chest pain.

Patients and methods

Study design and population

The present study protocol was complied with Declaration of Helsinki and was approved by the hospital ethics review board (Fu Wai Hospital & National Center for Cardiovascular Diseases, Beijing, China). Every patient signed the informed written consent before enrolled in this study.

The flowchart of the current study was presented in supplementary Fig. S1. We consecutively recruited 2583 patients with angina-like chest pain from October 2012 to April 2018 and 2433 patients who completed the determination of PCSK9 and routine coagulation tests including APTT, PT and TT.

Because lipid-lowering medications could increase circulating PCSK9 concentration and anti-coagulation drugs could prolong clotting time, confounding study results, patients taking any lipid-lowering agents within 3 months and taking any anti-coagulation agents within 1 month prior to entering the study were excluded from the present study. In addition, patients with acute or heart failure (left ventricular ejection fraction, left ventricular ejection fraction $< 45\%$), acute coronary syndrome, significant hematologic disorders (white blood cell count $\leq 3.0 \times 10^9$/L or $\geq 20 \times 10^9$/L), infectious or systematic inflammatory disease, thyroid dysfunction, severe liver and/or renal insufficiency and malignant disease were excluded from this study. 2348 patients were followed-up for MACEs. During a follow-up with a mean of 38.3 months, 91 patients lost to follow-up. Finally, a total of 2293 patients with angina-like chest pain were included in this study. All patients were divided according to the median of PCSK9 concentration (low/high PCSK9 groups) and further stratified by the mean of PT levels (low/high PT groups).

In the current study, 1447 patients were proven stable CAD according to following diagnostic criteria. Stable CAD was defined as typical angina-like chest pain, a positive treadmill exercise test (> 1 mm ST-segment depression), and stable obstructive lesion > 50% in at least 1 of the 3 major coronary arteries or major branches assessed by at least two independent senior interventional cardiologists who had no knowledge of the patients' clinical characteristics and biochemical data. 1418 patients were diagnosed with hypertension. The definition of hypertension was repeated systolic and/or diastolic blood pressure ≥ 140 and/or ≥ 90 mmHg on 2 different occasions or if patients were currently taking antihypertensive drugs. 538 patients with diabetes was diagnosed as fasting serum glucose levels ≥ 6.99 mmol/L in multiple determinations or patients were being treated with oral hypoglycemic agents or insulin.

Blood sample measurement

Fasting blood samples were obtained for all patients at admission and collected into EDTA-containing tubes. Plasma samples were prepared by centrifugation at 3500×g twice for 10 min each at 15–18 °C and were stored at − 80 °C until analysis. Plasma PCSK9 concentration was measured using a high-sensitivity, quantitative sandwich enzyme immunoassay (Quantikine ELISA, R&D Systems Europe Ltd) according to our previous study [11]. The lower limit of detection was 0.096 ng/mL. APTT testing was performed by the aPTT-SP® reagent with synthetic phospholipids and silica as activators (Instrumentation Laboratory, Bedford, USA) and PT testing was performed by the PT-Fibrinogen HS Plus® reagent (HemosIL® Instrumentation Laboratory. Bedford, USA) [12]. TT was performed by thrombin reagent. Plasma D dimer level was measured by Stago evolution (France). The plasma samples used to determine coagulation function test were not diluted and the results were automatically measured by the instruments of the Fu Wai hospital laboratory. The plasma levels of fibrinogen were quantitatively measured by the method of Clauss and a Stago autoanalyzer with STA Fibrinogen kit (Diagnostic Stago, Taverny, France). The concentrations of the plasma triglyceride (TG), total cholesterol (TC), high density lipoprotein cholesterol (HDL-C), LDL-C, apolipoprotein (apo) B, apoA-I and glucose were measured by automatic biochemistry analyser (Hitachi 7150, Japan). Hemoglobin A1C (HbA1C) was measured using Tosoh Automated Glycohemoglobin Analyser (HLC-723G8, Tokyo, Japan). The concentrations of high-sensitivity C-reactive protein (hsCRP) were determined using immunoturbidimetry (Beckmann Assay 360, Bera, CA, USA).

Follow-up for MACEs

Every patient was followed-up by professional technicians through telephones every six month. They were blinded to the clinical data of all patients and the purpose of this study until death occurred or the last day of follow-up period. The present study was followed to the end of June 30, 2019. The following MACEs were defined as nonfatal myocardial infarction (MI), coronary revascularization, hospitalization for unstable angina, ischemic stroke and cardiovascular death. Nonfatal MI was diagnosed as typical angina-like chest pain with increased cardiac troponins or typical electrocardiogram changes of MI. Coronary revascularization included percutaneous coronary intervention and coronary artery bypass grafting later than 90 days after their discharge. Unstable angina was confirmed if patients appeared new-onset severe angina or rest angina with normal serum levels of cardiac enzymes that required admission. Ischemic stroke was described by acute cerebral infarction symptoms and cerebral diagnostic imaging.

Statistical analysis

Clinical and laboratory data are expressed as mean ± standard deviation (normally distributed continuous data) or median with interquartile range (skewed distributed continuous data). Categorical variables were expressed as frequencies and percentages. Comparisons between categorical data were performed with Chi Squared tests, while continuous variables were assessed by unpaired t test (for normal distribution) or nonparametric Mann-Whitney test (for skewed distribution). To evaluate the association between log-transformed PCSK9 and other parameters, Pearson correlation analysis or spearman correlation analysis was used. Univariate linear regression analysis was used to analyze the relationship between APTT, PT and TT and lipid parameters including TC, TG, LDL-C and HDL-C. Stepwise multivariable linear regression analysis was performed to determine the relationship between PCSK9 and PT. To examine the relationship of PCSK9, coagulation-related indexes with MACEs, Kaplan-Meier curve and Cox regression analyses were used to calculate the event-free survival rates and hazard ratios (HR) for MACEs with 95% confidence interval (CI) of different PCSK9 and/ or PT subgroups. Statistical analysis was performed with Statistical Package for Social Sciences version 25.0. A $p < 0.05$ was considered to be statistically different.

Results

Baseline characteristics

In the present study, we consecutively enrolled 2293 patients (1387 males, mean age 55.6 ± 11.0 years) and the baseline characteristics including clinical data and laboratory parameters classified by the occurrence of MACEs were showed in Table 1. The circulating PCSK9 concentration ranged from 70.01 ng/mL to 551.97 ng/mL (median = 228.48 ng/mL). Additionally, the mean of APTT, PT and TT value were 36.25 ± 3.9 s, 12.75 ± 0.64 s and 16.40 ± 1.25 s. Patients with MACEs were older, had higher percentage of CAD and DM, lower percentage of family history of CAD, higher TC, LDL-C and HbA1C levels than that without MACEs (all $p < 0.05$). Meanwhile, a higher plasma of PCSK9 and fibrinogen concentration and a lower PT level were found in participants with MACEs compared to those without MACEs (all $p < 0.05$). There were no significant different regarding the proportion of male, the percentage of hypertension, smoking status, drinking status, the baseline levels of BMI, systolic and diastolic blood pressure, TG, HDL-C, glucose, hsCRP, APTT, TT, D dimer and platelet counts, and the usage of medications (all $p > 0.05$). Because hypercoagulability expresses itself in the short interval between the normal clotting time and the minimal clotting time and shortening of the PT is very sensitive to hypocoagulation but relatively insensitive to hypercoagulation, we defined the transformation of prothrombin time (PT-t) as the inverse of the difference between PT in patients and the minimal PT of normal

Table 1 The baseline characteristics in this study

	Overall	MACEs	non-MACEs	
	n = 2293	*n* = 186	*n* = 2107	*p*
Clinical data				
Age (years)	55.62 ± 11.01	57.73 ± 9.8	55.44 ± 11.09	0.006
Male sex n(%)	1387 (60.5)	111 (59.7)	1276 (60.6)	0.813
BMI (kg/m2)	25.63 ± 3.38	25.95 ± 3.37	25.6 ± 3.38	0.175
CAD n(%)	1447 (63.1)	142 (76.3)	1305 (61.9)	< 0.001
DM n(%)	538 (23.5)	60 (32.3)	478 (22.7)	0.003
Hypertension n(%)	1418 (61.8)	125 (67.2)	1293 (61.4)	0.116
Smoking n(%)	788 (34.4)	63 (33.9)	725 (34.4)	0.882
Drinking n(%)	468 (20.4)	44 (23.7)	424 (20.1)	0.252
Family history of CAD n(%)	514 (22.4)	30 (16.1)	484 (23)	0.032
SBP (mmHg)	128.05 ± 18.01	129.57 ± 16.49	127.92 ± 18.13	0.231
DBP (mmHg)	79.59 ± 11.19	80.25 ± 11.98	79.53 ± 11.12	0.398
Laboratory parameters				
TC (mmol/L)	4.9 ± 1.09	5.09 ± 1.08	4.88 ± 1.09	0.014
TG (mmol/L)	(1.15,2.3)	1.65 (1.17,2.36)	1.58 (1.14,2.29)	0.598
HDL-C (mmol/L)	1.11 ± 0.35	1.11 ± 0.34	1.16 ± 0.37	0.074
LDL-C (mmol/L)	3.2 ± 1.0	3.35 ± 1.01	3.18 ± 1.0	0.030
Glu (mmol/L)	5.65 ± 1.88	5.84 ± 2.44	5.63 ± 1.83	0.145
HbA1C (%)	6.02 ± 1.0	6.24 ± 1.06	6.0 ± 1.0	0.001
hsCRP (mg/L)	1.37 (0.72,2.46)	1.65 (0.77,2.89)	1.36 (0.72,2.46)	0.192
PCSK9 (ng/mL)	228.48 (189,275.5)	246.69 (208.92,297.11)	227.24 (187.33,274.18)	< 0.001
Coagulation indexes				
APTT (s)	36.25 ± 3.9	36 ± 3.91	36.27 ± 3.89	0.374
PT (s)	12.75 ± 0.64	12.66 ± 0.58	12.76 ± 0.64	0.032
PT-t (1/s)	0.83 (0.63.1.25)	0.91 (0.70,1.25)	0.83 (0.63,1.25)	0.028
TT (s)	16.4 ± 1.25	16.28 ± 1.55	16.41 ± 1.22	0.170
Fib (g/L)	3.06 ± 0.73	3.19 ± 0.85	3.05 ± 0.71	0.013
D dimer (μg/mL)	0.31 (0.24,0.41)	0.31 (0.23,0.45)	0.31 (0.24,0.41)	0.531
Platelet(10^12)	216.79 ± 55.66	212.69 ± 49.81	217.15 ± 56.14	0.295
Medication				
Aspirin/Clopidogrel n(%)	748 (32.6)	72 (38.7)	676 (32.1)	0.065
ACEI/ARB n(%)	383 (16.7)	34 (18.3)	349 (16.6)	0.548

BMI body mass index, *CAD* coronary artery disease, *DM* diabetes mellitus, *SBP* systolic blood pressure, *DBP* diastolic blood pressure, *TC* total cholesterol, *TG* triglyceride; HDL-C, high-density lipoprotein cholesterol, *LDL-C* low-density lipoprotein cholesterol, *Glu* glucose, *HbA1C* hemoglobin A1C, *hs-CRP* high-sensitivity C-reactive protein, *PCSK9* proprotein convertase subtilisin/kexin type 9, *APTT* activated partial thromboplastin time, *PT* prothrombin time, *PT-t* transformation of prothrombin time (the inverse of the difference between PT and the minimal PT of normal plasma), *TT* thrombin time, *Fib* fibrinogen, *ACEI* angiotensin converting enzyme inhibitors, *ARB* angiotensin receptor blockers. $p < 0.05$ suggested significant difference

plasma for further analysis. Interestingly, we found that PT-t levels were higher in patients with events than those without events ($p < 0.05$).

Next, we divided all patients into two groups according to PCSK9 median to analyze baseline characteristic data and coagulation parameters, as summarized in Table 2. The data showed that age, gender, smoking status, drinking status, diastolic blood pressure and family history of CAD were statistical difference between high and low PCSK9 subgroups (all $p < 0.05$). Furthermore, patients with high PCSK9 levels trended to have higher TC, TG, HDL-C, LDL-C, HbA1C and hsCRP levels (all $p < 0.05$). In addition, APTT and PT were lower and PT-t, fibrinogen, d dimer and platelet counts were higher in patients with high PCSK9 levels than those with low PCSK9 levels (all $p < 0.05$). However, no significant difference with regard to variables including BMI, the percentage of CAD, diabetes mellitus and hypertension,

Table 2 The clinical and biochemical data according to PCSK9 levels

Variables		PCSK9 (ng/mL)		*p*
	Overall	< 228.48	> 228.48	
	n = 2293	*n* = 1146	*n* = 1147	
Clinical data				
Age (years)	55.62 ± 11.01	54.92 ± 11.12	56.32 ± 10.86	0.002
Male sex n(%)	1387 (60.5)	795 (69.4)	592 (51.6)	< 0.001
BMI (kg/m^2)	25.63 ± 3.38	25.76 ± 3.39	25.49 ± 3.37	0.054
CAD n(%)	1447 (63.1)	723 (63.1)	724 (63.1)	0.987
DM n(%)	538 (23.5)	257 (22.4)	281 (24.5)	0.242
Hypertension n(%)	1418 (61.8)	710 (62.0)	708 (61.7)	0.910
Smoking n(%)	788 (34.4)	422 (36.8)	366 (31.9)	0.013
Drinking n(%)	468 (20.4)	261 (22.8)	207	0.005
Family history of CAD n(%)	514 (22.4)	236 (20.6)	278 (24.2)	0.036
SBP (mmHg)	128.05 ± 18.01	128.58 ± 17.97	127.52 ± 18.04	0.161
DBP (mmHg)	79.59 ± 11.19	80.08 ± 11.21	79.1 ± 11.16	0.035
Laboratory parameters				
TC (mmol/L)	4.9 ± 1.09	4.68 ± 0.96	5.12 ± 1.17	< 0.001
TG (mmol/L)	(1.15,2.3)	1.53 (1.11,2.23)	1.64 (1.19,2.35)	0.012
HDL-C (mmol/L)	1.11 ± 0.35	1.09 ± 0.36	1.14 ± 0.33	0.001
LDL-C (mmol/L)	3.2 ± 1	2.99 ± 0.88	3.41 ± 1.08	< 0.001
Glu (mmol/L)	5.65 ± 1.88	5.6 ± 2.1	5.69 ± 1.64	0.264
HbA1C (%)	6.02 ± 1.0	5.94 ± 0.94	6.09 ± 1.06	< 0.001
hsCRP (mg/L)	1.37 (0.72,2.46)	1.32 (0.71,2.46)	1.47 (0.73,2.63)	0.009
Coagulation indexes				
APTT (s)	36.25 ± 3.9	36.46 ± 3.86	36.03 ± 3.92	0.008
PT (s)	12.75 ± 0.64	12.84 ± 0.63	12.67 ± 0.63	< 0.001
PT-t (1/s)	0.83 (0.63.1.25)	0.77 (0.59,1.11)	0.83 (0.67,1.43)	< 0.001
TT (s)	16.4 ± 1.25	16.38 ± 1.08	16.42 ± 1.39	0.386
Fib (g/L)	3.06 ± 0.73	2.98 ± 0.64	3.15 ± 0.79	< 0.001
D dimer (μg/mL)	0.31 (0.24,0.41)	0.3 (0.24,0.39)	0.32 (0.24,0.43)	0.011
Platelet(10^12)	216.79 ± 55.66	211.32 ± 54.48	222.25 ± 56.31	< 0.001
Medication				
Aspirin/Clopidogrel n(%)	748 (32.6)	379 (33.1)	369 (32.2)	0.646
ACEI/ARB n(%)	383 (16.7)	193 (16.8)	190 (16.6)	0.859

PCSK9 proprotein convertase subtilisin/kexin type 9, *BMI* body mass index, *CAD* coronary artery disease, *DM* diabetes mellitus, *SBP* systolic blood pressure, *DBP* diastolic blood pressure, *TC* total cholesterol, *TG* triglyceride, *HDL-C* high-density lipoprotein cholesterol, *LDL-C* low-density lipoprotein cholesterol, *Glu* glucose, *HbA1C* hemoglobin A1C, *hs-CRP* high-sensitivity C-reactive protein, *APTT* activated partial thromboplastin time, *PT* prothrombin time, *PT-t* transformation of prothrombin time (the inverse of the difference between PT and the minimal PT of normal plasma), *TT* thrombin time, *Fib* fibrinogen, *ACEI* angiotensin converting enzyme inhibitors, *ARB* angiotensin receptor blockers. $p < 0.05$ suggested significant difference

systolic and diastolic blood pressure, glucose, TT, and the usage of medications (all $p > 0.05$).

Associations of PCSK9 and coagulation-related parameters

Pearson or spearman correlation analysis was performed in this study to clarify the association with log-transformed PCSK9 levels with parameters in all patients (Table S1). Consistent with previous results, our data showed that circulating PCSK9 concentration was associated with age, TC, HDL-C, LDL-C, glucose, HbA1C and hsCRP levels ($r = 0.073$, $p < 0.001$; $r = 0.269$, $p < 0.001$; $r = 0.111$, $p < 0.001$; $r = 0.259$, $p < 0.001$; $r = 0.065$, $p = 0.002$; $r = 0.113$, $p < 0.001$; $r = 0.107$, $p < 0.001$, respectively, Table S1). Moreover, we observed a negative correlation of APTT and PT, a positive correlation of fibrinogen and platelet counts with plasma levels of PCSK9 levels in the present study ($r = -0.075$, $p < 0.001$;

r = − 0.194, $p < 0.001$; r = 0.167, $p < 0.001$; r = 0.138, $p <$ 0.001, respectively, Table S1 and Fig. 1). Additionally, a positive relation of PT-t with PCSK9 was found in all patients (r = 0.180, $p < 0.001$, Table S1). However, no significant correlation between PCSK9 levels and body mass index (BMI), systolic and diastolic blood pressure, TG, TT and D dimer (all $p > 0.05$).

In order to eliminate impact of potential association with circulating PCSK9 concentration and PT with age, gender, hypertension, diabetes mellitus, smoking status, BMI, a stepwise multivariate linear regression analysis was used to determine the relationship between PCSK9 levels and PT after adjusting for these confounders (Table 3). The results indicated that a negative association with PCSK9 levels and PT remained significant after adjustment for age, gender, hypertension, diabetes mellitus, CAD, smoking status, BMI ($\beta = -0.189$, $p < 0.001$, Table 3). Even if adding TG, TC, HDL-C, LDL-C, glucose, HbA1C and hsCRP to multivariate linear regression model, the negative correlation of PCSK9 levels and PT remained statistically significant ($\beta = -0.135$, $p < 0.001$). Due to APTT, TT, fibrinogen and D dimer reflect the coagulation status in vivo, and then we further added these parameters to adjust. Similarly, it showed that plasma PCSK9 level and PT still remained significant correlation in all patients ($\beta = -0.115$, $p < 0.001$). Likewise, it was worth noting that PT-t levels were independently and positively associated with higher concentration of PCSK9 after adjusting for multiple confounders in stepwise multivariate linear regression analysis ($\beta = 0.085$, $p < 0.001$, Table 3). However, the significant difference between PCSK9 and APTT was disappeared in multivariable regression stepwise model (p = 0.367, Table S2).

Associations of PCSK9, PT and MACEs

One hundred eighy-six MACEs including 9 died of cardiovascular diseases, 55 underwent coronary revascularization, 3 suffered nonfatal MI, 16 had ischemic stroke and 103 experienced hospitalizations because of unstable angina pectoris, were developed in a mean follow-up of 38.3 months in the current study. Kaplan Meier curve indicated that patients in high PCSK9 or low PT groups had higher incidence of MACEs compared with patients in low PCSK9 or high PT groups (all $p < 0.05$, Fig. 2A and 2B). When the event-free survival rate classified into 4 subgroups by the combination of PCSK9 and PT, high PCSK9 + low PT group was more likely to have significantly lower event-free survival rate compared to low PCSK9 + high PT group (the reference group, Fig. 2C, $p <$ 0.05), whereas there was no significant difference in low PCSK9 + low PT and high PCSK9 + high PT groups compared with the reference group (all $p > 0.05$). Moreover, the incidence of MACEs was 5.4% (low PCSK9 + high PT), 7.5% (low PCSK9 + low PT), 8.1% (high PCSK9 + high PT group) and 11.4% (high PCSK9 + low PT group) in ascending order (Fig. 3A, p = 0.001). Multivariate Cox regression analysis showed that subjects in high PCSK9 or low PT groups had 1.393-fold (95%CI: 1.023–1.896) and 1.396-fold (95%CI: 1.029–1.895) higher risk of events than those in low PCSK9 or high PT groups (Table 4). Subsequently, we observed the combined impact of PCSK9 and PT on future cardiovascular events, and found that the multivariable-adjusted HR with 95%CI in high PCSK9 + low PT group was 1.815 (1.193–2.762) compared to the reference group. Similarly, we classified all patients into high or low PT-t groups based on the median of PT-t and found that patients in high PT-t group had higher risk of MACEs compared with those in low PT-t group (adjusted HR: 1.396, 95%CI: 1.029–1.895, p = 0.032, Table S3). When combined the PCSK9 levels and PT-t status, a higher incidence of cardiovascular events was occurred in high PCSK9 + high PT-t group compared with low PCSK9 + low PT-t group (adjusted HR: 1.815, 95%CI: 1.193–2.762, p = 0.005, Table S3).

Discussion

In the present study, we evaluated the association of circulating PCSK9 concentration with indexes of routine coagulation tests and cardiovascular events. The major findings of our study were that circulating PCSK9 concentration was independently and negatively correlated with PT, and the combination of high PCSK9 and low PT was associated with elevated cardiovascular outcomes, which might further provide novel information with regard to PCSK9 and hypercoagulability in cardiovascular risks.

As commonly recognized, PCSK9, a novel regulator of cholesterol metabolism, takes part in atherosclerosis, leading to the occurrence of CAD. Our previous studies had observed a higher circulating PCSK9 levels in patients with stable CAD patients and PCSK9 was significantly and positively associated with severity of coronary and adverse cardiovascular prognosis [13, 14]. Recently, FOURIER trial and ODYSSEY OUTCOMES trial have confirmed that PCSK9 inhibitors reduce major adverse cardiovascular and cerebrovascular events in patients with ASCVD compared with the placebo group [15, 16]. Interestingly, PCSK9 has been known to have various effects beyond LDL-C, which has been reported to be related to hypercoagulability and promote thrombosis to accelerate atherosclerosis [9]. Moreover, prior studies indicated that plasma PCSK9 levels were positively correlated with coagulation fibrinogen and platelet indices [10, 17]. Additionally, several animal studies using PCSK9 over expressing or PCSK9 knockout mice model found that an interesting phenomenon related to PCSK9 and hypercoagulable state, platelet activation and carotid artery thrombosis [18, 19]. However, there is no

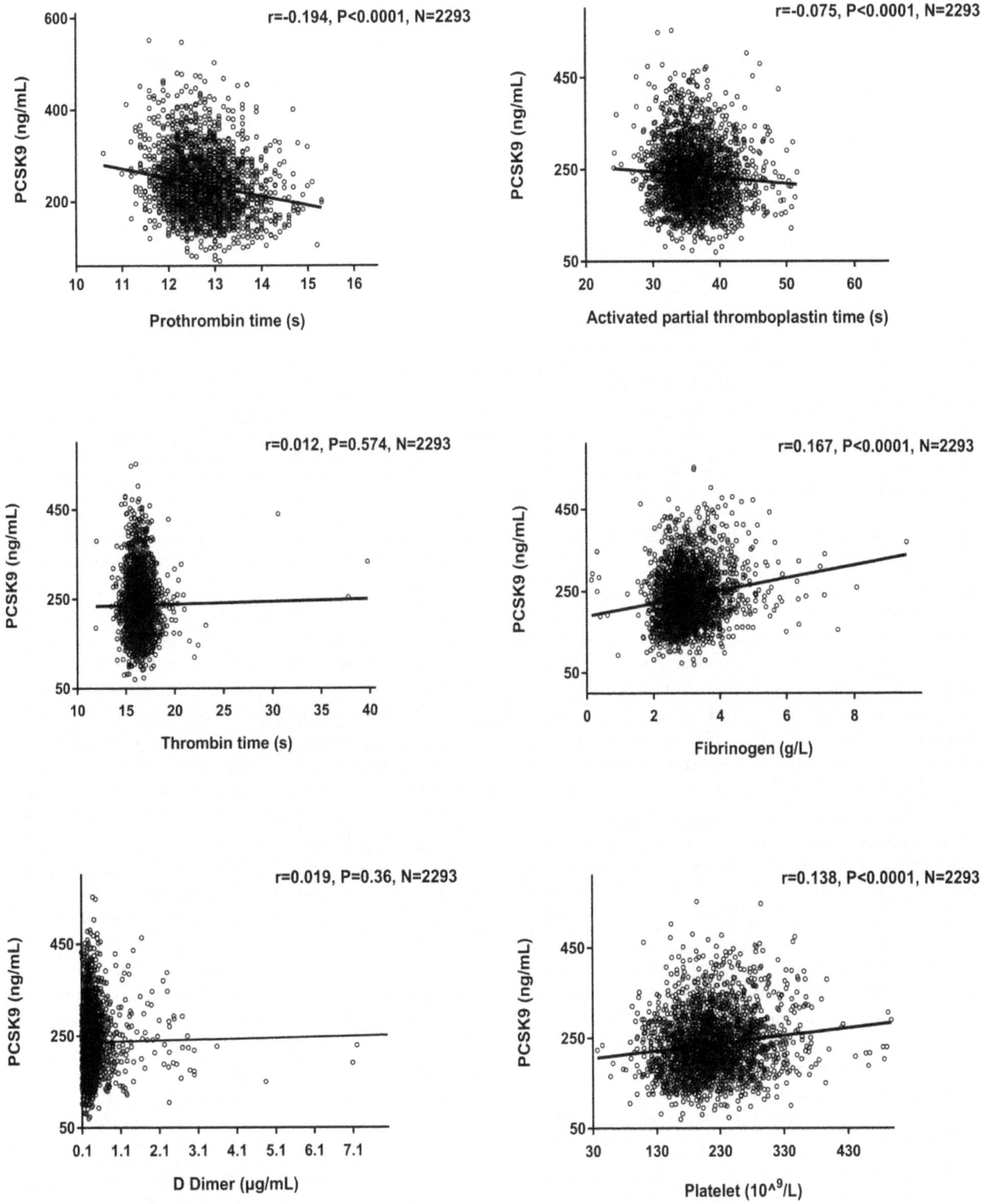

Fig. 1 Association of PCSK9 and coagulation-related indicators in all patients ($N = 2293$). $p < 0.05$, PCSK9, proprotein convertase subtilisin/Kexin type 9

Table 3 Independent determinants of PT or PT-t to log-transformed PCSK9

	Independent variable PT		Independent variable PT-t	
	Standardized regression coefficients β	*p*	Standardized regression coefficients β	*p*
Model 1[a]	−0.192	**< 0.001**	0.139	**< 0.001**
Model 2[b]	− 0.19	**< 0.001**	0.137	**< 0.001**
Model 3[c]	−0.189	**< 0.001**	0.136	**< 0.001**
Model 4[d]	−0.142	**< 0.001**	0.105	**< 0.001**
Model 5[e]	−0.135	**< 0.001**	0.100	**< 0.001**
Model 6[f]	−0.135	**< 0.001**	0.100	**< 0.001**
Model 7[g]	−0.115	**< 0.001**	0.085	**< 0.001**

The multivariable regression stepwise models are shown. The log-transformed PCSK9 is the dependent variable.
[a]Adjusted for age and sex
[b]Adjusted for age, sex, hypertension and diabetes, CAD
[c]Adjusted for age, sex, hypertension, diabetes, CAD, smoking status and BMI
[d]Adjusted for age, sex, hypertension, diabetes, CAD, smoking status, BMI, TG, TC, HDL-C and LDL-C
[e]Adjusted for age, sex, hypertension, diabetes, CAD, smoking status, BMI, TG, TC, HDL-C, LDL-C, glucose and HbA1C
[f]Adjusted for age, sex, hypertension, diabetes, CAD, smoking status, BMI, TG, TC, HDL-C, LDL-C, glucose, HbA1C and hsCRP
[g]Adjusted for age, sex, hypertension, diabetes, CAD, smoking status, BMI, TG, TC, HDL-C, LDL-C, glucose, HbA1C, hsCRP, fibrinogen, D dimer, platelet, APTT and TT.
PT, prothrombin time; PT-t, transformation of prothrombin time (the inverse of the difference between PT and the minimal PT of normal plasma), *PCSK9* proprotein convertase subtilisin/Kexin type 9, *CAD* coronary artery disease, *BMI* body mass index, *TG* triglyceride, *TC* total cholesterol, *HDL-C* high-density lipoprotein cholesterol, *LDL-C* low-density lipoprotein cholesterol, *HbA1C* hemoglobin A1C, *hsCRP* high-sensitivity C-reactive protein, *ESR* erythrocyte sedimentation rate, *APTT* activated partial thromboplastin time, *TT* thrombin time

clinical data for explore the relationship between the PCSK9 and indicators of regular coagulation including APTT, PT and TT.

In the current study, we, for the first time, found that PCSK9 was only independently correlated with lower PT levels in patients with angina-like chest pain who took no lipid-lowering therapy. In order to further support the association of PCSK9 wIthink hypercoagulable state, we analyzed the relation of PCSK9 with PT-t and found a similar result. An increasing study have provided that hypercoagulability plays a crucial role in atherosclerosis contributing to both atherosclerotic plaque development and acute thrombotic complications, which is considered as a primary cause of morbidity and mortality of patients with CAD [20–22]. Furthermore, it is well known that coagulation factors can trigger non-hemostatic proatherogenic effect [23]. PT, the major component of routine coagulation tests, is a measure of the integrity of the extrinsic and final common pathways of the pro-coagulant cascade, which is recognized as a risk factor of CAD [24, 25]. A GWAS study for PT conducted in 2583 participants and identified genome-wide significant associations of the *F7* and *PROCR/EDEM2* regions with PT, of which may relate to the risk of CAD by assessment of these gene expression and CAD database comprised 22,233 cases of CAD and 64,762 controls of European ancestry [5]. Nevertheless, the role of PT in predicting cardiovascular prognosis needs to further investigate in different population. What's more, whether there is an additive effect of two measures on MACEs remains to explore.

In this study, we evaluated the predictive ability of routine coagulation indexes including APTT, PT, and TT in MACEs. Firstly, we found that only lower PT levels (or higher PT-t levels), reflecting hypercoagulable state, were related to adverse cardiovascular outcomes in all patients. It is known that increasing or decreasing circulating concentration and activation or inhibition of clotting factors involved in extrinsic pathways of coagulation cascade will lead to a shortening or extension of PT. Activated of TF and factor VII (FVII) are the initial and pivotal step to trigger extrinsic coagulation pathway, which is different from intrinsic coagulation pathway reflected by APTT [26, 27]. When vascular injury exposes plasma to a variety of TF-expressing cells, zymogen FVII binds to TF and rapidly converts to FVIIa by limited proteolysis, thereby generating the active TF-FVIIa complex to greatly increase the enzymatic activity of FVIIa [28]. Moreover, it was showed that recombinant human FVIIa administration to individuals with liver disease resulted in a transient shortening of PT [29]. Therefore, circulating TF and FVII levels reduce or increase and TF and FVII activity is been inhibited or activated, the value of PT would be changed. Notably, tissue factor pathway inhibitor (TFPI), an important factor in the extrinsic pathway of coagulation cascade, could result in a negative feedback on the formation of TF/FVIIa complexes to shut down the extrinsic activation of coagulation in vivo. Furthermore, accumulating evidence of animal and clinical studies showed that TF and TFPI were closely associated with atherosclerosis and CAD [30–35]. Meanwhile, data on the prognostic value of TF activity or TF suggested that systemic TF activity had a harmful prognostic value in patients with AMI from a prospective study recruited 174 patients with unstable angina pectoris and 112 patients with acute myocardial infarction followed for a mean period of 3.26 years [35], and from a prognostic study with 1146 patients stable angina pectoris and 523

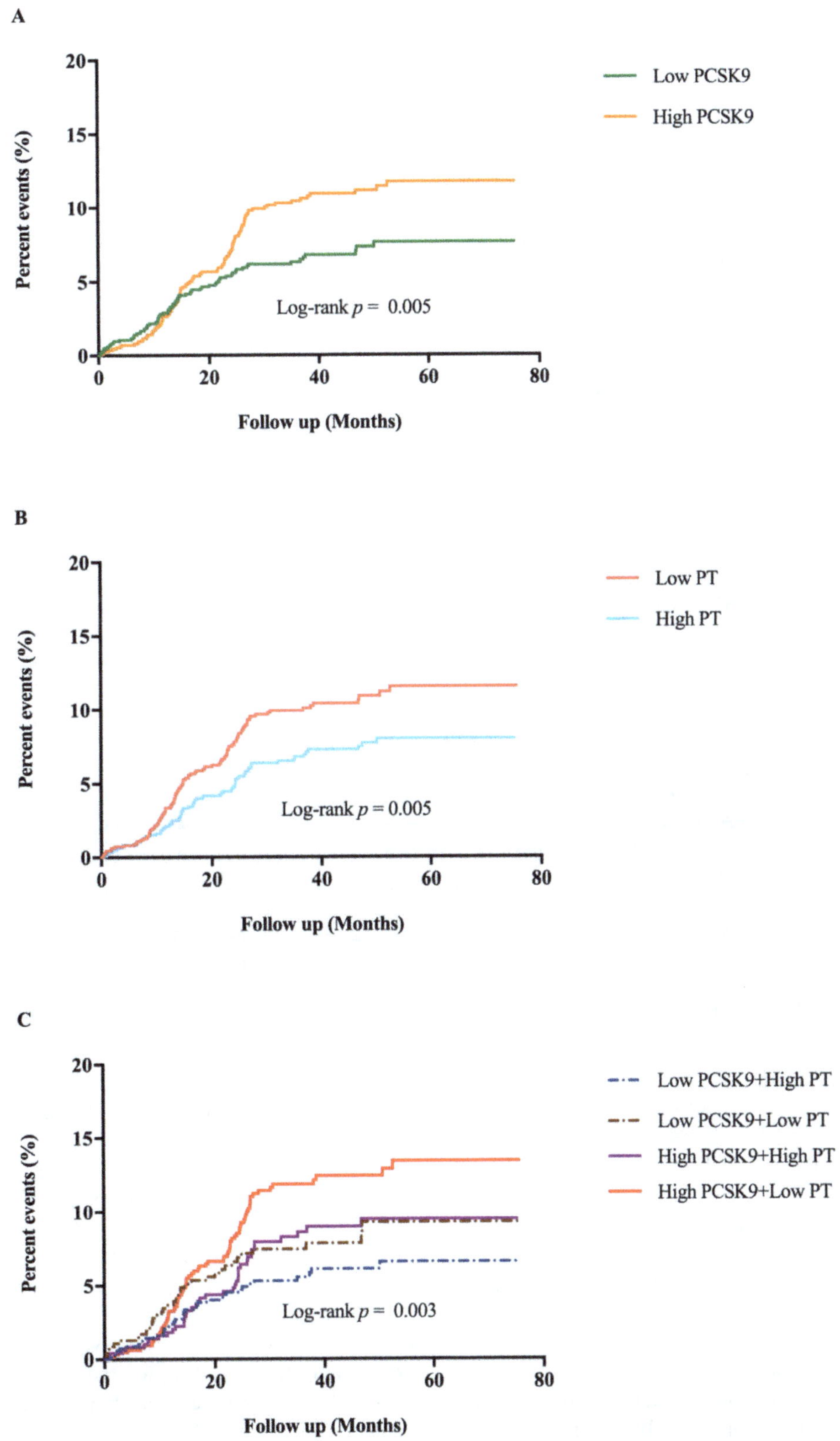

Fig. 2 Kaplan-Meier analysis according to different PCSK9, PT levels and the combination of PCSK9 and PT status. PCSK9, proprotein convertase subtilisin/kexin type 9; PT, prothrombin time

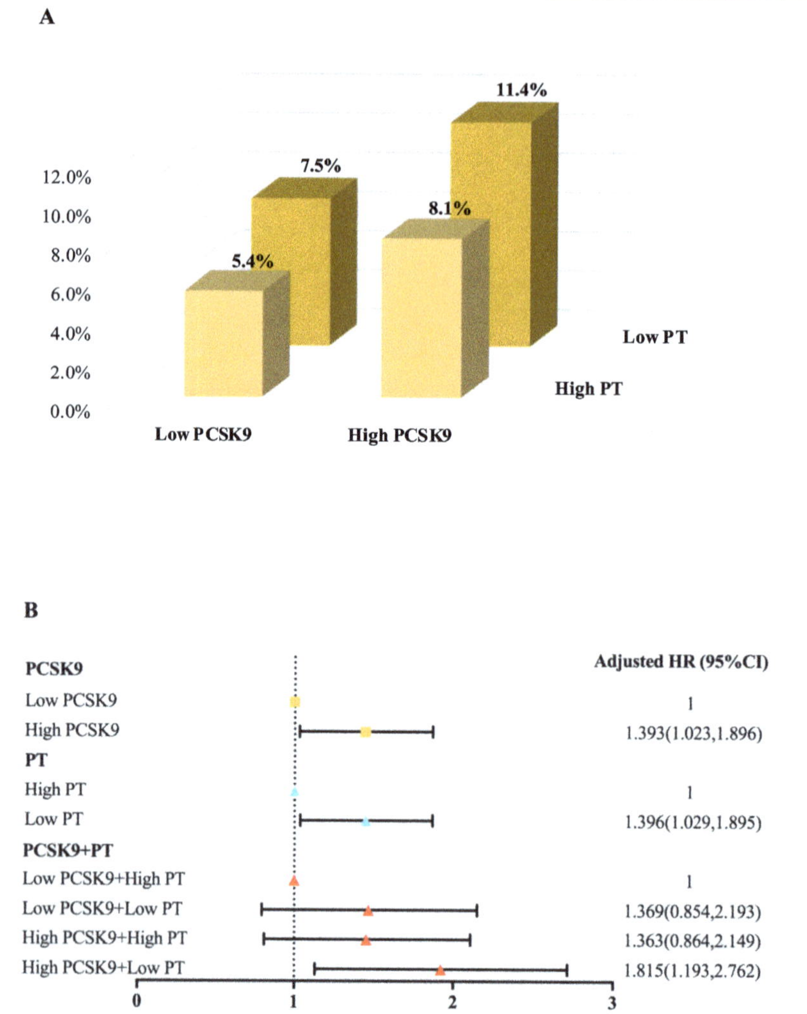

Fig. 3 **A**. The percentage of MACEs in different subgroups according to the combination of PCSK9 and PT. **B**. Multiple Cox regression analysis in different subgroups. Adjusted model was adjusted for age, gender, CAD, diabetes, family history of CAD, TC, LDL, HbA1C, fibrinogen. MACEs, major adverse cardiovascular events; PCSK9, proprotein convertase subtilisin/kexin type 9; PT, prothrombin time; HR, hazard ratio; CI, confidence interval; CAD, coronary artery disease; TC, total cholesterol; HDL-C, LDL-C, low-density lipoprotein cholesterol; HbA1C, hemoglobin A1C

patients with acute coronary syndrome followed over a mean period of 2.3 years [34]. These results supported our finding of lower PT or higher PT-t associated with MACEs.

Nonetheless, a large-scaled clinical trial with 2 years follow-up and revealed that elevated PT was an independent risk predictor for all-cause mortality in 2734 acute MI patients (adjusted HR, 4.04; 95%CI, 2.83–5.7) [36], which seemed to be inconsistent with our results. It was worth to noting that the median of PT in acute MI patients was 13.85 seconds which was larger than our patients and meant that they had a greater risk of bleeding. In addition, the endpoint event observed of this study was all-cause of death but did not further analyze the association of PT with cardiovascular death. Therefore, our study firstly found that the hypercoagulable state presented by low PT level or high PT-t level were an independently risk factor of cardiovascular events.

As well-known, PCSK9 levels have been proposed to predict cardiovascular outcomes in different population [37]. Similarly, our data also found that circulating levels of PCSK9 were significantly associated with MACEs in patients with chest pain. Of note, our study further revealed that the combination of high PCSK9 and low PT had better predictive ability in cardiovascular outcomes in entire population after adjusting for multiple risk factors, which provided a new connection of lipid metabolism and coagulation in ASCVD. PCSK9 may have impact on extrinsic coagulation cascade via altering the levels and activity of TF and/or FVII. Meanwhile, it has been reported that dyslipidemia and hypercoagulable state play critical role in atherosclerosis and cardiovascular risks [35, 37].

Table 4 Cox regression analysis of PCSK9, PT status with MACEs

Variables	Events/ subjects	HR(95%CI)			
		Crude model	*p*	Adjusted model	*p*
PCSK9					
Low PCSK9	72/1146	1 (Reference)	/	1 (Reference)	/
High PCSK9	114/1147	1.526 (1.136,2.049)	0.005	1.393 (1.023,1.896)	0.035
PT					
High PT	77/1178	1 (Reference)	/	1 (Reference)	/
Low PT	109/1115	1.512 (1.129,2.024)	0.006	1.396 (1.029,1.895)	0.032
PCSK9 + PT					
Low PCSK9 + High PT	37/682	1 (Reference)	/	1 (Reference)	/
Low PCSK9 + Low PT	35/464	1.415 (0.891,2.246)	0.141	1.369 (0.854,2.193)	0.192
High PCSK9 + High PT	40/496	1.43 (0.914,2.236)	0.117	1.363 (0.864,2.149)	0.183
High PCSK9 + Low PT	74/651	2.049 (1.381,3.041)	< 0.001	1.815 (1.193,2.762)	0.005

Adjusted model was adjusted for age, gender, CAD, diabetes, family history of CAD, TC, LDL, HbA1C, fibrinogen. MACEs, major adverse cardiovascular events; PCSK9, proprotein convertase subtilisin/kexin type 9; *PT* prothrombin time, *HR* hazard ratio, *CI* confidence interval, *CAD* coronary artery disease, *TC* total cholesterol, *HDL-C, LDL-C* low-density lipoprotein cholesterol, *HbA1C* hemoglobin A1C. $p < 0.05$ suggested significant difference

Furthermore, the link between the two abnormal states has been described, especially in the relation of LDL abnormality and extrinsic coagulation dysfunction [30, 38]. Importantly, PCSK9 directly and remarkably has currently reported to reduce circulating LDL-C levels by mediating lysosomal degradation of hepatic LDLR and has impacts on thrombosis [8]. Hence, the combination of PCSK9 and PT (or PT-t) had an additive impact on the incidence of cardiovascular events in patients with angina-like chest pain, which was benefited for cardiovascular risk stratification.

There were some limitations in this study. First, the sample size recruited in a single center had effect on the generalizability of the results. Second, the cross-sectional design of this study could not exclude residual confoundings. Third, the current study only observed the association between PCSK9 and PT, but did not investigate the relationship of PCSK9 with several important extrinsic clotting factors such as aforementioned TF and FVII. Additionally, the possible causal association of PCSK9 and PT was not been confirmed because this was an observational and prospective study. Finally, we could not examine the changes of PCSK9 and PT, and these impacts on predicting MACEs during follow-up.

Conclusions

The present study for the first time showed a negative relation of PCSK9 with PT and found that the combination of PCSK9 and PT was significantly associated with adverse cardiovascular outcomes, suggesting that PCSK9 may induce and/or promote hypercoagulability.The combination of these two measures may be useful to further identify cardiovascular risk stratification.

Abbreviations

ASCVD: Atherosclerotic cardiovascular disease; CAD: Coronary artery disease; APTT: Activated partial thromboplastin time; PT: Prothrombin time; TT: Thrombin time; PCSK9: Proprotein convertase subtilisin/kexin type 9; LDLR: Low density lipoprotein cholesterol receptor; LDL-C: Low density lipoprotein cholesterol; MACEs: Major adverse cardiovascular events; TG: Triglyceride; TC: Total cholesterol; HDL-C: High density lipoprotein cholesterol; HbA1C: Hemoglobin A1C; hsCRP: High-sensitivity C-reactive protein; MI: Myocardial infarction; HR: Hazard ratios; CI: Confidence interval; PT-t: The transformation of prothrombin time; TF: Tissue factor; TFPI: Tissue factor pathway inhibitor; FVII: Factor VII

Supplementary Information

Additional file 1: Table S1. Correlation analysis between log-transformed PCSK9 and related-parameters in all patients (N=2293). **Table S2.** Multiple linear analysis of PCSK9 and coagulation-related indexes. **Table S3.** Cox regression analysis of PCSK9, PT-t status with MACEs. **Figure S1.** The flowchart of this study. PCSK9, proprotein convertase subtilisin/kexin type 9; MACEs, major adverse cardiovascular events.

Acknowledgements

The authors thank all the staff and participants of this study for their important contributions.

Authors' contributions

PJ completed the project, analyzed the data, and wrote the manuscript. LJJ and ZCG designed the study, interpreted the data, and contributed to critically revising the article. LMM, LHH, GYL, WNQ and DQ contributed to data collection. QJ and DKF contributed to recruitment of patients. All authors have approved the final article.

References

1. Santos-Gallego CG, Bayón J, Badimón JJ. Thrombi of different pathologies: implications for diagnosis and treatment. Curr Treat Options Cardiovasc Med. 2010;12(3):274–91. https://doi.org/10.1007/s11936-010-0075-8.
2. Santos-Gallego CG, Picatoste B, Badimón JJ. Pathophysiology of acute coronary syndrome. Curr Atheroscler Rep. 2014;16(4):401. https://doi.org/10.1007/s11883-014-0401-9.

3. Corti R, Fuster V, Badimon JJ. Pathogenetic concepts of acute coronary syndromes. J Am Coll Cardiol. 2003;41:7s–14s.
4. Badimon L, Vilahur G. Thrombosis formation on atherosclerotic lesions and plaque rupture. J Intern Med. 2014;276(6):618–32. https://doi.org/10.1111/joim.12296.
5. Tang W, Schwienbacher C, Lopez LM, Ben-Shlomo Y, Oudot-Mellakh T, Johnson AD, et al. Genetic associations for activated partial thromboplastin time and prothrombin time, their gene expression profiles, and risk of coronary artery disease. Am J Hum Genet. 2012;91(1):152–62. https://doi.org/10.1016/j.ajhg.2012.05.009.
6. Horton JD, Cohen JC, Hobbs HH. PCSK9: a convertase that coordinates LDL catabolism. J Lipid Res. 2009;50(Suppl):S172–7. https://doi.org/10.1194/jlr.R800091-JLR200.
7. Cunningham D, Danley DE, Geoghegan KF, Griffor MC, Hawkins JL, Subashi TA, et al. Structural and biophysical studies of PCSK9 and its mutants linked to familial hypercholesterolemia. Nat Struct Mol Biol. 2007;14(5):413–9. https://doi.org/10.1038/nsmb1235.
8. Mach F, Baigent C, Catapano AL, Koskinas KC, Casula M, Badimon L, et al. ESC/EAS guidelines for the management of dyslipidaemias: lipid modification to reduce cardiovascular risk. Eur Heart J. 2019;2019(5):3826. https://doi.org/10.15829/1560-4071-2020-3826.
9. Paciullo F, Momi S, Gresele P. PCSK9 in Haemostasis and thrombosis: possible pleiotropic effects of PCSK9 inhibitors in cardiovascular prevention. Thromb Haemost. 2019;119(3):359–67. https://doi.org/10.1055/s-0038-1676863.
10. Zhang Y, Zhu CG, Xu RX, Li S, Guo YL, Sun J, et al. Relation of circulating PCSK9 concentration to fibrinogen in patients with stable coronary artery disease. J Clin Lipidol. 2014;8:494–500.
11. Yang SH, Li S, Zhang Y, Xu RX, Guo YL, Zhu CG, et al. Positive correlation of plasma PCSK9 levels with HbA1c in patients with type 2 diabetes. Diabetes Metab Res Rev. 2016;32(2):193–9. https://doi.org/10.1002/dmrr.2712.
12. Rassi AB, d'Amico EA, Tripodi A, Rocha T, Migita BY, Ferreira CM, et al. Fresh frozen plasma transfusion in patients with cirrhosis and coagulopathy: effect on conventional coagulation tests and thrombomodulin-modified thrombin generation. J Hepatol. 2019;72(1):85–94. https://doi.org/10.1016/j.jhep.2019.09.008.
13. Li S, Zhang Y, Xu R-X, Guo Y-L, Zhu C-G, Wu N-Q, et al. Proprotein convertase subtilisin-kexin type 9 as a biomarker for the severity of coronary artery disease. Ann Med. 2015;47(5):386–93. https://doi.org/10.3109/07853890.2015.1042908.
14. Cao Y-X, Liu H-H, Sun D, Jin J-L, Xu R-X, Guo Y-L, et al. The different relations of PCSK9 and Lp(a) to the presence and severity of atherosclerotic lesions in patients with familial hypercholesterolemia. Atherosclerosis. 2018;277:7–14. https://doi.org/10.1016/j.atherosclerosis.2018.07.030.
15. Sabatine MS, Giugliano RP, Keech AC, Honarpour N, Wiviott SD, Murphy SA, et al. Evolocumab and clinical outcomes in patients with cardiovascular disease. N Engl J Med. 2017;376(18):1713–22. https://doi.org/10.1056/NEJMoa1615664.
16. Schwartz GG, Steg PG, Szarek M, Bhatt DL, Bittner VA, Diaz R, et al. Alirocumab and cardiovascular outcomes after acute coronary syndrome. N Engl J Med. 2018;379(22):2097–107. https://doi.org/10.1056/NEJMoa1801174.
17. Li S, Zhu CG, Guo YL, Xu RX, Zhang Y, Sun J, et al. The relationship between the plasma PCSK9 levels and platelet indices in patients with stable coronary artery disease. J Atheroscler Thromb. 2015;22(1):76–84. https://doi.org/10.5551/jat.25841.
18. Camera M, Rossetti L, Barbieri SS, Zanotti I, Canciani B, Trabattoni D, et al. PCSK9 as a positive modulator of platelet activation. J Am Coll Cardiol. 2018;71(8):952–4. https://doi.org/10.1016/j.jacc.2017.11.069.
19. Dwivedi DJ, Grin PM, Khan M, Prat A, Zhou J, Fox-Robichaud AE, et al. Differential expression of PCSK9 modulates infection, inflammation, and coagulation in a murine model of Sepsis. Shock. 2016;46(6):672–80. https://doi.org/10.1097/SHK.0000000000000682.
20. Gao J, Ma X, Zhang Y, Guo M, Shi D. The role of microRNAs in prethrombotic status associated with coronary artery disease. Thromb Haemost. 2017;117(03):429–36. https://doi.org/10.1160/TH16-07-0503.
21. Tosi F, Micaglio R, Sandri M, Castagna A, Minguzzi D, Stefanoni F, et al. Increased plasma thrombin potential is associated with stable coronary artery disease: an angiographically-controlled study. Thromb Res. 2017;155:16–22. https://doi.org/10.1016/j.thromres.2017.04.021.
22. Roger VL, Go AS, Lloyd-Jones DM, Benjamin EJ, Berry JD, Borden WB, et al. Heart disease and stroke statistics--2012 update: a report from the American Heart Association. Circulation. 2012;125(1):e2–e220. https://doi.org/10.1161/CIR.0b013e31823ac046.
23. Borissoff JI, Spronk HM, ten Cate H. The hemostatic system as a modulator of atherosclerosis. N Engl J Med. 2011;364(18):1746–60. https://doi.org/10.1056/NEJMra1011670.
24. Hoffman M. Coagulation in liver disease. Semin Thromb Hemost. 2015;41(5):447–54. https://doi.org/10.1055/s-0035-1550435.
25. Kamal AH, Tefferi A, Pruthi RK. How to interpret and pursue an abnormal prothrombin time, activated partial thromboplastin time, and bleeding time in adults. Mayo Clin Proc. 2007;82(7):864–73. https://doi.org/10.4065/82.7.864.
26. Abbate R, Cioni G, Ricci I, Miranda M, Gori AM. Thrombosis and acute coronary syndrome. Thromb Res. 2012;129(3):235–40. https://doi.org/10.1016/j.thromres.2011.12.026.
27. ten Cate H. Tissue factor-driven thrombin generation and inflammation in atherosclerosis. Thromb Res. 2012;129(Suppl 2):S38–40. https://doi.org/10.1016/j.thromres.2012.02.028.
28. Gajsiewicz JM, Morrissey JH. Structure-function relationship of the interaction between tissue factor and factor VIIa. Semin Thromb Hemost. 2015;41(07):682–90. https://doi.org/10.1055/s-0035-1564044.
29. Van Thiel DH, Farr DE, Mindikoglu AL, Todo A, George MM. Recombinant human factor VIIa-induced alterations in tissue factor and thrombomodulin in patients with advanced liver cirrhosis. J Gastroenterol Hepatol. 2005;20(6):882–9. https://doi.org/10.1111/j.1440-1746.2005.03761.x.
30. Winckers K, ten Cate H, Hackeng TM. The role of tissue factor pathway inhibitor in atherosclerosis and arterial thrombosis. Blood Rev. 2013;27(3):119–32. https://doi.org/10.1016/j.blre.2013.03.001.
31. Li Q, Kuang Y, Qiu J, Zhang X, Ruan Y, Li Z. The correlation between plasma tissue factor and interleukin 18 and their significance in patients with acute coronary syndrome. Cardiovasc Toxicol. 2015;15(3):276–82. https://doi.org/10.1007/s12012-014-9296-5.
32. Crawley J, Lupu F, Westmuckett AD, Severs NJ, Kakkar VV, Lupu C. Expression, localization, and activity of tissue factor pathway inhibitor in normal and atherosclerotic human vessels. Arterioscler Thromb Vasc Biol. 2000;20(5):1362–73. https://doi.org/10.1161/01.ATV.20.5.1362.
33. Westrick RJ, Bodary PF, Xu Z, Shen YC, Broze GJ, Eitzman DT. Deficiency of tissue factor pathway inhibitor promotes atherosclerosis and thrombosis in mice. Circulation. 2001;103(25):3044–6. https://doi.org/10.1161/hc2501.092492.
34. Morange PE, Blankenberg S, Alessi MC, Bickel C, Rupprecht HJ, Schnabel R, et al. Prognostic value of plasma tissue factor and tissue factor pathway inhibitor for cardiovascular death in patients with coronary artery disease: the AtheroGene study. J Thromb Haemost. 2007;5(3):475–82. https://doi.org/10.1111/j.1538-7836.2007.02372.x.
35. Steppich BA, Braun SL, Stein A, Demetz G, Groha P, Schömig A, et al. Plasma TF activity predicts cardiovascular mortality in patients with acute myocardial infarction. Thromb J. 2009;7(1):11. https://doi.org/10.1186/1477-9560-7-11.
36. Wang X, Chen R, Li Y, Miao F. Predictive value of prothrombin time for all-cause mortality in acute myocardial infarction patients. Conf Proc IEEE Eng Med Biol Soc. 2018;2018:5366–9.
37. Peng J, Liu MM, Jin JL, Cao YX, Guo YL, Wu NQ, et al. Association of circulating PCSK9 concentration with cardiovascular metabolic markers and outcomes in stable coronary artery disease patients with or without diabetes: a prospective, observational cohort study. Cardiovasc Diabetol. 2020;19(1):167. https://doi.org/10.1186/s12933-020-01142-0.
38. Zawadzki C, Susen S, Richard F, Haulon S, Corseaux D, Jeanpierre E, et al. Dyslipidemia shifts the tissue factor/tissue factor pathway inhibitor balance toward increased thrombogenicity in atherosclerotic plaques: evidence for a corrective effect of statins. Atherosclerosis. 2007;195(2):e117–25. https://doi.org/10.1016/j.atherosclerosis.2006.10.012.

21

Prognostic value of characteristics of plaque combined with residual syntax score among patients with STEMI undergoing primary PCI: An intravascular optical coherence tomography study

Xiaoxiao Zhao[1], Ying Wang[1], Runzhen Chen[1], Jiannan Li[1], Jinying Zhou[1], Chen Liu[1], Peng Zhou[1], Zhaoxue Sheng[1], Yi Chen[1], Li Song[1], Hanjun Zhao[1*] and Hongbing Yan[2*]

Abstract

Aim: The present study aimed to explore these characteristics, particularly thin-cap fibroatheroma (TCFA), in relation to residual syntax score (rSS) in patients who presented with acute MI.

Methods and outcomes: A total of 434 consecutive patients with MI aged ≥18 years who had STEMI underwent primary PCI. Notably, compared with other subgroups, the presence of TCFA in culprit lesions and a higher level of rSS, were significantly associated with MACE. When rSS was divided into three groups, high rSS levels were associated with a higher incidence of MACE, in the subgroups of without TCFA ($P = 0.005$), plaque erosion ($P = 0.045$), macrophage infiltration ($P = 0.026$), and calcification ($P = 0.002$). AUC of ROC curve was 0.794 and 0.816, whereas the AUC of the survival ROC was 0.798 and 0.846.

Conclusion: The results of this study could be used in clinical practice to support risk stratification.

Keywords: Optical coherence tomography, Residual syntax score, Thin-cap fibroatheroma, Prognosis value

Introduction

The residual Synergy Between Percutaneous Coronary Intervention with Taxus and Cardiac Surgery (SYNTAX) score (rSS) is a quantitative, objective, and reliable measure developed to assess the complexity of residual stenosis and the degree of angiographic completeness of revascularization based on the recalculation of the SYNTAX score from coronary angiography after percutaneous coronary intervention (PCI) [1–3]. High rSS has been shown to be correlated with worse outcomes and adverse mortality in patients undergoing angiography-guided PCI [1, 2, 4, 5].

Optical coherence tomography (OCT) is a high-resolution, cross-sectional, intravascular imaging technique that enables detailed identification of coronary plaque characteristics [6, 7], including thin-cap fibroatheroma (TCFA), which is an important index of morphological characteristics with respect to vulnerable

* Correspondence: 15210020808@163.com; hbyanfuwai2018@163.com
Diagnosis and Treatment of Acute Coronary Syndrome Group of Yan Hongbing from Fuwai Hospital - Chinese Academy of Medical Sciences (CAMS).
[1]Department of Cardiology, Fuwai Hospital, National Center for Cardiovascular Diseases, Peking Union Medical College & Chinese Academy of Medical Sciences, No.167, Beijing 100037, China
[2]Fuwai Hospital, Chinese Academy of Medical Sciences, 12 Langshan Rd, Shenzhen 518000, China

plaques [8]. Nonetheless, the association between rSS and the morphological characteristics of vulnerable coronary plaques in patients with acute myocardial infarction (MI) has not been fully investigated using OCT. Therefore, the present study aimed to explore these characteristics, especially TCFA, in relation to rSS in patients who presented with acute MI in order to elucidate the effects of different rSS groups based on TCFA on the incidence of major adverse cardiovascular events (MACEs) in a prospective cohort consisting of patients who underwent OCT for culprit lesions (Optical Coherence Tomography Examination in Acute Myocardial Infarction [OCTAMI], ClinicalTrials.gov: NCT03593928).

Methods

Study population

For this study, a post hoc analysis of the OCTAMI registry, in which all enrolled patients were screened by OCT, was conducted. A total of 434 consecutive patients with MI aged ≥18 years who had ST-segment elevation myocardial infarction (STEMI) underwent primary PCI at Fuwai Hospital, the largest PCI center in China, between March 2017 and March 2019. Enrollment into this study required that the patients did not meet any of the following clinical exclusion criteria: (1) end-stage renal disease; (2) cardiac shock; (3) allergy to contrast media; (4) serious liver dysfunction; (5) contraindication to aspirin or ticagrelor; (6) congestive heart failure; and (7) lesions with characteristics that increased the difficulty in performing OCT (e.g., heavily calcified vessels, left main coronary artery diseases, and chronic total occlusion). STEMI was defined according to established criteria [9].

This study was conducted in accordance with the principles outlined in the Declaration of Helsinki and was approved by the Ethics Committee (Fuwai Hospital, BeiJing, China). Written informed consent was obtained prior to the inclusion of participants in this study. All enrolled patients who were examined using OCT had provided additional written informed consent specific to the OCT study (Fuwai Hospital OCTAMI Registry, clinical trials.gov: NCT03593928).

Calculation of rSS

Specific calculation of the SYNTAX score has been described in detail by previous studies [3, 10]. Dedicated interventional cardiologists carried out the procedure for calculating the baseline SYNTAX score and rSS. Briefly, each coronary lesion with ≥50% diameter stenosis in vessels with diameters ≥1.5 mm was obtained from the preprocedural angiogram and scored using the SYNTAX score algorithm from the website http://syntaxscore.com/. Two experienced observers who were blinded to other data (including baseline clinical presentations, coronary angiography characteristics, and clinical follow-up outcomes) anonymously and independently analyzed the calculated rSS in a core laboratory. From the post-procedural angiogram, the sum of individual SYNTAX scores (each coronary lesion with ≥50% diameter stenosis in vessels with diameters ≥1.5 mm that remained untreated) constituted the rSS [2].

OCT image acquisition

Intravascular OCT imaging was performed in accordance with a previous study [6]. Briefly, OCT images of culprit lesions were acquired using a frequency-domain OCT system (ILUMIEN OPTIS™; St. Jude Medical/Abbott, St. Paul, MN, USA) and a catheter (Dragonfly™; LightLab Imaging, Inc., Westford, MA, USA) after restoring the antegrade coronary blood flow and reducing the thrombus burden by pre-dilatation and/or thrombus aspiration. To remove blood from the field of view and thereby achieve a virtually blood-free environment, continuous flushing with contrast media via manual injection directly from the guiding catheter was performed in the coronary blood during image acquisition. Images of the entire length of culprit vessels were acquired using an automatic pullback device that moved at 36 mm/s, and cross-sectional images were generated at a rotational rate of 180 frames/s. The total length of the OCT pullback was 75 mm and digitally archived.

Quantitative OCT image analysis

Three independent observers who were blinded to clinical presentations and angiographic data analyzed all OCT images on an OCT offline review workstation (St. Jude Medical) in a core laboratory. When there was inconsistency among the investigators, a consensus reading was obtained. The entire segments of culprit plaques were identified by OCT analysis conducted with the entire OCT pullback. A culprit plaque was defined as a plaque centered on the culprit lesion and bilaterally extending to > 5 mm of the normal vessel segment [11]. Based on established criteria [6], TCFA, culprit plaques, lipid-rich plaques, calcification, white/ red thrombi, Cholesterol crystals and Macrophage infiltration were defined (Fig. 1).

Endpoints and follow-up

MACEs were defined as a composite of all-cause death, MI recurrence, revascularization, and ischemic cerebrovascular events. The follow-up questionnaire is presented in the supplement. These questions were involved the following questionnaire: If taking the following medicine, please clarify the dosage and Pharmaceutical specifications. Have you stopped taking the medicine? The time and the reason of stop taking medicine. The medicine involved in the follow up including

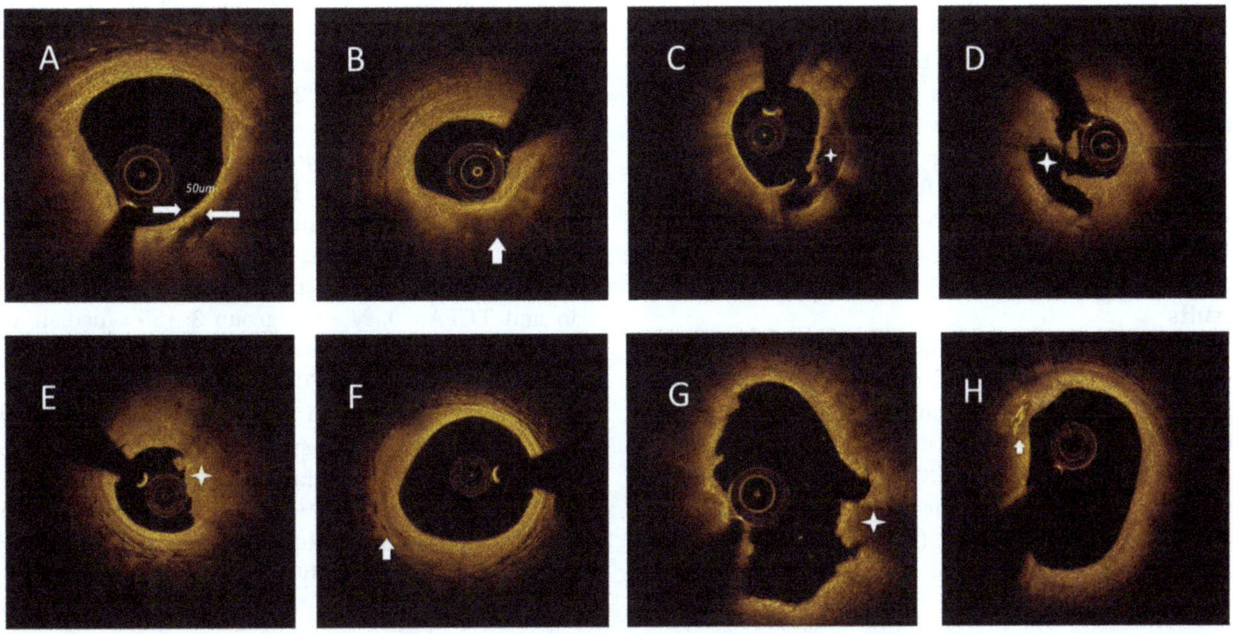

Fig. 1 Representative cross-sectional optical coherence tomography images. **A** Thin-cap fibroatheroma was defined as a lipid-rich plaque (lipid identified as signal poor and attenuating) of more than two quadrants of vessel lumen with a fibrous cap (identified as signal rich, or brightly reflecting, with low attenuation) thickness measuring 65 um or less. (arrow). **B** Lipid plaque (arrow) most often appears as diffusely bordered, signal-poor regions with overlying signal-rich bands. **C** Calcification identified by the presence of a well-delineated, low-backscattering heterogeneous region (asterisk). **D** Plaque rupture identified by disruption of the fibrous cap and cavity formation (asterisk). **E** Plaque erosion identified by the presence of attached thrombus (asterisk) overlying an intact plaque. **F** Microvessels defined as tubule luminal structures that do not generate a signal, with no connection to the vessel lumen (arrow). **G** Red thrombus consists mainly of red blood cells; relevant OCT images are characterized as high-backscattering protrusions with signal free shadowing (asterisk). H. Cholesterol crystal (arrow) identified by linear, highly backscattering structures without remarkable backward shadowing

antiplatelet drug usage (Aspirin, Clopidogrel, Ticagrelor), anticoagulant drugs (Warfarin, Rivaroxaban, Apixaban, Dabigatran, Edoxaban) and other cardiovascular medications (statins, nitrates, ACEI/ARB, β- receptor blockers, calcium channel blockers, diuretics). Well-trained nurses or cardiologists who were uninformed about the purpose of this study confirmed the events in the enrolled patients via telephone calls, direct interviews, and hospital discharge records or clinical notes in the event of death. The follow-up methods were approved by obtaining permission from the Institutional Review Board of Fuwai Hospital. Well-trained physicians in charge of the follow-up primary endpoints, including cardiac death, all-cause death, angina pectoris, revascularization, heart failure, and ischemic stroke, identified and extracted the primary endpoints from hospital records, laboratory reports, emergency records, medical records, and clinical notes (required to be sent to our centers). Clinical endpoints were confirmed by at least two professional physicians.

Statistical analysis

Continuous data are presented as mean ± standard deviation or as median (interquartile range). Between-group differences were analyzed using one-way analysis of variance. Categorical data are presented as number (%) and were compared using Pearson's χ^2 test or Fisher's exact test. Univariable and multivariable Cox proportional hazards regression models with adjustments for confounding factors were used to determine the association between rSS and TCFA determined by OCT with MACEs. The relationship between microstructural features of culprit lesions on OCT and follow-up outcomes stratified by rSS levels and TCFA was assessed using the Spearman correlation. Survival analysis was performed using the Kaplan–Meier method. Receiver operating characteristic (ROC) curves were created using MedCalc version 18.2.1 (MedCalc Software, Ostend, Belgium). For the assessment of the discriminatory value of rSS and TCFA, time-dependent ROC curves were plotted using R language version X64 4.0.4 (R Foundation for Statistical Computing, Vienna, Austria) in order to obviate the limitation of potential bias due to censoring. ROC curves were generated by incorporating the following four predictive values: (1) predictive value I: traditional risk factors; (2) predictive value II: traditional risk factors + rSS; (3) predictive value III: traditional risk factors + rSS + TCFA; and (4) predictive value IV: traditional risk factors + rSS + TCFA + microstructural features of culprit lesions. Models III and IV were dichotomized based on a cutoff determined by the Youden index (cutoff value). Kaplan–Meier curves were generated using R language, and cumulative event rates were compared using the log-rank test. Other analyses were performed using SPSS version 20.0 (IBM Corp., Armonk, NY, USA). All *P*-values were two-tailed, and statistical significance was set at $P < 0.05$.

Results

A total of 434 patients presented with STEMI and underwent OCT imaging of native culprit vessels between March 2017 and March 2019. After applying the inclusion criteria, 160 patients were excluded because of a lack of pre-intervention OCT examinations ($n = 8$), low-quality OCT images due to a massive thrombus ($n = 87$), in-stent restenosis ($n = 34$), coronary spasm ($n = 11$), coronary embolism ($n = 2$), calcified nodule ($n = 17$), and absence of follow-up data ($n = 1$). Consequently, a total of 274 patients were enrolled in this study. A flow diagram illustrating the study sample selection is presented in Fig. 2.

Baseline clinical and angiographic data

Table 1 summarizes the baseline clinical and angiographic characteristics stratified by rSS levels and TCFA (group 0: rSS ≤ median and TCFA = 0, $N = 108$; group 1: rSS ≤ median and TCFA = 1, $N = 32$; group 2: rSS > median and TCFA = 0, $N = 97$; group 3: rSS > median and TCFA = 1, $N = 37$). The mean age of the study participants was 58.0 years, and 80.7% were males. Most participants were considered to have traditional risk factors for cardiovascular disease such as hypertension (59.9%), hyperlipidemia (86.1%), and current smoking (68.2%), while only 28.5, 8, and 4.7% of the enrolled patients had a history of diabetes mellitus (DM), PCI, and peripheral atherosclerosis, respectively. The high rSS with TCFA

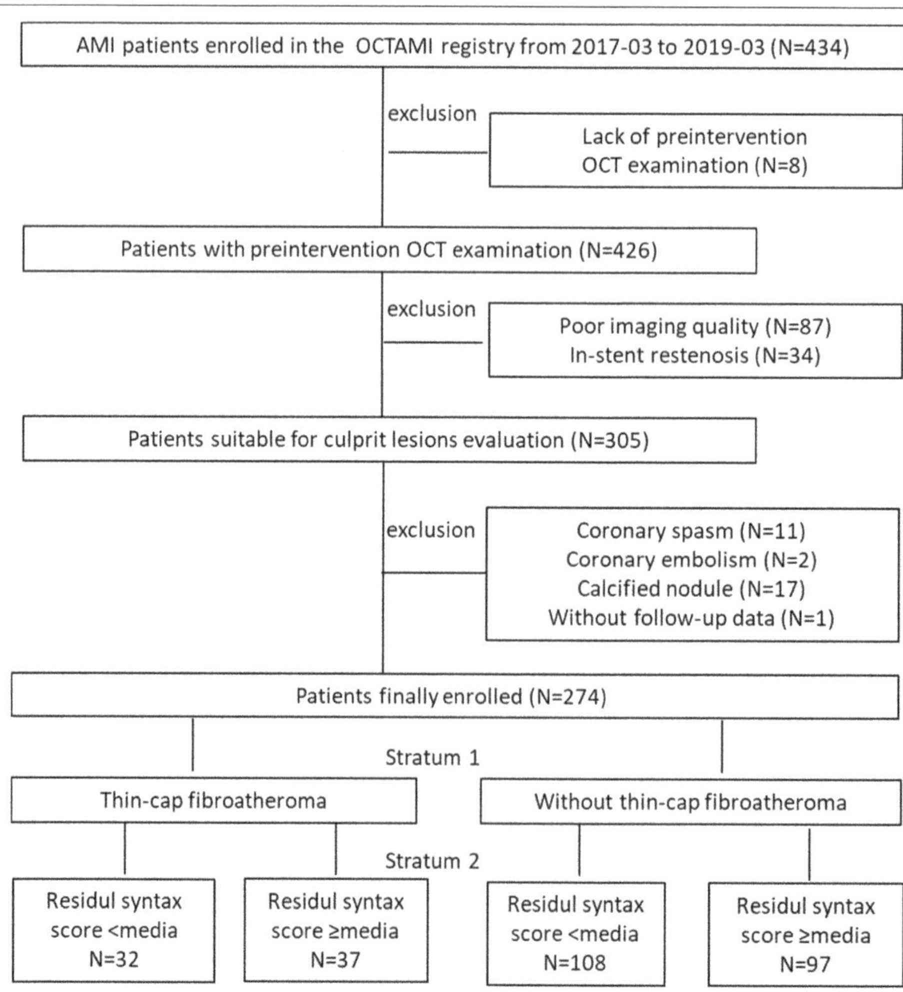

Fig. 2 Flow chart 2 Study flow chart. OCTAMI, Optical Coherence Tomography Examination in Acute Myocardial Infarction; OCT optical coherence tomography, AMI acute myocardial infarction

Table 1 Baseline clinical characteristics of the study population

Variables	Total ($N = 274$)	Group = 0 (TCFA absent &Rss ≤ 4)	Group = 1 (TCFA present &Rss ≤ 4)	Group = 2 (TCFA absent &Rss>4)	Group = 3 (TCFA present &Rss>4)	*P* value
Age (years)	58.0 (50.0, 67.0)	55.0 (49.0, 64.5)	61.5 (54.8, 72.0)	61.0 (51.0, 68.0)	59.0 (50.0, 63.0)	0.068
Male [%(n)]	221 (80.7)	92 (85.2)	23 (71.9)	71 (73.2)	35 (94.6)	0.011*
Height (cm)	170.0 (165.0, 173.0)	170.0 (165.0, 175.8)	169.0 (160.0, 172.0)	170.0 (165.0, 172.0)	170.0 (167.0, 172.0)	0.488
Weight (kg)	75.0 (67.0, 82.2)	75.0 (69.2, 82.9)	75.0 (69.0, 80.0)	72.0 (65.0, 83.0)	75.0 (65.0, 81.0)	0.751
Heart rate (beats per minute)	76.0 (65.0, 86.0)	80.0 (67.0, 90.0)	70.5 (65.0, 78.2)	74.0 (64.5, 83.0)	77.0 (66.0, 87.0)	0.091
SBP (mmHg)	121.0 (107.0, 134.0)	120.0 (106.0, 132.0)	111.0 (104.8, 126.0)	124.0 (110.0, 136.0)	123.0 (110.0, 135.0)	0.266
DBP(mmHg)	79.0 ± 12.3	79.4 ± 13.1	75.5 ± 10.2	78.4 ± 11.8	81.8 ± 13.0	0.266
Syntax score of base	16.0 (11.0, 22.5)	14.0 (9.0, 20.1)	11.5 (8.8, 16.0)	19.5 (15.0, 26.5)	20.0 (15.0, 26.0)	< 0.001
Residual syntax score	4.0 (0.0, 8.0)	0.0 (0.0, 2.0)	2.0 (0.0, 2.2)	8.0 (5.0, 12.0)	9.0 (6.0, 15.0)	< 0.001
Risk factors						
Hypertension[%(n)]	164 (59.9)	59 (54.6)	19 (59.4)	63 (64.9)	23 (62.2)	0.501
Diabetes[%(n)]	78 (28.5)	23 (21.3)	13 (40.6)	27 (27.8)	15 (40.5)	0.502
Hyperlipidemia[%(n)]	236 (86.1)	93 (86.1)	29 (90.6)	81 (83.5)	33 (89.2)	0.781
Smoking[%(n)]	165 (68.2)	60 (63.2)	19 (76)	58 (65.9)	28 (82.4)	0.160
Previous PCI[%(n)]	22 (8.0)	8 (7.4)	5 (15.6)	7 (7.2)	2 (5.4)	0.433
Peripheral atherosclerosis [%(n)]	12 (4.7)	5 (4.9)	1 (3.4)	4 (4.4)	2 (5.7)	0.977
CKD[%(n)]	4 (1.6)	2 (2)	2 (6.9)	0 (0)	0 (0)	0.076
Laboratory examinations						
HDL-cholesterol (mmol/L)	1.1 (0.9, 1.2)	1.1 (0.9, 1.2)	1.2 (1.0, 1.3)	1.0 (0.9, 1.2)	1.1 (0.8, 1.2)	0.215
LDL-cholesterol at (mmol/L)	2.8 ± 0.9	2.6 ± 0.8	3.1 ± 1.0	2.8 ± 0.9	3.0 ± 0.8	0.014*
Triglycerides (mmol/L)	1.4 (1.0, 2.0)	1.4 (0.9, 1.9)	1.4 (1.0, 1.8)	1.4 (1.0, 2.1)	1.7 (1.0, 2.5)	0.29
LPA (mg/L)	159.1 (71.5, 376.1)	166.5 (70.8, 378.8)	127.2 (84.1, 250.2)	159.2 (66.0, 389.6)	183.0 (75.0, 419.0)	0.841
hs-CRP (mg/L)	6.2 (2.7, 10.9)	6.2 (2.9, 11.1)	3.4 (1.7, 8.6)	5.9 (2.6, 10.9)	6.7 (3.2, 10.8)	0.194
D-dimer (ug/mL)	0.2 (0.1, 0.4)	0.2 (0.1, 0.4)	0.2 (0.1, 0.3)	0.2 (0.1, 0.4)	0.3 (0.2, 0.6)	0.268
TnI (ng/L)	0.9 (0.1, 5.2)	1.3 (0.1, 5.4)	0.8 (0.0, 3.4)	0.8 (0.2, 4.9)	0.3 (0.0, 3.8)	0.45
Peak level of TnI (ng/L)	23.9 (10.8, 46.5)	25.2 (9.6, 52.1)	18.2 (10.3, 32.5)	26.2 (11.3, 46.5)	19.2 (8.7, 42.8)	0.419
BNP (ng/L)	137.3 (47.9, 566.0)	182.0 (60.4, 626.5)	170.2 (47.7, 417.1)	131.7 (48.0, 571.1)	75.9 (33.7, 375.8)	0.300
Peak level of BNP (ng/L)	1606.0 (633.5, 3122.0)	1465.0 (602.4, 3164.0)	1598.0 (989.5, 2484.0)	1779.0 (511.3, 3113.0)	1190.0 (867.4, 3122.0)	0.955
WBC 10^9/L	9.8 (8.0, 11.9)	10.5 (7.9, 12.6)	10.0 (8.7, 11.6)	9.6 (8.1, 11.4)	9.2 (7.8, 10.9)	0.179
Hemoglobin	147.5 (136.0, 156.0)	149.0 (137.8, 156.0)	147.0 (136.2, 157.2)	147.0 (133.0, 154.0)	147.0 (137.0, 157.0)	0.635
Platelet	222.0 (191.2, 280.8)	222.0 (190.0, 285.2)	231.0 (186.5, 266.0)	230.0 (195.0, 281.0)	217.0 (190.0, 287.0)	0.909
Crea (umol/L)	79.0 (67.9, 91.8)	78.1 (67.1, 94.4)	83.1 (69.2, 91.7)	77.7 (66.0, 88.0)	82.2 (73.4, 92.4)	0.234
Glu	7.6 (6.3, 10.0)	7.1 (6.3, 9.0)	9.0 (7.4, 10.2)	7.7 (6.1, 10.3)	7.8 (6.5, 11.8)	0.082
ALC	6.0 (5.6, 7.1)	5.8 (5.5, 6.6)	6.2 (5.8, 7.9)	6.1 (5.6, 7.1)	6.2 (5.6, 7.7)	0.097
Discharge medication regimen						
Aspirin[%(n)]	265 (96.70)	105 (97.20)	31 (96.90)	93 (95.90)	36 (97.30)	0.952
Ticagrelor[%(n)]	139 (50.70)	50 (46.30)	22 (68.80)	51 (52.60)	16 (43.20)	0.113
Clopidogrel[%(n)]	135 (49.30)	58 (53.70)	10 (31.20)	46 (47.40)	21 (56.80)	0.113
ACEI/ARB[%(n)]	204 (74.50)	83 (76.90)	24 (75)	67 (69.10)	30 (81.10)	0.447
Beta-Blockers[%(n)]	240 (87.60)	95 (88)	28 (87.50)	84 (86.60)	33 (89.20)	0.988
Statin[%(n)]	266 (97.10)	104 (96.30)	32 (100)	93 (95.90)	37 (100)	0.638
Proton pump inhibitor[%(n)]	109 (39.80)	39 (36.10)	16 (50)	38 (39.20)	16 (43.20)	0.532

Table 1 Baseline clinical characteristics of the study population *(Continued)*

Variables	Total (*N* = 274)	Group = 0 (TCFA absent &Rss ≤ 4)	Group = 1 (TCFA present &Rss ≤ 4)	Group = 2 (TCFA absent &Rss>4)	Group = 3 (TCFA present &Rss>4)	*P* value
Oral anticoagulants[%(n)]	6 (2.20)	2 (1.90)	1 (3.10)	3 (3.10)	0 (0)	0.728
Procedural data						
Angiographic findings						
Culprit vessels						< 0.001*
LAD	131 (47.8)	69 (63.9)	15 (46.9)	37 (38.1)	10 (27)	
LCX	27 (9.9)	5 (4.6)	1 (3.1)	18 (18.6)	3 (8.1)	
RCA	116 (42.3)	34 (31.5)	16 (50)	42 (43.3)	24 (64.9)	
Coronary artery lesions						< 0.001*
SVD	66 (24.1)	53 (49.1)	9 (28.1)	3 (3.1)	1 (2.7)	
DVD	100 (36.5)	36 (33.3)	17 (53.1)	35 (36.1)	12 (32.4)	
TVD	108 (39.4)	19 (17.6)	6 (18.8)	59 (60.8)	24 (64.9)	
Pre-TIMI flow						0.793
0	172 (62.8)	71 (65.7)	19 (59.4)	62 (63.9)	20 (54.1)	
1	15 (5.5)	5 (4.6)	1 (3.1)	6 (6.2)	3 (8.1)	
2	25 (9.1)	9 (8.3)	5 (15.6)	9 (9.3)	2 (5.4)	
3	62 (22.6)	23 (21.3)	7 (21.9)	20 (20.6)	12 (32.4)	
AHA classification						0.793
A	2 (0.7)	0 (0)	0 (0)	1 (1)	1 (2.7)	
B1	25 (9.2)	11 (10.2)	3 (9.4)	6 (6.2)	5 (13.5)	
B2	38 (13.9)	16 (14.8)	4 (12.5)	13 (13.5)	5 (13.5)	
C	208 (76.2)	81 (75)	25 (78.1)	76 (79.2)	26 (70.3)	
Diameter of lesion	3.0 (2.8, 3.5)	3.0 (3.0, 3.5)	3.3 (3.0, 3.5)	3.0 (2.7, 3.5)	3.0 (3.0, 3.5)	0.033*
Length of lesion	26.0 (19.0, 37.0)	24.0 (17.8, 34.2)	29.0 (21.5, 42.8)	27.0 (21.0, 36.2)	30.0 (18.0, 35.0)	0.143
Endpoint events						
MACE [%(n)]	48 (17.5)	13 (12)	4 (12.5)	18 (18.6)	13 (35.1)	0.013*
Death [%(n)]	2 (0.70)	0 (0)	0 (0)	1 (10)	1 (2.70)	0.339
Recurrent MI [%(n)]	8 (2.90)	1 (0.90)	0 (0)	4 (4.10)	3 (8.10)	0.082
Stroke [%(n)]	9 (3.30)	4 (3.70)	2 (6.20)	2 (2.10)	1 (2.70)	0.618
Revascularization	37 (13.5)	9 (8.3)	2 (6.2)	15 (15.5)	11 (29.7)	0.012*
Heart failure [%(n)]	6 (2.20)	3 (2.80)	0 (0)	3 (3.1)	0 (0)	0.768

Continuous data are presented as median (interquartile range). Categorical data are presented as number (%)

DM diabetes mellitus, *SBP* systolic blood pressure, *DBP* diabetes blood pressure, *PCI* percutaneous coronary intervention, *CKD* chronic kidney disease, *HDL*, high density lipoprotein, *LDL* low density lipoprotein, *LPA* lipse activator, *hs-CRP* high sensitive C-reactive protein, *ACEI* angiotensin-converting enzyme inhibitor, *ARB* angiotensin receptor blocker, *TnI* troponin, *LAD* left anterior descending artery, *LCX* left circumfex artery, *RCA* right coronary artery, *DVD* double vessel disease, *SVD* single vessel disease, *TVD* triple vessel disease, *AHA* American Heart Association, *MACE* major adverse cardiovascular events, *MI* myocardial infarction, *TCFA* thin-cap fibroatheroma, *rSS* residual syntax score

**P* < 0.05

group (rSS > median and TCFA = 1) consisted of more male patients (94.6% vs. 85.2%/71.9%/73.2%) and had a higher MACE incidence (35.1% vs. 12.0%/12.5%/18.6%) at a median follow-up of 1.98 years (712.52 days). Other baseline characteristics were not statistically different among the four groups. Representative OCT images are shown in Fig. 1.

Baseline OCT findings

A comparison of plaque characteristics based on OCT findings among the four groups is presented in Table 2. The rate of plaque rupture in culprit lesions was higher among patients with high rSS and TCFA (group 3) than in those with low rSS without TCFA (group 0) (91.9% vs. 42.6%, $P < 0.001$). Similarly, the rates of lipid-rich plaques (91.9% vs. 37.0%, $P < 0.001$) and macrophage infiltration (94.6% vs. 40.7%, $P < 0.001$) were higher in group 0 than in group 3. However, the rates of fibrous plaques (5.4% vs. 28.2%, $P = 0.003$) and mixed plaques (2.7% vs. 21.9%, $P = 0.004$) were lower in the high rSS with TCFA group than in the low rSS without TCFA group. The frequencies of microstructural features such

Table 2 Optical coherence tomography characteristics

Variables	Total (N = 274)	Group = 0 (TCFA absent &Rss ≤ 4)	Group = 1 (TCFA present &Rss ≤ 4)	Group = 2 (TCFA absent &Rss>4)	Group = 3 (TCFA present &Rss>4)	P value						
						$P^{\#}_{for\ overall}$	$P_{0\ vs\ 1}$	$P_{0\ vs\ 2}$	$P_{0\ vs\ 3}$	$P_{1\ vs\ 2}$	$P_{1\ vs\ 3}$	$P_{2\ vs\ 3}$
Plaque morphology						< 0.001*	0.007*	0.940	< 0.001*	0.161	0.953	< 0.001*
Plaque rupture[%(n)]	155 (56.6)	46 (42.6)	24 (75)	51 (52.6)	34 (91.9)							
Intact fibrous cap[%(n)]	119 (43.4)	62 (57.4)	8 (25)	46 (47.4)	3 (8.1)							
Lipid-rich plaque[%(n)]	141 (51.5)	40 (37)	25 (78.1)	42 (43.3)	34 (91.9)	< 0.001*	< 0.001 *	1.000	< 0.001 *	0.004*	1.000	< 0.001 *
Fibrous plaque[%(n)]	78 (28.5)	38 (35.2)	2 (6.2)	36 (37.1)	2 (5.4)	< 0.001*	0.009*	1.000	0.003*	0.005*	1.000	0.002*
Mixed plaque [%(n)]	60 (21.9)	32 (29.6)	4 (12.5)	23 (23.7)	1 (2.7)	0.004*	0.240	1.000	0.004*	1.000	1.000	0.052
Healing plaque[%(n)]	55 (20.1)	15 (13.9)	6 (18.8)	26 (26.8)	8 (21.6)	0.145						
Calcification[%(n)]	140 (51.1)	48 (44.4)	17 (53.1)	54 (55.7)	21 (56.8)	0.354						
Micro-calcification[%(n)]	136 (49.6)	47 (43.5)	17 (53.1)	52 (53.6)	20 (54.1)	0.445						
Macrophage[%(n)]	149 (54.4)	44 (40.7)	31 (96.9)	39 (40.2)	35 (94.6)	< 0.001*	< 0.001 *	1.000	< 0.001 *	< 0.001*	1.000	< 0.001 *
Microvessels[%(n)]	48 (17.5)	20 (18.5)	9 (28.1)	13 (13.4)	6 (16.2)	0.290						
Cholesterol crystal[%(n)]	22 (8.0)	7 (6.5)	3 (9.4)	7 (7.2)	5 (13.5)	0.520						
Thrombus[%(n)]	271 (98.9)	106 (98.1)	32 (100)	96 (99)	37 (100)	1.000						
Minimal FCT, um	100.0 (60.0, 120.0)	100.0 (90.0, 150.0)	60.0 (50.0, 60.0)	110.0 (90.0, 140.0)	60.0 (50.0, 60.0)	< 0.001*	< 0.001 *	1.000	< 0.001 *	< 0.001 *	1.000	< 0.001 *
Maximal lipid arc, °	360.0 (248.0, 360.0)	360.0 (242.0, 360.0)	360.0 (360.0, 360.0)	293.0 (230.0, 360.0)	360.0 (360.0, 360.0)	< 0.001*	0.031*	1.000	0.005*	0.001*	1.000	< 0.001*
MLA, mm2	1.7 (1.4, 2.2)	1.6 (1.4, 2.2)	2.0 (1.6, 2.7)	1.6 (1.3, 2.1)	1.9 (1.6, 2.3)	0.022*	0.088	1.000	0.742	0.043*	1.000	0.418

Continuous data are presented as median (interquartile range). Categorical variables are presented as number (%)
TCFA thin-cap fibroatheroma, *rSS*, residual syntax score, *FCT* fibrous cap thickness, *MLA* minimal lumen area
*$P < 0.05$, # P for overall means statistical analysis among four groups

Table 3 Association between separate endpoints survival and groups which divided by TCFA and rSS in all enrolled patients

	Crude model		Adjust model I		Adjust model II		Adjust model III	
Group	**crude HR(95%CI)**	**crude P value**	**Adj I. HR(95%CI)**	**Adj. P value**	**Adj II. HR(95%CI)**	**Adj. P value**	**Adj III. HR(95%CI)**	**Adj. P value**
MACE								
0	1 (reference)	1 (reference)	1 (reference)	1 (reference)	1 (reference)	1 (reference)	1 (reference)	1 (reference)
1	1.09 (0.35,3.34)	0.884	0.94 (0.3,2.91)	0.915	1.14 (0.35,3.72)	0.832	1.28 (0.38,4.29)	0.692
2	1.53 (0.75,3.12)	0.244	1.36 (0.66,2.80)	0.404	1.50 (0.68,3.31)	0.315	1.62 (0.73,3.60)	0.233
3	3.21 (1.49,6.93)	0.003*	3.20 (1.47,6.96)	0.003*	3.79 (1.55,9.26)	0.003*	4.19 (1.69,10.41)	0.002*
Trend test	1.44 (1.1,1.87)	0.007*	1.42 (1.08,1.86)	0.011*	1.49 (1.1,2.02)	0.010*	1.53 (1.13,2.08)	0.006*
Stroke								
0	1 (reference)	1 (reference)	1 (reference)	1 (reference)	1 (reference)	1 (reference)	1 (reference)	1 (reference)
1	1.84 (0.34,10.05)	0.483	1.38 (0.24,7.83)	0.713	1.26 (0.19,8.32)	0.808	1.52 (0.21,11.21)	0.682
2	0.52 (0.09,2.84)	0.449	0.41 (0.07,2.27)	0.304	0.37 (0.06,2.17)	0.27	0.38 (0.06,2.40)	0.303
3	0.68 (0.08,6.11)	0.733	0.62 (0.07,5.62)	0.674	0.61 (0.06,6.34)	0.682	0.83 (0.08,8.95)	0.879
Trend test	0.8 (0.44,1.47)	0.477	0.74 (0.4,1.39)	0.349	0.71 (0.36,1.38)	0.314	0.75 (0.38,1.47)	0.406
Angina								
0	1 (reference)	1 (reference)	1 (reference)	1 (reference)	1 (reference)	1 (reference)	1 (reference)	1 (reference)
1	1.34 (0.36,5.07)	0.663	1.13 (0.29,4.36)	0.857	1.3 (0.3,5.5)	0.726	1.25 (0.28,5.60)	0.768
2	0.79 (0.27,2.27)	0.659	0.67 (0.23,1.97)	0.467	0.69 (0.22,2.21)	0.533	0.62 (0.19,2.06)	0.434
3	1.39 (0.42,4.61)	0.594	1.51 (0.44,5.1)	0.511	1.45 (0.38,5.46)	0.586	1.41 (0.36,5.52)	0.621
Trend test	1.02 (0.7,1.5)	0.914	1.00 (0.67,1.50)	0.983	0.99 (0.65,1.54)	0.998	0.98 (0.63,1.52)	0.915

Data presented are HRs and 95% CI. Adjust I model adjusts for sex and age; Adjust II model adjusts for adjust I plus ejection fraction, smoke, hypertension, hyperlipidemia, diabetes mellitus; Adjust III model adjusts for adjust II + white blood cell, hemoglobin, platelet, creatine kinase, glucose, glycosylated hemoglobin, C-reactive protain

TCFA thin-cap fibroatheroma, *rSS* residual syntax score, *Adj.* adjusted, *MACE* major adverse cardiovascular events

*$P < 0.05$

as healing plaques, calcification, microcalcification, microvessels, cholesterol crystals, and thrombus were similar among all three groups, as were quantitative parameters such as the minimal lumen area.

Findings with cox regression models in subgroups

Cox regression models indicated that the hazard ratio (HR) for MACEs was higher in patients with high rSS and TCFA than in patients with low rSS without TCFA (Table 3). The Kaplan–Meier curves for the crude prediction of revascularization, MACE and MACEs plus heart failure are presented in Supplementary Fig. 1. The high rSS with TCFA group had a higher incidence of MACEs (HR, 1.45; 95% confidence interval [CI], 1.13–2.08; $P = 0.002$) than the low rSS without TCFA group, and additional adjustment for other variables such as sex, age, ejection fraction, smoking, hypertension, hyperlipidemia, DM, WBC count, hemoglobin, platelet count, creatine kinase, glucose, glycosylated hemoglobin, and C-reactive protein did not alter the significant difference. However, a similar significant difference among the other subgroups was not observed. Further, multiple comparisons revealed that the incidences of stroke and angina pectoris were not significantly different among the subgroups. While the HR increased with an increase in rSS among patients without TCFA (Supplemental Fig. 2A), this tendency was not observed with an increase in rSS among patients with TCFA (curve fitting with Cox regression models; Supplementary Fig. 2B).

Table 4 shows the crude and adjusted multivariable relationships between MACEs stratified according to levels of rSS divided into subgroups according to characteristics on OCT. In patients without TCFA, increasing tertiles of rSS levels were associated with a higher cumulative incidence of MACEs over time (P for trend = 0.005). Nevertheless, in those with TCFA, increasing tertiles of rSS levels were not associated with a higher incidence of MACE risk over time in a stepwise manner (P for trend = 0.947). In the group without TCFA, the HR for MACEs among patients with high rSS was 5.85-fold higher than that among patients with low rSS in the fully adjusted Cox regression models ($P = 0.004$). Similarly, in the group with plaque erosion, the HR for MACEs among patients with high rSS was 3.63-fold higher than

Table 4 Association of rSS with MACE in enrolled patients according to subgroup of characteristics by OCT

Variables	MACE /Total	Crude model		Adjusted model I		Adjust model II		Adjust model III	
		crude HR(95%CI)	crude P value	Adj I. HR(95%CI)	Adj. *P* value	adj. HR(95%CI)	Adj. *P* value	adj. HR(95%CI)	Adj. *P* value
TCFA = 0									
rSS_{low}	7 (12.10)	1(reference)	1(reference)	1(reference)	1(reference)	1(reference)	1(reference)	1(reference)	1(reference)
rSS_{mid}	13 (13.10)	1.03 (0.41,2.59)	0.944	0.98 (0.39,2.46)	0.963	1.04 (0.38,2.86)	0.942	1.32 (0.45,3.88)	0.613
rSS_{high}	11 (22.90)	1.99 (0.77,5.15)	0.153	1.96 (0.76,5.07)	0.164	2.86 (0.99,8.27)	0.053	5.85 (1.78,19.28)	0.004*
Trend test	31 (15.1)	1.46 (0.88,2.42)	0.139	1.46 (0.88,2.43)	0.145	1.79 (1,3.21)	0.049	2.52 (1.32,4.81)	0.005*
TCFA = 1									
rSS_{low}	1 (7.10)	1(reference)	1(reference)	1(reference)	1(reference)	1(reference)	1(reference)	1(reference)	1(reference)
rSS_{mid}	9 (25.70)	4.28 (0.54,33.82)	0.168	4.20 (0.53,33.58)	0.176	6.97 (0.78,62.52)	0.083	11.14 (0.44,279.13)	0.142
rSS_{high}	7 (35.00)	5.51 (0.68,44.83)	0.110	5.94 (0.72,48.76)	0.097	3.94 (0.45,34.81)	0.217	2.3 (0.13,40.85)	0.570
Trend test	17 (24.6)	1.81 (0.89,3.68)	0.100	1.96 (0.93,4.14)	0.078	1.41 (0.68,2.9)	0.356	1.04 (0.34,3.18)	0.947
Plaque erosion									
rSS_{low}	5 (12.50)	1(reference)	1(reference)	1(reference)	1(reference)	1(reference)	1(reference)	1(reference)	1(reference)
rSS_{mid}	6 (10.90)	0.83 (0.25,2.71)	0.752	0.71 (0.21,2.43)	0.591	0.95 (0.25,3.69)	0.945	1.86 (0.29,11.92)	0.512
rSS_{high}	4 (16.70)	1.4 (0.38,5.22)	0.615	1.16 (0.3,4.51)	0.834	2.92 (0.6,14.18)	0.184	14.57 (1.22,173.3)	0.034*
Trend test	15 (12.60)	1.16 (0.57,2.36)	0.681	1.06 (0.51,2.22)	0.879	1.7 (0.71,4.05)	0.234	3.63 (1.03,12.86)	0.045*
Plaque rupture									
rSS_{low}	3 (9.40)	1(reference)	1(reference)	1(reference)	1(reference)	1(reference)	1(reference)	1(reference)	1(reference)
rSS_{mid}	16 (20.30)	2.26 (0.66,7.77)	0.194	2.15 (0.63,7.41)	0.223	1.69 (0.47,6.07)	0.421	1.36 (0.34,5.44)	0.663
rSS_{high}	14 (31.80)	3.8 (1.09,13.23)	0.036*	3.81 (1.09,13.38)	0.037*	3.06 (0.82,11.34)	0.095	2.65 (0.62,11.22)	0.186
Trend test	33 (21.30)	1.84 (1.10,3.10)	0.021*	1.88 (1.11,3.20)	0.020*	1.77 (0.98,3.2)	0.059	1.73 (0.88,3.4)	0.111
Without Macrophage									
rSS_{low}	5 (14.7)	1(reference)	1(reference)	1(reference)	1(reference)	1(reference)	1(reference)	1(reference)	1(reference)
rSS_{mid}	10 (15.4)	0.98 (0.33,2.87)	0.971	0.94 (0.32,2.8)	0.912	0.78 (0.22,2.8)	0.708	0.67 (0.17,2.62)	0.568
rSS_{high}	6 (23.1)	1.53 (0.47,5.02)	0.483	1.55 (0.47,5.1)	0.471	1.74 (0.43,7.03)	0.435	1.84 (0.36,9.43)	0.462
Trend test	21 (16.8)	1.25 (0.67,2.35)	0.485	1.26 (0.67,2.39)	0.470	1.36 (0.62,2.96)	0.443	1.3 (0.52,3.25)	0.577
With Macrophage									
rSS_{low}	3 (7.9)	1(reference)	1(reference)	1(reference)	1(reference)	1(reference)	1(reference)	1(reference)	1(reference)
rSS_{mid}	12 (17.4)	2.31 (0.65,8.20)	0.194	2.4 (0.67,8.64)	0.179	3.37 (0.83,13.61)	0.088	4.99 (1.05,23.72)	0.043*
rSS_{high}	12 (28.6)	4.12 (1.16,14.62)	0.028*	4.26 (1.2,15.13)	0.025*	4.76 (1.19,18.97)	0.027*	6.6 (1.24,35.02)	0.027*
Trend test	27 (18.1)	1.95 (1.12,3.38)	0.017*	1.97 (1.13,3.42)	0.016*	1.96 (1.08,3.56)	0.027*	2.39 (1.11,5.13)	0.026*
Without Calcification									
rSS_{low}	6 (13.6)	1(reference)	1(reference)	1(reference)	1(reference)	1(reference)	1(reference)	1(reference)	1(reference)
rSS_{mid}	9 (14.1)	0.99 (0.35,2.78)	0.982	0.86 (0.3,2.45)	0.776	0.95 (0.3,2.96)	0.93	1.13 (0.34,3.74)	0.847

Table 4 Association of rSS with MACE in enrolled patients according to subgroup of characteristics by OCT *(Continued)*

Variables	MACE /Total	Crude model		Adjusted model I		Adjust model II		Adjust model III	
		crude HR(95%CI)	crude *P* value	Adj I. HR(95%CI)	Adj. *P* value	adj. HR(95%CI)	Adj. *P* value	adj. HR(95%CI)	Adj. *P* value
rSS_{high}	9 (34.6)	2.87 (1.02,8.05)	0.046*	2.77 (0.98,7.81)	0.054	2.72 (0.76,9.8)	0.126	2.41 (0.6,9.67)	0.214
Trend test	24 (17.9)	1.79 (1,3.18)	0.049*	1.79 (0.99,3.23)	0.055	1.72 (0.84,3.49)	0.135	1.55 (0.75,3.2)	0.235
With Calcification									
rSS_{low}	2 (7.1)	1(reference)	1(reference)	1(reference)	1(reference)	1(reference)	1(reference)	1(reference)	1(reference)
rSS_{mid}	13 (18.6)	2.72 (0.61,12.07)	0.189	2.83 (0.63,12.65)	0.172	3.68 (0.75,18.01)	0.107	6.88 (1.02,46.59)	0.048*
rSS_{high}	9 (21.4)	3.15 (0.68,14.59)	0.142	3.31 (0.71,15.37)	0.127	5.06 (1,25.61)	0.05	23.25 (2.81,192.71)	0.004*
Trend test	24 (17.1)	1.53 (0.84,2.76)	0.162	1.55 (0.86,2.81)	0.144	1.92 (1.01,3.67)	0.048	4.18 (1.72,10.16)	0.002*
Without Micro-calcification									
rSS_{low}	6 (13.6)	1(reference)	1(reference)	1(reference)	1(reference)	1(reference)	1(reference)	1(reference)	1(reference)
rSS_{mid}	9 (13.4)	0.93 (0.33,2.62)	0.895	0.79 (0.28,2.26)	0.663	0.85 (0.27,2.65)	0.779	0.92 (0.28,3)	0.894
rSS_{high}	10 (37)	3.03 (1.1,8.35)	0.032	2.81 (1.01,7.8)	0.047*	2.67 (0.75,9.43)	0.128	2.44 (0.62,9.62)	0.201
Trend test	25 (18.1)	1.89 (1.06,3.35)	0.03	1.87 (1.03,3.37)	0.038*	1.74 (0.86,3.52)	0.126	1.56 (0.75,3.26)	0.234
With Micro-calcification									
rSS_{low}	2 (7.1)	1(reference)	1(reference)	1(reference)	1(reference)	1(reference)	1(reference)	1(reference)	1(reference)
rSS_{mid}	13 (19.4)	2.94 (0.66,13.07)	0.156	3.09 (0.69,13.78)	0.140	3.92 (0.81,19.08)	0.09	6.82 (1.06,44)	0.044
rSS_{high}	8 (19.5)	2.93 (0.62,13.8)	0.174	3.14 (0.66,14.86)	0.150	4.39 (0.85,22.76)	0.078	16.84 (2.03,139.54)	0.009*
Trend test	23 (16.9)	1.44 (0.8,2.6)	0.229	1.48 (0.82,2.68)	0.193	1.76 (0.91,3.37)	0.091	3.46 (1.41,8.48)	0.007*
Without lipid plaque									
rSS_{low}	5 (11.6)	1(reference)	1(reference)	1(reference)	1(reference)	1(reference)	1(reference)	1(reference)	1(reference)
rSS_{mid}	10 (16.4)	1.35 (0.46,3.94)	0.586	1.32 (0.45,3.88)	0.613	1.71 (0.51,5.65)	0.383	3.16 (0.71,14.08)	0.132
rSS_{high}	6 (20.7)	1.8 (0.55,5.91)	0.331	1.72 (0.52,5.69)	0.373	3.7 (0.97,14.09)	0.055	10.48 (1.68,65.48)	0.012*
Trend test	21 (15.8)	1.34 (0.74,2.43)	0.330	1.31 (0.72,2.38)	0.372	1.93 (0.98,3.83)	0.059	3.24 (1.29,8.11)	0.012*
With lipid plaque									
rSS_{low}	3 (10.3)	1(reference)	1(reference)	1(reference)	1(reference)	1(reference)	1(reference)	1(reference)	1(reference)
rSS_{mid}	12 (16.4)	1.67 (0.47,5.93)	0.426	1.6 (0.45,5.7)	0.465	1.27 (0.33,4.82)	0.728	1.25 (0.29,5.34)	0.767
rSS_{high}	12 (30.8)	3.39 (0.96,12.02)	0.059	3.45 (0.97,12.25)	0.056	2.64 (0.69,10.13)	0.158	2.33 (0.48,11.26)	0.291
Trend test	27 (19.1)	1.9 (1.07,3.4)	0.029*	1.95 (1.08,3.52)	0.026	1.75 (0.91,3.37)	0.094	1.62 (0.75,3.47)	0.216
Without mixed plaque									
rSS_{low}	4 (8.7)	1(reference)	1(reference)	1(reference)	1(reference)	1(reference)	1(reference)	1(reference)	1(reference)
rSS_{mid}	18 (17.3)	2.01 (0.68,5.94)	0.207	1.22 (0.5,2.96)	0.667	1.81 (0.6,5.44)	0.294	2.03 (0.64,6.46)	0.232
rSS_{high}	13 (28.3)	3.56 (1.16,10.92)	0.026*	2.5 (1.04,6.05)	0.041*	2.46 (0.76,7.96)	0.132	2.91 (0.8,10.65)	0.106
Trend test	35 (17.9)	1.85 (1.12,3.06)	0.017*	1.67 (1.07,2.62)	0.025*	1.52 (0.89,2.59)	0.126	1.65 (0.9,3.01)	0.105
With mixed plaque									
rSS_{low}	4 (15.4)	1(reference)	1(reference)	1(reference)	1(reference)	1(reference)	1(reference)	1(reference)	1(reference)

Table 4 Association of rSS with MACE in enrolled patients according to subgroup of characteristics by OCT *(Continued)*

Variables	MACE /Total	Crude model		Adjusted model I		Adjust model II		Adjust model III	
		crude HR(95%CI)	crude P value	Adj I. HR(95%CI)	Adj. *P* value	adj. HR(95%CI)	Adj. *P* value	adj. HR(95%CI)	Adj. *P* value
rSS_{mid}	4 (13.3)	0.81 (0.2,3.26)	0.772	2.94 (0.35,24.81)	0.321	1.07 (0.18,6.23)	0.941	1.24 (0.06,26.5)	0.891
rSS_{high}	5 (22.7)	1.48 (0.4,5.52)	0.558	1.12 (0.07,19.32)	0.937	5.05 (0.95,26.95)	0.058	14.66 (0.65,330.23)	0.091
Trend test	13 (16.7)	1.24 (0.61,2.5)	0.553	1.08 (0.37,3.14)	0.881	2.44 (0.99,6.01)	0.054	4.67 (0.85,25.7)	0.076

Adjust I model adjusts for sex and age; Adjust II model adjusts for adjust I plus ejection fraction, smoke, hypertension, hyperlipidemia, diabetes mellitus and killip classification; Adjust III model adjusts for adjust II + white blood cell, hemoglobin, platelet, creatine kinase, glucose, glycosylated hemoglobin, C-reactive protein, low density lipoprotein

rSS_{low} represent rSS = 0; rSS_{mid} represent $0 < rSS \leq 8$, rSS_{high} represent rSS > 8. rSS, residual syntax score

*$P < 0.05$

that among patients with low rSS in the fully adjusted Cox regression models ($P = 0.034$). Furthermore, among patients with macrophage infiltration, the HR for MACEs in the high rSS group was 4.12-fold higher than that in the low rSS group in the crude model, and additional adjustment for other variables did not change the significance of high rSS with respect to MACEs (HR, 6.6; 95% CI, 1.24–35.02; $P = 0.027$). Further comparisons revealed that increasing tertiles of rSS levels were associated with a higher cumulative incidence of MACEs over time (*P* for trend = 0.026) in the subgroup with macrophage infiltration in culprit plaques. However, no significant difference between subgroups without macrophage infiltration was noted. In patients with calcification, microcalcification, and absence of lipid-rich plaques, increasing tertiles of rSS levels were associated with a higher cumulative incidence of MACEs over time (*P* for trend = 0.002, 0.007, and 0.012, respectively). In those with plaque rupture, lipid-rich plaques, and mixed plaques, increasing tertiles of rSS levels were not associated with a higher cumulative incidence of MACEs over time (*P* for trend = 0.111,0.126, and 0.076, respectively).

Table 5 and Supplementary Fig. 3 present the stratified analysis of MACEs at a median follow-up of 1.98 years in all enrolled patients, divided according to TCFA and rSS levels. In the non-DM subgroup, the incidence of MACEs increased by 54% among patients with high rSS and TCFA (group 3), as compared to group 0 (HR: 1.54 [1.06, 2.26]). The tendency was similar in the subgroups of age < median (HR: 6.88 [1.37, 34.63]), ejection fraction ≥50% (HR: 3.25 [1.19, 8.84]), current smoking (HR: 4.11 [1.51, 11.19]), platelet count $< 300 \times 10^9$/L (HR: 4.02 [1.55, 10.45]), and absence of healing plaques (HR: 5.6 [2.11, 14.87]). Notably, in the subgroups of hypertension (*P* for interaction = 0.012) and WBC count $< 10 \times 10^9$/L (*P* for interaction = 0.030), the incidence of MACEs was significantly higher in group 3 than in group 0.

Diagnostic value of rSS in combination with TCFA

ROC curves were plotted to evaluate the diagnostic value of rSS in combination with morphological characteristics on OCT (particularly TCFA) for predicting MACEs, as compared to traditional risk factors (Fig. 3). The area under the ROC curve for traditional risk factors (including sex, age, ejection fraction, smoking, hypertension, hyperlipidemia, DM, Killip classification, WBC count, hemoglobin, platelet count, creatine kinase, glucose, glycosylated hemoglobin, C-reactive protein, low-density lipoprotein, triglyceride, and lipase activator) was 0.771 (95% CI, 0.716–0.819).

ROC and survival ROC curves for the discriminatory value of MACEs shown in Fig. 3 A and B. The area under the ROC curve was 0.794 (95% CI, 0.741–0.840) and 0.816 (95% CI, 0.765–0.860), respectively, whereas the area under the survival ROC curve was 0.798 and 0.846, respectively. The best cutoff values for model III (traditional risk factors + rSS + TCFA) and model IV (traditional risk factors + rSS + TCFA+ microstructural features of culprit lesions on OCT) according to the Youden index were 0.5970 and 0.6493, respectively. Therefore, the entire study population was categorized into two groups based on model III: model III ≤0.5970 (low model III, $n = 257$) and model III > 0.5970 (high model III, $n = 17$). The high model III group had a significantly higher incidence of MACEs for up to a median of 1.98 years than the low model III group ($P < 0.001$; Fig. 3C). When the entire study population was categorized into two groups based on model IV (model IV ≤0.6493 [low model IV, $n = 260$] and model IV > 0.6493 [high model IV, $n = 14$]), the high model IV group showed a significantly higher incidence of MACEs than the low model IV group ($P < 0.001$) (Fig. 3D).

Figure 4 shows the Kaplan–Meier curves for the cumulative incidence of MACEs for up to a median of 1.98 years stratified by rSS levels and TCFA among the subgroups. Among patients without hypertension, the high rSS with TCFA group showed a significantly higher incidence of MACEs than the low rSS without TCFA group ($P = 0.0059$). However, no significant differences were observed among the other subgroups.

Table 5 Stratified Analysis of MACE at median Follow-up of 1.98 yr in all enrolled patients divided by the status of TCFA and level of rSS

	Status					
Confounding factor category	Group = 0 (TCFA absent &Rss ≤ 4)	Group = 1 (TCFA present &Rss ≤ 4)	Group = 2 (TCFA absent &Rss>4)	Group = 3 (TCFA present &Rss>4)	P for trend	P for interaction
DM						
without	1(reference)	1.62 (0.64,4.1)	4.13 (1.35,12.61)	1.54 (1.06,2.26)	0.025*	0.226
with	1(reference)	2.48 (0.43,14.38)	1.89 (0.36,10)	4.28 (0.75,24.44)	0.156	
Age						
< media	1(reference)	2.93 (0.26,33.31)	0.86 (0.13,5.65)	6.88 (1.37,34.63)	0.088	0.490
≥ media	1(reference)	0.86 (0.21,3.54)	1.75 (0.68,4.46)	3.09 (0.97,9.83)	0.039	
EF						
< 50%	1(reference)	3.69 (0.01,1086.65)	15.65 (0.22,1091.81)	21.82 (0.23,2112.96)	0.113	0.724
≥ 50%	1(reference)	0.83 (0.21,3.19)	1.33 (0.54,3.27)	3.25 (1.19,8.84)	0.037*	
Smoke						
without	1(reference)	3.65 (0.49,27.06)	4.73 (1.07,20.9)	–	0.019*	0.191
with	1(reference)	0.82 (0.16,4.11)	1.18 (0.43,3.24)	4.11 (1.51,11.19)	0.012*	
Hypertension						
without	1(reference)	–	4.94 (1.48,16.5)	10.46 (1.94,56.45)	0.002*	0.012*
with	1(reference)	1.08 (0.28,4.23)	0.33 (0.09,1.25)	2.01 (0.62,6.57)	0.826	
History of PCI						
without	1(reference)	0.46 (0.06,3.73)	1.97 (0.84,4.6)	4.84 (1.82,12.88)	0.002*	0.192
with	1(reference)	–	–	–	0.986	
CRP						
< 10	1(reference)	1.76 (0.47,6.66)	1.47 (0.56,3.9)	6.06 (1.87,19.64)	0.017*	0.296
≥ 10	1(reference)	–	2.29 (0.46,11.5)	3.77 (0.59,23.96)	0.131	
LPA						
< 300	1(reference)	0.92 (0.17,5.02)	1.54 (0.52,4.61)	7.42 (2.16,25.53)	0.006*	0.192
≥ 300	1(reference)	4.73 (0.69,32.42)	1.78 (0.5,6.37)	1.02 (0.21,4.94)	0.768	
WBC						
< 10	1(reference)	3.8 (0.84,17.27)	2.15 (0.7,6.6)	8.37 (2.19,31.99)	0.011*	0.030*
≥ 10	1(reference)	–	2.02 (0.57,7.21)	6.53 (1.37,31.14)	0.027*	
Plt						
< 300	1(reference)	0.85 (0.22,3.24)	1.34 (0.58,3.13)	4.02 (1.55,10.45)	0.013*	0.499
≥ 300	1(reference)	14.11 (0.51,388.76)	5.78 (0.11,300.43)	6.95 (0.11,451.72)	0.280	
TMAO						
< media	1(reference)	–	0.72 (0.16,3.35)	4.09 (0.34,49.59)	0.848	0.474
≥ media	1(reference)	7.18 (0.89,58.24)	2.6 (0.42,16.11)	18.33 (2.92,115.1)	0.005*	
Healing plaque						
without	1(reference)	0.85 (0.23,3.2)	1.55 (0.68,3.52)	5.6 (2.11,14.87)	0.004*	0.197
with	1(reference)	–	–	–	0.580	

Confounding factors including sex, age, ejection fraction, smoke, hypertension, hyperlipidemia, diabetes mellitus, white blood cell, hemoglobin, platelet, creatine kinase, glucose, glycosylated hemoglobin, C-reactive protein

TCFA thin-cap fibroatheroma, *rSS* residual syntax score, *DM* diabetes mellitus, *EF* ejection fraction, *CRP, PCI* percutaneous coronary intervention, *CRP, C* reactive protein, *LPA* lipse activator, *WBC* white blood cell, *PLT* platelet, *TMAO* trimethylamine N-oxide, *Adj.*, adjusted

MACE, major adverse cardiovascular events

*$P < 0.05$

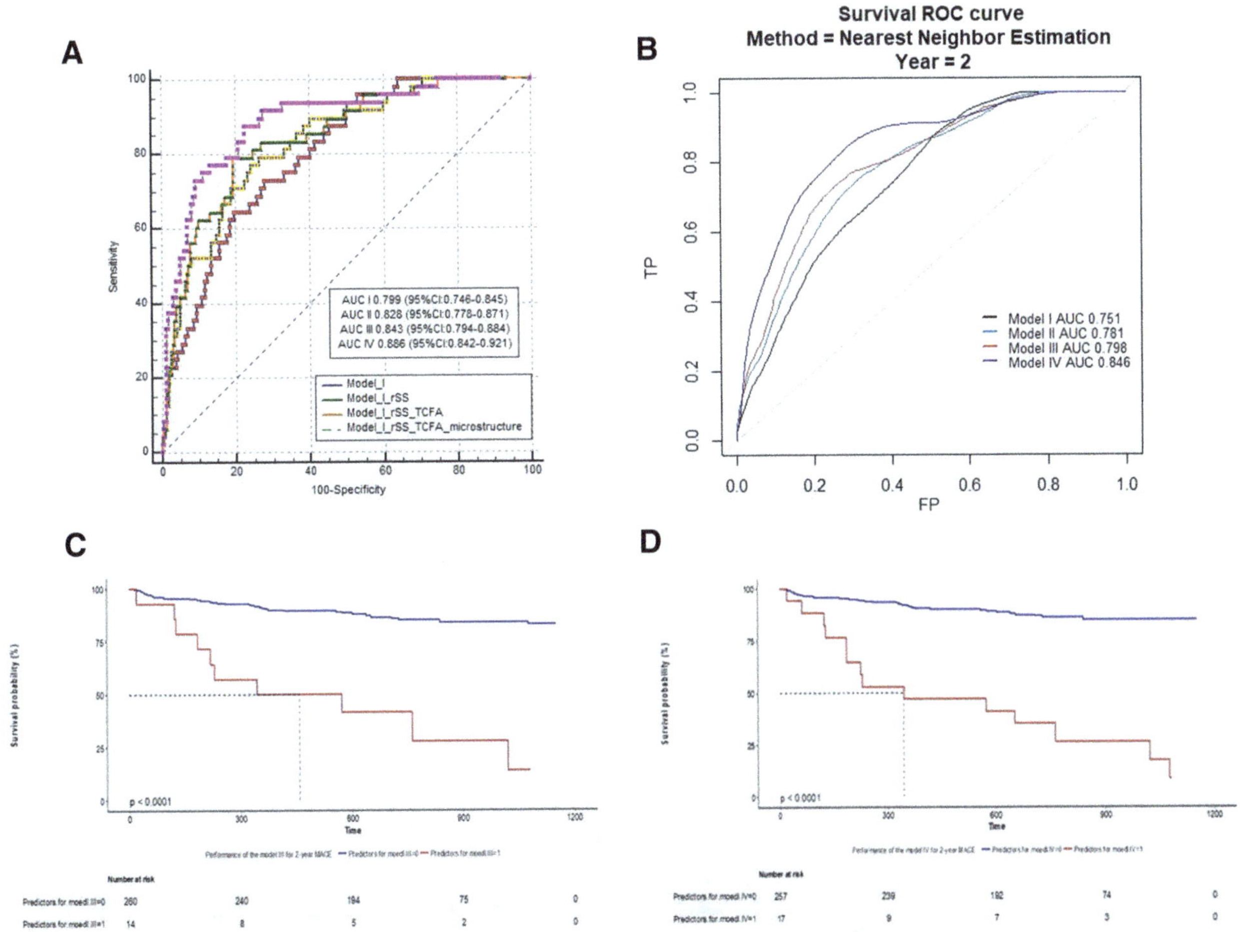

Fig. 3 ROC curve, survival ROC curve for rSS with traditional risk factors, TCFA and microstructure of culprit lesion by OCT in predicting 2-year MACE and K-M curve of performance of the model III and IV. **A**, Model I, predictor of traditional risk factors including sex, age, ejection fraction, hypertension, hyperlipidemia, diabetes mellitus, history of myocardial infarction, history of PCI, history of CABG, Killip classification, cTnI of baseline, peak level of cTnI, brain natriuretic peptide (BNP) of baseline, peak level of BNP, white blood cell, hemoglobin, platelet, creatine kinase, glucose, glycosylated hemoglobin, C-reactive protein, total cholesterol, triglyceride, low density lipoprotein, high density lipoprotein, triglyceride/ low density lipoprotein, lipse activator, aspirin, Ticagrelor, clopidogrel. Model II, Model I plus rSS. Model III, Model II plus TCFA. Model IV, Model III plus microstructure of culprit lesion by OCT including macrophage, thrombus, plaque rupture or erosion, mixed plaque, lipid plaque, fibrous plaque, calcification, max lipid-arc, fibrous cap thickness, minimal lumen area, micro-vessels. AUC, areas under the ROC curve; CI, 95% confidence interval. **B** Survival ROC curve, the confounding factors of model I, II, III, IV are as same as the (**A**). **C** Model III cutoff value=0.5970; 0, predictors of model III< cutoff value; 1, predictors of model III≥ cutoff value; **D** Model IV cutoff value=0.6493. 0, predictors of model III< cutoff value; 1, predictors of model III≥ cutoff value

Discussion

To the best of our knowledge, the present study is the first post hoc analysis exploring the association of rSS with morphological characteristics (particularly TCFA) of culprit plaques using OCT in patients with STEMI. The main findings of this study are as follows: **(1)** Notably, the presence of TCFA in culprit lesions and a higher level of rSS, which assesses the degree and complexity of residual stenosis, were significantly associated with future incidence of MACEs, as compared to other subgroups. **(2)** In particular subgroups of microstructural features of culprit lesions, high rSS levels were associated with a higher cumulative MACE incidence over time than low and medium rSS levels after full adjustment for other variables. **(3)** The ROC curve analysis showed that rSS in combination with TCFA by OCT could serve as a novel predictor of composite cardiovascular events.

Association of high rSS with MACEs

Généreux et al. [12] were the first to confirm that the rSS is a strong independent predictor of cardiovascular outcomes in patients with acute coronary syndrome. The CULPRIT-SHOCK trial [13], which enrolled 587 patients, reported a strong significant correlation between rSS and 30-day and 1-year mortality in a large

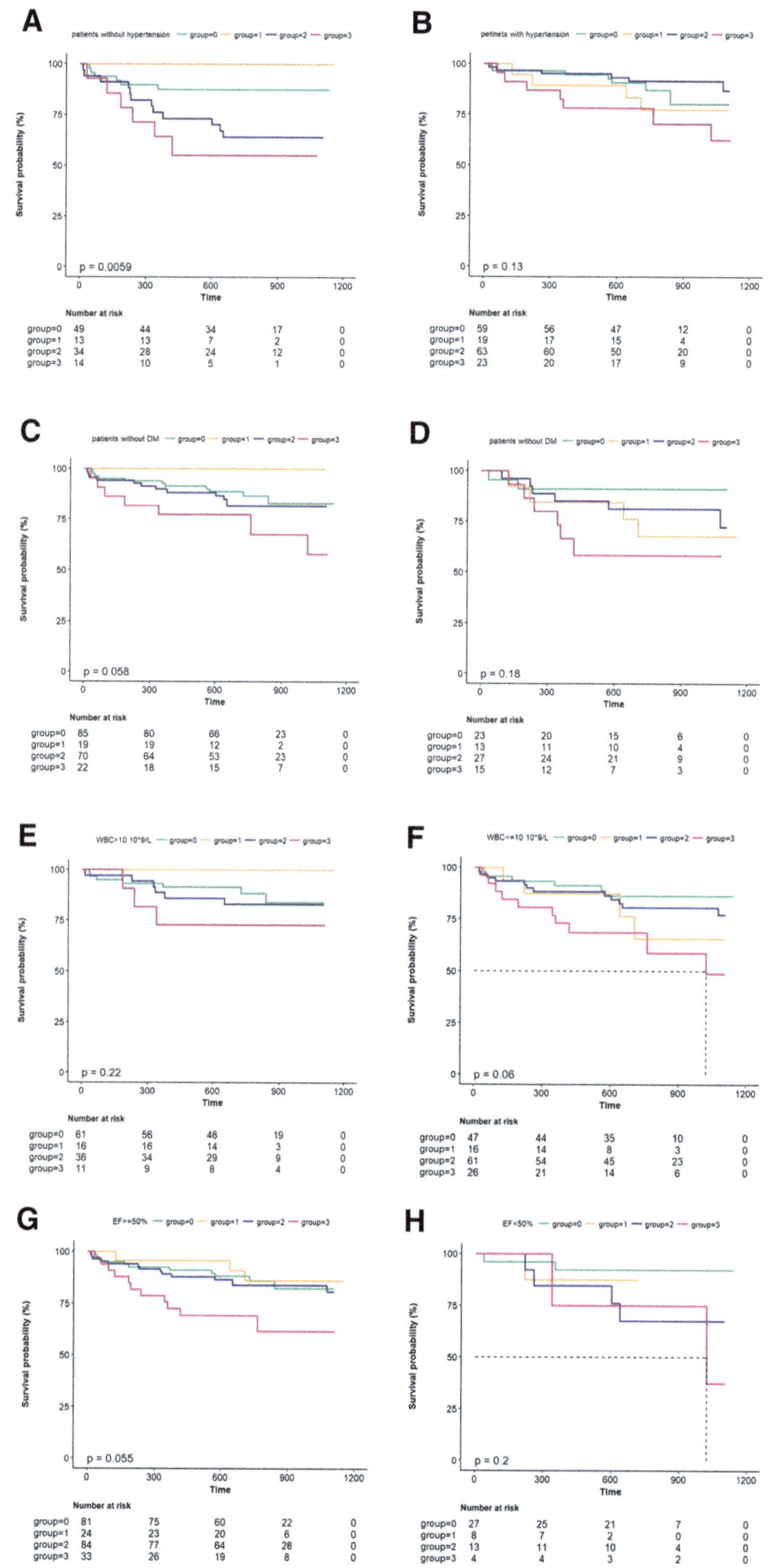

Fig. 4 (See legend on next page.)

(See figure on previous page.)
Fig. 4 Kaplan-Meier curves showing cumulative MACE rates for up to median 1.98 years stratified by the level of rSS and TCFA characteristic among subgroups. Group=0 represent the patients with low level of rSS (rSS≤4) and without characteristic of TCFA in the culprit lesion. Group=1 represent the patients with low level of rSS (rSS≤4) and characteristic of TCFA in the culprit lesion. Group=2 represent the patients with low level of rSS (rSS>4) and without characteristic of TCFA in the culprit lesion. Group=3 represent the patients with low level of rSS (rSS>4) and characteristic of TCFA in the culprit lesion. *DM, diabetes mellitus; WBC, white blood cell; EF, ejective fraction.* **A** Kaplan-Meier curves showing cumulative MACE rates stratified by the level of rSS and TCFA among subgroups without hypertension. **B** Kaplan-Meier curves showing cumulative MACE rates stratified by the level of rSS and TCFA among subgroups with hypertension. **C** Kaplan-Meier curves showing cumulative MACE rates stratified by the level of rSS and TCFA among subgroups without DM. **D** Kaplan-Meier curves showing cumulative MACE rates stratified by the level of rSS and TCFA among subgroups with DM. **E** Kaplan-Meier curves showing cumulative MACE rates stratified by the level of rSS and TCFA among subgroups WBC>10 10*9/L. **F** Kaplan-Meier curves showing cumulative MACE rates stratified by the level of rSS and TCFA among subgroups WBC≤10 10*9/L. **G** Kaplan-Meier curves showing cumulative MACE rates stratified by the level of rSS and TCFA among subgroups of EF≥50%. **H** Kaplan-Meier curves showing cumulative MACE rates stratified by the level of rSS and TCFA among subgroups of EF<50%

group of patients with cardiac stroke. A previous study showed that plaque morphology was significantly correlated with rSS and that rSS and plaque burden ≥70% independently predicted MACEs based on intravascular ultrasound [14]. OCT for the identification of neointimal microstructures such as TCFA, macrophage accumulation, calcified deposits, microvessels, and cholesterol crystals may be more useful than intravascular ultrasound in determining the optimal treatment strategy [6, 15]. Another previous study reported that lipid-rich plaques, thinner fibrous caps, TCFA, stents with irregular protrusions, and dissections were more frequent among patients with higher SS, indicating that higher SS may reflect higher plaque vulnerability and worse cardiovascular response to stenting [16]. In our study, the third tertile of rSS was associated with a higher incidence of MACEs over time in the subgroups of plaque erosion, macrophage infiltration, calcification, and microcalcification than the first tertile.

Using OCT for the coronary artery tree and left anterior descending artery in 165 patients with stable angina, Bryniarski et al. [17] reported that typical pathological features of plaque vulnerability were more frequent in patients with high rSS. Specifically, the main features of vulnerable plaques were TCFA and a large lipid pool [18], which could influence post-stent outcomes, as reported by a clinical study [19]. Ueda et al. [20] identified that lipid-rich plaques underlying stent edges were strong predictors of uncovered stent struts and that TCFA and large calcification at the proximal stent edge were strong predictors of uncovered stent struts at follow-up. In post-PCI OCT assessing 1002 lesions, suboptimal stent deployment, including in-stent minimal lumen area, distal reference lumen area, and dissection at the distal stent edge, was associated with an increased incidence of MACEs, which are a composite of all-cause death, MI, and target lesion revascularization during follow-up [21]. A one-year follow-up study from a multicenter registry observed that irregular protrusion after stent deployment was an independent and strong predictor of device-oriented clinical endpoints [22]. In combination with our results, these might explain the association between high rSS and MACEs. The number of patients involved is relatively small and the number of patients in 4 subgroups is only from 32 to 108. In order to clarify the validity of subgroup analysis, we calculated the sample power by chi-square test (IBM SPSS Sample Power 3.0.1) and the results indicated the validity of the results.

Discriminatory value of follow-up MACEs

Gao et al. [23] reported that rSS integrated with some traditional risk factors such as age, creatinine, and ejection fraction improved the prognostic value and predictive ability for 2-year cardiac mortality in a large-scale PCI population (N = 10,072). In the pooled analysis of a consecutive series of cohorts (N = 1608) after coronary artery bypass grafting, patients with an increase in rSS were shown to be at a higher risk for cardiovascular events at 1-year follow-up [24]. The present study not only evaluate the prognostic value of rSS in combination with plaque characteristics on OCT, but also the results of this study may be particularly useful for the risk stratification of patients with STEMI who are undergoing primary PCI. Adding microstructural features of culprit lesions by OCT to the rSS, together with the traditional cardiovascular risk factors, could improve the predictive power for clinical outcomes [25].

Limitations

Several limitations of this study should be noted. First, selection bias may exist because this study had a relatively small sample size with retrospective analysis of the data and was conducted at a single center. Although this study is a single center retrospective study with rigorous design in the real world, it has a good homogenization level due to its rigorous design, standardized implementation, long observed time, real research data, detailed and accurate records, demographic characteristics and disease type characteristics of cases. Therefore, the results of this study are relatively reliable and can become high-quality evidence to guide treatment decision-making. However, single center research will lead to bias inevitably which will affect the universality and popularization of the conclusion. Therefore, it is necessary to carry out a large sample, prospective randomized controlled study to confirm the results of the present study to explore the efficacy of the research and expand the treatment benefit population. The bias of single center observational clinical study is as follows: 1. Disclosure of researcher bias: The researchers of the present study have declared that the conflict of interest different from the study had been approved by the ethics committee. 2. Bias occurred in the process of data collection. We have recorded the types and definitions of variables in detail to collect medical records before data collection. Therefore, this type of bias can be ignored in this study. 3. Bias of data collection system: The observational study may lead to misclassification bias. In this study, we use standard data collection system to minimize data errors. Formatted and standardized electronic data report forms are used. 4. The extractor bias. Data extractors and researchers are trained to collect data independently, and they are double-blind for research purposes and research assumptions. Therefore, the bias from extractor in this study can be ignored. 5. The bias from target population of the study: Due to our study site is a typical representative site of the target population, each patient has the same probability to enter into the study. The inclusion and exclusion criteria of research objects have been set before data collecting, and the flow chart has been used to screen process of research objects. Thus, the bias from target population in the present study can be ignored. Therefore, more prospective and large cohort study should be conducted in the future. Furthermore, the study population is largely represented by males (80.7%) which might cause selected bias. The study is underpowered for the sub-groups evaluated. Once we get into subgroup analyses related to OCT characteristics, total number becomes small. Therefore, it is necessary to verify our results using a larger sample size. Furthermore, although data on the microstructural features of culprit lesions by OCT were prospectively collected, we conducted a retrospective analysis. Third, although the coronary plaque features measured by OCT ensured effective and reliable quantification and qualification, it is necessary to validate the findings of the present study in a wider population. Finally, the application in clinical practice may be difficult since further contrast and radiological exposure of patients and the routine use of OCT may be not available in the all Cardiac Catheterization lab.

Conclusion

The results of this study suggest that microstructural features of culprit lesions on OCT in combination with rSS, which assesses the angiographic completeness of revascularization, could be used in clinical practice to support risk stratification and predict a poorer prognosis.

Acknowledgments

The authors gratefully acknowledge all individuals who participated in this study.

Authors' contributions

Substantial contributions to conception and design, data acquisition, or data analysis and interpretation: Hongbing Yan, Xiaoxiao Zhao, Ying Wang, Runzhen Chen, Jiannan Li, Jinying Zhou, Chen Liu, Peng Zhou, Zhaoxue Sheng, Yi Chen, Li Song, Hanjun Zhao. Drafting the article or critically revising it for important intellectual content: Hongbing Yan, Xiaoxiao Zhao, Ying Wang, Runzhen Chen, Jiannan Li, Jinying Zhou, Chen Liu, Peng Zhou, Zhaoxue Sheng, Yi Chen, Li Song, Hanjun Zhao. Final approval of the version to be published: Hongbing Yan, Xiaoxiao Zhao, Ying Wang, Runzhen Chen, Jiannan Li, Jinying Zhou, Chen Liu, Peng Zhou, Zhaoxue Sheng, Yi Chen, Li Song, Hanjun Zhao. Agreement to be accountable for all aspects of the work in ensuring that questions related to the accuracy or integrity of the work are appropriately investigated and resolved: Hongbing Yan, Xiaoxiao Zhao, Ying Wang, Runzhen Chen, Jiannan Li, Jinying Zhou, Chen Liu, Peng Zhou, Zhaoxue Sheng, Yi Chen, Li Song, Hanjun Zhao.

References

1. Genereux P, Palmerini T, Caixeta A, et al. Quantification and impact of untreated coronary artery disease after percutaneous coronary intervention: the residual SYNTAX (synergy between PCI with Taxus and cardiac surgery) score. J Am Coll Cardiol. 2012;59:2165–74.
2. Farooq V, Serruys PW, Bourantas CV, et al. Quantification of incomplete revascularization and its association with five-year mortality in the synergy between percutaneous coronary intervention with taxus and cardiac surgery (SYNTAX) trial validation of the residual SYNTAX score. Circulation. 2013;128:141–51.
3. Serruys PW, Morice MC, Kappetein AP, et al. Percutaneous coronary intervention versus coronary-artery bypass grafting for severe coronary artery disease. N Engl J Med. 2009;360:961–72.
4. Malkin CJ, George V, Ghobrial MS, et al. Residual SYNTAX score after PCI for triple vessel coronary artery disease: quantifying the adverse effect of incomplete revascularisation. EuroIntervention. 2013;8:1286–95.
5. Park KW, Kang J, Kang SH, et al. The impact of residual coronary lesions on clinical outcomes after percutaneous coronary intervention: residual SYNTAX score after percutaneous coronary intervention in patients from the efficacy of Xience/ Promus versus cypher in rEducing late loss after stENTing (EXCELLENT) registry. Am Heart J. 2014;167:384–92.e5.
6. Tearney GJ, Regar E, Akasaka T, et al. Consensus standards for acquisition, measurement, and reporting of intravascular optical coherence tomography studies: a report from the international working Group for Intravascular Optical Coherence Tomography Standardization and Validation. J Am Coll Cardiol. 2012;59(12):1058–72.
7. Kubo T, Imanishi T, Takarada S, et al. Assessment of culprit lesion morphology in acute myocardial infarction: ability of optical coherence tomography compared with intravascular ultrasound and coronary angioscopy. J Am Coll Cardiol. 2007;50(10):933–9.
8. Naghavi M, Libby P, Falk E, et al. From vulnerable plaque to vulnerable patient: a call for new defnitions and risk assessment strategies: part I. Circulation. 2003;108(14):1664–72.
9. Ibanez B, James S, Agewall S, et al. 2017 ESC guidelines for the

management of acute myocardial infarction in patients presenting with ST-segment elevation: the task force for the management of acute myocardial infarction in patients presenting with ST-segment elevation of the European Society of Cardiology (ESC). Eur Heart J. 2018;39:119–77.

10. Serruys PW, Onuma Y, Garg S, et al. Assessment of the SYNTAX score in the syntax study. EuroIntervention. 2009;5:50–6.
11. Tian J, Ren X, Vergallo R, et al. Distinct morphological features of ruptured culprit plaque for acute coronary events compared to those with silent rupture and thin-cap fbroatheroma: a combined optical coherence tomography and intravascular ultrasound study. J Am Coll Cardiol. 2014; 63(21):2209–16.
12. Généreux P, Palmerini T, Caixeta A, et al. Quantification and impact of untreated coronary artery disease after percutaneous coronary intervention. J Am Coll Cardiol. 2012;59:2165–74.
13. Barthélémy O, Rouanet S, Brugier D, et al. Predictive value of the residual SYNTAX score in patients with cardiogenic shock. J Am Coll Cardiol. 2021; 77:144–55.
14. Fujino A, Kadohira T, Redfors B, et al. Significant association among residual SYNTAX score, non-culprit major adverse cardiac events, and greyscale and virtual histology intravascular ultrasound findings: a substudy from the PROSPECT study. EuroIntervention. 2019;14:1676–84.
15. Maehara A, Matsumura M, Ali ZA, et al. IVUS-guided versus OCT-guided coronary stent implantation: a critical appraisal. JACC Cardiovasc Imaging. 2017;10(12):1487–503.
16. Bryniarski KL, Walters DL, Kim C-J, et al. SYNTAX score and pre- and post stent optical coherence tomography findings in the left anterior descending coronary artery in patients with stable angina pectoris. Am J Cardiol. 2017;120(6):898–903.
17. Bryniarski KL, Walters DL, Kim C-J, et al. SYNTAX score, and pre- and post-stent optical coherence tomography findings in the left anterior descending coronary artery in patients with stable angina pectoris. Am J Cardiol. 2017;120(6):898.
18. Vancraeynest D, Pasquet A, Roelants V, et al. Imaging the vulnerable plaque. J Am Coll Cardiol. 2011;57:1961–79.
19. Farb A, Weber DK, Kolodgie FD, Burke AP, Virmani R. Morphological predictors of restenosis after coronary stenting in humans. Circulation. 2002; 105:2974–80.
20. Ueda T, Uemura S, Watanabe M, et al. Thin-cap fibroatheroma and large calcification at the proximal stent edge correlate with a high proportion of uncovered stent struts in the chronic phase. Coron Artery Dis. 2016;27:376–84.
21. Prati F, Romagnoli E, Burzotta F, et al. Clinical impact of OCT findings during PCI: the CLI-OPCI II study. JACC Cardiovasc Imaging. 2015;8:1297–305.
22. Soeda T, Uemura S, Park S-J, et al. Incidence and clinical significance of Poststent optical coherence tomography findings: one-year follow-up study from a multicenter registry. Circulation. 2015;132:1020–9.
23. Gao G, Dong Z, Song C, et al. Integrating the residual SYNTAX score to improve the predictive ability of the age, creatinine, and ejection fraction (ACEF) score for cardiac mortality in percutaneous coronary intervention patients[J]. Catheter Cardiovasc Interv. 2020;95:534–41.
24. Melinaa G, Angelonia E, Refice S, et al. Residual SYNTAX score following coronary artery bypass grafting. Eur J Cardiothorac Surg. 2017;51:547–53.
25. Kang J, Park KW, Han J-K, Yang H-M, Kang H-J, Koo B-K, et al. Usefulness of the baseline syntax score to predict 3-year outcome after complete revascularization by percutaneous coronary intervention. Am J Cardiol. 2016; 118:641–6.

22

A catastrophic seronegative anti-phospholipid syndrome

Vanda Pinto[1,2], Augusto Ministro[1,2,3*], Nuno Reis Carreira[4], Ana Cardoso[4], Catarina Sousa Gonçalves[4], Mickael Henriques[1,2], João Rato[1,2], Emanuel Silva[1,2] and Luís Mendes Pedro[1,2,3]

Abstract

Background: Antiphospholipid Syndrome (APS) is a multisystemic autoimmune disease characterized by arterial and venous thrombosis and / or obstetric morbidity in the presence of at least one circulating anti-phospholipid antibody. The spectrum of vascular events varies from deep venous thrombosis to catastrophic APS, a rare form characterized by acute multiorgan thrombosis and high mortality.

Case report: We present the case of a 32-week pregnant woman arriving in the hospital emergency room with bilateral acute lower limb ischemia. In the obstetric evaluation, fetal death was declared. Computerized Tomography angiography showed pulmonary embolism of both pulmonary arteries, areas of splenic and right renal infarction and multiple arterial and venous thrombosis. The patient underwent urgent caesarean section and axillary-bifemoral bypass. No events registered. In the postoperative period, in an intensive care unit, treatment with rituximab and plasmapheresis were added to anticoagulant therapy. The laboratorial investigation was negative for thrombophilia and autoimmune diseases.

Conclusion: Catastrophic APS develops quickly, with multiorgan involvement and high mortality rate. The presented case poses a multidisciplinary challenge, with the surgical approach of extra-anatomical revascularization being less invasive and guaranteeing immediate perfusion of the lower limbs. Although the serological tests were negative for anti-phospholipid antibodies, this case hardly fits into another diagnosis. Therefore, it was treated as a catastrophic APS, having shown a favorable evolution.

Keywords: Antiphospholipid syndrome, Aortic thrombosis, Renal thrombosis

Introduction

Pregnancy is characterized by a hypercoagulable state which confers protection against hemorrhagic challenges such as childbirth or miscarriage. Nonetheless, it simultaneously increases 4- to 5-fold the risk of thrombotic events [1], with the majority (75–80%) of pregnancy-related thrombotic events being venous. The most important risk factors are a previous history of thrombosis and thrombophilia, the most significant of which is antiphospholipid syndrome (APS) [1].

APS is a systemic autoimmune disorder (AID) characterized by recurrent arterial or venous thrombosis and/ or pregnancy morbidity (fetal loss and stillbirth) in the presence of anti-phospholipid (aPL) antibodies, typically lupus anticoagulant (LA), anticardiolipin (aCL) or anti-β2 glycoprotein-I (β2GPI) [2–6]. APS can be secondary (associated with other diseases, mainly systemic lupus erythematosus) or can be found in patients with neither

* Correspondence: Augusto.ministro@gmail.com
[1]Vascular Surgery Department, Heart and Vessels Division, Hospital Santa Maria (CHULN), Av. Prof. Egas Moniz s/n, 1649-035 Lisbon, Portugal
[2]Lisbon Academic Medical Center, Lisbon, Portugal

clinical or laboratory evidence of another condition (primary APS) [2, 5]. The APS presentation spectrum varies in severity and ranges from asymptomatic "carrier" for aPL to a life-threatening form, catastrophic APS (CAPS) [5, 7].

Catastrophic APS, also known as Asherson's syndrome, is a rare condition (less than 1% of APS patients) which includes multiple organ system thromboses and develops over a short period with high mortality [6]. CAPS classification criteria (Table 1) requires thrombotic events in three or more organs, developing in less than a week; microthrombosis evidence in at least one organ; and persistent aPL positivity [5, 6]. Most cases of CAPS present as a microangiopathic storm rather than large-vessel thrombosis, however any combination of vascular occlusive events may occur in the same patient leading to multiorgan failure with diverse primary clinical manifestations, depending on the organ systems involved [5, 6, 8].

Because CAPS is so uncommon, an international registry was formed by the European Forum on Anti-Phospholipid Anti-bodies in 2000 and most recent reported data (2016) includes 500 patients [7].

Mortality rate has decreased over time mainly due to triple therapy (anticoagulation, corticotherapy and therapeutic plasma exchange - TPE - or intravenous immune globulin IVIG), but it remains still above 30% [7].

Table 1 Criteria for the classification of catastrophic APS[5]

1. Evidence of involvement of three or more organs, systems and/or tissues[a]
2. Development of manifestations simultaneously or in less than a week.
3. Confirmation by histopathology of small vessel occlusion in at least one organ or tissue[b]
4. Laboratory confirmation of the presence of antiphospholipid antibodies (lupus anticoagulant and/or anticardiolipin antibodies)[c]
Definite catastrophic APS: All 4 criteria.
Probable catastrophic APS:
– All 4 criteria, except for only two organs, systems and/or tissues involvement.
– All 4 criteria, except for the absence of laboratory confirmation at least 6 weeks apart due to the early death of a patient never tested for aPL before the catastrophic APS.
– Criteria 1, 2 and 4.
– Criteria 1, 3 and 4 and the development of a third event in more than a week but less than a month, despite anticoagulation.

[a] Usually, clinical evidence of vessel occlusions, confirmed by imaging techniques when appropriate. Renal involvement is defined by a 50% rise in serum creatinine, severe systemic hypertension (> 180/100 mmHg) and/or proteinuria (> 500 mg/24 h)

[b] For histopathological confirmation, significant evidence of thrombosis must be present, although vasculitis may coexist occasionally

[c] If the patient had not been previously diagnosed as having an APS, the laboratory confirmation requires that presence of antiphospholipid antibodies must be detected on two or more occasions at least 6 weeks apart (not necessarily at the time of the event), according to the proposed preliminary criteria for the classification of definite APS

Our objective is to report an extremely rare and potentially lethal condition.

Case report

A 38-year-old woman, 32^{+2} weeks pregnant, previous smoker with a past history of one miscarriage and livedo reticularis was admitted to the emergency department (ED) of her local hospital due to a sudden onset of pain, cold and functional impotence of the lower limbs. During the obstetric evaluation, fetal death was observed.

Given the suspicion of lower limb ischemia, low weight molecular heparin was started, and the patient was transferred to our hospital, which has vascular surgery. On admission in our ED, she was alert and oriented, hemodynamically stable and presented with tachypnea. Absence of pulses, cold and pallor of the lower limbs, with minimal neurosensory deficit and muscle weakness were observed. Laboratory workup showed hypocapnia, thrombocytopenia, elevation of liver and pancreatic enzymes, elevated total creatinine kinase (CK) and lactate dehydrogenase (LDH). Table 2 resumes clinical and laboratory evolution during hospitalization. The Computed Tomography angiography (Angio CT) showed bilateral (central and lobar) pulmonary embolism (PE), deep venous thrombosis of the inferior vena cava and left iliac axis, areas of splenic and right kidney infarction and multiple arterial and venous thrombosis. Juxta-renal aortic thrombosis (Fig. 1) was also observed as well as thrombosis of the left renal artery (with hypocaptation of the left kidney), right common iliac artery, left hypogastric artery, left common femoral artery, right deep femoral artery and right tibioperoneal trunk (Fig. 2).

As lower limb ischemia was tolerated (acute limb ischemia - grade IIA), surgery was postponed. The patient was admitted to the intensive care unit (ICU) where presumptive CAPS diagnosis was made and anticoagulation with unfractioned heparin infusion was started. Despite anticoagulation, the patient presented worsening of neurosensory deficit and muscle weakness (acute limb ischemia - grade IIB), with the need of urgent revascularization surgery. Under general anesthesia, a cesarean section was performed to extract the dead fetus, and intrauterine balloon tamponade was placed for control of postpartum hemorrhage, followed by bilateral thromboembolectomy of the lower limbs and axillary-bifemoral bypass with synthetic prosthesis. Surgery was uneventful. Fetus had no anatomical abnormalities and weighed 1540 g. The patient recovered both lower limb perfusion as well as bilateral femoral, popliteal and distal pulses and was extubated the next day. During her stay in the ICU, the patient maintained therapeutic anticoagulation, underwent a total of six sessions of

Table 2 Evolution of CAPS in the described patient

Organ manifestation	Clinical signs	Laboratory abnormalities	(reference range)	Laboratory tests which were normal (negative)
Kidney	Polypnea	Hemoglobin: 11,1 g/dL	12.0–15.3	Peripheral blood smear (showed no
Renal Failure	Absence of pulses in the	WBC: 12,20 × 10^9/L	4.0–11.0	schizocytes)
Renal infarction	lower limbs	Platelet count 78 × 10^9/L	150–450 ×	INR: 0,97
Renal artery thrombosis	Minimal neurosensory deficit	pH 7.37	10^9/L	aPTT: 32,4/29
Lung	Moderate muscle weakness	pCO_2 20,5 mmHg	7,35 - 7,45	Fibrinogen: 397 mg/dL (200–400)
Bilateral Pulmonary		HCO_3^- 18,5 mmol/L	35–45 mmHg	Lupic anticoagulant
Embolism		Serum creatinine 1,09 mg/dL	22–26 mmol/L	aCL IgG; aCL IgM
Liver		AST 106 U/L	0,5–9,0 mg/dL	aβ2GPI IgG; aβ2GPI IgM
Elevated liver enzymes		ALT 34 U/L	0–32 U/L	Antinuclear antibodies
Peripheral vessel		Pancreatic amylase 98 U/L	0–33 U/L	Anti-DS-DNA antibodies
Venous thrombosis		LDH 950 U/L	13–53 U/L	Anti-cytoplasm (MPO; PR3) antibodies
Arterial thrombosis		Total Creatinine Kinase (CK)	100–250 U/L	Anti-mitochondria antibody (AMA)
Spleen		1217 U/L	26–192 U/L	Anti-smooth muscle antibody (ASMA)
Splenic infarction		D-dimers (DD) 4,72 µg/ml	0–0,5 µg/ml	anti-citrulline antibody (anti-CCP)
Heart		T-Troponin 2137 ng/L	< 14 ng/L	Rheumatoid factor
Obstetric		NT-proBNP 4041 pg/mL	< 300 pg/mL	HLA - B27 normal
fetal death		Proteinuria 75 mg / dL	NEGATIVE	Complement count (C3; C4)
		Leukocyturia 100 cel / uL	NEGATIVE	Absence of Leiden Factor V mutation
		Erythrocyturia 150 cel / uL	NEGATIVE	Absence of prothrombine mutation
				PT20210A
				Protein C and protein S
				Funcional Antithrombin III
				Anti-HIV 1/2 (CHIV Ag/Ab)
				Ag-HBs
				Anti-HCV
				SARS-CoV-2

plasmapheresis and the first dose of rituximab (1000 mg) was administered. Under this treatment, an evident improvement was observed: the platelet count, hepatic enzymes and serum creatinine normalized. On the sixth day of hospitalization, she was transferred to an intermediate care unit at the hospital of her residence area where she continued TPE until the 14th day, when the second dose of rituximab was administered. After those treatments, the patient was discharged with a vitamin K antagonist. Regarding the initial laboratory workup, before plasmapheresis or rituximab infusions, antiphospholipid antibodies were negative (LA, aCL and β2GPI) as well as screening for thrombophilia (including protein C and protein S deficiency, antithrombin III deficiency, Leiden Factor V mutation and prothrombin mutations), and other autoimmune diseases. Histological examination of the placenta showed areas of small vessel infarction.

Six months after discharge, the patient has resumed her day-to-day life activities. She remains under warfarin therapy and the bypass is functional, with distal pulses maintained and without intermittent claudication. Additional workup was repeated and continued to be negative for aPL (even with the patient taking warfarin, which could cause a false positive lupus anticoagulant) and other autoimmune diseases (including SLE, vasculitis and sarcoidosis), with normal complement counts (C3, C4 and CH50) as well as negative for thrombophilia, cryoglobulinemia, cold agglutinin disease, autoimmune hemolytic anemia, paroxysmal nocturnal hemoglobinuria and infectious diseases (negative for hepatitis B virus, hepatitis C virus, cytomegalovirus, Epstein Barr and toxoplasmosis). CD19 positive cells are still depleted (0,1%; normal 7–23%), due to previous rituximab infusions. Other extra-criteria antibodies testing was not available in the laboratory and was not performed [Table 3].

Discussion

The initial diagnosis of CAPS was clinical, given the sudden onset of thrombosis in large and small vessels, and across multiple organs, as clearly shown on Angio CT. Her previous miscarriage, livedo reticularis and thrombocytopenia might support a previous undiagnosed APS and the initial trigger might have been the pregnancy, that culminated in fetal death, which is the precipitating factor in 8% of CAPS registry cases [7].

Differential diagnoses included other entities, such as HELLP syndrome, disseminated intravascular coagulation (DIC) and malignancy. HELLP syndrome was not suspected since hyperbilirubinemia was not present and peripheral blood smear did not show signs of microangiopathy, including the absence of schizocytes. There was no evidence of DIC because coagulation times were not prolonged, fibrinogen was not reduced (397 mg/dL [200–400]). There was no suspicion of malignancy since she had no signs or symptoms of neoplastic disease, and no suspected features were found in the CT scan.

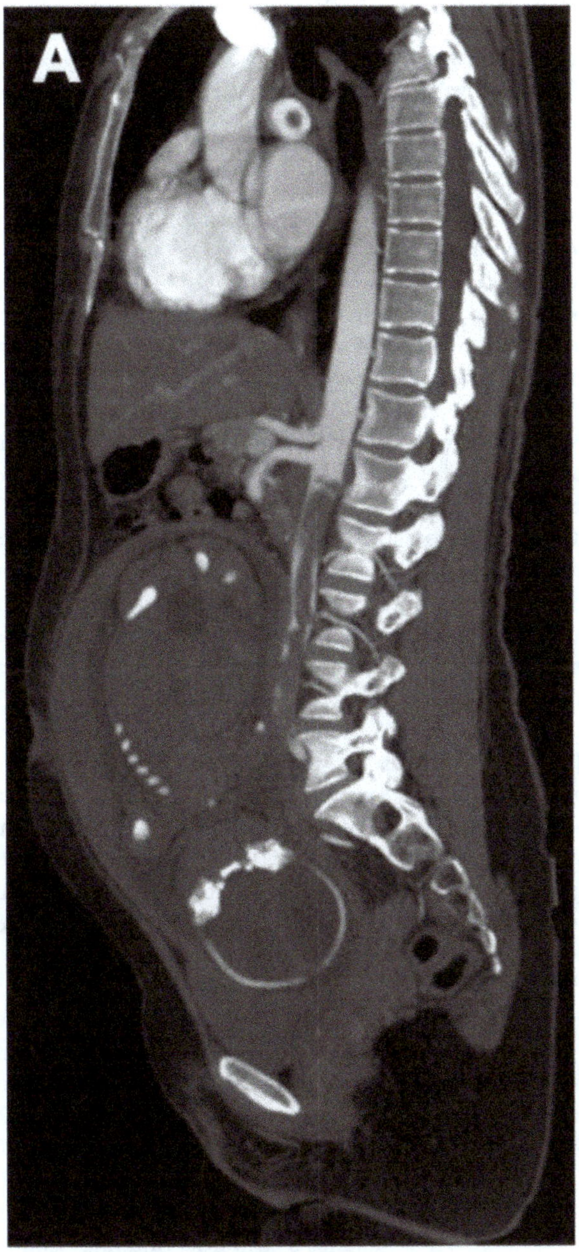

Fig. 1 Angio-CT - sagittal view - showing juxta renal aortic thrombosis

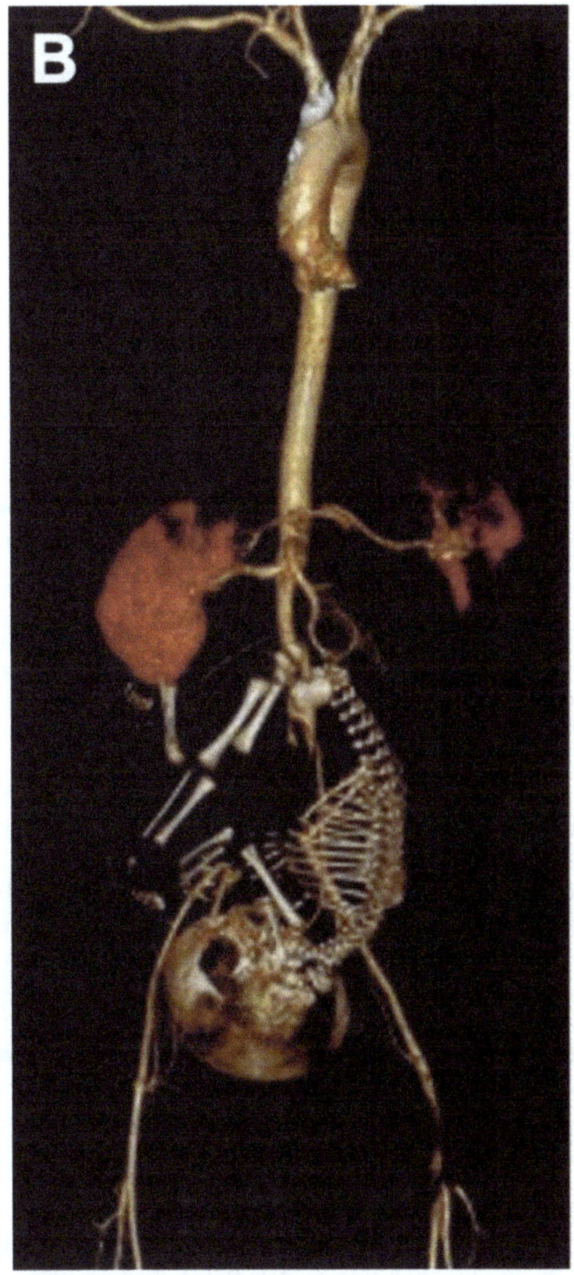

Fig. 2 3D reconstruction of CT angiography showing areas of splenic and right renal infarction, thrombosis of the juxta renal aorta and left renal artery, the distal segment of the right deep femoral artery and the left common femoral artery and its bifurcation

As a condition that is both rare and potentially lethal, there are no randomized clinical trials to guide CAPS treatment with the recommendations being empiric: based on analysis of CAPS registry and expert consensus [6, 10]. "Triple therapy" is the most accepted treatment at date and consists of anticoagulation, corticotherapy and therapeutic plasma exchange (TPE/plasmapheresis) or intravenous immune globulin (IVIG). New therapeutic modalities such as rituximab may have a role as a second-line therapy in the treatment of complicated, refractory/relapsing CAPS patients [6, 10]. Additionally, potential initiating factors or "triggers" must be identified and treated, and supportive care must be given as for any critically ill patient [6, 10, 11].

In the present case report, thrombolysis wasn't indicated as treatment for the PE, since the patient was hemodynamically stable and would probably need surgery in a few hours. Anticoagulation with unfractioned heparin infusion was started in the

Table 3 Suggested extra-criteria antibodies in seronegative antiphospholipid syndrome and its clinical manifestations. (Adapted from [9])

Extra-criteria antibodies	Clinical manifestations
Anti-prothrombin/ phosphatidylserine antibodies	Thrombosis
Anti-annexin V antibodies/annexin A5 resistance	Thrombosis and/or pregnancy complications
Antibodies to vimentin/CL complex	Arterial thrombosis
Phosphatidylethanolamine	Fetal loss and/or thrombosis
Phosphatidic acid	Fetal loss
Phosphatidylserine	Fetal loss
Phosphatidylinositol	Fetal loss

ICU, to allow rapid reversal if surgery was required and, for its additional anti-inflammatory effects (especially inhibition of complement activation and inhibition of aPL binding) [6, 10, 12]. Despite all efforts, lower limb ischemia continued to worsen, and revascularization became urgent. Several surgical options were considered. Endovascular surgery was excluded due to the high risk of in-stent thrombosis. Anatomical revascularization surgery, despite presenting better long-term permeability, presented a high hemorrhagic risk and the presence of a gravid uterus was an anatomical concern. Therefore, we opted for a less invasive extra-anatomical revascularization (axillary-bifemoral bypass) to ensure immediate perfusion of the lower limbs, postponing an eventual anatomical revascularization for a second time (after stabilization). Considering the risk of anastomotic blow out and bypass thrombosis with an induction of labor (due to effort and anatomical position of the delivery), a cesarean section was performed. An intrauterine balloon tamponade was placed to minimize the bleeding risk after cesarean section and was removed after 48 h.

Immunosuppression with corticosteroids inhibits the cytokine cascade, which plays a major role in CAPS [6, 11], but it also delays the healing process and increases the risk of surgical wound and bypass prosthesis infection. For this reason, rituximab, a chimeric monoclonal antibody against CD20 that reduces the number of B- cells and therefore the production and concentration of harmful cytokines, was initiated instead. TPE was used for additional immunosuppression since it removes circulating free antibodies (aPL), immune complexes, cytokines, TNF- α, and complement products [11, 13].

During hospitalization, the laboratorial results for aPL were negative, and it was assumed that were false negatives due to consumption [8] or the presence of other aPL antibodies not usually tested [14].

During the six-month follow-up after discharge, laboratory workup persisted negative for autoimmune diseases, thrombophilia or infectious disease. However, CD19 positive cells remained depleted (0,1%; normal 7–23%) due to rituximab infusions, which could explain a negative aPL, with or without other autoimmune disease. Another possibility is the existence of other aPL besides LA, aCL and β2GPI, that aren't routinely measured in most laboratories.

Given the rapid development of manifestations, the number of organs involved and the histopathological confirmation of small vessel occlusion in the placenta, this case undoubtedly fulfills criteria 1, 2 and 3 for CAPS diagnosis (Table 1). However, the absence of positive aPL prevents this diagnosis, even though this case hardly fits any other known coagulopathy, or diagnosis.

In clinical practice, there are often discrepancies between antibody levels and clinical disease expression. Routine screening tests for aPL may miss some cases and it is also possible that previously positive aPL titers become negative - either acutely by "consumption" during an acute thrombotic episode, or slowly, over time [8, 15]. In 2003, Hughes and Khamashta introduced seronegative APS (SNAPS) to describe patients with clinical manifestations highly suggestive of APS but with persistently negative aPL [15]. Since then, other reviews recognizing this entity were published [8, 9, 14, 16, 17] and some new antigenic targets for aPL in APS have been recently investigated, some of them associated with thrombosis and/or fetal loss [9] (Table 3 [9]).

SNAPS is usually a diagnosis of exclusion and should be suspected in patients with a clinical history suggestive of APS, such as those with recurrent arterial venous thrombotic events, recurrent miscarriage, or unexplained thrombocytopenia, with persistent negativity of aPL tested on at least two occasions, and when other causes of thrombosis are excluded, such as thrombophilia, active cancer, trauma, major surgery, or prolonged bed rest [9]. SNAPS diagnosis implies fulfilling clinical criteria, plus "non-criteria" manifestations, with persistently negative aPL [18]. "Non-criteria" manifestations are described in Table 4 [9, 18]. In this case, it stands out the presence of livedo reticularis and thrombocytopenia as a "non-criteria" manifestation of antiphospholipid syndrome.

This patient could be either a truly SNAPS (in the absence of extra-criteria antibodies [Table 3], but in the presence of "extra-criteria" manifestations [Table 4]) or a "Laboratory non-criteria APS", given the presence of clinical criteria with persistently negative or low titer criteria aPL, but positive "extra-criteria" aPL [18].

Considering the above, the clinical team assumed a Catastrophic SNAPS diagnosis and the patient was

Table 4 "Non-criteria" manifestations of antiphospholipid syndrome (adapted from [9, 18])

Nervous system	Dementia
	Seizures
	Multiple sclerosis–like illness
	Chorea
	Myelitis
	Brain MRI white matter lesions
	Cognitive impairment
	Migraine
Skin	Livedo reticularis
	Livedoid vasculopathy
	Raynaud's phenomenon
	Splinter hemorrhages
	Skin ulcers
Heart	Valve vegetations or thickening (Libman-Sacks Endocarditis) Diastolic dysfunction
Blood	Thrombocytopenia
	Hemolytic anemia
	Coombs´ test positivity
Kidney	Microangiopathy
	Chronic vaso-occlusive lesions (atherosclerosis, glomerular ischemia, interstitial fibrosis, arterial fibrous intimal hyperplasia)
Obstetric	Late intrauterine growth restriction (after 34 weeks)
	Late pre-eclampsia (after 34 weeks)
	Placental abruption
	Placental hematoma
	Preterm birth (> 34 to < 37 weeks)
	Puerperal pre-eclampsia
	Two or more unexplained in vitro fertilization failures
	Two unexplained spontaneous abortions < 10 weeks
Other	Superficial vein thrombosis
	Amaurosis fugax
	Sensorineural hearing loss
	Ischemic necrosis of bone
	Pulmonary hypertension

treated accordingly, with good results. The patient will be kept under warfarin treatment indefinitely and will perform follow-up laboratorial tests, to look for positive aPL or other laboratorial changes that that confirms CAPS or evidence another diagnosis.

Conclusion

CAPS is a rare form of APS that develops quickly, with multiorgan involvement, high mortality rate, and its approach often poses a multidisciplinary challenge.

This patient presented with fetal loss and multiple arterial and venous thrombosis, clinical manifestations highly suggestive of CAPS, that hardly fits into another diagnosis, but with persistently negative aPL.

Some APS patients may present with negative aPL due to either consumption or presence of other anti-phospholipid antibodies, not routinely tested and are referred to as SNAPS or "Laboratory non-criteria APS".

We believe that this is a rare case of catastrophic SNAPS, that presented a favorable evolution under therapy with anticoagulation, plasmapheresis and rituximab.

Acknowledgements

I would like to express my deep gratitude to Dr. Inês Donas Boto for her help in revising the manuscript and language editing.

Authors' contributions

All authors contributed to the preparation of the manuscript and case report. All authors read and approved the final manuscript.

Author details
[1]Vascular Surgery Department, Heart and Vessels Division, Hospital Santa Maria (CHULN), Av. Prof. Egas Moniz s/n, 1649-035 Lisbon, Portugal. [2]Lisbon Academic Medical Center, Lisbon, Portugal. [3]Faculty of Medicine, University of Lisbon, Lisbon, Portugal. [4]Department of Internal Medicine (Medicina 2), Hospital Santa Maria (CHULN), Lisbon, Portugal.

References

1. James AH. Thrombosis in pregnancy and maternal outcomes. Birth Defects Research Part C: Embryo Today: Reviews. 2015;105(3):159–66. https://doi.org/10.1002/bdrc.21106.
2. Bundhun PK, Soogund MZS, Huang F. Arterial/venous thrombosis, fetal loss and stillbirth in pregnant women with systemic lupus erythematosus versus primary and secondary antiphospholipid syndrome: a systematic review and meta-analysis. BMC Pregnancy Childbirth. 2018;18(1):212. https://doi.org/10.1186/s12884-018-1850-x.
3. Miyakis S, Lockshin MD, Atsumi T, et al. International consensus statement on an update of the classification criteria for definite antiphospholipid syndrome (APS). J Thromb Haemost. 2006;4(2):295–306. https://doi.org/10.1111/j.1538-7836.2006.01753.x.
4. Tektonidou MG, Andreoli L, Limper M, Tincani A, Ward MM. Management of thrombotic and obstetric antiphospholipid syndrome: a systematic literature review informing the EULAR recommendations for the management of antiphospholipid syndrome in adults. RMD Open. 2019;5(1):e000924. https://doi.org/10.1136/rmdopen-2019-000924.
5. Cervera R. Antiphospholipid syndrome. Thromb Res. 2017;151:S43–7. https://doi.org/10.1016/s0049-3848(17)30066-x.
6. Carmi O, Berla M, Shoenfeld Y, Levy Y. Diagnosis and management of catastrophic antiphospholipid syndrome. Expert Rev Hematol. 2017;10(4):365–74. https://doi.org/10.1080/17474086.2017.1300522.
7. Rodríguez-Pintó I, Moitinho M, Santacreu I, Shoenfeld Y, Erkan D, Espinosa G, et al. Catastrophic antiphospholipid syndrome (CAPS): descriptive analysis of 500 patients from the international CAPS registry. Autoimmun Rev. 2016;15(12):1120–4. https://doi.org/10.1016/j.autrev.2016.09.010.
8. Nayfe R, Uthman I, Aoun J, Saad Aldin E, Merashli M, Khamashta M. Seronegative antiphospholipid syndrome. Rheumatology. 2013;52(8):1358–67. https://doi.org/10.1093/rheumatology/ket126.
9. Pignatelli P, Ettorre E, Menichelli D, Pani A, Violi F, Pastori D. Seronegative antiphospholipid syndrome: refining the value of non-criteria antibodies for the diagnosis and clinical management. Haematol. 2020;105(3):562–72. https://doi.org/10.3324/haematol.2019.221945.
10. Silver RM. Catastrophic antiphospholipid syndrome and pregnancy. Semin Perinatol. 2018;42(1):26–32. https://doi.org/10.1053/j.semperi.2017.11.006.
11. Cervera R. Update on the diagnosis, treatment, and prognosis of the catastrophic antiphospholipid syndrome. Curr Rheumatol Rep. 2010;12(1):70–6. https://doi.org/10.1007/s11926-009-0073-6.
12. Girardi G, Redecha P, Salmon JE. Heparin prevents antiphospholipid antibody-induced fetal loss by inhibiting complement activation. Nat Med. 2004;10(11):1222–6. https://doi.org/10.1038/nm1121.
13. Uthman I, Shamseddine A, Taher A. The role of therapeutic plasma exchange in the catastrophic antiphospholipid syndrome. Transfus Apher Sci. 2005;33(1):11–7. https://doi.org/10.1016/j.transci.2004.10.025.
14. Conti F, Capozzi A, Truglia S, Lococo E, Longo A, Misasi R, et al. The mosaic of "seronegative" antiphospholipid syndrome. J Immunol Res. 2014;2014:1–7. https://doi.org/10.1155/2014/389601.
15. Hughes G, Khamashta M. Seronegative antiphospholipid syndrome. Ann Rheum Dis. 2003;62(12):1127. https://doi.org/10.1136/ard.2003.006163.
16. Cervera R, Conti F, Doria A, Iaccarino L, Valesini G. Does seronegative antiphospholipid syndrome really exist? Autoimmun Rev. 2012;11(8):581–4. https://doi.org/10.1016/j.autrev.2011.10.017.
17. Pengo V, Tripodi A, Reber G, Rand JH, Ortel TL, Galli M, et al. Update of the guidelines for lupus anticoagulant detection. J Thromb Haemost. 2009;7(10):1737–40. https://doi.org/10.1111/j.1538-7836.2009.03555.x.
18. da Rosa GP, Bettencourt P, Rodríguez-Pintó I, et al. "Noncriteria" antiphospholipid syndrome: a nomenclature proposal. Autoimmun Rev. 2020;19(12):102689. https://doi.org/10.1016/j.autrev.2020.102689.

23

COVID19 infection in a patient undergoing treatment for Paroxysmal Nocturnal Hemoglobinuria (PNH) with Ravulizumab

Sufana Shikdar[1,3*], Azra Borogovac[1], Elabdallah Mohamad[2] and Mohamad Khawandanah[1]

Abstract

Background: In the recent COVID19 pandemic, patients with hematological disorders were considered at high risk for severe disease. Limited data is available regarding the course of COVID19 infection in this subgroup.

Case Presentation: We describe a case of a 32-year-old man with paroxysmal nocturnal hemoglobinuria (PNH) undergoing treatment with ravulizumab (Ultomiris) who presented with COVID19 infection. He experienced only mild symptoms and had a rapid recovery from COVID19 infection.

Conclusion: This case may demonstrate the beneficial effects of ravulizumab on complement mediated inflammatory damage linked with COVID19 infection especially in PNH patients.

Keywords: COVID19, Paroxysmal nocturnal hemoglobinuria, Complement inhibitor

Background

Coronavirus disease 2019 (COVID-19) has become a global pandemic with at least 229.3 million confirmed cases and a total of 4,700,000 deaths worldwide as of September 2021 [1]. In December 2019, an outbreak of COVID-19 disease was detected in China caused by the Severe Acute Respiratory Syndrome Coronavirus-2 (SARS-CoV-2). The clinical manifestation of COVID-19 is characterized by respiratory distress, and in more severe cases can progress towards acute respiratory distress syndrome (ARDS) and death [2]. COVID-19 infection carries a potentially fatal risk, especially with an immunocompromised state and multiple comorbidities [3]. Several mutations of SARS-CoV-2 have been reported so far, and most recently a new mutation in the Delta variant (B.1.617.2 lineage) was found which seems to be highly contagious and is now the dominant variant globally [4]. Meanwhile, on December 11, 2020, FDA approval of the Pfizer-BioNTech in individuals 16 years of age and older vaccine has opened a new door to fight against the global pandemic; currently, we have three FDA approved vaccines available in the US [4]. Even though the COVID vaccine is highly effective at preventing severe illness, they do not give full protection in preventing and transmitting the COVID-19 infection.

COVID-19 infection causes hyperactivation of the complement system and excessive inflammatory response leading to worsening lung injury and poor clinical outcomes [2, 5]. The interaction between the complement system and COVID-19 infection raises the possibility that immunosuppression could be a promising approach to inhibit the consequences of complement mediated inflammatory destruction in COVID-19 infection. Moreover, patients with PNH may be vulnerable to COVID-19 complications due to impaired immune status [6]. Based on this immunological rationale, it was

* Correspondence: Sufana.shikdar@gmail.com
[1]Department of Hematology/Oncology, Stephenson Cancer Center, University of Oklahoma Health Sciences Center, 73104 Oklahoma City, United States, OK
[3]Hematology/Oncology fellow, Department of Medicine, Division of Hematology-Oncology Stephenson Cancer Center, University of Oklahoma Health Sciences Center, 800 NE 10th St., 6th Floor, OK 73104 Oklahoma City, United States

speculated that the therapeutic use of complement inhibitors might be an effective strategy to control systemic inflammation in COVID-19 infection.

Although complement blockade strategies are being prospectively studied in clinical trials and reported in case reports, no cases of PNH with COVID-19 infection managed with complement blocker agents have been reported [7, 8]. Herein, we report the first case of COVID-19 pneumonia in a patient with PNH on treatment with intravenous ravulizumab, a complement component C5 inhibitor. He had a favorable clinical course linked to COVID19 infection and was discharged without any complications.

Case presentation

Our patient was a 32-year-old Nigerian immigrant male who presented around September 2018 with a clinical picture of severe aplastic anemia. The patient received one cycle of Horse antithymocyte globulin (ATG; 40 mg/kg once daily for 4 days); two weeks of prednisone (100 mg orally twice a day, then tapered), and six months of eltrombopag (150 mg orally daily) and cyclosporin A (10 mg/kg orally daily). The diagnosis of combined PNH and aplastic anemia due to bone marrow failure, hemolysis, and detection of PNH clone in addition to aplastic hypocellular marrow was made, and the patient was started with eculizumab for 5 cycles, then switched to ravulizumab around March 2019 with the last dose in February 2020. He remained profoundly pancytopenic and he was waiting for an allogeneic transplant.

He presented in March 2020 with fever, runny nose, dry cough, and altered taste (dysgeusia) for 4 days. Physical examination revealed normal blood pressure, fever (38.3 °C), tachypnea (30 breaths per min) with baseline oxygen saturation of 95 % in room air. The COVID19 test using targeted rich multiplex polymerase chain reaction of a nasopharyngeal swab came back positive for SARS-CoV-2 infection. A chest radiography did not show infiltrates (Fig. 1). Infectious workup including blood and urine cultures were negative. Respiratory viral panel was negative for influenza A and B. Laboratory tests revealed WBC 1.93 cells/mm3, absolute neutrophil count (ANC) 950 cells/mm3, Hb 8 gm/l, Platelet 37,000/mm3; increased levels of acute phase reactants, including CRP (108 mg/l; normal range <5 mg/l), ferritin (3355 ng/ml; normal range 10–322 ng/ml), serum lactate dehydrogenase (364 U/l; normal range 112–236 U/l), and fibrinogen (615 mg/dl; normal value 150-450 mg/dl). The patient was treated with azithromycin, hydroxychloroquine, and prophylactic enoxaparin. He required no oxygen, remained afebrile, and oxygen saturation was maintained around 95 % in room air. He demonstrated a rapid and progressive improvement in his symptoms and was discharged from the

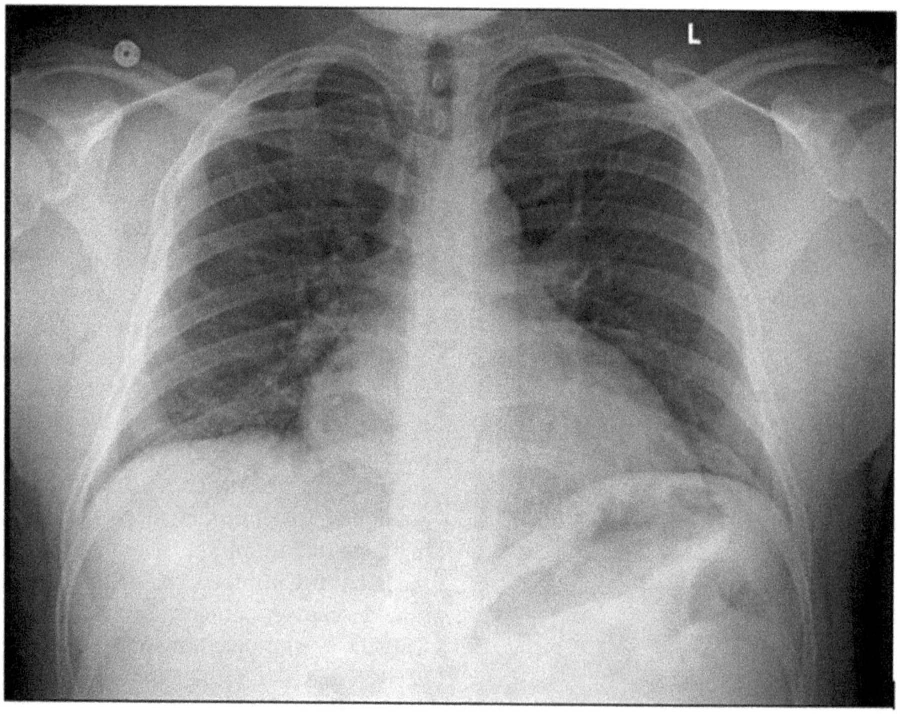

Fig. 1 Chest Xray on admission: No infiltrates noted with COVID19 infection

hospital 4 days after diagnosis with no immediate complications and no evidence of breakthrough hemolysis.

Discussion and conclusions

PNH is a clonal disorder of hematopoietic progenitor cells caused by an acquired mutation of the X-linked phosphatidylinositol glycans class A (PIG-A) gene [9]. The absence of glycosylphosphatidylinositol (GPI) anchored complement regulatory proteins CD55 and CD59 from the membrane of circulatory cells is responsible for the activation of the complement system on the surface of the red cell membrane. This leads to complement mediated intravascular hemolysis, activation of platelets, and the coagulation cascade resulting in a hypercoagulable state [9]. PNH, although rare, can be fatal and includes an increased risk of thromboembolism and severe end-organ damage. Approximately, 35 % of patients die within five years if untreated due to thrombosis and related complications [10].

There is a close relationship between PNH and aplastic anemia (AA) especially when PNH evolves into bone marrow hypoplasia, which is a hallmark of AA. An overlap entity can be the presenting symptom i.e., dual diagnosis. Three presentations lead to overlap or dual diagnosis: (1) aplastic anemia on original presentation then the discovery of PNH clone, (2) PNH presentation then evolution to aplastic anemia, and (3) Aplastic anemia and PNH dual diagnosis on presentation [11]. Our patient presented with the dual diagnosis of PNH manifested by hemolysis and jaundice in addition to profoundly aplastic bone marrow.

Ravulizumab (ALXN1210; Alexion Pharmaceuticals, Inc) is a second generation humanized monoclonal antibody that prevents complement protein 5 (C5) cleavage and activation, ultimately blocking membrane attack complex (MAC) formation in the complement pathway [12]. Ravulizumab is now approved by the FDA to treat PNH. It has an extended 8-week maintenance dosing interval and reduces the need for frequent drug administration with subsequent improvement in symptom control and better quality of life.

The complement system activation is a critical component in the sequelae of COVID19 infection. Evidence suggests that severe outcomes in COVID19 infection are attributed to the excessive activation of the complement cascade leading to acute lung injury and associated with an increased prothrombotic state [2, 5, 13, 14]. Notably, C5a concentration was noted to be higher in patients with COVID19 infection [2, 14]. Based on these observations, complement component blockers could be used as potential therapeutic targets in COVID-19 patients.

Several clinical trials have been ongoing to target complement mediated inflammatory response in the emerging COVID19 outbreak. An anti C3 agent, compstatin analog Cp40/AMY-101 has shown efficacy in complement mediated severe ARDS in COVID19 patients, and a phase II clinical trial is ongoing [7]. In addition, a multicenter phase II/III trial using a monoclonal neutralizing anti-C5a antibody (IFX-1) is recruiting patients with severe COVID19 pneumonia [8]. Preliminary PK/PD analysis of ALXN1210-COV-305 phase 3 trial found that patients with severe COVID-19 infection treated with modified ravulizumab dosing regimen resulted in improved clinical outcomes [15, 16]. Alexion also initiated a clinical trial in critical COVID19 patients on a related drug, eculizumab (NCT04288713) [17]. A proof-of-concept study by Annane et al. found survival benefits with eculizumab in patients with severe COVID-19 [18]. Clinical and experimental research is ongoing to optimize therapeutic interventions targeting the complement system [19–22]. For example, zilucoplan, an anti-C5 drug, is being evaluated in a phase 2 ACCORD trial for hospitalized COVID-19 patients [19]. Also, the TACTIC-R trial is currently assessing the efficacy of ravulizumab among Pre-ICU COVID-19 patients [20]. In addition, Multi-center Pilot Trial (PROTECT-COVID-19) is evaluating the efficacy of conestat alpha, the C1 esterase inhibitor in severe COVID-19 infection [21], and I-SPY COVID-19 trial is investigating the benefit of anti-MASP-2 antibody Narsoplimab in critically ill COVID-19 patients [22]. While these trials posit a new potential treatment strategy, the therapeutic use of complement inhibitors in COVID-19 immunocompromised patients is limited. Few case reports have shown a promising effect of complement inhibitors in COVID-19 patients. Eculizumab used in the patients with thrombotic microangiopathic anemia in the setting of COVID19 showed dramatic improvement in kidney function [23]. Another patient with a transplanted kidney who was on Eculizumab for the atypical hemolytic uremic syndrome (HUS), was treated for COVID19 infection and had a full recovery [24]. Similarly, a patient with PNH diagnosed with COVID-19 pneumonia showed fast recovery with the initiation of eculizumab [25].

Immunocompromised patients are at higher risk for severe COVID19 infections and may experience prolonged hospitalization due to COVID19-related morbidity, and mortality. Additionally, administration of most scheduled anti-cancer treatments may be delayed or interrupted. In our case, the continuation of ravulizumab during COVID19 infection may have assisted a prompt recovery by attenuating complement activation.

The CDC recommends adopting strategies to minimize the risk of COVID19 exposure, such as limiting contacts between patients and healthcare providers. Ravulizumab has a longer therapeutic window and therefore a less frequent dosing schedule than eculizumab. We recommend against interrupting or holding the dose of ravulizumab even during systemic inflammation to combat complement mediated tissue damage and multiorgan failure. We also recommend switching the every 8-weeks dosing schedule of eculizumab with ravulizumab to minimize the exposure to COVID19 and other infections and reduce the economic burden on hospital systems due to less frequent dosing.

Given the worldwide COVID19 pandemic, specific clinical and economically cost-effective therapeutic options should be explored and prioritized. Treatment with ravulizumab during COVID19 pneumonia was safe, cost-effective, and found to have a favorable clinical course in a patient with PNH. A systemic prospective trial is warranted to demonstrate the utility and usefulness of ravulizumab in patients with PNH in the COVID-19 outbreak.

Acknowledgements
None.

Authors' contributions
SS made substantial contributions to the conception and design, drafting of the manuscript, analysis, and interpretation of data, and revising the manuscript and gave final approval for publication. AB, and EM, provided clinical care for the patient and critically revised the manuscript for important intellectual content. MK served as primary consultant in the management of the patient and made substantial contributions to the conception and design; analysis and interpretation of data; drafting of the manuscript; and revising the manuscript critically for important intellectual content; and gave final approval of the version to be published. All authors read and approved the final manuscript.

Author details
[1]Department of Hematology/Oncology, Stephenson Cancer Center, University of Oklahoma Health Sciences Center, 73104 Oklahoma City, United States, OK. [2]Department of Internal Medicine, University of Oklahoma Medical Center (OUMC), 73104 Oklahoma City, United States, OK. [3]Hematology/Oncology fellow, Department of Medicine, Division of Hematology-Oncology Stephenson Cancer Center, University of Oklahoma Health Sciences Center, 800 NE 10th St., 6th Floor, OK 73104 Oklahoma City, United States.

References
1. World Health Organization. Coronavirus [internet]. https://www.who.int/data. Accessed 22 September 2021.
2. Bosmann M. Complement activation during critical illness: Current findings and an outlook in the era of COVID-19. Am J Respir Crit Care Med. 2020;202: 163–5.
3. Najjar S, Najjar A, Chong DJ, Pramanik BK, Kirsch C, Kuzniecky RI, et al. Central nervous system complications associated with SARS-CoV-2 infection: integrative concepts of pathophysiology and case reports. J Neuroinflammation. 2020;17:231.
4. Aleem A, AB AS, Slenker AK. Emerging Variants of SARS-CoV-2 And Novel Therapeutics Against Coronavirus (COVID-19).
5. Fletcher-Sandersjöö A, Bellander B-M. Is COVID-19 associated thrombosis caused by overactivation of the complement cascade? A literature review. Thromb Res. 2020;194:36–41.
6. Malard F, Genthon A, Brissot E, van de Wyngaert Z, Marjanovic Z, Ikhlef S, et al. COVID-19 outcomes in patients with hematologic disease. Bone Marrow Transplant [Internet]. 2020; Available from: https://doi.org/10.1038/s41409-020-0931-4.
7. Mastaglio S, Ruggeri A, Risitano AM, Angelillo P, Yancopoulou D, Mastellos DC, et al. The first case of COVID-19 treated with the complement C3 inhibitor AMY-101. Clin Immunol. 2020;215:108450.
8. Vlaar A.Open-label. Randomized Study of IFX-1 in Patients With Severe COVID-19 Pneumonia (PANAMO) 2020. [accessed 2020 July]Available from: https://clinicaltrialsgov/ct2/show/NCT04333420 [Ref list].
9. Rosti V. The molecular basis of paroxysmal nocturnal hemoglobinuria. Haematologica. 2000;85:82–7.
10. Gembillo G, Siligato R, Cernaro V, Santoro D. Complement inhibition therapy and dialytic strategies in paroxysmal nocturnal hemoglobinuria: The nephrologist's opinion. J Clin Med. 2020;9:1261.
11. Olson TS. Aplastic anemia: Pathogenesis, clinical manifestations, and diagnosis. UpToDate. Accessed 22 September 2021 from https://www.uptodate.com/contents/aplastic-anemia-pathogenesis-clinical-manifestations-and diagnosis.
12. Stern RM, Connell NT. Ravulizumab: a novel C5 inhibitor for the treatment of paroxysmal nocturnal hemoglobinuria. Ther Adv Hematol. 2019;10: 2040620719874728.
13. Porfidia A, Valeriani E, Pola R, Porreca E, Rutjes AWS, Di Nisio M. Venous thromboembolism in patients with COVID-19: Systematic review and meta-analysis. Thromb Res. 2020;196:67–74.
14. Risitano AM, Mastellos DC, Huber-Lang M, Yancopoulou D, Garlanda C, Ciceri F, et al. Complement as a target in COVID-19? Nat Rev Immunol. 2020;20:343–4.
15. Efficacy and Safety Study of IV Ravulizumab in Patients With COVID-19 Severe Pneumonia. - Full Text View - ClinicalTrials.Gov [Internet]. Clinicaltrials.gov. [cited 2020 Aug 29]. Available from: http://clinicaltrials.gov/ct2/show/NCT04369469.
16. McEneny-King AC, Monteleone JP, Kazani SD, Ortiz SR. Pharmacokinetic and pharmacodynamic evaluation of ravulizumab in adults with severe Coronavirus Disease 2019. Infectious Diseases Therapy. 2021 ;10(2):1045–54.
17. Eculizumab. (Soliris) in covid-19 infected patients (SOLID-C19). Available at: https://clinicaltrials.gov/ct2/show/NCT04288713. Published February 28, 2020. Updated March 30, 2020. Accessed 20 July 2020.
18. Annane D, Heming N, Grimaldi-Bensouda L, Frémeaux-Bacchi V, Vigan M, Roux AL, Marchal A, Michelon H, Rottman M, Moine P. Eculizumab as an emergency treatment for adult patients with severe COVID-19 in the intensive care unit: a proof-of-concept study. EClinicalMedicine. 2020 Nov 1; 28:100590.
19. Wilkinson T, Dixon R, Page C, Carroll M, Griffiths G, Ho LP, De Soyza A, Felton T, Lewis KE, Phekoo K, Chalmers JD. ACCORD: a multicentre, seamless, phase 2 adaptive randomisation platform study to assess the efficacy and safety of multiple candidate agents for the treatment of COVID-19 in hospitalised patients: a structured summary of a study protocol for a randomised controlled trial. Trials. 2020 ;21(1):1–3.
20. Kulkarni S, Fisk M, Kostapanos M, Banham-Hall E, Bond S, Hernan-Sancho E, Norton S, Cheriyan J, Cope A, Galloway J, Hall F. Repurposed immunomodulatory drugs for Covid-19 in pre-ICu patients-mulTi-Arm Therapeutic study in pre-ICu patients admitted with Covid-19–Repurposed Drugs (TACTIC-R): A structured summary of a study protocol for a randomised controlled trial. Trials. 2020 ;21(1):1–3.
21. Urwyler P, Charitos P, Moser S, Heijnen IA, Trendelenburg M, Thoma R, Sumer J, Camacho-Ortiz A, Bacci MR, Huber LC, Stüssi-Helbling M. Recombinant human C1 esterase inhibitor (conestat alfa) in the prevention of severe SARS-CoV-2 infection in hospitalized patients with COVID-19: A structured summary of a study protocol for a randomized, parallel-group, open-label, multi-center pilot trial (PROTECT-COVID-19). Trials. 2021 ;22(1):1–3.
22. I-SPY, COVID-19. TRIAL: an adaptive platform trial for critically ill patients full text view. Available from: ClinicalTrials.gov. Accessed May23, 2021.
23. Boudhabhay I, Rabant M, Roumenina LT, Coupry LM, Poillerat V, Marchal A, Frémeaux-Bacchi V, El Karoui K, Monchi M, Pourcine F. Case Report: Adult Post-COVID-19 Multisystem Inflammatory Syndrome and Thrombotic Microangiopathy. Front Immunol. 2021;23:2284.
24. Mentese IB, Velioglu A, Aykent B, Gunay DS, Arikan H, Tuglular S. Course of COVID-19 Pneumonia in a Kidney Transplant Patient Receiving Eculizumab. Progress in Transplantation. Jun. 2021;18:15269248211024629.
25. Sokol J, Nehaj F, Mokan M, Lisa L, Stasko J. COVID19 infection in a patient with paroxysmal nocturnal hemoglobinuria: A case report. Medicine. 2021 May 21;100(20).

The disulfide bond Cys2724-Cys2774 in the C-terminal cystine knot domain of von Willebrand factor is critical for its dimerization and secretion

Yuxin Zhang[1,2], Fengwu Chen[2], Aizhen Yang[2], Xiaoying Wang[1], Yue Han[2], Depei Wu[2], Yi Wu[1,2*] and Jingyu Zhang[1*]

Abstract

Background: Type 3 von Willebrand disease (VWD) exhibits severe hemorrhagic tendency with complicated pathogenesis. The C-terminal cystine knot (CTCK) domain plays an important role in the dimerization and secretion of von Willebrand factor (VWF). The CTCK domain has four intrachain disulfide bonds including Cys2724-Cys2774, Cys2739-Cys2788, Cys2750-Cys2804 and Cys2754-Cys2806, and the single cysteine mutation in Cys2739-Cys2788, Cys2750-Cys2804 and Cys2754-Cys2806 result in type 3 VWD, demonstrating the crucial role of these three disulfide bonds in VWF biosynthesis, however, the role of the remaining disulfide bond Cys2724-Cys2774 remains unclear.

Method and results: In this study, by the next-generation sequencing we found a missense mutation a c.8171G>A (C2724Y) in the CTCK domain of *VWF* allele in a patient family with type 3 VWD. In vitro, VWF C2724Y protein was expressed normally in HEK-293T cells but did not form a dimer or secrete into cell culture medium, suggesting that C2724 is critical for the VWF dimerization, and thus for VWF multimerization and secretion.

Conclusions: Our findings provide the first genetic evidence for the important role of Cys2724-Cys2774 in VWF biosynthesis and secretion. Therefore, all of the four intrachain disulfide bonds in CTCK monomer contribute to VWF dimerization and secretion.

Keywords: von Willebrand factor (VWF), von Willebrand disease (VWD), cystine knot domain, multimerization, disulfide bond

Introduction

VWF is a large-molecular multimerized glycoprotein synthesized and secreted by endothelial cells and megakaryocytes. This protein has multiple contributions to the hemostatic process: it mediates platelet adhesion and aggregation at sites of vascular injury and carries coagulation factor VIII (FVIII) in the circulation[1]. Functional and/or quantitative deficiencies of VWF are known as von Willebrand disease (VWD), a disorder affecting 0.01–1% of the population[1]. These patients with VWF deficiency manifest a severe hemorrhagic phenotype, originating from defective formation of platelet-rich thrombi and a secondary deficiency of FVIII impairing the generation of a fibrin network[1]. Quantitative deficiencies of VWF result from changes in biosynthesis, secretion, and/or clearance of the protein.

VWF processor contains multiple domains in the order of D1-D2-D9-D3-A1-A2-A3D4-B1-B2-B3-C1-C2-

* Correspondence: yiwu99@gmail.com; zjyhbsjz@163.com
[1]Department of Hematology, Key Laboratory of Hematology of Hebei Province, The Second Hospital of Hebei Medical University, 050000 Shijiazhuang, China

CK[2]. The VWF sequence contains an unusually high content of cysteine residues (8.3%), a percentage fourfold higher than the average in human proteins. In the biosynthesis of VWF, its multimerization is a critical step and involves the pairing of cysteines. pro-VWF monomers are linked pairwise through interchain disulfide bond(s) at the C-terminal cystine knot (CTCK) domain[3]. The CTCK domain has 11 cysteines, 8 of which form 4 intrachain disulfide bonds, Cys2724-Cys2774, Cys2739-Cys2788, Cys2750-Cys2804 and Cys2754-Cys2806, the other 3 cysteines form 3 interchain disulfide bonds [4] ensuring the long-term stability of the dimeric conformation of VWF. In the endoplasmic reticulum (ER), pro-VWF subunits first engage into a covalent connection, involving the formation of 3 interchain cysteine pairs located in the C-terminal cysteine knot (CK) domains. Importantly, the structural location of these 3 intermolecular pairs protects them from disulfide reduction, ensuring the long-term stability of the dimeric conformation of VWF. Homozygous mutations of C2739Y[5], C2804Y[6], C2754W[7, 8], and C2806R[9] caused type 3 VWD. These mutations impair C-terminal dimerization and consequently, preventing the formation of long multimers, demonstrating that these three disulfide bonds Cys2739-Cys2788, Cys2750-Cys2804, and Cys2754-Cys2806 are critical for VWF biosynthesis. However, the functional role of the remaining disulfide bond of Cys2724-Cys2774 in VWF biosynthesis remains unknown.

In this study, we diagnosed a patient family with type 3 VWD, next-generation sequencing revealed that the proband had a *VWF* allele with a c.3814delT deletion mutation and the other *VWF* allele with a c.8171G>A (C2724Y) missense mutation in CK domain. In a cell expression system, we found that the VWF C2724Y mutation did not affect VWF monomer expression but caused defective VWF dimerization and secretion. These data provide the first evidence for the critical role of the disulfide bond Cys2724-Cys2774 in CTCK domain in VWF biosynthesis and secretion.

Materials and methods

Blood samples and laboratory tests

This study was approved by the Ethics Committee of the Second Hospital of Hebei Medical University. All patients were informed about the experimental nature of this study and gave their consent to participation. Venous blood collected using 105 mM sodium citrate as anti-coagulant was centrifuged at 4000 g for 10 min at room temperature (RT), followed by collection of plasma. Within 2 h after sample collection, activated partial thromboplastin time (APTT) and FVIII coagulant activities (FVIII:C) were tested by an automatic coagulation instrument (ACLTOP700, Spanish Wolfen Group). Plasma VWF antigen (VWF:Ag) was measured using an enzyme-linked immunosorbent assay (ELISA) kit according to the manufacturer's instructions (HemosIL® von Willebrand Factor Antigen, Spanish Wolfen Group).

VWF multimer analysis

Analysis of VWF multimers in plasma from patients, cell lysate, and cell cultural medium was performed using 1.5% SDS-agarose gel electrophoresis, as previously described with slight modification[10, 11]. Briefly, the plasma was diluted 1: 5 and cell lysate and cultural medium were diluted 1: 3 with sample dilution buffer (0.5 M Tris/HCl, pH 6.8, 0.5 M EDTA, 0.1% SDS, 9 M Urea) and heated at 60 °C for 30 minutes. Fifteen μL of sample was loaded and VWF multimer was separated by electrophoresis at 3 mA for 10 h. The gel was washed with double distilled (dd) H_2O, air-dried and blocked with 5% skimmed milk. VWF multimers were detected by immunoblotting with a rabbit anti-human VWF antibody (Dako).

Screening for mutations

Genomic DNA of the blood cells from the proband was screened by next-generation sequencing. Two mutations c.3814delT deletion and c.8171G>A mutation in *VWF* gene of the proband were discovered, the first-generation sequencing was used to verify the mutations. DNA sequences containing the c.3814delT deletion mutation and c.8171G>A mutation in exon 28 and exon 52 of the *VWF* gene were amplified by polymerase chain reaction (PCR) using the primers of VWF-6059034-F: 5'-GGATAGGTATCCGAACACGGAG-3', VWF-6,059,034-R: 5'- ACAAGAGGGTTGCTTTAGCCAT-3', VWF-6,128,770-F: 5'- CAGCTCTGACGGTCGCTTC-3', and VWF-6,128,770-R: 5'- TCTGTGGGAATATGGA AGTCATTG-3'. The amplified DNA fragments were sequenced directly.

Plasmid construction

The plasmid pSVHVWF containing the full-length wild-type human *VWF* cDNA was kindly provided by Dr. Evan Sadler (Washington University School of Medicine, St Louis, USA). Plasmid of VWF C2724Y was constructed by PCR-based mutagenesis using the pSVHVWF plasmid expressing VWF-WT (wild-type) as a template. The sequence of site-directed mutation primers is 5'- GTGAGG AGCCTGAGTACAACGACATCACTGC-3'. PCR amplification conditions: pre-denaturation at 95℃ for 30 s; denaturation at 98℃ for 10 s, annealing at 65℃ for 30 s, extension at 72℃ for 10 min, repair extension at 72℃ for 15 min after 22 cycles. PCR products were digested at 37℃ by the enzyme of Dpn I for 3 h and transformed into *E. coli* DH5α competent cells by the method of heat shock. Plasmids of VWF WT and VWF C2724Y were purified with the endotoxin-free plasmid extraction kit from Qiagen, and verified by sequencing.

Expression of recombinant VWF protein in HEK-293T cells

HEK-293T cells were cultured in Dulbecco's modified Eagle's medium (DMEM) with high glucose supplemented with 10% fetal bovine serum. Cells were seeded in 6well plate to reach 50-70% confluence at transfection. Transient transfection was performed with a total of 2 μg of WT or C2427Y mutant VWF plasmid, or mixture of WT and C2427Y mutant plasmids using PolyJet™ transfection reagent according to the manufacturer's instructions (SignaGen@ Laboratories). After 48 h, cells and culture supernatant were harvested, and the cells were lysed with a buffer containing 100 mM Tris/HCl, pH 7.5, 1% Triton X-100 and proteinase inhibitor cocktail (Sigma). Cell lysate and culture supernatant was concentrated to 1/10 of the starting volume using an ultrafiltration cassette (Millipore), and analyzed for VWF expression and multimerization.

Results

Diagnosis of a patient family with type 3 VWD

The proband was a 12-year-old girl, suffered frequently from large ecchymosis in bump injury since childhood. She was diagnosed as type 3 VWD for intermittent petechiae and coagulopathy when she was 5 years old. She had a history of admitting to hospital with severe menorrhagia and was treated with transfusion of cryoprecipitated FVIII when she was 11 years old. During the next year, she experienced several times of excessive menstrual bleeding. Neither her parents nor her sister at 20-year-old had a bleeding tendency. The results of laboratory tests showed that the proband had a prolonged activated partial thromboplastin time (APTT, 66.8 s), low plasma VWF Antigen level (VWF:Ag, 2%) and markedly reduced FVIII coagulant activities (FVIII:C, 2%). As shown in Fig. 1, the multimer analysis of plasma VWF showed that the VWF multimer was almost missing in the proband, while VWF from the proband's parents had a normal concentration and multimer distribution. This result explained the abnormal coagulation activity of the plasma from the proband and was consistent with the diagnosis of type 3 VWD.

Identification of candidate VWF gene mutations

To understand the genetic basis underlying the VWD in this family, we isolated genomic DNA from the blood cells of the proband, with which the next-generation genetic sequencing was performed. Sequencing analysis revealed that the proband had a *VWF* allele from her mother with a c.3814delT deletion mutation in exon 28, predicting a frameshift-mutations involving the loss of Cys1272; and the other *VWF* allele from her father had

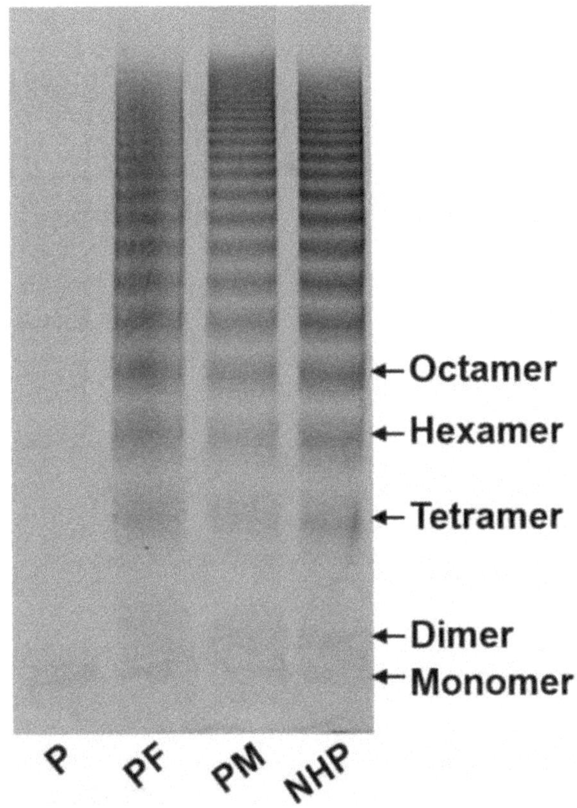

Fig. 1 VWF multimer analysis of plasma from the family with type 3 VWD. Plasma VWF multimers were assessed by 1.5% SDS-agarose gel non-reducing electrophoresis and Western blotting. All plasma samples were diluted 1:5 with sample dilution buffer. NHP, normal human plasma; P, proband; PF, proband's father; PM, proband's mother

a c.8171G>A missense mutation in exon 51, predicting a substitution of cysteine with tyrosine at amino acid 2724. The accuracy of the results of next-generation genetic sequencing was verified by the first-generation sequencing (Fig. 2 A). Cys2724 locates in the CK domain (Fig. 2B).

Expression of recombinant WT and mutant VWF in mammalian cells

To determine the mechanism of C2724Y mutation leading to type 3 VWD, we constructed a C2724Y mutant *VWF* plasmid by PCR-based site-directed mutagenesis. The results of genetic sequencing indicated a successful mutation of Cys2724 in VWF cDNA (Fig. 3 A). To characterize the effect of the C2724Y mutation on VWF synthesis and secretion, HEK-293T cells were transfected with plasmids of VWFWT, VWF-C2724Y, and mixture of VWF-WT and VWF-C2724Y. After 72 h, the transfected cells and culture supernatant was tested for VWF antigen level by reduced SDS-PAGE and western

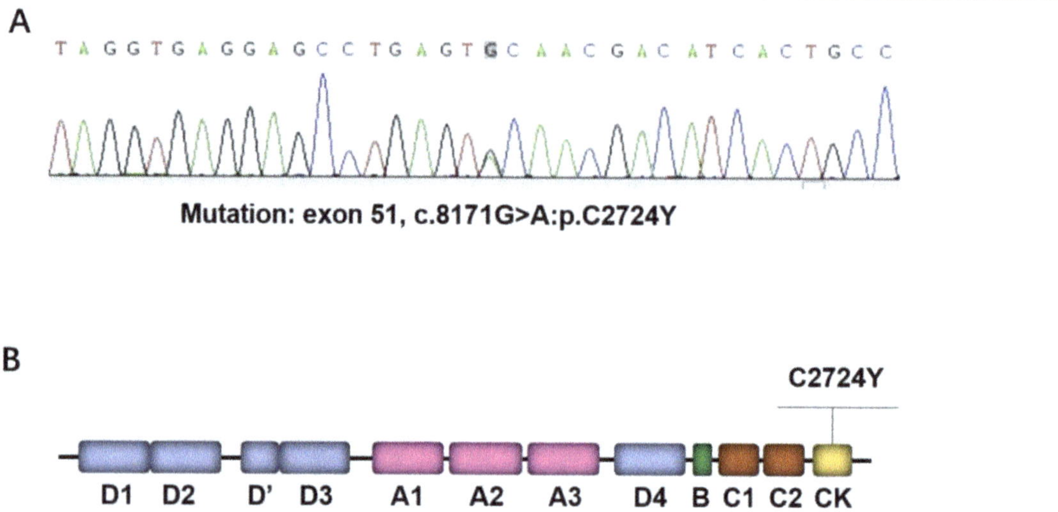

Fig. 2 Identification of candidate VWF gene mutations. **A** Results of first-generation sequencing showed that one *VWF* allele of the proband had a c.8171G>A:p.C2724Y mutation in exon 51. **B** The location of the C2724Y mutation site in the CK domain of VWF molecular

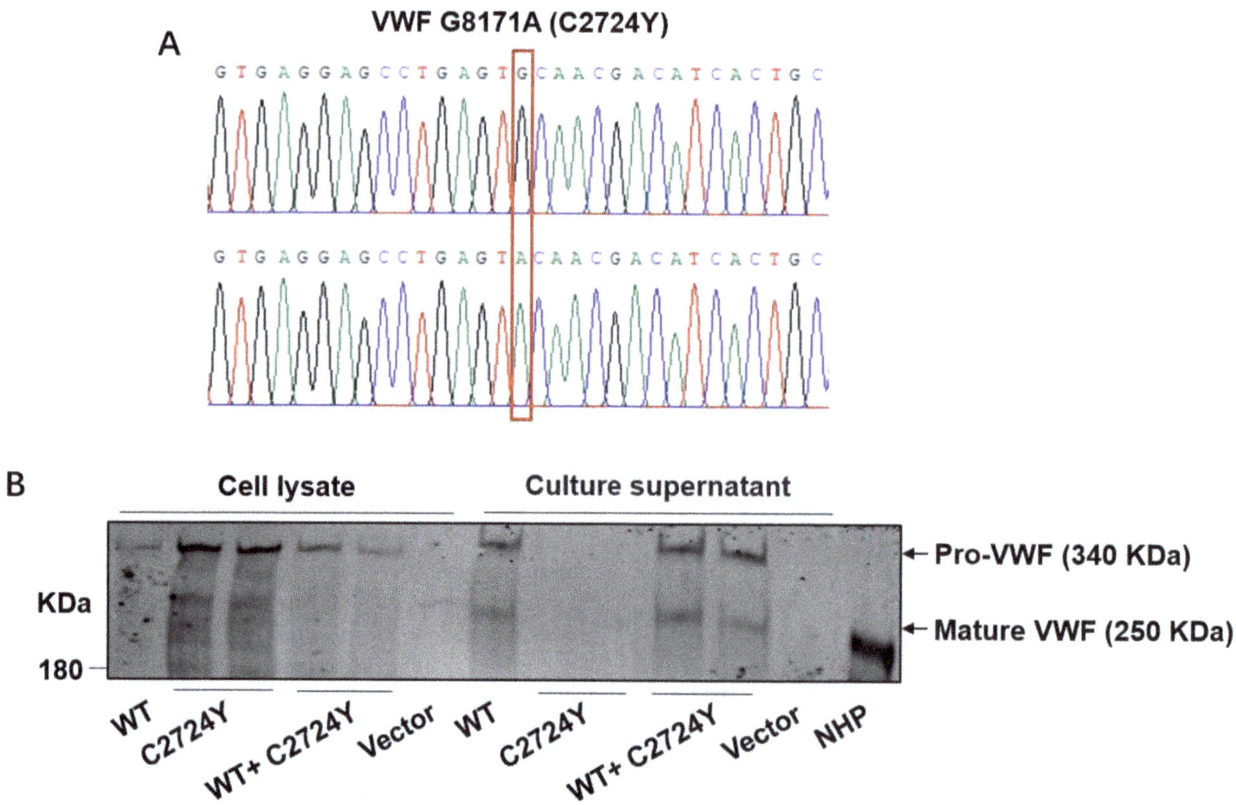

Fig. 3 Expression of recombinant VWF protein in HEK-293T cells. **A** The results of genetic sequencing showed a G >A mutation at position 8171 of VWF. **B** Western blotting analysis of concentrated lysate and supernatant from cultured cells transfected with the plasmids of VWF WT, VWF C2724Y, and mixture of VWF WT and VWF C2724Y. Protein in the lysate and supernatant was separated by 8% reducing SDS-PAGE and immunoblotted with anti-VWF antibody

blotting. As shown in Fig. 3B, recombinant VWF C2724Y protein was expressed normally in HEK-293T cells, but it could not be secreted into cell culture medium, compared with VWF-WT protein. This result, which is consistent with the reduced VWF antigen level in plasma of the proband with the C2724Y mutant, suggests that C2724-C2774 disulfide bond is critical for the VWF secretion.

Multimer analysis of recombinant VWF-C2724Y protein expressed in HEK293T cells

To further determine whether C2724Y mutation affects VWF multimerization, we analyzed the multimer pattern of the lysate and culture supernatant of cells transfected with the plasmid of VWF-WT, VWF-C2724Y, and mixture of VWF-WT and VWFC2724Y. As shown in Fig. 4 A, both recombinant VWF-WT and VWF-C2724Y were expressed in HEK-293T cell, however, dimerized product was observed only with the recombinant VWF-WT, while VWF-C2724Y only had a single band of monomer. In cell culture supernatant, there was no expression of VWF C2724Y, although normal expression and multimer pattern of VWF WT and co-expression of VWF WT and VWF C2724Y were detected (Fig. 4-B), consistent with the immunoblotting in the reduced condition. These results indicated that mutation of C2724Y causes defective VWF dimerization, which further leads to dysfunction of VWF multimerization and secretion.

Discussion

Cys2724 has been reported to form a disulfide bond with Cys2774. In this study, we found a new type 3 VWD family with the proband having almost no VWF antigen and markedly reduced activity of VWF:RCo and FVIII:C (<5%) [12]. The proband experienced several times of severe menorrhagia, had a prolonged APTT, low level of plasma VWF Antigen (2%), and markedly reduced FVIII coagulant activities (2%). The proband had a *VWF* allele with a c.3814delT deletion mutation in exon 28, and the other *VWF* allele with a c.8171G>A missense mutation in exon 51. The latter mutation causes a substitution of cysteine 2724 to tyrosine. These data provide new evidence revealing the critical role of the disulfide bond Cys2724-Cys2774 in VWF biosynthesis.

There are 11 cysteines contained in VWF CK domain, 8 of them form 4 intrachain disulfide bonds, Cys2724-Cys2774, Cys2739-Cys2788, Cys2750-Cys2804, and Cys2754-Cys2806, the other 3 cysteines form 3 interchain disulfide bonds, Cys2771- Cys2773', Cys2771'-Cys2773, and Cys2811-Cys2811'[4]. Mutations of C2739Y[5], C2754W[7, 8], C2804Y[6], and C2806R[9] have also been proven to cause type 3 VWD phenotype, indicating a critical role of disulfide bonds Cys2739-Cys2788, Cys2750-Cys2804, and Cys2754-

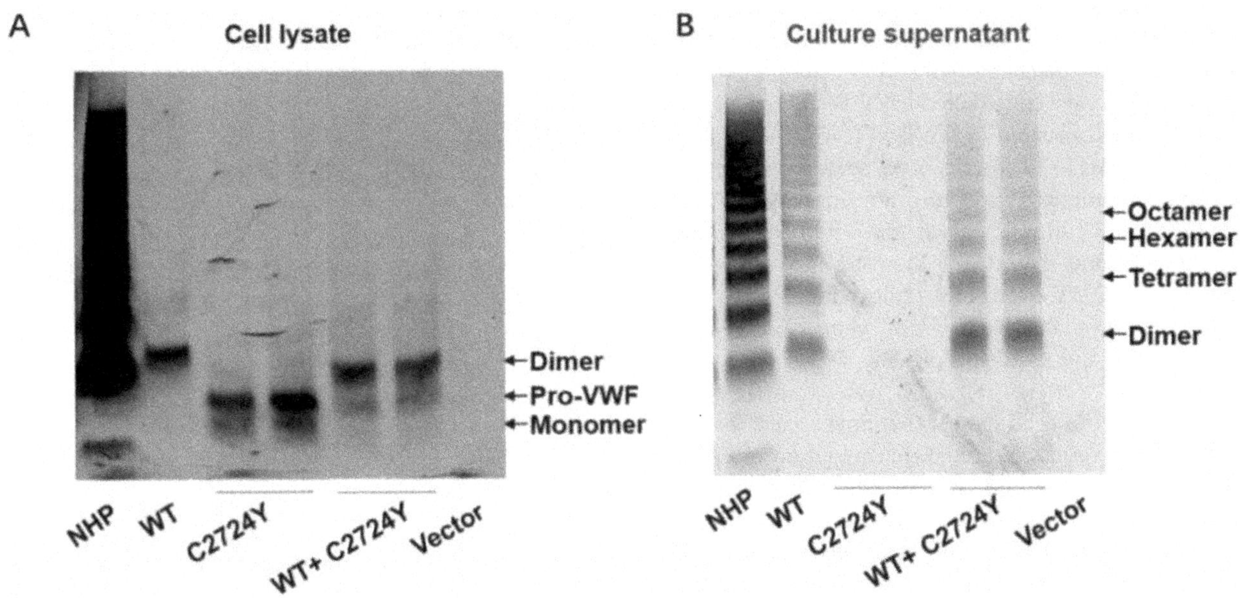

Fig. 4 Multimer analysis of recombinant VWF protein in HEK-293T cells. Multimer analysis of concentrated lysate (**A**) and supernatant (**B**) of cultured cells transfected with the plasmid of vector, VWF WT, VWF C2724Y, and mixture of VWF WT and VWF C2724Y (1:2). Protein in the lysate and culture supernatant was separated by non-reducing electrophoresis on a 1.5% agarose gel and immunoblotted with anti-VWF antibody. NHP, normal human plasma

Table 1 Mutations of disulfide bond in VWF CK domain reported in the literatures

	Disulfide bond	Mutation	Phenotype	Reference
Intrachain	Cys2724-Cys2774	C2724Y	Type 3 VWD	This paper
	Cys2739-Csy2788	C2739Y	Type 3 VWD	[5]
	Cys2750-Csy2804	C2804Y	Type 3 VWD	[6]
	Cys2754-Cys2806	C2754W, C2806R	Type 3 VWD	[7–9]
Interchain	Cys2771-Cys2773′	C2771S/C2771Y, C2773S	Type 2 A/IID VWD	[13–15]
	Cys2771′-Cys2773	C2771S/C2771Y, C2773S	Type 2 A/IID VWD	[13–15]
	Cys2811-Cys2811′	C2811A	Normal VWF multimerization and secretion, but occurrence of odd-numbered multimer	[15–17]

Cys2806 in VWF multimerization and secretion. Compared with the mutations of cysteines forming intrachain disulfide bonds, the mutations of cysteines in interchain disulfide bonds in CK domains did not cause serious phenotypes. Homozygous mutations of C2771S/C2771Y[13] and C2773S[14, 15] did not affect secretion of VWF protein, manifested as type 2 A VWD, subtype IID (VWD 2 A/IID). Mutation of Cys2811 affects neither VWF dimerization nor VWF secretion, but leads to the occurrence of odd-numbered multimer[15–17] (Table 1). These results indicate that the intrachain disulfide bonds in CK domain are much more important than the interchain disulfide bonds in VWF dimerization and secretion. Up to now, mutations of VWF Cys2750, Cys2774, or Cys2788 have not yet been reported.

Cys2724 locates at the N-terminal of VWF CK domain, forms an intrachain disulfide bond with Cys2774[4]. In this study, we provided the evidence showing that the disruption of this Cys2724-CysC2774 caused defective VWF multimerization and secretion in cells, a potential new mechanism underlying the pathogenesis of type 3 VWD. To determine the mechanism of C2724Y mutation leading to type 3 VWD, we constructed a VWF-C2724Y plasmid, then transfected plasmid of VWF-WT, VWF-C2724Y, or together into HEK-293T cells, and analyzed the expression and multimerization of recombinant VWF in transfected cells and cultural supernatant. The results showed that recombinant VWF-C2724Y protein expressed normally in HEK-293T cells, however, it cannot form a dimer or secrete into cell culture medium, while VWF-WT protein expressed and secreted normally, as well had a normal multimer pattern (Fig. 3B). We transfected the plasmids into Hela cells and get the same results (data not shown). These results indicated that mutation of C2724Y causes defective VWF dimerization, which further leads to defective VWF multimerization and secretion, which interprets the reduction of VWF antigen level in plasma from the proband. Based on our new finding of the mutation of C2724Y in new family of type 3 VWD, all of the four intrachain disulfide bonds (Cys2724-Cys2774, Cys2739-Cys2788, Cys2750-Cys2804, and Cys2754-Cys2806) in CK monomer are critical for VWF dimerization and secretion, the disruption of any of these disulfide bonds may lead to the significant reduction of VWF antigen in plasma and development of type 3 VWD.

Although Cys2754, Cys2773, Cys2739, and Cys2724 are cysteines of interchain disulfide bonds in CK domains, and mutations of them disrupt the dimerization of VWF and result in abnormal multimerization, however, there are odd-numbered multimers in plasma from patients with heterozygous C2754W[7, 8]and C2773S[14, 15] mutations, as well as the medium of co-expression of VWF WT and C2754W or C2773S protein, while the plasma from patients with heterozygous C2724Y, and medium of co-expression of VWF WT and C2739Y[18] or C2724Y protein had no odd-numbered multimers. The underlying mechanisms remain further study. As shown in the VWF multimer analysis of cell lysate, VWF with C2739Y mutation cannot form a dimer and exist in the form of pro-VWF(Fig. 4 A), supporting that the dimer formation of pro-VWF through the N-terminus in Golgi apparatus is dependent on the formation of CK-linked dimer in ER[19].

Conclusions

In summary, we have identified a novel missense C2724Y mutation in VWF CK domain in a family of patients with type 3 VWD. This C2724Y mutation caused defective VWF dimerization and secretion, providing the first evidence showing critical role of the disulfide bond Cys2724-Cys2774 in VWF biosynthesis.

Acknowledgements
Not applicable.

Authors' contributions
JZ and YW conceived the project and designed the experiments; YZ, FC, AY and XW performed the experiments and analyzed the data with supervision from JZ and YW; YH and DW assisted with experimental reagents and interpretation of the data; FC, YW and JZ wrote the manuscript. All authors have read and approved the final manuscript.

Author details
[1]Department of Hematology, Key Laboratory of Hematology of Hebei Province, The Second Hospital of Hebei Medical University, 050000

Shijiazhuang, China. [2]National Clinical Research Center for Hematologic Diseases, the First Affiliated Hospital, Collaborative Innovation Center of Hematology, State Key Laboratory of Radiation Medicine and Prevention, Cyrus Tang Medical Institute, Soochow University, 215123 Suzhou, China.

References

1. Lenting PJ, Christophe OD, Denis CV. von Willebrand factor biosynthesis, secretion, and clearance: connecting the far ends. Blood. 2015;125:2019–28.
2. Voorberg J, Fontijn R, van Mourik JA, Pannekoek H. Domains involved in multimer assembly of von willebrand factor (vWF): multimerization is independent of dimerization. EMBO J. 1990;9:797–803.
3. Katsumi A, Tuley EA, Bodo I, Sadler JE. Localization of disulfide bonds in the cystine knot domain of human von Willebrand factor. J Biol Chem. 2000; 275:25585–94.
4. Zhou YF, Springer TA. Highly reinforced structure of a C-terminal dimerization domain in von Willebrand factor. Blood. 2014;123:1785–93.
5. Zhang ZP, Blomback M, Egberg N, Falk G, Anvret M. Characterization of the von Willebrand factor gene (VWF) in von Willebrand disease type III patients from 24 families of Swedish and Finnish origin. Genomics. 1994;21:188–93.
6. Baronciani L, Cozzi G, Canciani MT, Peyvandi F, Srivastava A, Federici AB, Mannucci PM. Molecular characterization of a multiethnic group of 21 patients with type 3 von Willebrand disease. Thromb Haemost. 2000;84: 536–40.
7. Schneppenheim R, Budde U, Obser T, Brassard J, Mainusch K, Ruggeri ZM, Schneppenheim S, Schwaab R, Oldenburg J. Expression and characterization of von Willebrand factor dimerization defects in different types of von Willebrand disease. Blood. 2001;97:2059–66.
8. Tjernberg P, Vos HL, Castaman G, Bertina RM, Eikenboom JC. Dimerization and multimerization defects of von Willebrand factor due to mutated cysteine residues. J Thromb Haemost. 2004;2:257–65.
9. Montgomery RR, Jozwiak MA, Hutter JJ, Endres JL, Foster PA, Friedman KD. A homozygous variant of von Willebrand factor (vWF) that fails to C-terminal dimerize resulting in loss of vWF multimers larger than dimer. Blood. 1999;94:443a–443a.
10. Chen J, Hinckley JD, Haberichter S, Jacobi P, Montgomery R, Flood VH, Wong R, Interlandi G, Chung DW, Lopez JA, Di Paola J. Variable content of von Willebrand factor mutant monomer drives the phenotypic variability in a family with von Willebrand disease. Blood. 2015;126:262–9.
11. Chen J, Hobbs WE, Le J, Lenting PJ, de Groot PG, Lopez JA. The rate of hemolysis in sickle cell disease correlates with the quantity of active von Willebrand factor in the plasma. Blood. 2011;117:3680–3.
12. Branchford BR, Di Paola J. Making a diagnosis of VWD. Hematology Am Soc Hematol Educ Program. 2012;2012:161–7.
13. Enayat MS, Guilliatt AM, Surdhar GK, Jenkins PV, Pasi KJ, Toh CH, Williams MD, Hill FGH. Aberrant dimerization of von Willebrand factor as the result of mutations in the carboxy-terminal region: identification of 3 mutations in members of 3 different families with type 2A (phenotype IID) von Willebrand disease. Blood. 2001;98:674–80.
14. Schneppenheim R, Brassard J, Krey S, Budde U, Kunicki TJ, Holmberg L, Ware J, Ruggeri ZM. Defective dimerization of von Willebrand factor subunits due to a Cys-> Arg mutation in type IID von Willebrand disease. Proc Natl Acad Sci U S A. 1996;93:3581–6.
15. Tjernberg P, Vos HL, Spaargaren-van Riel CC, Luken BM, Voorberg J, Bertina RM, Eikenboom JC. Differential effects of the loss of intrachain- versus interchain-disulfide bonds in the cystine-knot domain of von Willebrand factor on the clinical phenotype of von Willebrand disease. Thromb Haemost. 2006;96:717–24.
16. Lippok S, Kolsek K, Lof A, Eggert D, Vanderlinden W, Muller JP, Konig G, Obser T, Rohrs K, Schneppenheim S, et al. von Willebrand factor is dimerized by protein disulfide isomerase. Blood. 2016;127:1183–91.
17. Lof A, Konig G, Schneppenheim S, Schneppenheim R, Benoit M, Budde U, Muller JP, Brehm MA. Advancing multimer analysis of von Willebrand factor by single-molecule AFM imaging. PLoS One. 2019;14:e0210963.
18. Wang JW, Valentijn KM, de Boer HC, Dirven RJ, van Zonneveld AJ, Koster AJ, Voorberg J, Reitsma PH, Eikenboom J. Intracellular storage and regulated secretion of von Willebrand factor in quantitative von Willebrand disease. J Biol Chem. 2011;286:24180–8.
19. Leebeek FW, Eikenboom JC. Von Willebrand's Disease. N Engl J Med. 2016; 375:2067–80.

25

Low FXIII activity levels in intensive care unit hospitalized COVID-19 patients

Yael Lichter[1], Tanya Badelbayov[2], Irina Shalev[2], Reut Schvartz[3], Yishay Szekely[4], Dan Benisty[2], Ilana Goldiner[5], Maxim Kagarlyk[6], Keren Asraf[6], Ram Doolman[6], Efrat Luttwak[2], Ilya Kirgner[2,7], Irit Avivi[2,7], Nimrod Adi[1,7] and Ben-Zion Katz[2,7*]

Abstract

Background: COVID-19 infection is associated with a hypercoagulable state. Severe COVID-19 patients present with high plasma fibrinogen levels, continuous deposition of fibrin and the presence of microthrombi in their lungs, accompanied by significant fibrinolysis, resulting in high D-dimer levels. Due to the role of FXIII in fibrin crosslinking and clot stabilization, we analyzed its activity levels and dynamics in COVID-19 patients hospitalized in the intensive care unit (ICU).

Methods: FXIII levels were measured in thirty four COVID-19 patients hospitalized in the ICU and in fourteen non-severe COVID-19 patients. FVIII levels were measured for comparison. Laboratory data and clinical variables were recorded.

Results: The average FXIII activity level in 34 ICU hospitalized COVID-19 patients was 69.9±33 %, significantly lower compared to an average of 120±20.9 % FXIII activity in 14 non-severe COVID-19 patients. FXIII activity levels were below the low normal value (< 79 % FXIII activity) in 74 % of the ICU hospitalized COVID-19 patients. In contrast, high FVIII activity was measured among all severe COVID-19 patients. Consecutive measurements, performed in fourteen ICU hospitalized COVID-19 patients, pointed to a significant decrease in FXIII activity from the average of 85.7±28.2 %, (which is in the normal range), to an average of 68.0±20.4 %, below the low normal range, within 6.4±3.4 days of ICU hospitalization. Liver functions did not differentiate between patients with low and normal FXIII activity. No inhibitor to FXIII activity was found in the plasma of severe COVID-19 patients. Levels of FXIII-A antigen correlated with FXIII activity, and were low in severe COVID-19 patients.

Conclusions: Low FXIII activity levels were found in COVID-19 patients hospitalized in the ICU, with gradual decline during their hospitalization. A mechanism of consumption may account for the low FXIII activity in these patients.

Keywords: COVID-19, FXIII, FVIII

Background

In December 2019, a novel Coronavirus, with person-to-person transmission emerged as a human pathogen [1]. Severe acute respiratory syndrome coronavirus-2 (SARS-CoV-2), causes coronavirus disease 2019 (COVID-19), which has a range of manifestations from asymptomatic to critical illness. SARS-CoV-2 affects mostly the respiratory system, causing viral pneumonitis that may lead to severe acute respiratory distress syndrome (ARDS) [2, 3], however, disease course may result in multi-organ involvement, inducing renal dysfunction, myocardial injury, and hemodynamic instability [4–6].

Early observations revealed a hypercoagulable state in COVID-19 patients, accompanied by elevated D-dimer and fibrinogen levels [3, 7, 8]. These findings correlated

* Correspondence: benzik@tlvmc.gov.il
[2]The Hematology Institute, Tel Aviv Sourasky Medical Center, 6 Weizman St, Tel Aviv, Israel
[7]Sackler Faculty of Medicine, Tel Aviv University, Tel Aviv, Israel

with a higher rate of intensive care admissions, as well as mortality [2, 6, 7, 9]. The rate of thrombotic complications appears to be higher amongst COVID-19 patients compared with other critically ill patients. Venous thromboembolic events (VTE) were found in 27 %- 69 % of these severe patients [10, 11]. Of the patients with VTE, deep vein thrombosis (DVT) was reported with an incidence of 23 % [12] (12.7 % in other non COVID-19 ICU patients [13]), and pulmonary embolism (PE) with an unusually high incidence of up to 81 % in some series. [10].

The mechanism underlying COVID-19 coagulopathy has yet to be fully elucidated, in order to obtain better control of this severe manifestation. High levels of FVIII were found in the plasma of COVID-19 patients [14], and vWF levels were higher in the plasma of ICU hospitalized compared with non-severe COVID-19 patients [15]. Reports have linked the hypercoagulable state with a hyperinflammatory state, as it appears that higher fibrinogen level were associated with higher IL-6 and CRP levels [16, 17]. Inflammatory cytokines are established modulators of coagulation and fibrinolysis activation [18]. The concept of immune thrombosis was coined, as cytokines were found to change the normal anticoagulant and profibrinolytic properties of the endothelium to an activated state [19], induce tissue factor (TF) gene expression in endothelial cells and monocytes, fibrinogen synthesis, and platelet production [20]. Autopsy findings indicated diffuse alveolar damage, coupled with microvascular involvement with intra- and extravascular fibrin deposition, and the frequent formation of microthombi in lung arterioles of COVID-19 patients [21]. Lung tissues autopsies of 33/38 (83 %) COVID-19 patients reveled platelet-fibrin thrombi [22]. Hence, fibrin deposition in damaged lung tissues is a prominent pathological aspect of the disease [21–23]. Coagulation factor FXIII plays a central role in the stabilization of the fibrin-based clot, and may also support platelet adhesion at sites of vascular damage [24]. Due to the significant presentations of fibrin deposition and platelets-fibrin microthrombi in the lungs of COVID-19 patients, we studied the levels of FXIII activity in the plasma of 34 severe COVID-19 patients. To the best of our knowledge this is a first report of low levels of FXIII in the plasma of severe COVID-19 patients. Possible mechanisms of FXIII deficiency involvement in COVID-19 morbidity are discussed.

Materials and methods

Patients and clinical assessment

This retrospective study was approved by the Tel Aviv Sourasky Medical Center local IRB. Consecutive COVID-19 patients, hospitalized in the ICU at the Tel Aviv Medical Center between March 10th 2020 and April 26th 2020 (7 patients, first outbreak in Israel), and January 5th to February 4th 2021 (27 patients, second outbreak in Israel) were included in the study. All patients were diagnosed with COVID-19, having a positive reverse-transcriptase–polymerase chain reaction assay for SARS-CoV-2 in a respiratory tract sample either prior to, or at admission. All patients were admitted to the ICU due to respiratory failure requiring ventilatory support (mechanical ventilation or high flow oxygen therapy). Demographic and clinical data of participating patients were obtained from the electronic medical records of each subject; these included: Age, gender, comorbid conditions, medications, laboratory findings, daily score of disease severity, invasive and noninvasive mechanical ventilation status, use of extracorporeal membrane oxygenation (ECMO), administration of hemodynamic support, acute cardiac injury, acute kidney injury, major bleeding events, thrombotic events and COVID-19 -related mortality. During their hospitalization, all patients underwent a comprehensive transthoracic echocardiography within 24 h of admission, being part of the routine baseline clinical assessment in ICU. Patients who then experienced clinical deterioration, determined as the need for intubation and mechanical ventilation, deterioration to severe level of hypoxemia (PaO2/FiO2<100), or new onset of circulatory shock, underwent repeated echocardiographic assessment as well as compression ultrasonography of femoral and popliteal veins of both legs.

Clinical definitions

Severe COVID-19 infection (WHO definition): SatO2< 93 on ambient air, RR>30, PF<300.

PE: Lacking a CTA, a diagnosis of PE was based on the combination of acute deterioration in hypoxemia severity without significant change in respiratory resistance or compliance, and the presence of echocardiographic signs suggestive of acute right ventricular strain due to elevated pulmonary vascular resistance (McConell sign, RV dilatation and dysfunction).

Laboratory assays

3.5 ml of whole blood was collected into vacuum tubes (Greiner, Kremsmunster, Austria) containing 1/10 volume of 3.2 % trisodium citrate. The samples were centrifuged for 8 min at room temperature at 2,500 g, and the plasma was utilized for analysis within two hours. Prothrombin Time assay was performed utilizing Innovin as a recombinant human tissue factor (Dade, Siemens, Marburg, Germany), and measured in seconds. Activated Partial Thrombin Time assay was performed utilizing FSL actin (Dade, Siemens, Marburg, Germany), and measured in seconds. All these assays were performed on either CS2100i or CS5100 instruments (Sysmex, Kobe, Japan). Factor VIII activity was measured by the one-stage clotting assay based on APTT and factor VIII-deficient plasma (Siemens) on a CS2500 instrument (Sysmex). FXIII activity was measured by a FXIII kit (Berichrom, Siemens, Marburg, Germany) on a CS2100i instrument (Sysmex). FXIII-A antigen levels were measured by the commercial automated latex enhanced immunoassay (Werfan, MA, USA) according to the manufacturer's instructions. Total neutrophils, monocytes and platelet counts were measured by Beckman coulter DxH800 CBC analyzers (Brea, CA, USA). All coagulation factor assays and CBC analyzers in the laboratory are subjected to the ECAT or CAP external quality control program, respectively, with excellent scores. The chemistry blood parameters: wide range CRP, alkaline phosphatase (ALP), Alanine Aminotransferase (ALT), Aspartate Aminotransferase (AST), Gamma-glutamyltransferase (GGT), Albumin and total bilirubin (TBIL) were measured by ADVIA system (Siemens Healthcare Diagnostics Inc., Tarrytown, NY 10591-5097 USA).

Statistics

Data collected included demographics, past medical history, clinical characteristics, and anticoagulation administered. Categorical variables are shown as frequencies and percentages, and continuous variables as means and standard deviations, or as medians and ranges in the cases of non-normal distributions of parameters. Student`s T-test was utilized to calculate statistical significance in continuous normal distributed variables, Mann Whitney for scale and continuous non-normal distributed variables and Chi square test for nominal variables, $p<0.05$ was considered significant. SPSS software (IBM SPSS Statistics for Windows, version 25, IBM corp., Armonk, NY, USA, 2017) was used for all statistical analyses.

Results

Patient characteristics

34 patients, diagnosed with respiratory failure caused by COVID-19 infection and admitted to ICU (defined as severe patients), were included in the study. 14 non-severe COVID-19 patients served as controls. All the severe patients presented with COVID19 pneumonia and required respiratory support in the form of mechanical ventilation or HFOT. The median age of our cohort of patients was 57 years (range, 22-76) and 29 % (n=10) were female. None of the patients had a history of respiratory disease, chronic liver disease, inflammatory or immuno-suppressive disease. None of the patients had a prior history of VTE or peripheral vascular disease (Table 1).

Table 1 Characteristics, clinical background and medications of severe COVID-19 patients. HTN, Hypertension; DM, Diabetes Mellitus; IHD, Ischemic Heart Disease; CKD. Chronic Kidney Disease; CVA. Cerebro Vascular Accident; TIA, Transient Ischemic Attack; VTE, Venous Thrombo Embolism; Hx, History; NOAC, Novel Anti-Coagulant; ACEi, Angiotensin II converting enzyme inhibitor; ARB, Angiotensin II Receptor Blocker. None of the differences between the groups of normal or low FXIII was statistically significant. Normal FXIII activity was defined as activity level >79 %. Low FXIII levels were levels were defined as activity level <79 %

FXIII activity	Overall (N=34)	Normal (>79 %) (N=9)	Low (<79 %) (N=25)
Age, median (range)	57 (22-76)	54 (42-67)	59 (22-76)
Female gender	10 (29 %)	2 (22 %)	8 (32 %)
HTN	15 (44 %)	6 (67 %)	9 (36 %)
DM	16 (47 %)	6 (67 %)	10 (40 %)
IHD	4 (12 %)	0	4 (16 %)
CKD	3 (9 %)	1 (11 %)	2 (8 %)
Obesity	17 (50 %)	7 (78 %)	10 (40 %)
Hx of CVA/TIA	0	0	0
Hx of VTE	0	0	0
Hx of Malignancy	1(3 %)	0	1 (4 %)
Acetylsalicylic acid	6 (18 %)	1 (11 %)	5 (20 %)
P2Y12 inhibitors	0	0	0
NOACs	0	0	0
ACEi/ARB	5 (15 %)	1 (11 %)	4 (16 %)

FXIII activity in ICU hospitalized COVID-19 patients

The average FXIII activity level among COVID-19 patients hospitalized in the ICU was 69.9±33 %, median 62.7 %, range 29-180 % with 74 % of the patients (25/34) below the low normal range (79 %) (Fig. 1). The average FVIII activity levels at the same time point were 404.8±95.1 %, median 434 %, range 210-500 % with all patients above the upper normal value (177 %) (Fig. 1). In contrast, in 14 non-severe COVID-19 patients, FXIII activity levels were significantly ($p<0.0005$) higher, with an average of 120.0±20.9 %, median 120 %, range 91-158 %, all within the normal range (Fig. 1). Also, FVIII activity was measured in 5 of these non-severe patients, with an average of 287.8±101.7 %, median 249 %, range 193-450 %, significantly ($p<0.02$) lower compared with the severe COVID-19 patients (Fig. 1). PT values at the time of FXIII measurement were within the normal range (median 11.2; range 10.1-19.8 s; normal range 10.03-12.43 s) in 85 % (29/34) of patients, and the aPTT values at the time of FXIII measurement were also within the normal range (median 28.2; range 20.5-54.3 s; normal range 25-34 s) in 59 % (20/34) of patients (Table 2).

Levels of FXIII activity varied significantly among the severe patients. As shown in Fig. 2 A, FXIII activity tends to decrease with prolongation of hospitalization. Severe patients with FXIII activity below the normal level had a significantly ($p<0.02$) longer hospitalization period (13.8±7.1 days) than severe patients with levels

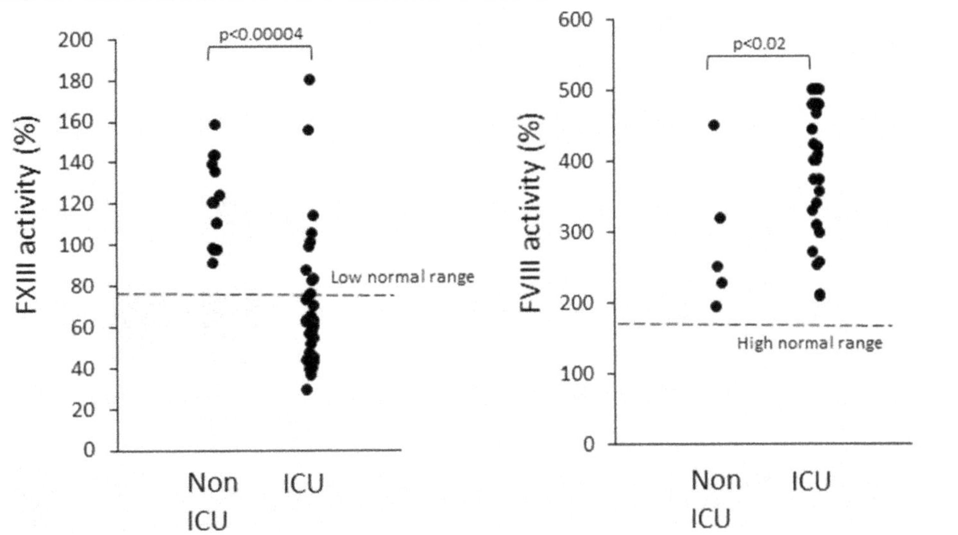

Fig. 1 FXIII activity levels of 34 severe ICU hospitalized and 14 non-severe COVID-19 patients (left), and FVIII activity levels of 34 severe ICU hospitalized and 5 non-severe COVID-19 patients (Right). Data are presented in % of activity for both factors. Dashed lines represent the low normal range of FXIII activity (left), and the high normal range of FVIII activity (right). Significant P values are presented

within the normal range (6.4±4.5 days) (Fig. 2B). Late recovery of FXIII activity levels may occur towards the end of hospitalization, as observed in a single patient at day 34 (Fig. 2 A). Consecutive FXIII activity measurements of 14 ICU hospitalized COVID-19 patients indicated a significant ($p<0.03$) decrease in FXIII activity from an average of 85.7±28.2 % to an average of 68.0±20.4 % within an average of 6.1±3.4 days (Fig. 2 C). No such decrease was observed in FVIII levels (Fig. 2 C).

FXIII activity in four ICU hospitalized COVID-19 patients in a mixing assay with 50 % normal plasma was significantly increased from the average of 46±6.2 % (all below the normal value) to 85.0±4.2 % (all within the normal range) (Fig. 3 A). Analysis of FXIII-A antigen in the plasma correlated well with FXIII activity measurements (Fig. 3B). The average levels of FXIII-A antigen in severe COVID-19 patients were 42±18 %, significantly lower ($p<0.004$) compared with the levels found in non-severe COVID-19 patients (90±18 %, Fig. 3B).

Laboratory parameters

No differences were found in CRP levels and total neutrophil counts (inflammation associated parameters) at

Table 2 Laboratory parameters of ICU hospitalized COVID-19 patients. Low FXIII, activity level <79 %; Normal FXIII, activity level >79 %. Median and ranges are presented. Statistical significance was established by Student`s T test (NS, not significance). PT, prothrombin time; PTT, partial thromboplastin time; Neut, total neutrophils count; CRP, C-reactive protein; ALB, albumin, GGT, gamma-glutamyl transferase; ALP, alkaline phosphatase; ALT, alanine transaminase; AST, aspartate aminotransferase; TBIL, total bilirubin. Normal FXIII activity was defined as activity level >79 %. Low FXIII levels were levels were defined as activity level <79 %

Parameter	Normal range	Overall (*N*=34)	Low FXIII (<79 %) (*N*=25)	Normal FXIII (>79 %) (*N*=9)	Significance
PT (sec)	10.03-12.43	11.2 (10.1-19.8)	11.15 (10.1-19.8)	11.3 (10.3-12.9)	NS
PTT (sec)	25-34	28.2 (20.5-54.3)	27.9 (21.4-54.3)	28.7 (20.5-33.4)	NS
Neut X10^3/µl	1.4-6	8.4 (3.2-27.5)	9.2 (3.2-27.5)	8.3 (5-13.5)	NS
CRP (mg/L)	0.03-5	101.2 (0.3-499.4)	102.33 (1.35-499.4)	81.13 (0.3-293.2)	NS
ALB (mg/dL)	35-50	29.3 (15.2-38.5)	26 (15.2-38.5)	32 (24-34.8)	*P*<0.05
GGT (U/L)	6-42	149.5 (18-1204)	158 (39-1204)	81 (18-567)	NS
ALP (U/L)	46-116	108 (45-412)	111 (49-412)	75 (45-372)	NS
ALT (U/L)	<40	46.5 (45.5-967)	45 (10-967)	46 (14-293)	NS
AST (U/L)	<41	48.5 (16-1344)	46 (18-1344)	57 (16-130)	NS
TBIL (mg/dL)	<1.2	0.36 (0.1-5.24)	0.31 (0.1-5.24)	0.37 (0.24-0.86)	NS

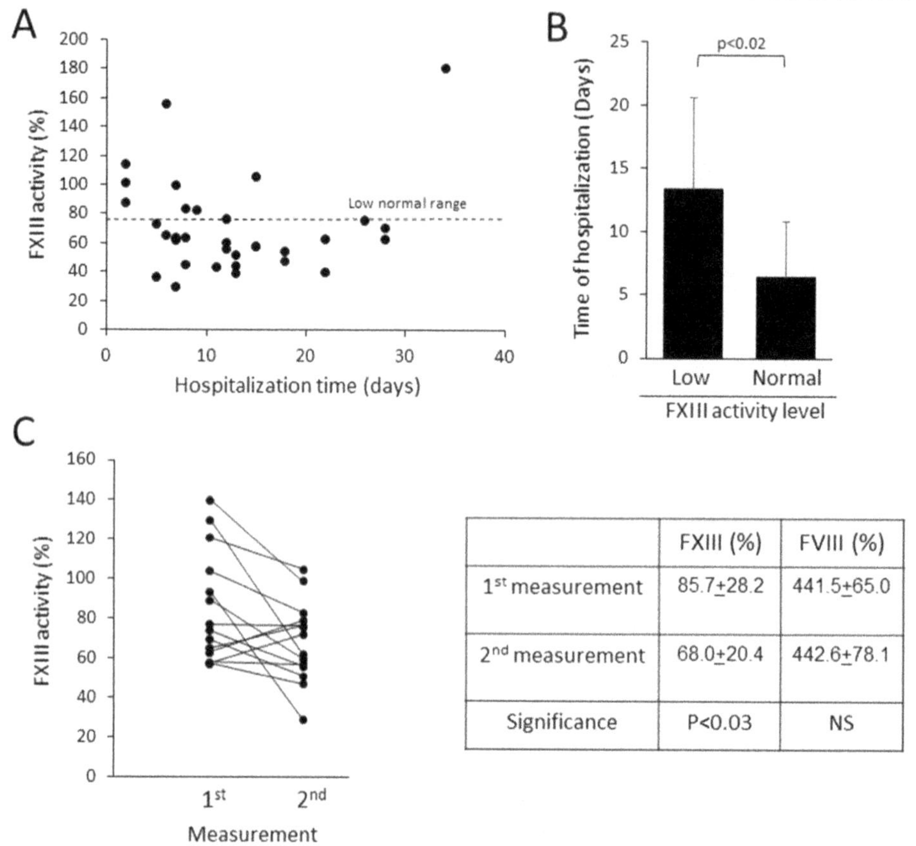

	FXIII (%)	FVIII (%)
1st measurement	85.7±28.2	441.5±65.0
2nd measurement	68.0±20.4	442.6±78.1
Significance	P<0.03	NS

Fig. 2 Dynamics of FXIII activity levels in severe COVID-19 patients. **A** FXIII activity levels as a function of time of hospitalization (in days). Dashed line, the lower threshold of normal FXIII activity range. **B** Duration of hospitalization In relation to FXIII measurement in severe COVID-19 patients with normal or with low FXIII levels (p<0.02). Normal FXIII activity was defined as activity level >79%. Low FXIII levels were levels were defined as activity level <79%. **C** Consecutive measurements of FXIII activity in 14 severe COVID-19 patients. Individual patients dynamics are shown (left), average FXIII and FVIII levels and significance are presented (right). The average interval between the two measurements is 6.1±3.4 days

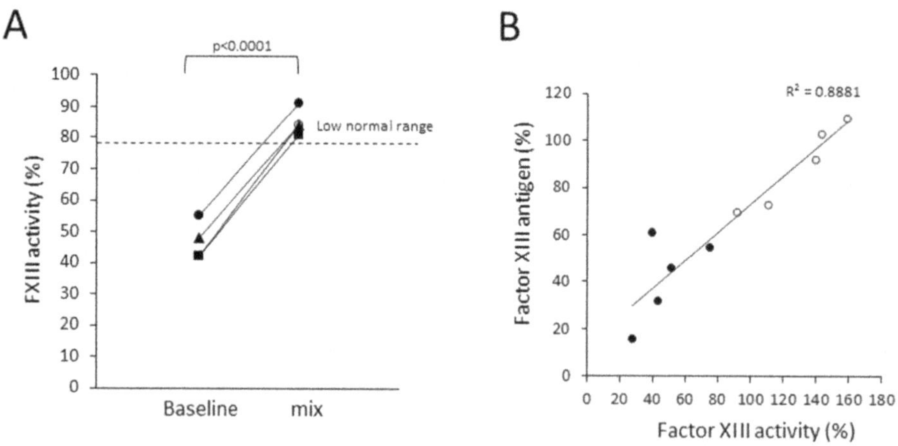

Fig. 3 **A** Mixing FXIII activity assay performed on plasma of four severe COVID-19 patients with low FXIII activity levels show significant increase to normal range values. Baseline and mix (1:1 with normal plasma) results are shown (p<0.0001). Dashed line, the lower threshold of normal FXIII activity range. **B** FXIII-A antigen levels in COVID-19 patients. FXIII-A antigen levels were determined, and correlated with FXIII activity in the same samples. R^2 value of the regression comparison between the antigen and activity levels are indicated. Empty circles, non-severe COVID-19 patients; Full circles, severe ICU-hospitalized COVIED-19 patients

the time of FXIII activity measurement, between the ICU hospitalized COVID-19 patients with normal FXIII activity, compared with patients with low levels of FXIII activity (Table 2). Abnormal liver function parameters were measured in most of our patients at the time of FXIII activity measurement, with no significant difference between the groups, except for reduced albumin levels in the patients with low FXIII activity (Table 2). In the peripheral blood, FXIII-A is predominantly stored in monocytes and platelets. The average absolute monocyte counts in the severe COVID-19 patients were 640± 279.9/μl in the patients with low FXIII levels, and 611.1± 279.9/μl in the patients with normal FXIII levels, within the normal range (0-1300/μl), without a significant difference between the groups. The average platelets concentrations in the severe COVID-19 patients were $218.4 \pm 108.3 \times 10^3/\mu l$ in the patients with low FXIII levels, and $287.2 \pm 101.5 \times 10^3/\mu l$ in the patients with normal FXIII levels, within the normal range ($150-450 \times 10^3/\mu l$), without a significant difference between the groups.

Clinical parameters

In 6/34 (18 %) ventilated patients, ECMO support was employed, of whom four expressed low FXIII activity levels. Bleeding events were recorded in 8/34 patients (24 %), all with low FXIII activity levels (Table 3). DVT events were recorded in 5/34 (15 %) of our patients, and PE events were recorded in 4/34 (12 %) of our patients (Table 3). Mortality rates were overall 13/34 (38 %); 3/9 (33 %) in the group with normal FXIII activity levels, and 10/24 (40 %) in the group with low FXIII activity (Table 3). No clinical variables reached statistical significance among the groups.

Discussion

The high D-dimer levels and possibly systemic procoagulant state of COVID-19 patients prompted the postulation of a novel pulmonary intravascular coagulopathy [25]. This theory is supported by autopsies performed on the lungs of COVID-19 patients, demonstrating small, firm thrombi and fibrin deposition in sections of the peripheral parenchyma in some of the cases [21–23]. As previously shown, aberrant fibrinolysis may occur locally in tissues affected by the disease [26], with no effects on global fibrinolysis. In spite of ongoing consumption, the levels of plasma fibrinogen are above the normal range in most of these patients. This may stem from parallel persistent fibrinogen production, driven by the substantial inflammation typical to severe COVID-19 [27]. Due to the coagulopathy in COVID-19 patients, comprehensive studies mapped various coagulation functions in these patients. For example, a recent study provided a comprehensive outlook of the coagulation system in 206 COVID-19 patients, but the levels of FXIII and its possible role in COVID-19 have not yet been examined [28].

We found low FXIII activity in most of our ICU hospitalized COVID-19 patients, but not in non-severe COVID-19 patients. Extensive serum (not plasma) proteomic analysis of COVID-19 patients pointed to the possibility of decrease in FXIII-B in the sera of COVID-19 patients, in a correlation to increase in IL-6 levels [29].

Table 3 Morbidity of severe COVID-19 patients. DVT, deep vein thrombosis. PE, pulmonary embolism, VTE, venous thromboembolism, NIV, non-invasive ventilation, ECMO, extracorporeal membrane oxygenation, AKI, acute kidney injury, LOS, length of stay, ICU, intensive care unit. The difference between the groups were not significant. Normal FXIII activity was defined as activity level >79 %. Low FXIII levels were levels were defined as activity level <79 %

FXIII activity	Overall (*N*=34)	Normal (>79 %) (*N*=9)	Low (<79 %) (*N*=25)
DVT	5 (15 %)	2 (22 %)	3 (12 %)
PE	4 (12 %)	3 (33 %)	1 (4 %)
Time from diagnosis to VTE (days)	14.5 (4-23)	17 (4-23)	13 (11-17)
Time from admission to VTE (days)	11 (0-24)	16 (12-24)	7 (0-13)
Major Bleed	8 (23.5 %)	0	8 (32 %)
NIV	23 (68 %)	8 (89 %)	15 (60 %)
ECMO	6 (18 %)	2 (22 %)	4 (16 %)
Medical Hemodynamic support	24 (71 %)	6 (67 %)	18 (72 %)
AKI	14 (41 %)	2 (22 %)	12 (48 %)
Mortality during follow up period	13 (38 %)	3 (33 %)	10 (40 %)
Follow up duration (days)	18 (5-45)	13 (5-35)	18 (8-45)
LOS ICU (days)	25 (9-45)	35.5 (35-36)	18 (9-45)

In our study, we did not find a correlation between low FXIII activity and inflammation associated parameters (CRP, total neutrophils count). Three possible mechanisms may account for the low levels of FXIII activity in such patients: (1) Inhibition, (2) Reduced production (mostly due to hepatic failure), 3.Consumption. The first mechanism may stem from inhibitory antibodies against FXIII, as autoantibodies are a common finding in COVID-19 patients [30], and the emergence of autoantibodies is a well-established mechanism in acquired FXIII deficiency [31]. While the targets of such antibodies in COVID-19 are diverse and include components of the immune system, some may be associated with coagulopathy, such as anti-phospholipid autoantibodies [30]. However, this mechanism is not supported by our mixing test that complemented the levels of FXIII activity to a normal level, with no evidence of inhibitors in the plasma of the patients. Hepatic dysfunction has been reported in 14-53 % of COVID-19 patients [32], and since FXIII-B is produced in the liver we examined liver functions in our severe COVID-19 patients. We recorded abnormal liver functions in most of our ICU hospitalized COVID-19 patients, but with no significant difference between patients with low or normal levels of FXIII activity. We found lower albumin levels in patients with low FXIII activity, in agreement with previous studies that demonstrated hypoalbuminemia in severe COVID-19 patients [33]. It was suggested that the mechanism underlying hypoalbuminemia in COVID-19 patients is albumin excretion into damaged organs [33]. Since the major cellular storage of FXIII-A in the circulation is within monocytes and platelets [34], we examined their concentrations in our severe COVID-19 patients, and did not find any significant differences between patients with low or normal FXIII activity levels. Hence, our data indicate that production difficulties may not account for the low FXIII we observed in severe COVID-19 patients, but rather a consumption-based mechanism. This approach is supported by the concomitant reduction in FXIII-A (the catalytic subunit) antigen with the decreased FXIII activity in the severe patients. Consumption accompanies conditions such as inflammation and activation of the coagulation system, both relevant to COVID-19. We show herein that the levels of FXIII activity in the severe COVID-19 patients, are not stable, but rather decline with prolongation of hospitalization, and may be associated with continuous consumption due to the ongoing fibrin deposition in the lungs of these patients.

More data is needed to establish whether low levels of FXIII are involved in mechanisms underlying coagulopathy in severe COVID-19 patients, but previously published experimental data may point to such possibilities; Increased embolism was found in FXIII-/- compared with wild type mice in acute DVT model, apparently due to the effects of FXIII deficiency on clot stability [35]. Moreover, it was shown that FXIII supplementation stabilizes venous thrombi, and reduces embolism [36]. In humans, a weak protective effect of increased FXIII activity against VTE was demonstrated [37]. Moreover, the combination of high D-dimer and low FXIII concentrations was found to be associated with PE, and a threshold of 69 % of FXIII concentration was set to distinguish between confirmed PE and other serious diseases with similar symptoms [38]. In our cohort, the average level of FXIII activity in the severe patients was similar, 69.8 %, combined with high D-dimer levels in most of our patients. Hence, low FXIII levels may alter thrombi properties, resulting in an increased risk for embolism. The predominant manifestation of FXIII deficiency is bleeding [39]. We recorded bleeding events in 8/34 (24 %) of our patients which all occurred in patients with low FXIII activity (10/25, 32 % of these patients). Despite considerable coagulopathy in COVID-19, a high prevalence of bleeding has not been reported in this disease [40]. The overall hypercoagulable state in COVID-19 may overlay bleeding risk factors discussed before [40], or the low levels of FXIII activity presented in this study.

Conclusions

Low FXIII activity levels were found in most of our ICU hospitalized COVID-19 patients. In contrast, the levels in most of non-severe COVID-19 patients examined in this study were within normal ranges. The levels of FXIII activity in the severe COVID-19 patients decline with prolongation of hospitalization. Our data indicate that low production or circulating inhibitors may not account for the low FXIII we observed in severe COVID-19 patients, but rather a consumption-based mechanism. FXIII deficiency may be involved in COVID-19 morbidity.

Abbreviations

ALP: alkaline phosphatase; ALT: alanine aminotransferase; aPTT: activated partial thromboplastin time; AST: aspartate aminotransferase; ARDS: acute respiratory distress syndrome; CBC: complete blood count; COVID-19: coronavirus disease 2019; CRP: C reactive protein; CTA: computed tomography angiography; DVT: deep vein thrombosis; ECMO: extracorporeal membrane oxygenation; FVIII: coagulation factor 8; FXIII: coagulation factor 13; GGT: Gamma-glutamyltransferase; HFOT: high flow oxygen therapy; ICU: intensive care unit; IL-6: interleukin 6; PE: pulmonary embolism; PT: prothrombin time; SARS-CoV-2: Severe acute respiratory syndrome coronavirus-2; TBIL: total bilirubin; TF: tissue factor; VTE: venous thromboembolic events; vWF: von Wilebrand factor

Acknowledgements

NA.

Authors' contributions

YL, KBZ, AN, IA- Contribution to concept and design, analysis and/or interpretation of data; critical writing or revising the intellectual content; final approval of the version to be published. RS, YS, TB, IS, DB, KA, MK, RD, EL, IK-providing clinical or laboratory data and/or interpretation of data.

Author details
[1]The Intensive Care Unit, Tel Aviv Sourasky Medical Center, Tel Aviv, Israel. [2]The Hematology Institute, Tel Aviv Sourasky Medical Center, 6 Weizman St, Tel Aviv, Israel. [3]Division of anesthesiology, Tel Aviv Sourasky Medical Center, Tel Aviv, Israel. [4]The Division of cardiology, Tel Aviv Sourasky Medical Center, Tel Aviv, Israel. [5]The Central Laboratory, Tel Aviv Sourasky Medical Center, Tel Aviv, Israel. [6]The Dworman Automated-Mega Laboratory, Sheba Medical Center, Tel-Hashomer, Ramat-Gan, Israel. [7]Sackler Faculty of Medicine, Tel Aviv University, Tel Aviv, Israel.

References

1. Li Q, Guan X, Wu P, Wang X, Zhou L, Tong Y, et al. Early transmission dynamics in Wuhan, China, of novel coronavirus infected pneumonia. N Engl J Med. 2020;382:1199–207.
2. WHO Coronavirus. disease 2019 (COVID-19) Situation Report – 95. https://www.who.int/docs/default-source/coronaviruse/situation-reports/20200424-sitrep-95-covid-19.pdf?sfvrsn=e8065831_4;.
3. Zhu N, Zhang D, Wang W, Li X, Yang B, Song J, et al. A novel coronavirus from patients with pneumonia in China, 2019. N Engl J Med. 2020;382:727–33.
4. Wang D, Hu B, Hu C, Zhu F, Liu X, Zhang J, et al. Clinical characteristics of 138 hospitalized patients with 2019 novel coronavirus infected pneumonia in Wuhan, China. 323: JAMA; 2020. pp. 1061–9.
5. Chen N, Zhou M, Dong X, Qu J, Gong F, Han Y, et al. Epidemiological and clinical characteristics of 99 cases of 2019 novel coronavirus pneumonia in Wuhan, China: a descriptive study. The Lancet. 2020;395:507–13.
6. Richardson S, Hirsch JS, Narasimhan M, Crawford JM, McGinn T, Davidson KW, et al. Presenting characteristics, comorbidities, and outcomes among 5700 patients hospitalized with COVID-19 in the New York City area. 323: JAMA; 2020. pp. 2052–9.
7. Arentz M, Yim E, Klaff L, Lokhandwala S, Riedo FX, Chong M, et al. Characteristics and outcomes of 21 critically ill patients with COVID-19 in Washington State. 323: JAMA; 2020. pp. 1612–4.
8. Zhou F, Yu T, Du R, Fan G, Liu Y, Liu Z, et al. Clinical course and risk factors for mortality of adult inpatients with COVID-19 in Wuhan, China: a retrospective cohort study. The Lancet. 2020;395:1054–62.
9. Han H, Yang L, Liu R, Liu F, Wu KL, Li J, et al. Prominent changes in blood coagulation of patients with SARS-CoV-2 infection. Clin Chem Lab Med; 2020;58:1116–20.
10. Klok FA, Kruip MJHA, van der Meer NJM, Arbous MS, Gommers DAMPJ, Kant KM, et al. Incidence of thrombotic complications in critically ill ICU patients with COVID-19. Thromb Res;2020;191:145–7.
11. Llitjos JF, Leclerc M, Chochois C, Monsallier JM, Ramakers M, Auvray M, Merouani K. High incidence of venous thromboembolic events in anticoagulated severe COVID-19 patients. J Thromb Haemost;2020;18:1743–6.
12. Spiezia L, Boscolo A, Poletto F, Cerruti L, Tiberio I, Campello E, et al. COVID-19-Related Severe Hypercoagulability in Patients Admitted to Intensive Care Unit for Acute Respiratory Failure. Thromb Haemost;2020; 120:998–1000.
13. Malato A, Dentali F, Siragusa S, Fabbiano F, Kagoma Y, Boddi M, et al. The impact of deep vein thrombosis in critically ill patients: a meta-analysis of major clinical outcomes. Blood transfusion. 2015;10:559–68.
14. Panigada M, Bottino N, Tagliabue P, Grasselli G, Novembrino C, Chantarangkul V, et al. Hypercoagulability of COVID-19 patients in Intensive Care Unit. A Report of Thromboelastography Findings and other Parameters of Hemostasis. J Thromb Haemost;2020;18:1738–42.
15. Goshua G, Pine AB, Meizlish ML, Chang CH, Zhang H, Bahel P, et al. Endotheliopathy in COVID-19-associated coagulopathy: evidence from a single-centre, cross-sectional study. Lancet Haematol. 2020;7:e575-82.
16. Ranucci M, Ballotta A, Di Dedda U, Bayshnikova E, Dei Poli M, Resta M, et al. The procoagulant pattern of patients with COVID-19 acute respiratory distress syndrome. J Thromb Haemost. 2020;18:1747–51.
17. Wu C, Chen X, Cai Y, Xia J, Zhou X, Xu S, et al. Risk Factors Associated With Acute Respiratory Distress Syndrome and Death in Patients With Coronavirus Disease 2019 Pneumonia in Wuhan, China. JAMA Intern Med. 2020;180:934–43.
18. Vazquez-Garza E, Jerjes-Sanchez C, Navarrete A, Joya-Harrison J, Rodriguez D. Venous thromboembolism: thrombosis, inflammation, and immunothrombosis for clinicians. J Thromb Thrombolysis. 2017;44:377–85.
19. Libby P, Crea F. Clinical implications of inflammation for cardiovascular primary prevention. Eur Heart J. 2010;31:777–83.
20. Kerr R, Stirling D, Ludlam CA. Interleukin 6 and haemostasis. Br J Haematol; 2001;;115:3-12.
21. Buja LM, Wolf DA, Zhao B, Akkanti B, McDonald M, Lelenwa L, et al. The emerging spectrum of cardiopulmonary pathology of the coronavirus disease 2019 (COVID-19): Report of 3 autopsies from Houston, Texas, and review of autopsy findings from other United States cities. Cardiovasc Pathol. 2020;48:107233.
22. Carsana L, Sonzogni A, Nasr A, Rossi RS, Pellegrinelli A, Zerbi P, et al. Pulmonary post-mortem findings in a series of COVID-19 cases from northern Italy: a two-centre descriptive study. Lancet Infect Dis. 2020;20: 1135–40.
23. Fox SE, Akmatbekov A, Harbert JL, Li G, Quincy Brown J, Vander Heide RS. Pulmonary and cardiac pathology in African American patients with COVID-19: an autopsy series from New Orleans. Lancet Respir Med. 2020;8:681–6.
24. Magwenzi SG, Ajjan RA, Standeven KF, Parapia LA, Naseem KM. Factor XIII supports platelet activation and enhances thrombus formation by matrix proteins under flow conditions. J Thromb Haemost;201;9:820–33.
25. Fogarty H, Townsend L, Ni Cheallaigh C, Bergin C, Martin-Loeches I, Browne P, et al. COVID-19 Coagulopathy in Caucasian patients. Br J Haematol;2020; 189:1044–9.
26. Whyte CS, Morrow GB, Mitchell JL, Chowdary P, Mutch NJ. Fibrinolytic abnormalities in acute respiratory distress syndrome (ARDS) and versatility of thrombolytic drugs to treat COVID-19. J Thromb Haemost;2020;18:1548–55.
27. Felsenstein S, Herbert JA, McNamara PS, Hedrich CM. COVID-19: Immunology and treatment options. Clin Immunol;2020;215:108448.
28. Martín-Rojas RM, Pérez-Rus G, Delgado-Pinos VE, Domingo-González A, Regalado-Artamendi I, Alba-Urdiales N, et al. COVID-19 coagulopathy: An in-depth analysis of the coagulation system. Eur J Haematol. 2020;105:741–50.
29. D'Alessandro A, Thomas T, Dzieciatkowska M, Hill RC, Francis RO, Hudson KE, et al. Serum Proteomics in COVID-19 Patients: Altered Coagulation and Complement Status as a Function of IL-6 Level. J Proteome Res. 2020;19:4417–27.
30. Khamsi R. Rogue antibodies could be driving severe COVID-19. Nature;2021; 590:29-31.
31. Ichinose A, Japanese Collaborative Research Group on AH13. Autoimmune acquired factor XIII deficiency due to anti-factor XIII/13 antibodies: A summary of 93 patients. Blood Rev. 2017;31:37–45.
32. Jothimani D, Venugopal R, Abedin MF, Kaliamoorthy I, Rela M. COVID-19 and the liver. J Hepatol. 2020;73:1231–40.
33. Hariyanto TI, Japar KV, Kwenandar F, Damay V, Siregar JI, Lugito NPH, et al. Inflammatory and hematologic markers as predictors of severe outcomes in COVID-19 infection: A systematic review and meta-analysis. Am J Emerg Med. 2021;41:110–9.
34. Poon MC, Russell JA, Low S, Sinclair GD, Jones AR, Blahey W, et al. Hemopoietic origin of factor XIII A subunits in platelets, monocytes, and plasma. Evidence from bone marrow transplantation studies. J Clin Invest. 1989;84:787–92.
35. Shaya SA, Saldanha LJ, Vaezzadeh N, Zhou J, Ni R, Gross PL. Comparison of the effect of dabigatran and dalteparin on thrombus stability in a murine model of venous thromboembolism. J Thromb Haemost;2016;14:143–52.
36. Shaya SA, Gani DM, Weitz JI, Kim PY, Gross PL. Factor XIII Prevents Pulmonary Emboli in Mice by Stabilizing Deep Vein Thrombi. Thromb Haemost;2019;119:992–9.
37. Van Hylckama Vlieg A, Komanasin N, Ariëns RA, Poort SR, Grant PJ, Bertina RM, Rosendaal FR. Factor XIII Val34Leu polymorphism, factor XIII antigen levels and activity and the risk of deep venous thrombosis. Br J Haematol; 2002;119:169–75.
38. Tang N, Sun Z, Li D, Yang J, Yin S, Guan Q. Combined measurement of factor XIII and D-dimer is helpful for differential diagnosis in patients with suspected pulmonary embolism. Clin Chem Lab Med;2017;55:1948–53.
39. Muszbek L, Katona É. Diagnosis and Management of Congenital and Acquired FXIII Deficiencies. Semin Thromb Hemost. 2016;42:429–39.
40. Connors JM, Levy JH. COVID-19 and its implications for thrombosis and anticoagulation. 135: Blood; 2020. pp. 2033–40.

Permissions

All chapters in this book were first published by BioMed Central; hereby published with permission under the Creative Commons Attribution License or equivalent. Every chapter published in this book has been scrutinized by our experts. Their significance has been extensively debated. The topics covered herein carry significant findings which will fuel the growth of the discipline. They may even be implemented as practical applications or may be referred to as a beginning point for another development.

The contributors of this book come from diverse backgrounds, making this book a truly international effort. This book will bring forth new frontiers with its revolutionizing research information and detailed analysis of the nascent developments around the world.

We would like to thank all the contributing authors for lending their expertise to make the book truly unique. They have played a crucial role in the development of this book. Without their invaluable contributions this book wouldn't have been possible. They have made vital efforts to compile up to date information on the varied aspects of this subject to make this book a valuable addition to the collection of many professionals and students.

This book was conceptualized with the vision of imparting up-to-date information and advanced data in this field. To ensure the same, a matchless editorial board was set up. Every individual on the board went through rigorous rounds of assessment to prove their worth. After which they invested a large part of their time researching and compiling the most relevant data for our readers.

The editorial board has been involved in producing this book since its inception. They have spent rigorous hours researching and exploring the diverse topics which have resulted in the successful publishing of this book. They have passed on their knowledge of decades through this book. To expedite this challenging task, the publisher supported the team at every step. A small team of assistant editors was also appointed to further simplify the editing procedure and attain best results for the readers.

Apart from the editorial board, the designing team has also invested a significant amount of their time in understanding the subject and creating the most relevant covers. They scrutinized every image to scout for the most suitable representation of the subject and create an appropriate cover for the book.

The publishing team has been an ardent support to the editorial, designing and production team. Their endless efforts to recruit the best for this project, has resulted in the accomplishment of this book. They are a veteran in the field of academics and their pool of knowledge is as vast as their experience in printing. Their expertise and guidance has proved useful at every step. Their uncompromising quality standards have made this book an exceptional effort. Their encouragement from time to time has been an inspiration for everyone.

The publisher and the editorial board hope that this book will prove to be a valuable piece of knowledge for researchers, students, practitioners and scholars across the globe.

List of Contributors

Norah S. Alsubaie, Shahad M. Al Rammah, Reema A. Alshouimi, Mohammed Y. Alzahrani and Majed S. Al Yami
Department of Pharmacy Practice, College of Pharmacy, King Saud bin Abdulaziz University for Health Sciences, Riyadh, Saudi Arabia

Abdulaali R. Almutairi
Saudi Food and Drug Authority, Riyadh, Saudi Arabia

Osamah M. Alfayez
Department of Pharmacy Practice, College of Pharmacy, Qassim University, Qassim, Buraydah, Saudi Arabia

Ghazwa B. Korayem
Department of Pharmacy Practice, College of Pharmacy, Princess Nourah bint Abdulrahman University, Riyadh, Saudi Arabia

Omar A. Almohammed
Department of Clinical Pharmacy, College of Pharmacy, King Saud University, Riyadh 11451, Saudi Arabia

Hiroyuki Fukase
Clinical Research Hospital, Tokyo, Japan

Gregory Calligaro
Division of Pulmonology, Department of Medicine, University of Cape Town, Groote Schuur Hospital, Cape Town, South Africa

Jessica J. S. Opie
Division of Haematology, Department of Pathology, University of Cape Town & National Health Laboratory Service, Groote Schuur Hospital, Cape Town, South Africa

Noppacharn Uaprasert, Krissana Panrong, Ponlapat Rojnuckarin and Thita Chiasakul
Division of Hematology, Department of Medicine, Faculty of Medicine, Chulalongkorn University and King Chulalongkorn Memorial Hospital, Thai Red Cross Society, Bangkok, Thailand
Research Unit in Translational Hematology, Faculty of Medicine, Chulalongkorn University and King Chulalongkorn Memorial Hospital, Thai Red Cross Society, Bangkok, Thailand

Yuu Oda and Ikuro Maruyama
Department of Systems Biology in Thromboregulation, Kagoshima University Graduate School of Medical and Dental Sciences, Kagoshima, Japan

Takashi Ito
Department of Systems Biology in Thromboregulation, Kagoshima University Graduate School of Medical and Dental Sciences, Kagoshima, Japan
Department of Biomedical Laboratory Sciences, Faculty of Life Sciences, Kumamoto University, 4-24-1 Kuhonji, Kumamoto 862-0976, Japan

Yoichiro Yamada
PPD-SNBL K.K., Kagoshima, Japan

Tadashi Koga
Clinical Study Support, Inc., Nagoya, Japan

Tomoka Nagasato, Tomoko Ohnishi-Wada and Kazuya Hosokawa
Research Institute, Fujimori Kogyo Co, Ltd., Yokohama, Japan

Colette Neethling and Malcolm Miller
Department of Anaesthesia & Perioperative Medicine, University of Cape Town, Groote Schuur Hospital, Anzio Drive, Observatory, Cape Town 7925, South Africa

Teruto Hashiguchi
Department of Laboratory and Vascular Medicine, Kagoshima University Graduate School of Medical and Dental Sciences, Kagoshima, Japan

Maofeng Gong, Xu He, Boxiang Zhao, Jie Kong, Jianping Gu and Guoping Chen
Department of Interventional and Vascular Radiology, Nanjing First Hospital, Nanjing Medical University, Jiangsu 210006 Nanjing, People's Republic of China

Tanapong Panpikoon, Wisanu Phattharaprueksa, Tharintorn Treesit, Chinnarat Bua-ngam, Kaewpitcha Pichitpichatkul and Apichaya Sriprachyakul
Department of Diagnostic and Therapeutic Radiology, Faculty of Medicine Ramathibodi Hospital, Mahidol University, 270 Rama VI Rd. Phyathai, Ratchathewi, 10400 Bangkok, Thailand

Flavio Giuseppe Biccirè
Department of Clinical Internal, Anesthesiological, and Cardiovascular Sciences, Sapienza University of Rome, Viale del Policlinico 155, 00161 Rome, Italy
Department of General and Specialized Surgery "Paride Stefanini", Sapienza University of Rome, Viale del Policlinico 155, 00161 Rome, Italy

Carlo Gaudio, Pasquale Pignatelli, Gaetano Tanzilli and Daniele Pastori
Department of Clinical Internal, Anesthesiological, and Cardiovascular Sciences, Sapienza University of Rome, Viale del Policlinico 155, 00161 Rome, Italy

Alessio Farcomeni
Department of Economics and Finance, University of Rome "Tor Vergata", Via Columbia 2, 00133 Rome, Italy

M. Müller-Knapp
Department of Pediatrics, Interdisciplinary Pediatric Intensive Care Medicine, University Medical Center Rostock, Rostock, Germany

C. F. Classen
Department of Pediatrics, Oncology and Hematology Unit, University Medical Center Rostock, Rostock, Germany

R. Knöfler
Department of Pediatrics, Division of Pediatric Hemostaseology, University Hospital Carl Gustav Carus, Technical University Dresden, Dresden, Germany

C. Spang and J. Ehler
Department of Pediatrics, Interdisciplinary Pediatric Intensive Care Medicine, University Medical Center Rostock, Rostock, Germany
Department of Anesthesiology and Intensive Care Medicine, Interdisciplinary Pediatric Intensive Care Medicine, University Medical Center Rostock, Rostock, Germany

D. A. Reuter
Department of Anesthesiology and Intensive Care Medicine, Interdisciplinary Pediatric Intensive Care Medicine, University Medical Center Rostock, Rostock, Germany

C. Hauenstein
Institute of Diagnostic and Interventional Radiology, Paediatric Radiology and Neuroradiology, University Medical Center Rostock, Rostock, Germany

T. Heinrich
MVZ für Humangenetik und Molekularpathologie GmbH, Rostock, Germany

F. L. P. Gabriel
Institute for Clinical Chemistry and Laboratory Medicine, University Medical Center Rostock, Rostock, Germany

J. Däbritz
Department of Pediatrics, University Medical Center Rostock, Rostock, Germany

Nancy Glober, Lauren Stewart and JangDong Seo
Indiana University, Indianapolis, Indiana, United States

Carlos Camargo and Christopher Kabrhel
Harvard Medical School, Boston, Massachusetts, United States

Kristen Nordenholz
University of Colorado Anschutz Medical Campus, Colorado, Aurora, United States

Jeffrey Kline
Department of Emergency Medicine, Wayne State University School of Medicine, 4201 St. Antoine, 48201 Detroit, Michigan, United States

Pall T. Onundarson
Central Laboratory/Hematology, Landspitali National University Hospital of Iceland and University of Iceland Faculty of Medicine, Hringbraut, 101 Reykjavik, Reykjavik, Iceland

Ragnar Palsson
Nephrology Division, Department of Medicine, Massachusetts General Hospital, Boston, MA, USA

Daniel M. Witt
Department of Pharmacotherapy, University of Utah College of Pharmacy, Salt Lake City, UT, USA

Brynja R. Gudmundsdottir
Central Laboratory/Hematology, Landspitali National University Hospital of Iceland, Reykjavik, Iceland

Chiao-Chin Lee, Chiao-Hsiang Chang, Yuan Hung, Chin-Sheng Lin, Shih-Ping Yang, Shu-Meng Cheng, Fan-Han Yu and Wei-Shiang Lin
Division of Cardiology, Department of Medicine, Tri-Service General Hospital, National Defense Medical Center, Taipei, Taiwan

Wen-Yu Lin
Division of Cardiology, Department of Medicine, Tri-Service General Hospital, National Defense Medical Center, Taipei, Taiwan
Division of Cardiology, Department of Internal Medicine Tri-Service General Hospital, National Defense Medical Center, No. 325, Cheng-Gong Road, Section 2, Neihu 114, Taipei, Taiwan

Jie Ge, Peipei Zhou, Yifei Yang, Tianshu Xu and Xu Yang
Department of stomatology, Changzhou First People's Hospital, Juqian Street, Changzhou 185, Jiangsu, China

Mariana Fragão-Marques and Adelino Leite-Moreira
Cardiovascular Research and Development Center, Faculty of Medicine of the University of Porto, 4200 Porto, Portugal
São João University Hospital Center, Porto, Portugal
Faculty of Medicine of the University of Porto, Porto, Portugal

Francisco Teixeira
Faculty of Medicine of the University of Porto, Porto, Portugal

Jennifer Mancio and Inês Falcão-Pires
Cardiovascular Research and Development Center, Faculty of Medicine of the University of Porto, 4200 Porto, Portugal
Faculty of Medicine of the University of Porto, Porto, Portugal

João Rocha-Neves
São João University Hospital Center, Porto, Portugal
Faculty of Medicine of the University of Porto, Porto, Portugal

Nair Seixas
Vila Nova de Gaia Hospital Center, Vila Nova de Gaia, Portugal

Guina Liu and Sirui Zhang
West China School of Medicine, Sichuan University, 610041 Chengdu, China

Yupei Li
Department of Nephrology, Med+ Biomaterial Institute, West China Hospital, Sichuan University, 610041 Chengdu, China
Institute for Disaster Management and Reconstruction, Sichuan University, 610207 Chengdu, China

Baihai Su
West China School of Medicine, Sichuan University, 610041 Chengdu, China
Department of Nephrology, Med+ Biomaterial Institute, West China Hospital, Sichuan University, 610041 Chengdu, China
Institute for Disaster Management and Reconstruction, Sichuan University, 610207 Chengdu, China
The first People's Hospital of Shuangliu District, 610200 Chengdu, China
Med-X Center for Materials, Sichuan University, 610041 Chengdu, China

Ping-Yen Liu
Institute of Clinical Medicine, College of Medicine, National Cheng Kung University, Tainan, Taiwan

Wei-Chieh Lee
Institute of Clinical Medicine, College of Medicine, National Cheng Kung University, Tainan, Taiwan
Division of Cardiology, Department of Internal Medicine, Kaohsiung Chang Gung Memorial Hospital, Chang Gung University College of Medicine, 123 Ta Pei Road, Niao Sung District, Kaohsiung City 83301, Taiwan

Po-Jui Wu, Yen-Nan Fang, Huang-Chung Chen, Hsiu-Yu Fang and Mien-Cheng Chen
Division of Cardiology, Department of Internal Medicine, Kaohsiung Chang Gung Memorial Hospital, Chang Gung University College of Medicine, 123 Ta Pei Road, Niao Sung District, Kaohsiung City 83301, Taiwan

Pai-Wei Lee and Shang-Hung Chang
Center for Big Data Analytics and Statistics, Chang-Gung University and Hospital, Taipei, Taiwan

Yu-Sheng Lin
Division of Cardiology, Chang Gung Memorial Hospital, Chiayi, Taiwan

Jing Wang
Departments of Cardiology, the First Affiliated Hospital of Nanjing Medical University, 300 Guangzhou Road, Nanjing 210029, Jiangsu, China
Department of Cardiology, the Affiliated Huaian No.1 People's Hospital of Nanjing Medical University, Huai'an, Jiangsu, China

Zhou Dong, Jiazheng Ma, Jianzhen Teng, Qian Gu, Zekang Ye, Inam Ullah, Chuchu Tan, Samee Abdus, Lu Shi, Xiaoxuan Gong and Chunjian Li
Departments of Cardiology, the First Affiliated Hospital of Nanjing Medical University, 300 Guangzhou Road, Nanjing 210029, Jiangsu, China

Tong Wang
Departments of Cardiology, the First Affiliated Hospital of Nanjing Medical University, 300 Guangzhou Road, Nanjing 210029, Jiangsu, China
Department of Cardiology, the First People's Hospital of Yancheng, Yancheng, Jiangsu, China

Xiaofeng Zhang
Departments of Cardiology, the First Affiliated Hospital of Nanjing Medical University, 300 Guangzhou Road, Nanjing 210029, Jiangsu, China
Department of Cardiology, the Second Hospital of Nanjing, Nanjing University of Chinese Medicine, Nanjing, Jiangsu, China

Yang Zhang, Rui Peng, Xiaojuan Li, Gaowa Cheng, Ximing Wang, Jinxing Yu, Xi Chen and Zhou Zhou
Diagnostic Laboratory Service, State Key Laboratory of Cardiovascular Disease, Fuwai Hospital, National Center for Cardiovascular Diseases, Chinese Academy of Medical Sciences, Peking Union Medical College, No.167, Beilishi Road, Xicheng District, Beijing 100037, China

Muxing Hua
Department of Laboratory Medicine, Yunnan Fuwai Cardiovascular Hospital, Kunming 650000, China

Makoto Shoji, Taiju Matsui, Hideaki Tanaka, Kosuke Nomura, Hiroaki Tsujita, Yusuke Kodama, Shinji Koba, Youichi Kobayashi and Toshiro Shinke
Department of Medicine, Division of Cardiology, Showa University School of Medicine, 1-5-8 Hatanodai, Shinagawa-ku, Tokyo 142-8666, Japan

Liqin Ling, Xunbei Huang, Chaonan Liu, Juan Liao and Jing Zhou
Department of Laboratory Medicine, West China Hospital, Sichuan University, No. 37 Guo Xue Alley, Sichuan 610041 Chengdu, China

Jia Peng, Ming-Ming Liu, Hui-Hui Liu, Yuan-Lin Guo, Na-Qiong Wu, Qian Dong, Jie Qian, Ke-Fei Dou, Cheng-Gang Zhu and Jian-Jun Li
Cardiometabolic Medicine Center, State Key Laboratory of Cardiovascular Disease, Fu Wai Hospital, National Center for Cardiovascular Diseases, Chinese Academy of Medical Sciences and Peking Union Medical College, No 167 BeiLiShi Road, XiCheng District, Beijing 100037, China

Zhao, Ying Wang, Runzhen Chen, Jiannan Li, Jinying Zhou, Chen Liu, Peng Zhou, Zhaoxue Sheng, Yi Chen, Li Song and Hanjun Zhao
Department of Cardiology, Fuwai Hospital, National Center for Cardiovascular Diseases, Peking Union Medical College & Chinese Academy of Medical Sciences, No.167, Beijing 100037, China

Hongbing Yan
Fuwai Hospital, Chinese Academy of Medical Sciences, 12 Langshan Rd, Shenzhen 518000, China

Vanda Pinto, Mickael Henriques, João Rato and Emanuel Silva
Vascular Surgery Department, Heart and Vessels Division, Hospital Santa Maria (CHULN), Av. Prof. Egas Moniz s/n, 1649-035 Lisbon, Portugal
Lisbon Academic Medical Center, Lisbon, Portugal

Augusto Ministro and Luís Mendes Pedro
Vascular Surgery Department, Heart and Vessels Division, Hospital Santa Maria (CHULN), Av. Prof. Egas Moniz s/n, 1649-035 Lisbon, Portugal
Lisbon Academic Medical Center, Lisbon, Portugal
Faculty of Medicine, University of Lisbon, Lisbon, Portugal

Nuno Reis Carreira, Ana Cardoso and Catarina Sousa Gonçalves
Department of Internal Medicine (Medicina 2), Hospital Santa Maria (CHULN), Lisbon, Portugal

Sufana Shikdar
Department of Hematology/Oncology, Stephenson Cancer Center, University of Oklahoma Health Sciences Center, 73104 Oklahoma City, United States
Hematology/Oncology fellow, Department of Medicine, Division of Hematology-Oncology Stephenson Cancer Center, University of Oklahoma Health Sciences Center, 800 NE 10th St., 6th Floor, OK 73104 Oklahoma City, United States

Azra Borogovac and Mohamad Khawandanah
Department of Hematology/Oncology, Stephenson Cancer Center, University of Oklahoma Health Sciences Center, 73104 Oklahoma City, United States

Elabdallah Mohamad
Department of Internal Medicine, University of Oklahoma Medical Center (OUMC), 73104 Oklahoma City, United States

Xiaoying Wang and Jingyu Zhang
Department of Hematology, Key Laboratory of Hematology of Hebei Province, The Second Hospital of Hebei Medical University, 050000 Shijiazhuang, China

Yuxin Zhang and Yi Wu
Department of Hematology, Key Laboratory of Hematology of Hebei Province, The Second Hospital of Hebei Medical University, 050000 Shijiazhuang, China
National Clinical Research Center for Hematologic Diseases, the First Affiliated Hospital, Collaborative Innovation Center of Hematology, State Key Laboratory of Radiation Medicine and Prevention, Cyrus Tang Medical Institute, Soochow University, 215123 Suzhou, China

Fengwu Chen, Aizhen Yang, Yue Han and Depei Wu
National Clinical Research Center for Hematologic Diseases, the First Affiliated Hospital, Collaborative Innovation Center of Hematology, State Key Laboratory of Radiation Medicine and Prevention, Cyrus Tang Medical Institute, Soochow University, 215123 Suzhou, China

Yael Lichter
The Intensive Care Unit, Tel Aviv Sourasky Medical Center, Tel Aviv, Israel

Tanya Badelbayov, Irina Shalev, Dan Benisty and Efrat Luttwak
The Hematology Institute, Tel Aviv Sourasky Medical Center, 6 Weizman St, Tel Aviv, Israel

Reut Schvartz
Division of anesthesiology, Tel Aviv Sourasky Medical Center, Tel Aviv, Israel

Yishay Szekely
The Division of cardiology, Tel Aviv Sourasky Medical Center, Tel Aviv, Israel

Ilana Goldiner
The Central Laboratory, Tel Aviv Sourasky Medical Center, Tel Aviv, Israel

Maxim Kagarlyk, Keren Asraf and Ram Doolman
The Dworman Automated-Mega Laboratory, Sheba Medical Center, Tel-Hashomer, Ramat-Gan, Israel

Ilya Kirgner, Irit Avivi and Ben-Zion Katz
The Hematology Institute, Tel Aviv Sourasky Medical Center, 6 Weizman St, Tel Aviv, Israel
Sackler Faculty of Medicine, Tel Aviv University, Tel Aviv, Israel

Nimrod Adi
The Intensive Care Unit, Tel Aviv Sourasky Medical Center, Tel Aviv, Israel
Sackler Faculty of Medicine, Tel Aviv University, Tel Aviv, Israel

Index

A

Acute Coronary Syndrome, 57-59, 64, 66, 68-69, 92-93, 95-96, 100-101, 147, 158-159, 172, 180-183, 195

Acute Kidney Injury, 13, 64, 68, 130-131, 133-139, 219, 223

Acute Limb Ischemia, 39-40, 43, 48-49, 82

Aggregometry, 140-141, 146, 148-150, 152-153, 158-159

Amputation, 39, 41, 45-47

Anticoagulant Treatment, 10, 50-51, 54-56, 101

Anticoagulation, 6-7, 9-10, 12-13, 18, 20, 33, 50-52, 54-55, 66-68, 71, 73, 75-76, 82-86, 88, 90-91, 93-94, 96, 98-108, 110, 113-114, 116-122, 124-129, 131, 135, 138-139, 159, 201, 203, 205, 220, 225

Antigen, 74-75, 85, 91, 165, 212-213, 215-216, 218, 220-222, 224-225

Antiphospholipid Syndrome, 72, 91, 200, 204-206

Antiplatelet, 33, 38, 41, 58, 66-67, 69, 93-94, 99-100, 140-142, 146-150, 152, 154-155, 157-159, 185

Antiplatelet Effect, 149, 157, 159

Aortic Thrombosis, 200-201, 203

Artificial Uniform Capillaries, 33

Atherosclerosis, 2, 36, 38, 163-165, 171, 176, 178, 180, 182, 186-187, 205

Atrial Fibrillation, 43, 84, 87, 90-93, 95, 99-101, 107-108, 114-116, 130-131, 138-139

B

Baseline Characteristics, 13, 16, 23-26, 42-43, 95, 117, 120, 125-126, 132-137, 145, 151, 161, 173-174, 188

C

Cardiac Surgery, 107-108, 112, 114-115, 158, 183, 198

Cardiovascular Risk, 32-38, 66, 68-69, 127, 145, 158, 172, 181-182, 197

Catheter-based Thrombectomy, 39-40, 42-44, 46

Chronic Thrombi, 50, 55-56

Clinical Events, 140, 142-146, 159

Clot Formation, 19, 77, 167

Clot Strength, 11-14, 16, 18-20, 147

Coagulopathy, 11-12, 14-16, 20, 23, 29, 31, 117, 125-127, 129, 170, 182, 204, 213, 219, 223-225

Cohort, 14, 18-20, 29, 31, 38, 40-41, 46, 50-51, 55, 61, 69, 76, 81-82, 88, 91-101, 107-110, 117-120, 124-131, 138-139, 146, 159, 164, 171, 182, 184, 198, 220, 224-225

Complement Inhibitor, 207

D

Deep Vein Thrombosis, 4, 47, 50, 54, 56, 76, 106, 127-128, 223-225

Diabetes Mellitus, 38, 43, 68, 95, 132-137, 139, 157, 159, 161, 163, 165, 174-176, 186, 188, 190, 193-195, 197

Direct Oral Anticoagulants, 1-2, 7, 10, 84, 91, 130-134, 139

Disease Severity, 12-18, 125-126, 170

Disulfide Bond, 211-212, 215-216

Drinking Status, 173-174

Dual Antiplatelet Therapy, 41, 58, 93, 100, 140-141, 147-149, 152, 154-155, 157-159

E

Endovascular Techniques, 39, 41

Endovascular Treatment, 40, 48

F

Fetal Loss, 200, 204-206

Fibrinogen Level, 41

Fibrinolysis, 12, 14, 20, 31, 38, 69, 166-170, 218-219, 223

G

Gene Mutation, 72

Genetic Analysis, 72, 74

Glomerular Filtration Rate, 130, 132-134, 136-139, 144-145

H

Hemodialysis, 95, 97, 99, 131-137, 139, 161-162

Hemorrhage, 22-24, 26-30, 44-45, 47, 84, 128-129, 138-139, 167, 201

Hypercoagulability, 11-13, 16, 18, 20, 172-173, 176, 181, 225

Hypercoagulable State, 11-14, 16, 20, 58, 81-82, 176, 178, 180, 200, 218-219, 224

Hypertension, 13, 15-16, 25, 38, 43, 79-81, 93-95, 132-139, 144-146, 151, 154, 157, 160-162, 164-165, 172, 174-176, 178, 186-187, 190, 193-195, 197, 201, 205, 220

I

Immunoassay, 169, 173, 220

Infectious Disease, 102, 204

Ischemia, 23, 39-49, 61, 82, 109, 112, 114, 149, 159, 200-201, 204-205

Ischemic Event, 93, 147

Ischemic Stroke, 29, 33, 63, 77, 79, 81, 91, 108, 112-115, 159, 173, 176, 185

L

Lemierre Syndrome, 102, 105-106

Limb Salvage, 39-41, 44-47

Liver Functions, 218, 224

M
Mean Platelet Volume, 148-149, 151-152, 154-155, 158-159
Mechanical Ventilation, 11-12, 219
Meta-analysis, 1-10, 20, 22-24, 28-31, 58-59, 64, 69-70, 76, 87, 90, 98-101, 108-109, 113-118, 122, 124-127, 158, 206, 225
Morphologic Findings, 52, 55
Mortality, 1-2, 12, 20, 23, 29, 33, 48, 50, 56-64, 68-69, 72, 74, 81-82, 84, 92-94, 97, 100-101, 105, 107-109, 111-122, 124-129, 135, 153, 159, 166, 172, 178, 180, 182-183, 195, 197-201, 205, 209, 219, 223, 225
Multimerization, 211-213, 215-217
Myocardial Infarction, 20, 29, 33, 38, 57-59, 64, 66-70, 77, 84, 92-93, 95, 98, 100-101, 115, 119, 140, 142, 144, 147, 151, 153, 157-159, 173, 178, 181-182, 186, 188, 195, 198-199

N
No-reflow Phenomenon, 57-58, 60, 64-65, 67, 69-70

O
Optical Coherence Tomography, 183, 185-186, 189, 198-199
Oral Anticoagulation, 67-68, 71, 73, 83, 90, 93, 96, 99-101, 107-108, 139

P
Peripheral Blood, 164, 202, 223
Plaque Erosion, 157, 159, 183, 185, 190-191, 197
Platelet Activation, 38, 118, 149, 176, 182, 225
Platelet Function Tests, 147-149, 157-158
Platelet Reactivity, 140-144, 146-149, 152-159
Popliteal Vein, 51-54, 56, 72
Prognosis, 20, 40, 48, 57-59, 62, 66, 68-69, 81, 128-129, 143, 161, 169, 171, 176, 178, 183, 198, 206
Propensity Score Matching, 130, 132-137, 139
Prothrombin Time, 12, 15-16, 18-19, 83, 85-86, 89-91, 167, 170-172, 174-175, 178-182, 221, 224

R
Renal Death, 131, 133-137
Renal Outcomes, 132-137
Residual Syntax Score, 183, 187-190, 193-194, 198-199
Residual Thrombus, 40, 45, 55-56
Revascularization, 39-40, 46-48, 60, 62-64, 69, 92, 94, 98, 140, 142, 144, 173, 183-184, 188, 190, 197-200, 204
Risk Stratification, 57-58, 66, 68-69, 100, 159, 164, 181, 183, 198
Rivaroxaban, 2-4, 6-10, 63, 66-67, 69, 87, 89-91, 93-94, 96, 98, 100, 130-131, 133, 135, 137-139, 185
Rotarex Catheters, 39, 41-44

S
Smoking Status, 173, 174, 176, 178

T
Therapeutic Window, 84, 140, 142-143, 146-147, 209
Thin-cap Fibroatheroma, 183, 185, 188-190, 194, 199
Thrombomodulin, 69, 160-165, 182
Thromboprophylaxis, 1-10, 79, 117-119, 125-129
Thrombus Thickness, 50-56

V
Venous Thromboembolism, 1-2, 4, 10, 20, 23, 27, 31, 50, 56, 76, 78, 82, 84, 90, 118, 128, 170, 172, 223, 225
Von Willebrand Factor, 38, 69, 211-212, 217

W
Warfarin, 6-7, 10, 83-91, 96, 100-101, 103, 110, 116, 130-136, 138-139, 185, 202, 205

www.ingramcontent.com/pod-product-compliance
Lightning Source LLC
LaVergne TN
LVHW082156200926
848484LV00008B/2173